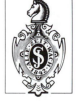

Dorothy C. Wertz    John C. Fletcher (Eds.)

# Ethics and Human Genetics

A Cross-Cultural Perspective

Springer-Verlag Berlin Heidelberg New York
London Paris Tokyo Hong Kong

Dorothy C. Wertz, Ph. D.
Health Services Section
Boston University School of Public Health
80 East Concord Street, Boston
MA 02118-2394, U.S.A.

John C. Fletcher, Ph. D.
Department of Medicine
University of Virginia
School of Medicine, Box 348
Charlottesville, VA 22908
U.S.A.

ISBN 3-540-19224-7 Springer-Verlag Berlin Heidelberg New York
ISBN 0-387-19224-7 Springer-Verlag New York Berlin Heidelberg

Library of Congress Cataloging-in-Publication Data
*Ethics and human genetics:* a cross cultural perspective / Dorothy C. Wertz, John C. Fletcher (eds.).
p. cm. Bibliography: p. Includes index.
ISBN 0-387-19224-7 (U.S. : alk. paper) 1. Medical genetics – Moral and ethical aspects – Cross-cultural studies. I. Wertz, Dorothy C. II. Fletcher, John C., 1931-   . RB 155.E82 1989 174'.2–dc19

The use of general descriptive names, registered names, trademarks, etc. in this publication does not imply, even in the absence of a specific statement, that such names are exempt from the relevant protective laws and regulations and therefore free for general use.

Product Liability: The publisher can give no guarantee for information about drug dosage and application thereof contained in this book. In every individual case the respective user must check its accuracy by consulting other pharmaceutical literature.

Typesetting: Appl, Wemding
2127/3145-543210   Printed on acid-free paper

*We dedicate this book to the memory
of our parents:*

*Helen Leggett Corbett · William Joseph Corbett*
*Estelle Caldwell Fletcher · Robert Capers Fletcher*

# Preface

Medical geneticists are facing important social and ethical issues in most countries. The nature of these issues and their similarity or dissimilarity among nations or regions probably reflect the total social and ethical setting within which the medical geneticist works. The way the social and ethical questions are handled may be of considerable importance for the availability and delivery of medical genetics services. The coping behavior and attitudes of medical geneticists and families with genetic disorders may reflect differences among regions with respect to values, religion, or laws. Medical geneticists are necessarily part of and influenced by the community in which they work. On the other hand, their genetic and scientific expertise, international involvement, and obligation to serve individuals and families with genetic problems will provide input from the international scientific and medical community on thinking, attitudes, and medical practices.

For the above and many other reasons, it is an important task that Drs. Dorothy C. Wertz and John C. Fletcher and their co-workers have taken on, attempting to identify similarities or dissimilarities among and within nations in attitudes, services offered, and practical performance in the area of medical genetics. The thoughtful design of the study has resulted in the accumulation of a wealth of information on the practices of individual doctorate-level genetic counselors that is truly unique. The workers who responded to this initiative tell us how the "grass roots work" is being conducted. These facts could not have been brought together in any other way. No similar survey has ever been undertaken.

With 682 respondents to the survey, the individual answers needed to be put into a broader perspective. In addition to responses from a great many workers, one or two medical geneticists and one ethicist from each country were recruited to draw an over-all picture of the national situation, reflecting responses from individual workers, as well as the authors' over-all evaluation of the present situation and long-term perspectives. The role of the national authors has not been one of "censoring" the answers from individual workers but one of trying to help create as correct a picture as possible of the total situation in each country and of helping to explain national peculiarities. Valuable comments are provided by the national authors on numerous situations where countries appear to differ in their perspectives.

The worries and scenarios that are often the subject of public debates and media interest are well known. Several elements of these scenarios are highly unrealistic. Nevertheless, they create worry, almost to an extent where certain circles would rather not have more progress in genetics or related areas. In one of the areas of medical genetics, prenatal diagnosis, the abortion issue used to dominate the debate. This debate is, at the international level, more or less past history. There is general agreement that important ethical issues are involved, but there is also widespread agreement that these issues are primarily problems that need to be solved by the couple in question, the people who would have to live with the consequences of having or not having prenatal diagnosis.

All 682 survey respondents felt that women must retain the right to abort the fetus with a defect or malformation, and most thought that it had to be the woman's decision whether the particular genetic disorder was serious enough to warrant abortion.

More complicated ethical problems are now surfacing, including those relating to predictive genetic testing. Authors from all 19 nations stressed the need to protect the privacy of tested people from institutional third parties, especially insurance companies and employers. The separate issue of "pre-clinical diagnosis" of a serious disorder such as Huntington disease is complicated and important and should interest legislators and lawyers even more than geneticists and physicians. In common disorders, the important point is that the traits predisposing to disease are normal ones. Thus, any individual person who has a given trait of this kind is not deemed to have the disease. In fact, most of the people with such traits will survive to old age and enjoy a healthy life. The predisposing traits increase an individual's risk of having a given disease (such as early coronary heart disease) compared to the population in general.

The rational response to being genetically predisposed to a common disease would be to initiate as efficient preventive efforts as scientific knowledge can offer. There is every reason to believe that if preventive efforts with respect to coronary heart disease are initiated early in life, in highly motivated individuals who continue to adhere strictly to the preventive measures, disease prevention would be much more effective than today.

The difficulty is that if information about a given person's genetic predisposition to disease were to become known, it could be used to the individual's disadvantage, for example in connection with purchasing life insurance, entering pension systems or employment or achieving promotion. Therefore, this must be an area for strict legislation. It should not cause problems to introduce such legislation. Until now, neither insurance companies nor employers have to any extent used predictive genetic tests (because few have been available). Accordingly, it could not be argued that such tests are necessary for insurers or employers. There should be decisive action in this matter before unfortunate practices become established and by their own momentum become impossible to control. The very fact that the traits predisposing to common disorders are normal genetic traits distinguish such tests in a significant way from diagnostic tests for existing or previous diseases. There should be no difficulty in establishing that normal traits predisposing to common disorders are so different from clinical and pathological findings that they are not covered in current laws, whose makers could not have foreseen them.

Another ethical question identified by the participants was giving access to family members and other private persons with a legitimate interest, to knowledge concerning a given person's condition, with particular reference to the risk of transmitting disease to future generations. This is a topic which in many instances has been met with a naive claim of a right not to know. However, there are many examples of situations where such an attitude would be highly unethical. For example, if a future spouse were to be put at risk of contracting a serious infection such as AIDS, few people would argue that a person's right to know should overrule all other considerations. Medical geneticists are frequently confronted with strong criticism from people who have married into families with autosomal dominant disorders occurring relatively late in life, particularly Huntington's chorea, who find that they have been betrayed by doctors as well as family members who have not given them relevant information. There is little doubt that people in this situation often feel that physicians have a moral duty to disclose information concerning a genetic disorder in the family, because of its vital importance. It may well be argued that a privilege not to know and not to let other people know has to be put aside if such a practice can hurt innocent third parties. A frequent result of not informing people who marry into families with a serious inherited disease such as Huntington's chorea is that the problems are passed on to other persons (the spouse who in mid-life may find himself or herself with a hopelessly ill companion, and the offspring).

Members of families with serious genetic disorders have a reasonable duty to act responsibly towards innocent third parties. By adequately informing the spouse or the spouse to be, they may help limit the spread of the disease gene, for example by having prenatal diagnosis. In this way, members of families with serious genetic disorders can contribute to improved conditions for the entire family. It may be argued that members of families with genetic diseases have a collective responsibility to their group that should not easily be ignored. This responsibility may include participation in research that could improve the health of future families. Although free and informed consent must be required in all cases where experiments are conducted on humans, the moral responsibility of members of families with hereditary diseases may justify an active attitude on the part of the researchers to achieve participation by the group members. It seems quite clear that an unconditional right not to know lacks ethical justification. Nevertheless, it goes without saying that information should not be forced on people who do not want it, if no benefit can be derived from the information and if third parties are not hurt by the withholding of information.

Although widely different health care systems exist in the nations covered, the overwhelming ethical issue faced by medical geneticists was the limitation in fair access to genetic services in a time of increasing demand. People working in the field simply could not manage to cope with the extensive needs expressed, and there were many shortcomings in health care systems with regard to coverage of the needs of families. Even in many developed countries, the majority of pregnant women over age 35 did not receive prenatal diagnosis, although they were more likely to receive it in nations with national health insurance than in nations with health care systems that are mainly private. Great inequalities exist. For example, in one study 60% of white women over 35 and 0.5% of black women over 35 had prenatal diagnosis (in the same state in the USA). Some respondents pointed to the dangers of allowing free market principles to operate in genetic services.

The survey fully confirmed the impression that practically everybody working in genetic counseling favors non-directive counseling and tries to conduct his or her work according to this ideal. This should provide a strong warranty against misuse of genetic counseling or related activities.

Worries expressed by media personalities have until now received great attention. This new book offers, I believe for the first time, views and thoughts of the professionals who work in the field and who in many ways are caught between the needs of patients and families on the one hand, and often misleading media debates on the other hand. This is what makes this book so uniquely interesting. The views of the people involved in caring for patients and families with genetic disorders are as legitimate as those of the mass media and the general public. The book shows that although attitudes and solutions vary between nations and regions, the problems that are felt by medical geneticists as the most pressing are surprisingly similar.

Kåre Berg
Institute of Medical Genetics, University of Oslo
March 1989

# Table of Contents

Table of Contents

XII

# List of Contributors

*Principal Authors*

Dorothy C. Wertz, Ph. D.
Research Professor
Health Services Section
School of Public Health
Boston University
80 E. Concord Street
Boston, MA 02118

John C. Fletcher, Ph. D.
Professor of Biomedical Ethics
Box 348
Medical Center
University of Virginia
Charlottesville, VA 22908

*Australia*

John Rogers, M. D.
Anna Marie Taylor, Ph. D.
Birth Defects Research Institute
Royal Children's Hospital
Flemington Road, Parkville
Victoria 3052, Australia

*Brazil*

Prof. Francisco M. Salzano, Ph. D.
Departamento de Genética
Instituto de Biociências
University Federal do Rio Grande do Sul
Caixa Postal 1953
Porto Alegre, RS, Brazil

Prof. Sergio D. J. Pena, M. D., Ph. D.
Departamento de Bioquimica
Instituto de Ciências Biologicas-UFMG
Caixa Postal 2486
30000 Belo Horizonte, MG, Brazil

## Canada

Prof. Judith G. Hall, M. D.
University of British Columbia
Clinical Genetics Unit
Grace Hospital
4490 Oak Street
Vancouver V6H 3V5, BC, Canada

David Roy, Ph. D.
Director, Center for Bioethics
Clinical Research Institute of Montreal
110 avenue des Pins ouest
Montreal, Quebec H2W 1R7, Canada

## Denmark

Prof. Aage J. Therkelsen, M. D.
Institute of Human Genetics
Aarhus University
DK-8000 Aarhus C, Denmark

Prof. Lars Bolund, M. D.
Institute of Human Genetics
University of Aarhus
DK-8000 Aarhus C, Denmark

Dr. Viggo Mortensen
Associate Professor
Institute of Ethics
University of Aarhus
DK-8000 Aarhus C, Denmark

## Federal Republic of Germany

Prof. Dr. Traute Schroeder-Kurth
Institut für Anthropologie u. Humangenetik
Im Neuenheimer Feld 328
6900 Heidelberg
Federal Republic of Germany

Prof. Dr. Juergen Huebner
Protestant Institute for Interdisciplinary Research
Schmeilweg 5, D-6900 Heidelberg
Federal Republic of Germany

*France*

Prof. Jean-François Mattei, M.D., Ph.D.
Centre de Genétique Médicale
Hôpital de la Timone
13385 Marseille Cedex 5, France

Prof. Marc Gamerre, M.D.
Gynecologie Rue Paradis
Maternité de la Belle de Mai
23 Rue François Simon
13003 Marseille, France


*German Democratic Republic*

Prof. Regine Ch. Witkowski, M.D.
Hannelore Koerner, Dr. sc. nat.
Bereich Medizin (Charité)
der Humboldt Universität zu Berlin
Nervenklinik
Abteilung für medizinische Genetik
1040 Berlin, Schumannstrasse 20/21, DDR

Herrmann Metzke, Dr. sc. med.
Department of Medical Genetics
Medical Academy
Erfurt, DDR


*Greece*

Labrini Velogiannis-Moutsopoulos, J.D.
14–16 Gynekon Pimdou
Ioannina, Greece

Christos S. Bartsocas, M.D.
Athens Children's Hospital
"P. & A. Kyriakou"
First Pediatric Service
47 Vasilissis Sofias Avenue
GR 107 76 Athens, Greece

*Hungary*

Andrew Czeizel, M.D.
National Institute of Hygiene
Gyáli ut 2-6
H-1097 Budapest, Hungary

Prof. Georg Adam, M.D.
Semmelweis Medical University
Budapest H-1089
Nagyvarad ter 4, Hungary

*India*

Ishwar C. Verma, F.R.C.P., F.A.M.S., F.A.A.P.
Professor and Officer-in-Charge
Genetics Unit, Department of Pediatrics
Old Operation Theatre Building
All India Institute of Medical Sciences
Ansari Nagar
New Delhi 110029, India

Balbir Singh, Ph.D.
Department of Philosophy
Hindu College
New Delhi, India

*Israel*

Prof. Juan Chemke, M.D.
Clinical Genetics Unit
Kaplan Hospital
76100 Rehovot, Israel

Avraham Steinberg, M.D.
Pediatric Neurology Unit
Bikur Holim Hospital
Jerusalem, Israel

*Italy*

Faustina Lalatta, M.D.
Istituto Ostetrico Ginecologico
Prima Clinica
Via Commenda, 12
20122 Milano, Italy

XVI

Gianni Tognoni, M.D., Ph.D.
Laboratorio di Farmacologia Clinica
Istituto Mario Negri
Via Eritrea 62
20157 Milano, Italy

*Japan*

Prof. Koji Ohkura, M.D., D.M.S.
Department of Human Genetics
Tokyo University of Medicine and Dentistry
Yushima 1-5-45, Bunkyo-Ku
Tokyo 113, Japan

Prof. Rihito Kimura, J.D.
Kennedy Institute of Ethics
Georgetown University
Washington, D.C. 20057, USA

*Norway*

Prof. Kåre Berg, M.D., Ph.D.
Institute of Medical Genetics
University of Oslo
P.O. Box 1036
Blindern, Oslo 3, Norway

Prof. Knut Erik Tranøy, Ph.D.
Institute for Philosophy
University of Oslo
P.O. Box 1024
Blindern, Oslo 3, Norway

*Sweden*

Erwin Bischofberger, S.J., S.T.D.
St. Johannesgatan 22 A
S-752 35 Uppsala, Sweden

Prof. Jan Lindsten
Kungl. Karolinska Instutet
Department of Clinical Genetics
Karolinska Sjukhuset
P.O. Box 60500
S-104 01 Stockholm, Sweden

Prof. Urban Rosenqvist, M. D.
Department of Endocrinology
Karolinska Hospital
S-104 01 Stockholm, Sweden

*Switzerland*

Prof. Eric Engel, M. D., Ph. D.
Celia Dawn DeLozier-Blanchet, Ph. D.
University Institute of Medical Genetics
1211 Geneve 4
CMU – 9, av. de Champel, Switzerland

*Turkey*

Prof. Işik Bökesoy, M. D., Ph. D.
Boğaz Sokak. 19/16
Gazi Osman Paşa
Ankara, Turkey

Prof. Fuat Göksel, M. D.
Head, Deontology Department
University of Ankara Faculty of Medicine
Sihhiye – Ankara, Turkey

*United Kingdom of Great Britain and Northern Ireland*

Prof. Rodney Harris, M. D.
Department of Medical Genetics
St. Mary's Hospital
Hathersage Road
Manchester M13 OJH, England

*United States*

John J. Mulvihill, M. D.
Chief, Clinical Genetics Section
Clinical Epidemiology Branch
National Cancer Institute
National Institutes of Health
Executive Plaza North
Room 400
Bethesda, MD 20892, USA

Prof. Leroy Walters, Ph. D.
Center for Bioethics
Kennedy Institute of Ethics
Georgetown University
Washington, DC 20057, USA

# Introduction

This book reports and discusses a collaborative cross-cultural study of the approaches of medical geneticists to ethical problems in genetic counseling, prenatal diagnosis and screening. In this introduction, I trace the study's roots in my long interest in adapting the methods of action research to the study of problems in applied ethics. Part 3 gives a fuller account of my views on the significance of the study and the ethical problems discussed in Part 2 by co-authors in medical genetics and medical ethics from 19 nations.

To begin directly with the study, a reader should go to Part 1, a complete overview by my esteemed colleague, Dorothy C. Wertz. She is first author because she did the greater share of work on the questionnaire, the analysis of data, writing, and editing. However, I am responsible for the idea and organization of the project, selection of co-authors, and most assuredly for the project's shortcomings.

My two basic aims for this study were: 1) to involve medical geneticists in a collaborative effort to describe the approaches they actually take to the major ethical problems in daily practice, and 2) to determine the degree of consensus and variation among geneticists about these approaches. With these aims reached, a third goal is now possible, namely, that medical geneticists and their colleagues in medical ethics will reflect critically upon these findings, consolidate their moral experience in this generation to transmit to the next, and prepare for predictably more complex ethical problems in the very near future.

I undertook this study with encouragement and pledges of support from medical geneticists in many nations. I consider medical geneticists collectively the "client" for the project and primary audience of the book. However, many others concerned with ethical problems in this field may be helped by reading it. These include health policy makers, members of organizations that help patients and families with genetic disorders, parents' groups, and scholars in medical ethics, law and the social sciences. It will require a multidisciplinary effort to study the central problem more fully described in Part 3 and to take steps to improve the situation for the better. Briefly, the central problem that now faces medical geneticists is that this study shows significant differences in moral views on some of the major contemporary ethical problems in this field. These differences exist to such a degree that chances are high that medical geneticists will be too conflicted and unprepared to meet the more complex ethical issues occasioned by new advances in molecular biology. Given profound disagreements on many current issues, it is difficult to imagine how practitioners in this field, who ought to be among the main teachers of its ethical considerations, can participate creatively in shaping the main ethical features of its future. Much work in serious ethical analysis of current and future problems remains to be done, if human genetics is not to be a house so seriously divided within itself.

## Origins: Action Research in Applied Ethics

My approach to these three aims was functional, i.e., to involve medical geneticists actively in a cross-cultural study of ethical problems in their field. Experience in teaching professionals has convinced me that disciplined study of vexing problems in practice is the doorway to more satisfying and deeper study of the ethical principles and concepts that should finally correct and guide practitioners and patients. Practice and theory should be in dynamic tension, but careful study of practice arouses need for guidance and theory. Medical geneticists are, by experience, the most qualified teachers about the ethical problems in their field, assuming that they clearly understand the problems and attain some critical distance and grasp of concepts of ethics that ought to guide medical practice. If the project contributes to this eventual goal, it will have been altogether worthwhile.

The origin of this study lies in my previous experience with action research projects between 1966 and 1977, at key points in my development as a teacher and researcher in medical ethics. Action research, in the hands of its founders (Lewin 1947; Sanford 1970), is the use of psychological and social research to identify social problems in a group, coupled with active participation of the investigator in group efforts to understand and resolve these problems. The key to action research is that those who "have" the problems being studied and the investigator work collaboratively through the following five steps: 1) analysis of problems, 2) fact-finding, 3) planning an approach to resolving or improving the problem(s), 4) execution of the plan, and 5) evaluation. The aim of action research is to leave those thus studied better off than they were before the study began. The field research (Fletcher 1984) described below and in Part 1 comprised steps 1, 2, and 3. The study fully described and reported in Part 1 is step 4, and this book embodies evaluations of the results of step 4 in each of 19 nations.

I first learned about action research in circles of social scientists and clergy-activists who worked on urban problems and racism in U.S. cities in the late 1960s. I found an adapted form of action research highly useful for studies in descriptive ethics, the factual investigation of moral problems, moral beliefs, and moral behavior (Beauchamp and Childress 1983). Clear and objective descriptions of ethical problems are vital for the most productive considerations of "normative" ethics, which deals with the question as to which "action guides are worthy of moral acceptance and for what reasons?" (Beauchamp and Childress 1983) and how these action guides ought to be applied, in this case, applied in the practice of medical genetics. Introduction to action research happily occurred when I needed it most, i.e., before dissertation research to study the major ethical problems of medical research.

From 1964 to 1966, I pursued graduate studies in Christian ethics at Union Theological Seminary in New York. Interested from childhood in medicine, I did field work with medical researchers in transplantation at New York Hospital-Cornell Medical School. Here a fledgling ethicist took first steps with cases that raised questions that persist today.

For example, in 1965 physicians asked me to help with ethical problems in the case of a man dying from a rare form of inherited kidney disease. Dialysis was no longer feasible due to complications. He had no living relatives. No cadaver kidney was available. The choices came down to an experiment with a chimpanzee kidney as a bridge to a human transplant or certain death. The literature showed that the few heterografts done to date had failed with one exception. In this case (Reemtsma, McCracken, Schlegel et al. 1964), after two reversals of rejection, a chimpanzee graft had functioned in a 43-year-old man with terminal uremia for two months. The patient died of pneumonia, but sections of the graft showed no signs of rejection. I discussed the choices and searched for guidance alone with physicians, with the patient, and then with both together. After a full explanation of the risks involved, the patient said clearly that he preferred the experiment that could benefit others, even with its very small chance of benefit to him and the high risk of death, to his prolonged dying. I witnessed the consent agreement. The patient died, due to cardiac arrest, less than an hour after surgery. The heterograft produced urine for about fifteen minutes.

This case became a paradigm for me linking the study of ethical problems in medical research with approaches to treatment of genetic disease. The resources that I and the physicians brought to consider the ethical questions raised by the case were, in retrospect, quite inadequate and doubtless self-serving. No impartial ethics committee was convened to review the merit of the experiment or the approach to consent, nor did it occur to me at the time to ask for such review.

The case raised three perennial ethical questions that apply to all new research, including today's research directed to diagnosis and treatment of genetic disease in humans. First, the experiment could be done, but *ought* it be done at all? And *who* should decide? In those days, researchers alone weighed this primary ethical "ought" with the best available technical information about benefits and risks. Many societies have since deemed these choices too important to be left to the most self-interested researchers alone. In my view, the same social approach will continue in decisions about new genetic interventions and prospects for wider family, workplace, and population screening.

Second, should *this patient* be offered the choice? Was any benefit whatsoever possible for him? And, given the desperate circumstances, concern about his capacity to understand, and with no relatives to help, could a "yes or no" be voluntary and informed? Again, *who* should decide? If one steps outside the context of research into contemporary

XXII

practice of human genetics, some of the most controversial ethical problems today concern whether geneticists should acquiesce to the wishes of patients for procedures that are not medically indicated.

Third, should society encourage or discourage the use, even experimentally, of animal organs in transplantation? What implications and long range consequences for society's well-being could be discerned? Again, by analogy, society's long-range interests are clearly involved in the process of research, diagnosis, and treatment of genetic disorders. Whether societies will generate the wisdom to discriminate between harmful and beneficial uses of genetic knowledge and exercise wise control is an open question.

Such experiences in the field, and the help I received from my adviser, Roger L. Shinn, encouraged me to plan a dissertation on the ethics of medical research. We sensed that medical research and human genetics as fields were rich with ethical problems needing study, but I was uncertain about how best to proceed. My most serious need was to understand the milieu of medical research. A library-based approach to the dissertation, at that point, would have yielded little of value, since the literature was meager with few exceptions. One was Fox's [1959] pioneering participant-observer study of the social milieu of clinical research. I found inspiration in Fox's fieldwork and practical guidance in the steps of action-research described above. I determined to follow her example and study the *moral* milieu of clinical research by involving clinical-investigators and patient-subjects in the study. Officials at the Clinical Center of the National Institutes of Health (NIH) answered my need. Dr. Jack Masur, the first Director of this 500-bed research hospital founded in 1953 opened doors for my further education and research.

Two goals guided my dissertation research. First, following Fox and using an action-research model, I enlisted the help of medical researchers, their patients, and science administrators to describe accurately the most difficult and frequent problems of moral choice in the research process from the idea-stage of a project to transmission of its findings to society. While observing and consulting with clinical investigators and patients in the Clinical Center, we noted the patterns, practices and moral turning points in the long process of clinical research. I was especially interested in practices of "informed consent" with research subjects. A small action-research project was done, with the participation of researchers and patients, to study the effectiveness of the involvement of a third party (myself) in improving the outcomes of the consent process. Data were also collected for me by science administrators showing that prior group review had reduced the number of projects involving serious risks to research subjects. These activities were the distant forerunners of the field research and questionnaire involved in this international study.

The second was a goal in social ethics, namely, to scan the future of ethical problems posed for society by discoveries in medical research. How could society be best prepared to reflect on such issues and make discriminating choices? I aimed this work *between* the clinical setting and society's resources for deliberation about the impacts of science and medicine on its morality and institutions. Scientists and officials of the NIH participated in a series of conferences to give their views of the most important ethical and social issues posed in the near future by their work. They were in a good position to scan the future. Concurrently, through the work of others, two new social resources for reflection on such problems came into being, the Hastings Center and the Kennedy Institute of Ethics. In the formative years of these new organizations, I was fortunate to be involved in efforts to focus research and reflection on ethical problems in research and medicine. My dissertation consequently described the moral milieu of medical research and discussed many of the issues posed by advances in organ transplantation and other life-sustaining technologies, brain research, behavior control, and human genetics (Fletcher 1969).

In 1966 at the NIH I met two pioneers in genetic studies, Marshall Nirenberg and W. French Anderson. They spoke presciently about the implications of their research for society. Nirenberg was a Nobelist for discoveries about the "language" of the genetic code. He was alternately thunderstruck by the implications of understanding the genetic code and skeptical about the depth of society's ethical wisdom to guide genetic knowledge and potential interventions in beneficent ways. Anderson envisioned genetic therapy at the autosomal level for hemoglobinopathies and predicted controversies about prospects of alteration of genes in the pre-implantation human embryo, or even in the gametes. These talks convinced me to study ethical problems and future issues in human genetics, using the action-research strategy.

Where to begin? Testing newborns to begin treatment for phenylketonuria (PKU) was already legally mandated in most states, but genetic screening controversies would not arise until the early 1970s. I became interested in prenatal diagnosis by amniocentesis, a controversial technique then in the research stage. No research in prenatal diagnosis occurred at the NIH. A clinical research unit in obstetrics and neonatology opened at the Clinical Center in 1963 but was unsuccessful for many reasons (Hill 1988). Mainly, a setting of clinical research involving adults was unattractive to pregnant women and impractical for the care of newborns.

In 1969-1970, Cecil Jacobsen, then chief of the genetics center of George Washington University School of Medicine, helped me shape a study to follow 25 couples in genetic counseling and prenatal diagnosis. Enlisting the help of each couple prior to the first interview, I asked them to note and report the moral and ethical problems they faced before, during, and following prenatal diagnosis and its consequences. I met them and Jacobsen for interviews before, during and after prenatal diagnosis and the subsequent birth of the infant or abortion of an affected fetus. My goals were the same as in the clinical research study, namely, to describe accurately the major moral choices faced by physicians and the couples, and to frame the issues posed by prenatal diagnosis for social-ethical reflection. I subsequently reported this descriptive study of one series of patients in one genetics center (Fletcher 1973).

Concurrently, serious social conflict arose about mandatory screening for sickle cell trait (Reilly 1973). I and other colleagues tried to help in the sickle cell screening controversy with a small action research project to study approaches to informed consent in six genetic screening programs (Fletcher, Roblin, Powledge 1974).

Between 1970 and 1980, I participated in some interdisciplinary groups and meetings to study the ethical problems faced by geneticists, obstetricians and their patients, as well as ethical, social, and legal issues posed by advances in human genetics for U.S. society. These groups were mainly a forum for communication that surfaced the issues and permitted central social values and reflections from religious and philosophical traditions to be applied to some of the conflicts arising in prenatal diagnosis, screening and counseling. In 1970 and 1973 the NIH sponsored the first national conferences on technical, ethical, legal and social aspects of prenatal diagnosis (Harris 1972), and uses of genetic knowledge in clinical genetics and society (Hilton, Callahan, Harris et al. 1973). Two research groups of the Hastings Center identified ethical, legal, and social problems in genetic screening programs (Research Group 1972) and prenatal diagnosis (Powledge and Fletcher 1979) and shaped guidelines for professionals and public policy makers. The National Institute of Child Health and Human Development's (NICHD 1979) consensus development conference on prenatal diagnosis was notable, as are other NICHD consensus conferences, for including serious inquiry into social and ethical implications of scientific advances. An international conference of medical geneticists on prenatal diagnosis that convened in Canada was the first to add social, legal, and ethical considerations to its agenda. (Fletcher, Hibbard, Miller et al. 1980). Reflection today on these early group efforts shows two serious weaknesses: 1) patient and family experiences of genetic services were almost never sought, and 2) almost no systematic study, with the exception of the NICHD conference, was devoted to the problem of fair distribution of genetic services in the population.

Also, in this period when the U.S. Supreme Court struck down state laws restricting abortion (Roe v. Wade 1973), even more conflict erupted about indications for genetic abortions, including debate of longstanding about whether abortion to avoid genetic disease was the wrong (Ramsey 1970) or right (Jos Fletcher 1974) precedent for euthanasia in newborns whose parents would have preferred screening and abortion. In the genetic abortion-euthanasia debate, my position was that genetic abortion, now permitted with no restrictions, was morally different from pediatric euthanasia, mainly because the newborn is a separate individual deserving of protection (Fletcher 1975).

By these studies and interdisciplinary activities, I gained a grasp on the major moral choices facing parents, physicians, and their advisers in the practice of medical genetics in the U.S. In 1977, Mortimer Lipsett, then

Director of the Clinical Center, asked me to return to the NIH to direct a new bioethics program. Gathering the threads of reflection on ethical problems in human genetics, I believed that a decade of work had shaped a consensus, in the circles described above, about some general and specific ethical guidance for screening, counseling and prenatal diagnosis. I described these ideas, organized under the themes of "freedom and fairness," in a review article and hoped to test them in a survey with U.S. medical geneticists (Fletcher 1981).

In 1982, the President's Commission for the Study of Ethical Problems in Medicine and Biomedical and Behavioral Research [1983] circulated its recommendations to Congress on screening and counseling for genetic disorders. These recommendations, unanimously adopted by the Commission, stand in clear continuity with the work of earlier groups listed in the previous section. But questions arose needing study, i.e., did U.S. medical geneticists agree and how closely were the Commission's recommendations followed in practice? I looked forward to studying these questions in an action research project.

## A Cross-Cultural Study in Applied Ethics

In 1982, a crucial turn began in my plans for a study of medical geneticists. At the invitation of Kåre Berg, Director of the University of Oslo's Institute for Medical Genetics and co-author of Chapter 2.14, I helped to plan and participated in a symposium on "Research Ethics" for the 125th anniversary of the Norwegian Academy of Science and Letters (Berg and Tranøy 1983). In preparing papers on several topics in research ethics for this event, I was struck by how much light was shed on ethical problems in research by taking an evolutionary and historical view. One could see something like progress, at least in understanding ethical problems. Concurrently, I read widely in works in philosophy (Toulmin 1972; Midgley 1978; Singer 1981) which demonstrated how evolutionary concepts illuminated the history and development of human ethical systems.

As I worked on papers in research ethics, from the vantage point of almost thirty years of development since the judgments at the war trials at Nuremberg, I asked myself what the same period of cultural and ethical evolution would bring in human genetics. These basic questions arose: What were the similarities and differences between the evolution of the problems and issues in the two fields? What had been learned about the evolution of the ethics of research, including cross-cultural issues, that might shed light on what could happen in the arena of human genetics? What would the problems be in five or ten years?

Participation in an international symposium on research ethics left me profoundly impressed with the differences between nations in this field, despite similar problems. Clearly, different cultures and political-economic systems had strong influences on practices in research ethics. What could be found in terms of cultural differences in approaches to the ethical problems in human genetics? Was there any "common ground" on which to stand in the face of great ethical differences between practitioners in various nations? But prior questions needed to be answered. Did medical geneticists in different nations even see the same ethical problems? And how did they assess their frequency and difficulty? What could be found by a cross-cultural study of medical geneticists and the ethical problems they face? During the symposium, I shared this budding dream with Kåre Berg and his predecessor, Jan Mohr. Both strongly encouraged me.

Dr. Jay Shapiro, then Acting Director of the Clinical Center, sponsored my application for a NIH work-study program to support six months of field work in 1984 in European genetic centers to plan a cross-cultural study. The University of Oslo and the Institute for Medical Genetics made office space and help with housing available. The medical geneticists and laboratory scientists in Oslo, especially Arvid Heiberg, C. B. van der Hagen, and Paul Moeller, helped to shape my research strategy for the field visits and pre-tested a list of questions to be asked in each center. The directors and staffs of 24 genetic centers in 11 European nations received me graciously, if not with some serious reservations, since for most it was their first visit with an "ethicist." Some of these hosts are co-authors of the essays in Part 2. I will always be grateful for their hospitality and cooperation.

Many persons and institutions helped me in this effort. Maxwell Boverman, M. D., psychiatric consultant to the Bioethics Program, NIH, travelled with me to several centers in 1984 and helped me and geneticists to face some of the emotional problems associated with genetic counseling and disputes about ethics. Recognition and gratitude must go to the Norwegian Marshall Fund, which supported my travel in Europe. The Medical Trust, one of the Pew Charitable Trusts, and the Maurice and Muriel Miller Foundation supported all of the costs of the survey, the data analysis, and support for Dr. Wertz during the writing and editing. No Federal funds were expended on the survey itself. The current Director of the Clinical Center, NIH, John L. Decker, M. D., continued to support and encourage the completion of this study and approved my involvement.

In 1985, James R. Sorenson, a sociologist then at Boston University, helped me begin a collaboration with Dorothy C. Wertz, who became the major force in the international survey. Her boundless energy and hard work saved the project many times and insured that it would be brought to a successful conclusion as I left the NIH to take up a new position at the University of Virginia. She has scrupulously edited each manuscript in close cooperation with the co-authors. My secretary, Margaret Sexton, deserves the credit for transcribing the manuscripts onto disks for ease and speed of publication.

**Personal Addendum**
The origins of my interest in ethics and human genetics also lie undoubtedly in my personal history. My first questions about genetic disease arose in my family. As a hearing son with three hearing sisters of deaf

parents very active in the Episcopal ministry to hearing-impaired persons throughout the southeastern United States, I saw but only later understood the genetic risks of deafness in the deaf community in Birmingham, Alabama. The choice to learn and disclose how my parents actually lost their hearing, and the degree of genetic risk involved, in time became a personal issue for me. This choice was especially difficult with regard to my father, a widely known and respected minister.

I and countless others were told that my father lost his hearing in 1904, when at age four, he was "struck by lightning" standing on the back porch of an Alabama farm home watching a storm. My mother's deafness, observed from earliest infancy in 1901, was unclear as to cause and later raised a question about genetic risks. However, a story circulated in her family gatherings that she had been "dropped" by a black servant in her Texas home. The story of my father's miraculous survival was literally a legend in his time. My grandfather was an evangelistic Southern Baptist preacher who offered my father at the age of eighteen to that denomination as a missionary to the deaf, only to be told that his handicap prevented his ordination. The Episcopalians had a long history of ordaining deaf persons and welcomed him while a student at Gallaudet College, where he met my mother. After seminary studies for the ministry, my father proved his missionary zeal by organizing more than forty small congregations in twelve states for the hearing-impaired and blind at a time when there was little social support for them.

By 1980, my growing involvement with medical geneticists, unanswered questions about the actual cause of my parents' deafness, and three maturing children led me to seek help from genetic counselors to assess the genetic risks of deafness in our family. Discussions with neurologists at the NIH raised serious doubts about the lightning story. They had not heard of a case where only nerve deafness accompanied by no other consequences followed a lightning strike. My mother's deafness could have possibly arisen as a fresh mutation causing autosomal dominant deafness, but this was unlikely since all of her children or grandchildren could hear. No past occurrence of deafness on paternal or maternal sides, other than my parents', could be found. Should I push for an answer? My parents were then in their mid-seventies. Would they be harmed emotionally? Would my relationship with them suffer? The need to clarify these causes, if possible, prevailed over these potential discomforts.

After discussing my needs and plans with my parents, in 1980 I traveled to Alabama and sought out my father's favorite cousin, who was eight years older. His memory was clear. He told me that the lightning story was false. He said that my father had become "very sick, was taken to the doctor for a long time, and came back deaf. They blamed it on the doctor." George Fraser, a geneticist who became a good friend, conducted the most thorough study [1976] of the causes of childhood deafness. I learned from him that among the actual causes could have been meningitis, encephalitis, a viral infection, or other reasons, but not lightning. Sur-

XXVIII

viving a disease like meningitis in the era before antibiotics was a "miracle" comparable to surviving lightning, if this was indeed the case. We will never know the real cause, but we do know that a contemporary said that the lightning story was untrue. Whether my mother's deafness was prenatally or perinatally acquired is also unknown.

When I returned to report his cousin's statements, my father was able to remember that his father had taken him to services and prayer meetings in many small rural Baptist churches. He recalled his father praying over him to ask for divine healing. Was the lightning story born in this setting, serving a need of my grandfather's to be a "healer?" Possibly my father had been watching a storm before he fell ill and the association was born. However, the feared interpersonal consequences did not occur. Finding a likely explanation of his handicap helped us both to learn and drew us closer in his remaining years. In fact, he took great pride in my interest in human genetics. My father died at 87 years as this introduction was being written.

Dorothy Wertz joins me in dedicating this volume and our hopes for it to the memory of our parents, whose lives gave us the chance for life and for work together.

J. C. Fletcher
Charlottesville, Virginia
March, 1989

# References

Beauchamp TL, Childress JF [1983] Principles of biomedical ethics, 2nd ed. Oxford University Press, New York, p 8

Berg K, Tranøy KE (eds) [1983] Research ethics. Alan R. Liss, New York

Fletcher JC [1969] A study of the ethics of medical research. Thesis, Union Theological Seminary, New York

Fletcher JC [1973] Parents in genetic counseling: The moral shape of decision-making. In: Hilton B, Callahan D, Harris M et al. (eds) Ethical issues in human genetics, Plenum, New York, pp 301-327

Fletcher JC, Roblin RO, Powledge TM [1974] Informed consent in genetic screening programs. In: Bergsma D (ed) Ethical, social, and legal dimensions of screening for human genetic disease. Birth Defects. Original Article Series. Vol X, No 6, pp 137-144

Fletcher JC [1975] Abortion, euthanasia, and care of defective newborns. N Engl J Med 292: 75-78

Fletcher JC, Hibbard B, Miller JR et al [1980] Ethical, legal, and societal considerations of prenatal diagnosis. In: Hamerton JL, Simpson NE (eds) Prenatal diagnosis past, present, and future (Report of an International Workshop) Prenat Diag (Special issue) pp. 43-53

Fletcher JC [1981] Ethical issues in genetic screening and antenatal diagnosis. In: Simpson JL (ed) Antenatal diagnosis of genetic disorders. Clin Ob Gyn 24: 1151-1168

Fletcher JC [1984] Report on Work-Study Program. Office of Associate Director for Intramural Affairs. National Institutes of Health, Bethesda, MD

Fletcher JF [1974] The ethics of genetic control. Anchor Press/Doubleday, Garden City NY, p.153

Fox R [1959] Experiment perilous. Free Press, New York

Fraser G [1976] The causes of profound deafness in childhood. Johns Hopkins University Press, Baltimore, p 268

Harris M (ed) [1971] Early diagnosis of human genetic defects. Scientific and ethical considerations. Fogarty International Center, Proceedings no 6, HEW Publication no (NIH) 72-25. Bethesda MD, NIH

Hill JG [1988] Personal communication. National Institute of Child Health and Human Development, Bethesda MD

Hilton B, Callahan D, Harris M et al. (eds) [1973] Ethical issues in human genetics. Fogarty International Center, Proceedings no 13, Plenum, New York

Lewin K [1947] Group decision and social change. In: Newcomb TM, Hartley EL (eds) Readings in social psychology. Holt, Rinehart, Winston, New York, pp 76-103

Midgley M [1978] Beast and man. Cornell University Press, Ithaca NY

NICHD [1979] Antenatal diagnosis. Report of a consensus development conference. US Dept of HEW, publ no (NIH) 79-173

Powledge TM, Fletcher JC [1979] Guidelines for the ethical, social, and legal issues in prenatal diagnosis. N Engl J Med 300: 168-172

President's Commission for the Study of Ethical Problems in Medicine and Biomedical and Behavioral Research [1983] Genetic screening and counseling. US Government Printing Office, Washington DC

Ramsey P [1970] Reference points on deciding on abortion. In: Noonan JT (ed) The morality of abortion. Harvard University Press, Cambridge, pp 60-100

Reemtsma K, McCracken BH, Schlegel JU et al. [1964] Reversal of early graft rejection after renal heterotransplantation in man. JAMA 187: 691-696

Reilly P [1973] Sickle cell anemia legislation. J Leg Med 1: 4-39

Research Group of Ethical, Social, and Legal Issues in Genetic Counseling and Genetic Engineering [1972] Ethical and social issues in screening for genetic disease. N Engl J Med 286: 1129-1132

Roe v. Wade [1973] 410 US 113

Sanford N [1970] Whatever happened to action research? J Soc Issues 26: 3-23

Singer P [1981] The expanding circle. Ethics and sociobiology. Farrar, Straus, and Giroux, New York

Toulmin S [1972] Human understanding. Princeton University Press, Princeton NJ

# 1 The 19-Nation Survey; Genetics and Ethics Around the World

## 1.1 Rationale

Medical or clinical genetics is "the aspect of human genetics that is concerned with the relation between heredity and disease" [14]. This growing medical specialty is concerned with all aspects of genetic disorders, including research, diagnosis, counseling, and treatment. The scientific basis for medical genetics is developing rapidly. Demonstration that DNA is the genetic material has led to a firm definition of the gene and to new diagnostic tests based on the DNA concept.

Patients are mainly the parents or prospective parents of children with genetic disorders, who seek genetic testing, prenatal diagnosis, or counseling in order to get information for making decisions about whether to have a(nother) child [20]. Parents may also visit geneticists in order to monitor a child's progress or to get information on prognosis, education, and treatment. Geneticists' patients also include adults with genetic disorders, family members concerned about carrier status, and persons who have been exposed to toxic substances that could cause genetic damage.

New tests, techniques, and treatments have increased the complexity of ethical decision-making in medical genetics. Medical geneticists' views and approaches clearly carry weight as clinicians, policy makers, and patients resolve ethical problems. Individual geneticists have set forth their ethical views in publications listed in the bibliographies for each chapter, but there has been no systematic study of the actual approaches of medical geneticists to ethical problems.

Fletcher, Berg, and Tranøy [7] proposed that medical geneticists around the world would benefit from collective reflection on their preferred approaches to the most frequent of the difficult moral choices in practical genetics, for three reasons. First, older bodies of guidance, such as codes of professional ethics in medicine, need to be supplemented by practical ethical statements based on clinical experience in order to be applied to current problems of moral choice. Second, there is a need to consolidate what geneticists have learned to date in the form of written guidelines, in order to assist in teaching younger colleagues and to help the specialty present itself clearly to other medical specialties. Thus far, the views and approaches of medical geneticists have mostly remained in an "oral tradition" passed from teacher to student. The time has come to clarify standards of practice and to establish normative guidelines. Third, medical genetics will become even more ethically complex in the future. For example, the potential for presymptomatic diagnosis of disorders of late onset and for screening persons whose genotypes make them more susceptible to common diseases will raise new issues of disclosure and public policy. Facing these issues with help from guidelines is better than facing them simply on the basis of personal opinion.

1

In order to provide a basis for discussion and the development of guidelines, we undertook a cross-national survey of geneticists' approaches to ethical dilemmas in 19 nations. We hypothesized that there was a widely supported consensus among medical geneticists about four key ethical principles and approaches to difficult choices: 1) respect for patient autonomy, including an obligation to respect patient requests with which the geneticist disagrees; 2) duty to reduce or prevent suffering from genetic disorders, conditional upon respect for parental autonomy (e. g., counseling should be non-directive); 3) full disclosure of test results, including colleague disagreements; and 4) a voluntary, not mandatory, approach to genetic screening, except for newborns when treatment is available.

## 1.2 Methods

### 1.2.1 Site Visits

To gather data on ethical problems frequently encountered in the practice of medical genetics, John C. Fletcher undertook field studies in 1984 at 25 genetic centers in 12 nations (Denmark, Federal Republic of Germany (FRG), France, Greece, Hungary, Italy, the Netherlands, Norway, Sweden, Switzerland, the United Kingdom, and the United States).

Each site visit included the following components:

1. A two hour conference with all staff who actually did genetic counseling, in which the same questions or cases were posed in each center.
2. Interviews with the chief of the center and selected others who did genetic counseling to ascertain:
   a) the most frequent of the difficult problems of moral choice faced by medical geneticists in their setting;
   b) the approaches taken to these problems;
   c) the resources used to formulate these approaches;
   d) how younger colleagues were instructed in the ethical practices of medical geneticists.
3. Whenever possible, and with the counselee's consent, observation of genetic counseling cases.
4. By invitation, a lecture or seminar on "Ethics and Trends in Applied Human Genetics."

Problems identified through the site visits became the basis of the survey questionnaires.

## 1.2.2 The 19 Survey Nations

### 1.2.2.1 Criteria for Selection

The rationale for choosing countries for final study was: a) ten or more practicing geneticists; b) geographical and cultural distribution; and c) the presence of a medical geneticist willing to distribute and collect questionnaires and to co-author, with a specialist in medical ethics, a chapter in this book. Most developing nations had too few geneticists for inclusion in the study. We originally attempted to enlist the participation of 23 nations. Four (Iran, the Netherlands, People's Republic of China, and U.S.S.R.) found participation logistically difficult at the time requested, but indicated willingness to participate in future surveys. In all, 19 nations participated.

### 1.2.2.2 Socio-economic Characteristics of Nations

Some economic and social characteristics of participating nations are described in Table 1.1, using data from the World Bank and from Sivard, *World Military and Social Expenditures,* a classic source in international studies of health [18]. Each country is ranked with regard to Gross National Product (GNP) per capita, public health expenditures per capita, population per physician, and infant mortality rate. Rank orders are based on 142 nations. In addition, the nations are ranked on a composite indicator of "economic-social standing" developed by Sivard. Of the 19 nations represented in this book, 15 are developed nations and four (Brazil, Greece, India and Turkey) are classed as developing nations in World Bank reports. The first two, Brazil and Greece, are not poor nations but have an unequal exchange with developed nations. Some medical sociologists describe them as economically "semi-peripheral" to the capitalist "core" nations rather than as "developing nations." Overall ranks for economic social standing ranged from one (Norway) to 112 (India) among 142 nations worldwide. GNP per capita ranged from $16,246 (Switzerland) to $262 (India), and infant mortality ranged from 6 (Japan) to 101 (India).

Infant mortality is frequently used as an indicator of a nation's overall health. Among developed nations it is also an indicator of equitable distribution of health and social welfare services. Infant mortality depends not only on how much wealth a nation has, but on how it is used.

We suggest that readers refer back to Table 1.1 as they peruse the chapters on individual countries.

In nations with limited resources, basic maternal and child health, such as prenatal care and nutritional supplements, must necessarily take precedence over genetics services. A nation that has $28 or $2 per capita to spend on public health cannot afford to provide many prenatal diagnoses or other genetics services. On the other hand, in some wealthy nations, such as the United States, infant mortality rates suggest that basic maternal and child health care is not being provided to the poor. The same is no doubt true of genetics services.

3

**Table 1.1.** Ranking of Countries, Economic and Health Indicators 1983[1]

| Country | Economic Social Standing[2] | GNP per Capita[3] | | Public Health Expenditures per Capita[4] | | Population per Physician[5] | | Infant Mortality Rate[6] | |
|---|---|---|---|---|---|---|---|---|---|
| | Rank | Rank | US$ | Rank | US$ | Rank | Number | Rank | Rate |
| Norway | 1 | 8 | 14,007 | 3 | 889 | 19 | 480 | 5 | 8 |
| Canada | 2 | 10 | 12,284 | 5 | 774 | 26 | 510 | 9 | 9 |
| Sweden | 3 | 9 | 12,444 | 1 | 1,122 | 19 | 480 | 4 | 7 |
| United States | 3 | 7 | 14,172 | 10 | 591 | 22 | 490 | 17 | 11 |
| Denmark | 6 | 12 | 11,538 | 9 | 670 | 10 | 410 | 5 | 8 |
| Australia | 8 | 13 | 11,514 | 11 | 580 | 23 | 500 | 13 | 10 |
| France | 8 | 16 | 10,481 | 7 | 694 | 17 | 460 | 9 | 9 |
| Federal Republic of Germany | 10 | 14 | 11,403 | 4 | 886 | 12 | 420 | 13 | 10 |
| Switzerland | 10 | 5 | 16,346 | 2 | 923 | 10 | 410 | 5 | 8 |
| United Kingdom | 12 | 22 | 9,171 | 15 | 499 | 32 | 600 | 13 | 10 |
| Japan | 16 | 19 | 19,154 | 14 | 510 | 38 | 710 | 1 | 6 |
| Israel | 20 | 35 | 5,420 | 29 | 188 | 4 | 350 | 33 | 19 |
| Italy | 22 | 30 | 6,549 | 20 | 407 | 2 | 300 | 21 | 12 |
| Hungary | 24 | 34 | 5,526 | 31 | 149 | 4 | 350 | 33 | 19 |
| German Democratic Republic | 25 | 26 | 7,427 | 26 | 221 | 17 | 460 | 17 | 11 |
| Greece | 33 | 41 | 3,932 | 32 | 143 | 6 | 360 | 27 | 15 |
| Brazil | 57 | 53 | 2,032 | 60 | 28 | 51 | 1,150 | 76 | 70 |
| Turkey | 82 | 71 | 1,210 | 90 | 8 | 63 | 1,500 | 93 | 96 |
| India | 112 | 122 | 262 | 118 | 2 | 78 | 2,620 | 101 | 106 |

Notes to Table 1.1
[1] All ranks based on 142 countries, using data from Ruth Leger Sivard, *World Military and Social Expenditures, 1986,* (Washington, DC: World Priorities, 1986). The rank order number is repeated if more than one country has the same figure.
[2] Summary rank among all nations in economic-social indicators. Three factors are combined: GNP per capita, education, and health. For education, a summary rank was first obtained for 5 indicators: public expenditures per capita, school-age population per teacher, % school-age population in school, % women in total university enrollment, and literacy rate. For health, a summary rank was first obtained for 4 indicators: public expenditures per capita, population per physician, infant mortality rate, and life expectancy. The indicators chosen for education and health represent both input of national effort (e.g. public expenditures, numbers of physicians) and output (e.g., literacy, infant mortality). Input factors give credit for effort, which will determine social progress but may not yet show in slower-acting indicators of results (Sivard, p. 43).
[3] Gross National Product is the economy's total output of goods and services, valued at current market prices paid by the ultimate consumer.
[4] *Public health expenditures represent current and capital expenditures by governments for medical care and other health services.* "WHO has cautioned that differences in budgetary concepts and definitions of health seriously qualify comparisons among countries." (Sivard, p. 43).
[5] *Physicians refer to fully qualified doctors practicing in the country.* National reporting, however, may reflect differences in definition, qualifications, and training. Some countries include physicians who are inactive or practicing elsewhere. Some, including Italy, count dentists as physicians. Some report only physicians in government service. According to Sivard, physicians are probably more reliable for inter-country comparisons than are expenditure figures.
[6] Deaths under 1 year of age per 1,000 live births.

## 1.2.2.3 Health Care Systems

Types of health care systems are described in Table 1.2, using a classification system devised by Elling [5]. Nations are listed by income, political system, and structure of health system. Income categories are classifications used by the World Bank and by Sivard [4]. Eleven countries are classified as high income (Australia, Canada, Denmark, Federal Republic of Germany, France, Japan, Norway, Sweden, Switzerland, United Kingdom, and United States). Six are classified as upper middle income (Brazil, German Democratic Republic, Greece, Hungary, Israel, and Italy). Two (India and Turkey) are classified as low income. Two nations (German Democratic Republic and Hungary) are socialist; the other 17 are capitalist.

The 19 nations are categorized according to five types of health care structures. Type I is a fee-for-service private pay system with some federal public programs, including compulsory national health insurance for those 65 and older (Medicare). There is no regionalization of services, and the Public Health Service is not targeted geographically to reach all segments of the population. Of the 19 nations, only the United States falls into this category. Type II is a national health insurance system with universal coverage, but with little regionalization of service and no targeting to reach all groups and areas. Some private, fee-for-service elements coexist with national health insurance. Australia, Federal Republic of Germany, France, Greece, and Japan fall within this category. Type III is a national health insurance system covering all who do not seek private care on their own. This is a dualistic public-private system, not well regionalized and not geographically targeted to reach the entire population. Brazil, India, Switzerland, and Turkey fall in-

**Table 1.2.** Countries Grouped by Category of Health System, Government and Economics[1]

| Structure of National Health Services | Socialist Countries | Capitalist Countries | | |
|---|---|---|---|---|
| | Upper Middle Income | Upper Middle Income | High Income | Low Income |
| I. Segmented national health insurance (Medicare) – primarily market oriented | | | USA | |
| II. National Health insurance – primarily market oriented | | Greece | Australia FRG France Japan | |
| III. Mixed public-private, planned market system | | Brazil | Switzerland | India Turkey |
| IV. National Health Service, regionalized and geographically targeted at periphery | GDR Hungary | | Denmark UK | |
| V. National Health Service, regionalized, but not targeted at periphery | | Israel Italy | Canada Norway Sweden | |

[1] Elling, Ray H. (1986) *The Struggle for Workers' Health.* Farmingdale, NY: Baywood, pp. 30, 73

5

to this category. Type IV is a national health service, as opposed to national health insurance. In a national health service, doctors are salaried government employees and there are almost no private elements. The national health service is regionalized and geographically targeted so as to reach all segments of the population, including those in rural areas. Denmark, the German Democratic Republic, Hungary, and the United Kingdom fall into this category. Although in the GDR private health care is nonexistent, Hungary has some private health care in outpatient clinics. In the UK cutbacks in the National Health Service have led to increasing privatization. Type V is also a national health service, but differs from Type IV in that it is not geographically targeted to reach all segments of the population. In a Type V system, a patient can enter the health care structure in several ways, for example through a clinic at work or through a neighborhood health center, while in a Type IV system s/he can enter the health system in only one, geographically ordered way. Canada, Israel, Italy, Norway, and Sweden fall into Type V, though Sweden is moving toward Type IV. Types IV and V are those most likely to reach the entire population equitably and to provide a just distribution of available services.

## 1.2.3 Survey Questionnaires

### 1.2.3.1 Development and Content

In developing the questionnaire, we composed 14 clinical cases involving ethical problems in clinical genetics. Respondents were asked *what* they would do, from a fixed list of possible responses, and *why*, in their own words, they had chosen this particular course of action. They were also asked which cases had given them the most and the least ethical conflict. There were four questions on screening for genetic disorders and access to results. Next, the respondents were asked to place two lists of ten issues each in rank order, beginning with the one of most ethical concern. The first list was ethical priorities (to geneticists) in their own nation; the second list was priorities for geneticists "around the world." Finally, there were questions about goals and approaches to counseling originally proposed by Fraser [9] because previous researchers [20] had surveyed geneticists' responses to them. All questionnaires were administered and answered in English. The questionnaire was pilot-tested twice, between April and June, 1985, on 11 and 10 geneticists respectively, and revised after each trial.

The questionnaires took approximately two hours to complete. We asked respondents to set them aside for a day after completing the first half, so that they might approach the second half freshly. Questionnaires were answered anonymously.

Eighteen of the participants in the pilot study were from the United States (eight from Massachusetts, six from the National Institutes of Health, and four from other areas), two were from Canada, and one was from Spain. There were eleven men, ten women, six chiefs of genetics units, four who were primarily counselors, and three whose duties consisted primarily of laboratory work. When possible, one of the authors observed them answering the questionnaire in order to see whether questions presented problems in comprehension. Afterword, we spoke with each person for an hour in order to get suggestions for clarifying phraseology.

## 1.2.3.2 Criteria for Inclusion of Geneticists

We selected geneticists who held an M. D., Ph. D., or equivalent degree, and were engaged in delivering or administering genetic services (testing, counseling, prenatal diagnosis, laboratory work). Although in some countries (notably the United States) counseling is sometimes done by specially-trained persons who do not hold a doctorate, we decided to omit these persons to control for consistency of training across the entire sample.

In each country, including the United States, our contact geneticists tried to include all qualified medical geneticists in the survey. Lists were compiled from certifying boards, genetics centers, and the National Foundation - March of Dimes *International Directory of Genetic Services* [15].

## 1.2.3.3 Distribution and Follow-up

Our colleagues in each country wrote cover letters to their compatriots explaining the purpose of the study and mailed these, together with the questionnaires, to all geneticists in their respective countries. Questionnaires were to be returned anonymously to our colleagues in envelopes provided. In order to permit follow-up while preserving anonymity, we provided postcards to be signed and returned to our colleagues separately from the questionnaires. We instructed our colleagues to follow up those who did not return questionnaires, either by mail or telephone, in order to maximize participation. Each contact geneticist was provided with enough questionnaires for two follow-ups, return envelopes and postcards addressed to him/her, and an optional form for hand-tallying the results if they chose. After looking over the questionnaires and taking notes for their own use, they were to send the questionnaires to the Boston University School of Public Health for entry into the computer. In the case of one country with few geneticists, respondents asked to send their questionnaires directly to us, rather than to our contact person, in order to insure anonymity.

Our colleagues received the questionnaires and other materials in July, 1985, with the exception of India and Turkey, where new contacts were established in July, 1986. Colleagues from 16 nations returned the questionnaires to Boston University by August 5, 1986. Questionnaires from India and Turkey arrived in February 1987. The questionnaires from the German Democratic Republic (GDR) could not be sent to us, for reasons of confidentiality, but our colleague provided us with a hand tally of responses. Although data from the German Democratic Republic could not be entered into the computer, we were able to include the

7

GDR in most of our tables by using this hand tally. In Hungary, the professional association of geneticists required that distribution be to centers rather than to individuals, with each center receiving one questionnaire and the individuals associated with that center each having input into the center's response. The unit of analysis for Hungary is therefore genetics centers rather than individual geneticists.

On account of the large numbers of geneticists involved, questionnaires in the United States were mailed directly from Boston University rather than by our geneticist colleague. The first mailing, on August 11, 1985, went to all persons with M.D.'s or Ph.D's listed in the 1982 Membership Directory of the American Board of Medical Genetics, which was the most recent list of board certified persons available at that time, and to directors of centers listed in the National Foundation - March of Dimes Birth Defects Foundation *International Directory of Genetic Services* for 1983. This mailing elicited 162 responses; follow-up mailings on September 15, 1985 and November 1, 1985 elicited 95 and 38 responses respectively.

## 1.2.4 Responses

### 1.2.4.1 Participation Rates

Of the 1098 geneticists asked to participate, 682 (62%) returned completed questionnaires by the close of the study in June, 1987 (Table 3). Ninety-five per cent of these answered all questions, and 80% gave reasons for all their choices of action. Reasons were stated in their own words. This represented a very good response rate for a questionnaire that took native speakers of English two hours to complete and that probably took longer for others.

### 1.2.4.2 Professional Characteristics of Respondents

Major professional characteristics of respondents are described by country in Table 1.4. Eighty-one per cent held M.D.'s, including 45% who were pediatricians, 6% internists, and 5% obstetricians; 16% were Ph.D.'s who did not hold an M.D., and 3% held other degrees. They had a median of 14 years in the practice of genetics, ranging from seven years in India to 15 in Canada and Greece. Eighty-two per cent were members of their national genetics society, and 77% were board certified or accredited in countries where certification or accreditation in genetics was possible. These countries were Canada (96%), Hungary (80%), the United Kingdom (61%), and the United States (82%). Respondents spent a median of 45 hours a week in genetics, ranging from 17 hours in Hungary to 49 in Norway. Those who specified their activities spent a median of seven hours per week seeing patients, six hours in clerical or administrative work, four hours reading professional journals, and four hours a week in laboratory work. In Australia, Federal

**Table 1.3.** Participating Nations

| Nation | Number Asked to Participate | Number of Persons Responding | Response Rate (%) |
|---|---|---|---|
| Australia | 14 | 12 | 86 |
| Brazil | 51 | 32 | 63 |
| Canada | 73 | 47 | 64 |
| Denmark | 28 | 15 | 58 |
| Federal Republic of Germany (FRG) | 55 | 47 | 85 |
| France | 35 | 17 | 49 |
| German Democratic Republic (GDR) | 25 | 21 | 80 |
| Greece | 11 | 7 | 64 |
| Hungary* | 18 | 15 | 83 |
| India | 72 | 27 | 38 |
| Israel | 17 | 15 | 88 |
| Italy | 26 | 11 | 42 |
| Japan | 74 | 51 | 69 |
| Norway | 10 | 6 | 60 |
| Sweden | 26 | 21 | 81 |
| Switzerland | 10 | 5 | 50 |
| Turkey | 13 | 5 | 38 |
| United Kingdom | 50 | 33 | 66 |
| United States | 490 | 295 | 60 |
| Total | 1,098 | 682 | 62 |

* Unit of analysis is genetics centers

**Table 1.4.** Professional Characteristics

| Country | Total % M.D.'s | % Pedia-tricians | % Ph.D.'s | Median Years in Genetics | Median Hours/wk in Genetics | Median Patients/ Week Counseled |
|---|---|---|---|---|---|---|
| Australia | 100 | 75 | 0 | 11 | 40 | 8 |
| Brazil | 56 | 38 | 38 | 13 | 40 | 4 |
| Canada | 72 | 38 | 26 | 15 | 45 | 3 |
| Denmark | 100 | 20 | 0 | 17 | 40 | 3 |
| Federal Rep. of Germany | 96 | 23 | 4 | 9 | 39 | 7 |
| France | 100 | 88 | 0 | 17 | 34 | 12 |
| German Dem. Republic | 95 | 48 | 0 | 10 | 40 | 8 |
| Greece | 71 | 57 | 14 | 15 | 38 | 8 |
| Hungary | 100 | 53 | 0 | 18 | 17 | 5 |
| India | 79 | 48 | 19 | 7 | 39 | 4 |
| Israel | 67 | 40 | 20 | 11 | 42 | 8 |
| Italy | 100 | 36 | 0 | 10 | 31 | 7 |
| Japan | 100 | 55 | 0 | 10 | 20 | 1 |
| Norway | 100 | 0 | 0 | 9 | 49 | 4 |
| Sweden | 90 | 43 | 10 | 8 | 38 | 4 |
| Switzerland | 80 | 20 | 20 | 13 | 41 | 4 |
| Turkey | 80 | 20 | 20 | 9 | 41 | 8 |
| United Kingdom | 91 | 27 | 9 | 13 | 39 | 9 |
| United States | 74 | 51 | 22 | 14 | 45 | 4 |
| Total | 81 | 45 | 16 | 14 | 45 | 4 |
| Total, Excluding U.S. | 86 | 39 | 12 | 12 | 40 | 5 |

Republic of Germany, France, German Democratic Republic and the United Kingdom the median number of hours in laboratory work was zero. Otherwise, there was little variation among nations in the numbers of hours spent on specific activities, and some did not specify how they distributed their time. They counseled a median of four genetics patients a week, ranging from one in Japan to 12 in France.

### 1.2.4.3 Personal Characteristics of Respondents

Personal data by country are listed in Table 1.5. The median age was 45, ranging from 38 in Brazil to 50 in France. Sixty-five per cent were male, ranging from 40% in Israel to 93% in Hungary, and 82% were married with a median of 1.5 children. Religious backgrounds were 40% Protestant, 18% Catholic, 17% Jewish, 12% none, 5% Buddhist, 4% Hindu, and 4% other. As a whole, they were nonpracticing, attending a median of one religious observance a year. Exceptions were France, with a median of 15–24 religious observances, and the United States and India, each with a median of 2–4 observances. In these three countries, 63%, 39%, and 35% respectively attended 15 or more observances a year, with 44%, 23%, and 32% attending 25 or more. Forty-nine per cent characterized themselves as politically liberal, 15% as conservative, and 36% as both equally.

### 1.2.4.4 Respondents and Non-respondents Compared

In the United States, a comparison between 274 respondents and 178 nonrespondents listed in the 1986 combined *Membership Directory* of the Genetics Society of America, American Society of Human Genetics, and American Board of Medical Genetics revealed no statistically significant differences between respondents and nonrespondents in type of degree, gender, geographical area, or subspecialty.

## 1.2.5 Data Analysis

### 1.2.5.1 Coding

Qualitative responses, including the responders' anticipation of the consequences of their choices, were quantified, using a coding system developed by the authors. Each questionnaire was coded independently by two persons with higher degrees in genetics or sociology, with a third coder making the final judgement in cases where the first two disagreed. Dr. Wertz examined the final coding of each questionnaire before entry into the computer. We coded the first two reasons given for each choice of action, using a list of the 98 reasons most frequently given. We also

**Table 1.5.** Personal Characteristics

| Country | Median Age | % Male | Median Number of Children | % Protestant | % Catholic | % Jewish | % Other | % None | Median Religious Observances/yr. | Liberal Politics | Conservative Politics |
|---|---|---|---|---|---|---|---|---|---|---|---|
| Australia | 42 | 67 | 3 | 58 | 0 | 25 | 0 | 17 | 1 | 33 | 33 |
| Brazil | 38 | 56 | 1 | 6 | 50 | 19 | 6 | 19 | 0 | 56 | 13 |
| Canada | 48 | 58 | 2 | 51 | 11 | 11 | 2 | 25 | 1 | 68 | 6 |
| Denmark | 47 | 87 | 2 | 73 | 0 | 0 | 0 | 27 | 0 | 57 | 7 |
| Federal Rep. of Germany | 42 | 52 | 1 | 60 | 32 | 0 | 2 | 6 | 1 | 41 | 9 |
| France | 50 | 60 | 3 | 0 | 100 | 0 | 0 | 0 | 15–24 | 31 | 19 |
| German Dem. Republic | 40 | 43 | 2 | 48 | 0 | 0 | 0 | 52 | 0 | 71** | 14 |
| Greece | 40 | 43 | 1 | 0 | 14 | 0 | 86* | 0 | 0 | 43 | 14 |
| Hungary | 49 | 93 | 1 | 13 | 67 | 0 | 0 | 20 | 0 | 27 | 13 |
| India | 43 | 54 | 1 | 8 | 4 | 0 | 88* | 0 | 2–4 | 40 | 0 |
| Israel | 48 | 40 | 2 | 0 | 0 | 100 | 0 | 0 | 0 | 67 | 7 |
| Italy | 41 | 64 | 1 | 0 | 91 | 0 | 0 | 9 | 0 | 46 | 0 |
| Japan | 46 | 82 | 2 | 6 | 2 | 0 | 65* | 27 | 1 | 35 | 18 |
| Norway | 47 | 80 | 0 | 40 | 0 | 0 | 0 | 60 | 0 | 50 | 25 |
| Sweden | 45 | 71 | 2 | 76 | 5 | 0 | 5 | 14 | 0 | 52 | 19 |
| Switzerland | 45 | 60 | 3 | 60 | 40 | 0 | 0 | 0 | 1 | 60 | 20 |
| Turkey | 41 | 60 | 1 | 0 | 0 | 0 | 100* | 0 | 0 | 40 | 0 |
| United Kingdom | 49 | 60 | 2 | 72 | 6 | 0 | 0 | 22 | 1 | 47 | 16 |
| United States | 45 | 67 | 2 | 46 | 14 | 28 | 7 | 5 | 2–4 | 51 | 18 |
| Total | 45 | 65 | 1.5 | 40 | 18 | 17 | 13 | 12 | 1 | 49 | 15 |
| Total, Excluding U.S. | 45 | 64 | 1.5 | 34 | 22 | 8 | 20 | 16 | 1 | 47 | 12 |

* Greece: Eastern Orthodox 86%; India: Hindu 81%; Japan: Buddhist 63%; Turkey: Moslem 80%.
** includes progressive

11

coded whether respondents envisioned or described specific consequences of their actions (such as the birth of a child with a genetic disorder), whether respondents described conflicts between the interests of different parties, and whose welfare the respondent considered most important. The coding system is described in detail in Section 1.7.1 below.

Responses were entered into a Statistical Package for the Social Sciences (SPSS-X) program. Cross-tabulations of all responses by country were performed, and the results were sent to our colleagues in 17 nations in August, 1986 and to India and Turkey in Spring, 1987.

### 1.2.5.2 Criteria for Consensus

Our criteria for consensus were those frequently used in legislative processes, in the absence of an accepted scientific criterion for consensus. We used a "3/4's rule" (3/4's of the respondents in each of 3/4's of countries) to define a "strong consensus," and a "2/3's rule" (2/3's of respondents in each of 2/3's of countries) to define a "moderate consensus." This method allows representation to each country. If we had used percentages of the total number of responses, the United States, with 43% of all respondents, would have been disproportionately represented.

### 1.2.5.3 Regression Analyses

In order to see whether geneticists' choices of actions were consistently related to factors in their professional or personal backgrounds, over and above their nationality, we entered all socio-demographic data, including degree, age, gender, years of experience, hours per week in genetics, patients per week, subspeciality, political inclination, religious background, religiosity, and nation into stepwise logistic regressions, with choice of action as the dependent variable. This method orders each background characteristic in terms of its strength of association with the dependent variable, while controlling for other variables that are statistically significant at the $p < 0.05$ level. In addition, this analysis provides an estimate of the "odds ratio," that is, the odds that a geneticist with a particular background characteristic will choose a particular course of action. A stepwise logistic regression was performed for responses to each question, using SAS (Statistical Analysis System). Wherever background characteristics were related to responses, over and above nationality, we have reported the odds ratios.

### 1.2.5.4 Internal and External Validity

Standard tests for internal validity were performed, comparing each individual's responses to related questions (e.g., approaches to clinical counseling cases versus statements about preferred counseling approaches). Results indicated that respondents answered in a consistent manner. There is no practical method of establishing external validity (relationships between responses and clinical practice) for such a large, geographically dispersed sample.

How accurately do the survey results reflect counselors' actual practices, as opposed to attitudes and beliefs? There is no practical way to assess this without extensive field observations in the 19 nations. There are inherent but unavoidable weaknesses in the questionnaire method, no matter how carefully contrived. No questionnaire of geneticists alone can validly assess the quality or efficacy of genetic services in different nations. In some nations the questionnaires may have elicited those responses that participants considered, whether consciously or unconsciously, most acceptable to their colleague who collected the questionnaires. The effects of having a senior person, usually a well-known and highly respected authority, disseminate and collect the questionnaires cannot be discounted entirely, even though responses were anonymous. The alternative, conducting the survey through unknown outsiders, would have produced a low response rate.

Some respondents trained in the U.S., U.K., or Canada may have responded in terms of the ethics learned in their post-graduate training rather than the ethics practiced in their own nations. As the questionnaires did not ask about training abroad, there is no way of assessing its effects upon ethical decision-making.

## 1.3 Results: Choices of Actions

### 1.3.1 Outline of Ethical Problems

The 14 clinical cases covered five types of ethical problems: 1) confidentiality versus duties to third parties (3 cases); 2) full disclosure of sensitive information (2 cases); 3) full disclosure of laboratory test results (3 cases), 4) indications for prenatal diagnosis (3 cases), 5) directive/nondirective counseling (3 cases). The cases are described, as presented in the questionnaires, in Table 1.6. The case numbers listed in Table 1.6 will be used hereafter to refer to cases.

### 1.3.2 Confidentiality versus Duties to Third Parties

Table 1.7 describes three cases of conflict between the physician's duty to preserve patient confidentiality and the duty to warn third parties, namely the husband or the relatives at risk for genetic disorders, of harm.

There was strong consensus on one case, false paternity (Case 1). In this case, genetic tests have revealed that the husband is not the biological father of the affected child. For 96% of respondents ($\geq$90% in all countries), protection of the mother's confidentiality overrode disclosure of true paternity. Eighty-one per cent said that they would tell the mother in private, without the husband present, and let her decide what to tell him; 13% would lie (*e.g.*, tell the couple that they are

**Table 1.6.** Clinical Cases by Type of Ethical Problem

| Ethical Problem | Clinical Situation |
| --- | --- |
| I. *Confidentiality vs. duties to third parties* | |
| 1. False paternity (Table 1.7) | You are evaluating a child with an autosomal recessive disorder for which carrier testing is possible and accurate. In the process of testing relatives for genetic counseling, you discover that the mother and half the siblings are carriers, whereas the husband is not. The husband believes that he is the child's biological father. |
| 2. Huntington disease (Table 1.7) | A client recently diagnosed as having Huntington disease (HD) refuses to permit disclosure of the diagnosis and relevant genetic information to siblings who may be at risk for Huntington disease. |
| 3. Hemophilia A (Table 1.7) | A client with a child recently diagnosed with hemophilia A refuses to permit disclosure of the diagnosis and relevant genetic information to her relatives who may be at risk for conceiving children with hemophilia A. |
| II. *Full disclosure of Sensitive information* | |
| 4. Parental translocation (Table 1.8) | You identify a parent of a Down syndrome child as having a balanced translocation. |
| 5. XY female (Table 1.8) | A woman undergoes diagnosis for infertility. Tests reveal that she is chromosomally male (XY). |
| III. *Full disclosure of laboratory results* | |
| 6. Conflicting test results (Table 1.9) | Maternal serum alpha-fetoprotein has been elevated in your patient on two occasions, but level II ultrasound discloses no abnormality, despite careful examination of the fetal head, spine, abdomen, and kidneys. The fetal karyotype is normal. Amniotic alpha-fetoprotein is elevated and acetylcholinesterase is borderline. These results raise the possibility of a small neural tube defect. What do you tell the patient? |
| 7. New/controversial interpretations (Table 1.9) | Repeated maternal serum alpha-fetoprotein tests reveal a value that is *below* the norm. Although some studies have found low maternal serum alpha-fetoprotein values to be associated with Down syndrome, geneticists are not in agreement about how a low value should be interpreted. |
| 8. Ambiguous/artifactual results, colleague disagreement (Table 1.9) | Laboratory analysis of amniotic fluid cells suggests that the fetus may be a trisomy 13 mosaic. There is disagreement among the medical geneticists responsible for the analysis as to whether or not these are artifacts of culture, in other words, false positives. Given the present state of knowledge, there is no way of resolving this disagreement scientifically within the legal time limit for termination of pregnancy, because the results of repeat tests will not be available until after 24 weeks gestational age. You were not responsible for the laboratory work in this case and have not taken one side or |

**Table 1.6.** (continued)

| Ethical Problem | Clinical Situation |
| --- | --- |
| | the other. You are, however, the medical geneticist responsible for dealing directly with the prospective mother. |
| IV. *Indications for Prenatal diagnosis* | |
| 9. Parents would refuse abortion (Table 1.11) | A 42 year-old woman requests prenatal diagnosis for Down syndrome. She and her husband already have a Down syndrome child. She tells you that they are opposed to abortion and that she will carry the fetus to term even if it is diagnosed as having Down syndrome. They would like to have prenatal diagnosis, however, in order to give themselves time to prepare for the birth of another affected child. |
| 10. Maternal anxiety (Table 1.11) | A 25 year-old woman with no family history of genetic disorders and no personal history of exposure to toxic substances requests prenatal diagnosis. There are no genetic or medical indications for its use. Nevertheless, she appears very anxious about the normalcy of the fetus, and persists in her demands for prenatal diagnosis even after being informed that in her case the potential medical risks for the fetus, in terms of miscarriage, may outweigh the likelihood of diagnosing an abnormality. |
| 11. Sex selection, in absence of X-linked disease (Table 1.11) | A couple requests prenatal diagnosis for purposes of selecting the sex of the child. They already have four girls and are desperate for a boy. They say that if the fetus is a girl, they will abort it and will keep trying until they conceive a boy. They also tell you that if you refuse to do prenatal diagnosis for sex selection, they will abort the fetus rather than run the risk of having another girl. |
| V. *Directive/Nondirective Counseling* | |
| 12. Fetuses with low burden disorders (Table 1.13) | Prenatal diagnosis has revealed an abnormal fetus. How would you counsel the prospective parents of an XO (Turner) or XYY fetus? Choices are advise carrying to term, advise abortion, give optimistically or pessimistically slanted information, counsel nondirectively, and counsel nondirectively but also describe difficulties of termination. |
| 13. and 14. Presenting reproductive options to male and female carriers of disorders diagnosable prenatally (Table 1.14) | Evaluation of a child produces findings consistent with a diagnosis of tuberous sclerosis. Upon examining the parents, you find evidence that one carries the tuberous sclerosis gene, even though intelligence seems normal. After a discussion of the risk of having another child with tuberous sclerosis who might be severely affected, the couple asks you whether recurrence of the disorder can be prevented. The options are; taking their chances, contraception, sterilization, adoption, artificial insemination by a donor, IVF with a donated egg, and insemination of a surrogate mother with the husband's sperm. |

15

**Table 1.7.** Patient Confidentiality Versus Duties to Third Parties

Per Cent Who Would Disclose Diagnosis to Husband or Relatives at Risk, Against Patient's Wishes

| Country | False Paternity (Case 1) | | Huntington disease (Case 2) | | Hemophilia A (Case 3) | |
|---|---|---|---|---|---|---|
| | (In parentheses: per cents who would disclose to mother alone without husband present) | | (In parentheses: per cents who would disclose even if relatives did not ask) | | | |
| Australia | 0+ | (50) | 75* | (0)+ | 75* | (17)+ |
| Brazil | 3+ | (78)* | 91* | (38) | 94* | (47) |
| Canada | 4+ | (87)* | 57 | (32) | 57 | (32) |
| Denmark | 0+ | (79)* | 87* | (33) | 87* | (53) |
| Federal Republic of Germany | 4+ | (79)* | 74 | (9)+ | 67 | (7)+ |
| France | 0+ | (100)* | 47 | (18)+ | 53 | (18)+ |
| German Democratic Republic | 0+ | (81)* | 57 | (43) | 67 | (33) |
| Greece | 0+ | (100)* | 14+ | (0)+ | 43 | (14)+ |
| Hungary | 0+ | (93)* | 47 | (40) | 73 | (67) |
| India | 4+ | (70) | 48 | (33) | 67 | (63) |
| Israel | 7+ | (73) | 73 | (27) | 73 | (40) |
| Italy | 0+ | (100)* | 82* | (36) | 73 | (27) |
| Japan | 4+ | (67) | 53 | (16)+ | 65 | (24)+ |
| Norway | 0+ | (100)* | 83* | (50) | 50 | (17)+ |
| Sweden | 10+ | (76)* | 48 | (14)+ | 48 | (10)+ |
| Turkey | 0+ | (80)* | 80* | (60) | 80* | (20)+ |
| Switzerland | 0+ | (80)* | 40 | (20)+ | 60 | (20)+ |
| United Kingdom | 3+ | (81)* | 58 | (32) | 50 | (16)+ |
| United States | 6+ | (84)* | 53 | (24)+ | 54 | (29) |
| Total | 4+ | (81)* | 58 | (24)+ | 60 | (29) |
| (95% Confidence limits) | (2,6) | (77, 85) | (53, 63) | (20, 28) | (55, 65) | (25, 33) |
| Total, Excluding U.S. | 3+ | (79)* | 63 | (25)+ | 66 | (30) |
| (95% Confidence limits) | (1,5) | (73, 85) | (57, 69) | (20, 30) | (60, 72) | (25, 35) |

* Strong consensus *for* disclosure
+ Strong consensus *against* disclosure

both genetically responsible); 4% would tell both husband and wife; and the remaining 2% would ascribe the child's disorder to a new mutation, a one-in-a-million occurrence. As their reasons for such answers, 58% cited preserving the family unit, 30% gave the mother's right to decide, and 13% gave the mother's right to privacy.

In Cases 2 and 3, the patient (with Huntington disease or hemophilia A) has refused to permit disclosure of the diagnosis to relatives at risk for the same disorder. The potential benefits of disclosure are very different for the two disorders. Huntington disease (HD) causes mental degeneration, is untreatable, and of late onset. Although it can now be diagnosed prenatally or presymptomatically in families where DNA analysis is possible, such tests are not widely available. The clinical diagnosis may occur too late for disclosure to affect the reproductive decisions of the patient's siblings or children, and disclosure may only cause psychological distress. In contrast, hemophilia A is diagnosable prenatally and is treatable; disclosure could help relatives in reproductive planning. We expected that significantly more would disclose a diagnosis of hemophilia A than of Huntington disease. This was not the case. Instead, 58% would tell the relatives of the Huntington patient, and 60% would tell the relatives of the hemophilia A patient. These percentages included 24% and 29% respectively who would seek out and tell the relatives even if they did not ask for information. Thirty-two per cent would preserve the confidentiality of the Huntington patient and 10% would refer the matter to the patient's family doctor for decision; 27% would respect the confidentiality of the hemophilia A patient and 12% would refer the decision to the family doctor. There was strong consensus for disclosure of both diagnoses in four nations, Australia, Brazil, Denmark and Turkey, and strong consensus for disclosure of the Huntington diagnosis in an additional two nations, Italy and Norway. In both cases, those who would disclose were significantly more likely (p < 0.0001) to envision and discuss the consequences of their actions than were those who would preserve patient confidentiality.

## 1.3.3 Full Disclosure of Sensitive Information

Table 1.8 describes two situations involving disclosure of psychologically sensitive information that may harm the patient (Cases 4 and 5). In Case 4, genetic testing reveals which parent carries a balanced translocation that has caused Down syndrome in their child. Disclosure of this information might enable the couple and relatives at risk to use reproductive options that would prevent the birth of another Down syndrome child, but could also cause guilt in the carrier or threaten the marriage. In Case 5, a phenotypic woman presents for infertility and is found to have XY genotype. Disclosure could severely damage her self-image, but could resolve doubts about fertility. Both cases involve conflicts between the clinician's duty to tell the truth (which may also be phrased in terms of the patient's right to know) and the duty to do no harm. In both cases, patients have asked for information about etiology, but they have not asked specific questions about their carrier status or genotype. Respondents were almost equally divided about disclosure, with 54% saying that they would disclose, unasked, which parent was a carrier and 51% disclosing XY genotype. In the balanced translocation case, an additional 43% would tell the couple that the information exists and give them the choice of knowing or not knowing. There was strong consensus in Switzerland and Turkey in favor of disclosure of carrier status, and strong consensus in seven countries, Brazil, France, German Democratic Republic, Greece, Hungary, Norway, and Switzerland, *against* disclosure of XY genotype. In three countries, Turkey, Canada, and the United States, a majority (100%, 68% and 64%, respectively) would disclose XY genotype. In both cases worldwide, those who would not disclose were significantly more likely (p < 0.00001) to envision and discuss the consequences of their actions than those who would disclose.

**Table 1.8.** Full Disclosure of Psychologically Sensitive Information

| Per Cent Who Would Disclose | Type of Information | |
|---|---|---|
| | Which parent carries a balanced translocation that has caused Down syndrome in their child, even if they do not ask (Case 4) | XY genotype in a female (androgen insensitivity syndrome) (Case 5) |
| Australia | 67 | 58 |
| Brazil | 63 | 9+ |
| Canada | 60 | 68 |
| Denmark | 67 | 40 |
| Federal Republic of Germany | 38 | 52 |
| France | 69 | 13+ |
| German Democratic Republic | 65 | 19+ |
| Greece | 72 | 14+ |
| Hungary | 27 | 20+ |
| India | 44 | 52 |
| Israel | 71 | 27 |
| Italy | 64 | 27 |
| Japan | 6+ | 40 |
| Norway | 67 | 17+ |
| Sweden | 29 | 52 |
| Switzerland | 100* | 0+ |
| Turkey | 80* | 100* |
| United Kingdom | 41 | 37 |
| United States | 62 | 64 |
| Total (95% Confidence limits) | 54 (49, 59) | 51 (46, 56) |
| Total, Excluding U.S. (95% Confidence limits) | 46 (40, 52) | 41 (35, 47) |

* Strong consensus for disclosure
+ Strong consensus against disclosure

## 1.3.4 Full Disclosure of Laboratory Test Results

Three of the 14 clinical situations (Cases 6, 7, and 8) dealt with the ethics of full disclosure of conflicting, new/controversial, or ambiguous, possibly artifactual results. There was strong consensus in all three cases (94%-98%) for telling patients that there might be an abnormality (Table 1.9). There was also strong consensus, in the two cases where we asked respondents how they would advise patients, that counseling should be nondirective. For a discussion of Case 6, see 1.3.6 below.

In Case 7, a new, controversial interpretation of low alpha-fetoprotein (AFP), 82% would tell patients that geneticists were not in agreement about the interpretation, but that some geneticists think there may be a possibility of Down syndrome, explain the relative risks of genetic abnormality and prenatal diagnostic

**Table 1.9.** Disclosure of Conflicting, Controversial, or Ambiguous Results

| Country | Per Cent Disclosing | | | | | |
|---|---|---|---|---|---|---|
| | Conflicting Results for Small NTD (in parentheses: % who would not give advice) | | New or Controversial Interpretation of Low AFP (in parentheses: % who would not give advice about PDX) | | Ambiguous or Artifactual Results[+] | Colleague Disagreement About the Meaning of Results |
| | (Case 6) | | (Case 7) | | (Case 8) | (Case 8) |
| Australia | 100* | (100)* | 100* | (83)* | 100* | 50 |
| Brazil | 97* | (84)* | 97* | (91)* | 91* | 72 |
| Canada | 100* | (94)* | 96* | (83)* | 98* | 66 |
| Denmark | 93* | (79)* | 100* | (73) | 93* | 47 |
| Federal Republic of Germany | 100* | (73) | 96* | (81)* | 91* | 77* |
| France | 94* | (56) | 88* | (65) | 100* | 47 |
| German Democratic Republic | 100* | (48) | 95* | (62) | 100* | 71 |
| Greece | 100* | (100)* | 100* | (100)* | 100* | 43 |
| Hungary | 93* | (47) | 87* | (53) | 93* | 60 |
| India | 89* | (63) | 92* | (50) | 100* | 56 |
| Israel | 100* | (100)* | 87* | (73) | 100* | 57 |
| Italy | 100* | (91)* | 100* | (100)* | 100* | 46 |
| Japan | 98* | (77)* | 86* | (75)* | 94* | 61 |
| Norway | 100* | (67) | 83* | (67) | 100* | 33 |
| Sweden | 100* | (86)* | 76* | (62) | 100* | 48 |
| Switzerland | 100* | (100)* | 100* | (100)* | 80* | 20 |
| Turkey | 100* | (100)* | 100* | (80)* | 100* | 100* |
| United Kingdom | 94* | (84)* | 84* | (78)* | 90* | 52 |
| United States | 98* | (95)* | 97* | (89)* | 99* | 75* |
| Total | 98* | (87)* | 94* | (82)* | 97* | 66 |
| (95% Confidence limits) | (96, 100) | (83, 91) | (91, 97) | (78, 86) | (95, 99) | (61, 71) |
| Total, Excluding U.S. | 97* | (80)* | 91* | (76)* | 96* | 60 |
| (95% Confidence limits) | (95, 99) | (74, 86) | (87, 95) | (70, 82) | (94, 98) | (54, 66) |

[+] 97% would tell patients that there might be an abnormality
* Strong consensus ($\geq 75\%$) in favor of disclosure or not giving advice

procedures, and then let the patients decide whether or not to have prenatal diagnosis; 9% would urge them to have prenatal diagnosis; 6% would not tell them about the test results; and 3% would tell them without mentioning prenatal diagnosis.

In Case 8, ambiguous, possibly artifactual, results, 97% would tell patients that there might be an abnormality. Fewer (66%) would also tell patients that their colleagues disagreed about how to interpret the results. In three nations, the Federal Republic of Germany, Turkey and the United States, there was $\geq 75\%$ consensus for disclosing colleague disagreements. In their reasoning, 50% said that they had an obligation to tell the truth, and 40% said that patients had a right to know or a right to decide. Those who would disclose colleague disagreements, cross-nationally, were 3.9 times more likely to be men, 3.87 times more likely to be single, 3.12

19

times less likely to be members of their own nation's genetics association, and 2.20 times more likely to have 20 or more years experience in genetics than those who would not disclose.

Fewer than 1% saw full disclosure as a possible source of harm in any of the three cases, including disclosure of colleague disagreements.

## 1.3.5 Prenatal Diagnosis

### 1.3.5.1 Diffusion of New Techniques

Of the total, 37% said that their genetics unit did chorionic villus sampling (CVS), and 28% said that their unit planned to do it as soon as they had resources (Table 1.10). A majority of units were already performing CVS in nine nations (Australia, Denmark, Federal Republic of Germany, France, Israel, Italy, Sweden, Switzerland, and United Kingdom). In the United States, 28% were performing CVS and 32% were planning to perform it. Fetoscopy was less widely used; 15% said that their units performed it and 6% were planning to do so.

**Table 1.10.** Use of Chorionic Villus Sampling (CVS) and Fetoscopy

| Country | CVS | | Fetoscopy | |
|---|---|---|---|---|
| | Do now (%) | Plan to do (%) | Do now (%) | Plan to do (%) |
| Australia | 83* | 0 | 58* | 0 |
| Brazil | 22 | 34 | 0 | 25 |
| Canada | 41 | 41 | 16 | 2 |
| Denmark | 73* | 0 | 13 | 0 |
| Federal Republic of Germany | 70* | 26 | 9 | 0 |
| France | 59* | 29 | 18 | 0 |
| German Democratic Republic | 14 | 52* | 38 | 10 |
| Greece | 43 | 14 | 43 | 29 |
| Hungary | 33 | 33 | 20 | 13 |
| India | 27 | 37 | 0 | 22 |
| Israel | 60* | 20 | 20 | 0 |
| Italy | 64* | 36 | 55* | 18 |
| Japan | 6 | 14 | 6 | 8 |
| Norway | 0 | 80* | 0 | 0 |
| Sweden | 60* | 35 | 44 | 6 |
| Switzerland | 60* | 40 | 0 | 20 |
| Turkey | 0 | 40 | 20 | 0 |
| United Kingdom | 72* | 9 | 25 | 3 |
| United States | 28 | 31 | 14 | 4 |
| Total | 37 | 28 | 15 | 6 |
| Total, Excluding U.S. | 45 | 26 | 17 | 8 |

* Majority

## 1.3.5.2 Indications

In 1979, a Consensus Development Conference sponsored by the National Institute of Child Health and Human Development in the United States recommended that amniocentesis be considered for patients with one or more of the following indications [23]:

1.) Maternal age of 35 years or more;
2.) A previous pregnancy that has resulted in the birth of a chromosomally abnormal offspring;
3.) A chromosome abnormality that is known to exist in either parent;
4.) History of Down syndrome or other chromosome abnormality in a family member;
5.) History of multiple (three or more) spontaneous abortions in this marriage or in a previous mating of either spouse;
6.) Previous birth of a child with multiple major malformations;
7.) Women with male relatives with Duchenne muscular dystrophy, severe hemophilia, or who are at risk of being carriers of other deleterious X-linked genes;
8.) Couples at risk for detectable inborn errors of metabolism (X-linked or autosomal recessive);
9.) Pregnancies at increased risk for fetal neural tube defects.

In drawing up these guidelines, conference participants called attention to the fact that "the age limit is arbitrarily decided by logistical concerns and is not the consequence of a sudden biological difference between women above and below any given age" [23]. In 1983, the President's Commission on Screening and Counseling for Genetic Conditions suggested more flexible standards for maternal age [16].

Performance of prenatal diagnosis for non-medical indications depends in part upon a nation's abortion laws. These are summarized in figure 1. Table 1.11 describes three cases (Cases 9, 10, and 11) in which patients either request prenatal diagnosis without medical indications or say that they will not abort an affected fetus. In Case 9, a couple aged 42 with a Down syndrome child requests prenatal diagnosis in order to prepare themselves for the possible birth of another Down syndrome child, but say that they will not terminate the pregnancy. Eighty-five per cent of respondents would either perform prenatal diagnosis for this couple (83%) or refer them to someone who would (2%). There was strong consensus in favor of actual performance in 10 nations (Australia, Brazil, Canada, Denmark, Federal Republic of Germany, Israel, Sweden, Switzerland, United Kingdom and United States). In their reasoning, 54% of all respondents stated that performance of prenatal diagnosis should not depend on the use that patients intend to make of the information. Thirty-four per cent stated that such patients may change their minds about termination and thereby justified performing prenatal diagnosis. Refusals were largely based on lack of resources.

In Case 10, a woman of 25 with no personal or family history of genetic disorder or toxic exposure requests prenatal diagnosis because she is extremely anxious about the health of the fetus. Seventy-three per cent of respondents would either perform prenatal diagnosis for maternal anxiety in the absence of other indica-

21

**Fig. 1.** Abortion Laws

| Country | Legal Grounds[a] | | | |
|---|---|---|---|---|
| | On Demand | Mother's Mental Health | Socio-Economic | Fetal Malformation |
| Australia | No | Yes | No | No[b] |
| Brazil | No | No | No | No |
| Canada | As of 28/1/88, Canada has no laws restricting abortion[c] | | | |
| Denmark | Yes (12 wks) | Yes | Yes (12 wks) | Yes (no limit) |
| Federal Republic of Germany | | Yes (12 wks) | Yes (12 wks) | Yes (22 wks) |
| France | Yes (12 wks) | | Yes (12 wks) | Yes (20 wks) |
| German Democratic Republic | Yes (12 wks) | Yes (no limit) | | Yes (no limit) |
| Greece | Yes | | Yes | Yes (24 wks) |
| Hungary | | Yes | Yes[d] | Yes (20 wks)[e] |
| India | | Yes (20 wks) | Yes (20 wks)[f] | Yes (20 wks) |
| Israel | | Yes | No | Yes |
| Italy | | Yes (12 wks) | Yes (12 wks) | Yes (24 wks) |
| Japan | | | Yes | Yes-limited[g] |
| Norway | Yes (12 wks) | Yes | Yes | Yes (no limit) |
| Sweden | Yes (18 wks) | Yes | Yes | Yes (to viability) |
| Switzerland | | Yes | | No[b] |
| Turkey | Yes (10 wks) | | | No[h] |
| United Kingdom | | Yes (28 wks) | Yes (28 wks)[i] | Yes (28 wks) |
| United States | Yes (24 wks) | | | |

[a] Abortion is legal in all 19 nations to save the mother's life, and in all nations, except Brazil, to preserve the mother's physical health. In all nations that do not have abortion on demand, rape is a legal ground (Brazil) or is included under "mental health".
[b] Abortions for fetal abnormality are performed on grounds of "mother's mental health," up to the limits to fetal viability.
[c] See Chapter 2.3.
[d] Includes maternal age ≥ 35, extramarital pregnancy, 3 or more children, inadequate housing.
[e] No time limit for disorders incompatible with life.
[f] Includes failure of contraception.
[g] Genetic abortions are performed only if a family member has 1 of 30 listed disorders; fetal malformation is not a legal ground. Abortions after prenatal diagnosis are performed on socio-economic grounds (financial harm to family).
[h] Abortions for fetal defect are performed on grounds of "preserving the mother's health."
[i] Includes effect of continuing the pregnancy on mother's ability to care for her other children or on health of existing children.

tions (63%) or refer the patient to someone who would perform it (10%). There was strong consensus in six nations (Denmark, Israel, Sweden, Switzerland, United Kingdom, and United States) in favor of actually performing prenatal diagnosis. Of those in favor, 56% mentioned patient autonomy and 46% mentioned the removal of anxiety. Among those opposed to prenatal diagnosis, 61% cited possible harm to the fetus from the procedure, and 70% cited wise use of resources.

Case 11 (Table 1.11), use of prenatal diagnosis solely for selecting the sex of the child, in the absence of an X-linked disease, was the case that geneticists reported

**Table 1.11.** Indications for Prenatal Diagnosis. Per Cent Who Would Perform Prenatal Diagnosis or Refer to Someone Who Would Perform It

| Country | Patients Who Refuse Abortion (Case 9) | | Maternal Anxiety Only (Case 10) | | Sex Selection, in Absence of X-Linked Disease (Case 11) | |
|---|---|---|---|---|---|---|
| | Perform | Refer | Perform | Refer | Perform | Refer |
| Australia | 92* | | 50 | 17 | 9+ | 8 |
| Brazil | 78* | 3 | 14+ | 30 | 21+ | 9 |
| Canada | 87* | 2 | 55 | 15 | 30 | 17 |
| Denmark | 87* | | 87* | | 13+ | |
| Federal Republic of Germany | 85* | | 73 | 7 | 2+ | 2 |
| France | 56 | | 38 | 19 | 7+ | 6 |
| German Democratic Republic | 54 | | 5+ | | 10+ | |
| Greece | 57 | | 43 | | 29 | |
| Hungary | 47 | | 20+ | | 60 | |
| India | 56 | 7 | 41 | 15 | 37 | 15 |
| Israel | 93* | | 80* | | 13+ | 20 |
| Italy | 73 | 18 | 73 | 9 | 18+ | |
| Japan | 44 | 4 | 16+ | 2 | 6+ | |
| Norway | 50 | | 50 | | 17+ | |
| Sweden | 91* | | 91* | | 28 | 10 |
| Switzerland | 100* | | 100* | | 0+ | |
| Turkey | 60 | | 20+ | 20 | 0+ | 20 |
| United Kingdom | 91* | | 79* | 9 | 9+ | 15 |
| United States | 96* | | 78* | 11 | 34 | 28 |
| Total (95% Confidence limits) | 83* (79, 87) | 2 | 63 (57, 69) | 10 | 25+ (19, 23) | 17 |
| Total, Excluding U.S. (95% Confidence limits) | 74 (68, 80) | 2 | 53 (47, 59) | 8 | 18+ (13, 23) | 8 |

* Strong consensus (≥75%) in favor of performing
+ Strong consensus (≥75%) against performing

as giving the greatest ethical conflict (see 1.3.7 below). In the case description, parents of four healthy daughters desire a son and threaten to terminate the pregnancy unless prenatal diagnosis is performed for sex selection, rather than risk having a fifth girl. If prenatal diagnosis is performed, they will terminate only if the fetus is female. Forty-two per cent would either perform prenatal diagnosis for sex selection (25%) or refer the couple to another medical geneticist or genetics unit offering the service (17%). There was strong consensus against actual performance in 13 nations (Australia, Brazil, Denmark, Federal Republic of Germany, France, German Democratic Republic, Israel, Italy, Japan, Norway, Switzerland, Turkey, and United Kingdom). The nations with the largest per cents who would actually perform prenatal diagnosis were Hungary (60%), India (37%), the United States (34%), Canada (30%), Greece (29%) and Sweden (28%). When referrals are added, however, a majority in the United States (62%), Hungary (60%) and India (52%)

would either perform prenatal diagnosis or refer. They would apparently do so for different reasons, however. In the United States, 68% of those who would perform prenatal diagnosis or refer would do so out of respect for parental autonomy; in Hungary, all 15 of those offering prenatal diagnosis would do so in order to prevent the otherwise certain abortion of a normal fetus. In their reasoning, 30% of all respondents said that they opposed the abortion of a normal fetus or that the interests of the fetus should be weighed equally with those of living persons. Those who would actually perform prenatal diagnosis were more likely ($p < 0.0001$) to set down the consequences of their actions, whereas those who would refuse or refer did not give their rationale. Stated consequences related to the fetus or parents, and not to society. Of the 605 persons who gave reasons for their action in this case, only 4.7% mentioned the position of women in society, 0.5% mentioned maintaining a balanced sex ratio, 0.6% mentioned limiting the population, and 4.9% mentioned setting a precedent that would harm the moral order. The exception was India, where 61% mentioned one of these social issues. Twenty-eight per cent of all respondents mentioned issues related to justice, such as wise use of medical resources or diversion of services away from patients at genetic risk.

Results of the stepwise logistic regression analyses showed that those with liberal politics were 3.9 times more likely than conservatives to perform prenatal diagnosis for patients who oppose abortion. Women were 3.96 times more likely than men to perform prenatal diagnosis for an anxious woman, in the absence of medical indications, and geneticists who saw more than ten patients per week were 1.9 times more likely than others to perform it.

No background variables were significantly related cross-nationally to performance of prenatal diagnosis for sex selection. In the United States, however, women were 2.01 times more likely than men to say that they would perform it, and those who attended no religious observances were 5.6 times more likely to perform it than those who attended 15 or more services a year. Where gender differences were significant, women's willingness to perform prenatal diagnosis was based on respect for the patient's absolute autonomy. In all, 39% of women and 31% of men cited patient autonomy in the maternal anxiety case. In the United States, 44% of women and 34% of men cited patient autonomy in the sex selection case, and 18% of both sexes said that they opposed the abortion of a normal fetus.

The regression analyses revealed significant interrelationships between the three cases. Those who would perform prenatal diagnosis for maternal anxiety were 7.31 times more likely than others to perform it for sex selection, cross-nationally, and 6.29 times more likely to perform it for parents who refuse abortion. Those who would perform it for parents who refuse abortion were 56.5 times more likely than others to perform it for maternal anxiety.

## 1.3.5.3 Regulating Commercial Laboratories

We asked whether commercial prenatal diagnostic laboratories should be prohibited by law from performing procedures for any of the three situations described in Table 1.11. The question was phrased as follows:

"A large commercial laboratory plans to open soon in your area. This lab has announced that it will have associated board certified obstetricians on the premises and that it intends to perform prenatal diagnosis for anyone who desires it and who is willing to pay the fee. Should there be any regulations prohibiting this lab from performing prenatal diagnosis *routinely?*"

In all, 83% (79% in the United States) said that there should be regulations prohibiting the existence of laboratories not associated with a medical genetics unit to interpret results (Table 1.12). In all, 71%, 34%, and 27% respectively, said that regulations should prohibit such laboratories from performing prenatal diagnosis for sex selection, for maternal anxiety, and for parents who refuse abortion.

In the United States, which is the only country likely to have substantial numbers of such commercial labs in the near future, 89%, 80%, and 50%, respectively,

**Table 1.12.** Regulating Commercial Prenatal Diagnostic Laboratories. Per Cent Agreeing that Regulations *Should* Prohibit

| Country | Labs Not Associated with a Medical Genetics Unit | Prenatal Diagnosis for Sex Selection | Prenatal Diagnosis for Maternal Anxiety | Prenatal Diagnosis for Parents Who Refuse Abortion |
|---|---|---|---|---|
| Australia | 73 | 100* | 42 | 33 |
| Brazil | 91* | 81* | 50 | 47 |
| Canada | 77* | 66 | 37 | 21+ |
| Denmark | 93* | 86* | 21+ | 21+ |
| Federal Republic of Germany | 87* | 98* | 30 | 34 |
| France | 100* | 100* | 56 | 53 |
| German Democratic Republic | 95* | 100* | 63 | 63 |
| Greece | 100* | 100* | 57 | 43 |
| Hungary | 93* | 100* | 67 | 80* |
| India | 92* | 81* | 58 | 44 |
| Israel | 87* | 86* | 27 | 27 |
| Italy | 91* | 91* | 0+ | 0+ |
| Japan | 86* | 100* | 90+ | 78* |
| Norway | 83* | 100* | 33 | 33 |
| Sweden | 83* | 90* | 17+ | 28 |
| Switzerland | 75* | 100* | 20+ | 20+ |
| Turkey | 100* | 100* | 75* | 75* |
| United Kingdom | 76* | 83* | 43 | 27 |
| United States | 79* | 50 | 20 | 11+ |
| Total | 83* | 71 | 34 | 27 |
| (95% Confidence limits) | (79, 87) | (66, 76) | (29, 39) | (22, 32) |
| Total, Excluding U.S. | 86* | 89* | 47 | 41 |
| (95% Confidence limits) | (81, 91) | (84, 94) | (41, 53) | (35, 47) |

* Strong consensus *in favor of* regulations
+ Strong consensus *against* regulations

25

said that there should be *no* regulations prohibiting performance for patients who refuse abortion, for maternal anxiety, or for sex selection. Overall, only 8% (2% in the United States) said that commercial laboratories should not exist at all or that "medicine should not be a business."

There was a tendency among medical geneticists to consider providing prenatal diagnosis on request, especially in the United States. Many geneticists saw their role as providing services without traditional medical indications. They said that the use that patients intended to make of the information should not be a precondition for prenatal diagnosis. There is an apparently new fairness towards patients who seek prenatal diagnosis but would not use the information for abortion. If the information will be used for sex selection, however, this viewpoint carries respect for patient autonomy to the extreme. Prenatal diagnosis on request, in the absence of medical indications, could soon become a routine part of all prenatal care. Sex selection is an emerging social issue, when viewed in terms of a growing trend in some nations to meet parents' requests for this purpose. Although differing methods of data collection make direct comparison difficult, responses from the United States and Canada contrast markedly with earlier findings between 1973 and 1975 that only 1% in a sample of 448 [10] and 21% of 149 geneticists [19] were willing to perform prenatal diagnosis for sex selection only.

As chorionic villus sampling becomes available, medical geneticists may become even more willing to comply with this request. The reasons given on the questionnaires reflected little awareness of the social consequences of sex selection. To some, it appeared to be an extension of families' self-evident right to determine the number, spacing and quality of their children. Others mentioned the ease with which patients desiring sex selection could conceal their real reasons for requesting prenatal diagnosis, for example, by claiming that they had been exposed to toxic substances. Although geneticists could prevent the use of prenatal diagnosis for sex selection by withholding information on fetal sex, this contravenes the practice of full disclosure and respect for patient autonomy. It is doubtful whether withholding this information would be tolerated by patients in the United States and other nations with fee-for-service health systems [13].

## 1.3.6 Directive/Nondirective Counseling

Modern genetic counseling has generally pursued the goals described by Fraser in 1974, including "helping clients to understand their options and to choose the course of action which seems most appropriate to them in view of their risk and their family goals and act in accordance with that decision" [9]. Counselors act as "decision facilitators", providing information without being directive. In a survey of 205 genetic counselors in the United States in 1979, Sorenson, Swazey, and Scotch [20] found widespread consensus about objectives and approaches. Most counselors claimed that they proceeded on the basis of respect for the patient's autonomy in decision-making; their stated approach was nondirective.

Our questionnaire included three cases focusing on counseling approaches (Cases 12, 13, and 14). In addition, Case 6 (disclosure of conflicting test results) in-

**Table 1.13.** Counseling about Fetuses with Low Burden Disorders

| Country | % Choosing Counseling Approach | | | | | | | | |
| --- | --- | --- | --- | --- | --- | --- | --- | --- | --- |
| | XYY (Case 12) | | | X0 (Turner syndrome) (Case 12) | | | Possible Small NTD (Case 6) | | |
| | Nondirective Counseling | Advise carry to Term[a] | Advise Abortion[b] | Nondirective Counseling | Advise Carry to Term[a] | Advise Abortion[b] | Nondirective Counseling | Advise Carry to Term[c,d] | Advise Abortion |
| Australia | 92* | 8 | 0 | 92* | 8 | 0 | 100* | 0 | 0 |
| Brazil | 84* | 13 | 3 | 85* | 9 | 6 | 84* | 13[c] | 3 |
| Canada | 91* | 9 | 0 | 98* | 2 | 0 | 94* | 2 | 2 |
| Denmark | 93* | 7 | 0 | 100* | 0 | 0 | 79* | 7[c] | 14 |
| Federal Republic of Germany | 76* | 24 | 0 | 74 | 26 | 0 | 73 | 20 | 2 |
| France | 35 | 65 | 0 | 82* | 12 | 6 | 56 | 38[c] | 6 |
| German Democratic Republic | 43 | 43 | 14 | 52 | 24 | 24 | 48 | 4 | 48 |
| Greece | 86* | 14 | | 100* | 0 | 0 | 100* | 0 | 0 |
| Hungary | 33 | 60 | 7 | 60 | 0 | 40 | 47 | 27[d] | 27 |
| India | 77* | 8 | 15 | 54 | 0 | 46 | 63 | 18[d] | 19 |
| Israel | 80* | 20 | 0 | 93* | 0 | 7 | 100* | 0 | 0 |
| Italy | 82* | 18 | 0 | 100* | 0 | 0 | 91* | 9 | 0 |
| Japan | 78* | 14 | 8 | 76* | 14 | 10 | 76* | 10 | 14 |
| Norway | 83* | 0 | 17 | 67 | 0 | 33 | 67 | 0 | 33 |
| Sweden | 90* | 10 | 0 | 95* | 5 | 0 | 86* | 5 | 9 |
| Switzerland | 80* | 20 | 0 | 80* | 20 | 0 | 100* | 0 | 0 |
| Turkey | 80* | 0 | 20 | 60 | 0 | 40 | 100* | 0 | 0 |
| United Kingdom | 91* | 9 | 0 | 97* | 3 | 0 | 84* | 10[d] | 6 |
| United States | 89* | 9 | 2 | 92* | 6 | 2 | 95* | 1[d] | 4 |
| Total (95% Confidence limits) | 84* (80, 88) | 14 | 2 | 88* (84, 92) | 7 | 5 | 87* (83, 91) | 5 | 8 |
| Total, Excluding U.S. (95% Confidence limits) | 80* (75, 85) | 17 | 3 | 84* (79, 89) | 8 | 8 | 80* (75, 85) | 8 | 11 |

* Strong consensus for nondirectiveness
[a] Includes giving optimistically slanted information [b] Includes giving pessimistically slanted information [c] Includes not telling parents about NTD [d] Includes telling parents that there is no major abnormality

27

cluded responses about counseling as well as disclosure. Cases 6 and 12 concern fetuses with "low burden" disorders; Cases 13 and 14 concern presenting reproductive options to carriers of genetic disorders. Table 1.13 summarizes the responses in three situations where prenatal diagnosis reveals or suggests a fetus with a disorder commonly viewed as having a low burden: XYY (Case 12), XO (Case 12), and a possible small neural tube defect (Case 6). There was ≥75% consensus in 75% of nations that counseling should be nondirective in all three situations. Eighty-four per cent would be nondirective for XYY and 88% for XO; 20% and 22%, respectively, would include a discussion of the emotional difficulties associated with terminating the pregnancy. Exceptions to the general consensus were France, Hungary, and the German Democratic Republic, where 65%, 60% and 43%, respectively, would advise carrying an XYY fetus to term or would give optimistically slanted information. In India, Hungary, Turkey, and Norway, 46%, 40%, 40%, and 33% respectively, would advise aborting an XO (Turner) fetus or give pessimistically slanted information. In India, geneticists cited the unmarriageability of an infertile girl and the consequent economic burden on the family. In the German Democratic Republic 48% would give purposively slanted information about XO (Turner), equally divided between optimistic and pessimistic. Fourteen per cent of all respondents would give optimistic information or advice about XYY, and 7% about XO (Turner). Twenty per cent considered a child with either disorder within the range of normal. Women were 5.63 times more likely than men to be nondirective for XO, and 3.45 times more likely than men to be nondirective for XYY.

In regard to a possible small neural tube defect, 98% (≥93% in each nation) would tell the couple that there might be a small neural tube defect; 87% would then counsel nondirectively, 5% would advise carrying to term, and 8% would advise abortion. Exceptions to the general consensus for nondirectiveness were the German Democratic Republic, Norway, Hungary, and India, where 48%, 33%, 27%, and 19%, respectively, would advise abortion, and France, where 38% would advise carrying to term or would tell parents that there was no major abnormality. In their reasoning, 40% of the total cited parents' right to know, 29% cited the geneticist's obligation to tell the truth, and 17% thought that the parents had a "duty to know," even if they did not want to know, and a duty to use the information in their decision-making. Six per cent said that the child would be in the normal range if a neural tube defect were present. Women were 5.97 times more likely than men to be nondirective.

Table 1.14 describes the presentation of reproductive options to carriers of tuberous sclerosis, a dominant disorder not diagnosable prenatally (Case 13, male carriers, Case 14, female carriers).

Options listed were adoption, artificial insemination by a donor (A. I. D.), taking their chances, contraception, tubal ligation, vasectomy, in vitro fertilization (IVF) with a donor egg, and insemination of a surrogate with the husband's sperm. The courses of action listed were 1) advise them to do this; 2) advise them *not* to do this; 3) explain that this is a possibility, without giving any advice; 4) explain that this is a possibility, and describe the risks and potential problems involved; 5) not discuss this; and 6) discuss this only if the clients ask you about it. Choice number 4 expresses nondirective and informative counseling to the fullest extent, but num-

**Table 1.14.** Presenting Reproductive Options

Per Cent Who Would Present Option, Without Giving Advice, in Cases Where One Parent Carries Tuberous Sclerosis, a Dominant Disorder Not Diagnosable Prenatally (Cases 13 and 14)

| Country | Option | | | | | | |
|---|---|---|---|---|---|---|---|
| | Adoption# | Artificial Insemination-Donor | Taking Their Chances# | Contraception# | Sterilization# | Donor Egg, IVF | Surrogate Mother |
| Australia | 100* | 100* | 64 (58) | 75* | 91* (75)* | 92* | 46 |
| Brazil | 78* | 50 | 66 | 63 | 69 | 59 | 34 |
| Canada | 98* | 98* | 86* | 82* | 89* | 59 | 37 |
| Denmark | 93* | 80* | 53 | 87* | 67 (60) | 80* | 47 |
| Federal Republic of Germany | 85* | 72 | 41 | 68 | 72 | 33 | 16+ |
| France | 77* (71) | 81* | 71 | 53 | 53 (47) | 44 | 0+ |
| German Democratic Republic | 35 (55) | 55 | 30 (80)* | 25+ (35) | 30 (0)+ | 25+ | 5+ |
| Greece | 80* | 67 | 40 (33) | 60 (50) | 50 | 80* | 25+ |
| Hungary | 57 (62) | 47 | 36 (43) | 73 (31) | 77* (39) | 46 | 31 |
| India | 54 | 54 | 44 | 50 (41) | 45 | 43 | 48 |
| Israel | 86* | 100* | 73 (69) | 67 (77)* | 67 | 80* | 39 |
| Italy | 91* | 80* | 82* | 82* | 64 (55) | 64 | 27 |
| Japan | 25+ (20)+ | 26 | 58 | 39 (36) | 19+ | 21+ | 10+ |
| Norway | 83* (50) | 83* | 67 | 50 (67) | 50 | 33 | 33 |
| Sweden | 86* | 90* | 68 | 85* (90)* | 84* | 55 | 30 |
| Switzerland | 80* | 100* | 60 | 60 | 60 | 80* | 20+ |
| Turkey | 60 | 60 | 80* | 75* (60) | 60 | 60 | 40 |
| United Kingdom | 93* | 94* | 94* | 90* | 90* | 63 | 27 |
| United States | 95* | 96* | 88* | 85* | 84* | 83* | 67 |
| Total | 85* (84)* | 83* | 75* | 74 | 74 (73) | 66 | 46 |
| (95% Confidence limits) | (81, 89) | (79, 87) | (70, 80) | (69, 79) | (69, 79) | (61, 71) | (41, 51) |
| Total, Excluding U.S. | 76* (75)* | 72 | 64 | 66 | 66 (64) | 52 | 28 |
| (95% Confidence limits) | (70, 82) | (66, 78) | (58, 70) | (60, 72) | (60, 72) | (46, 58) | (23, 33) |

* Strong consensus in favor of presenting
+ Strong consensus against presenting
# Questions asked for both male and female carriers. Per cents are for female carriers; per cents for male carriers given in parentheses in countries where these differed from those for females.

29

ber 3 can also be considered nondirective counseling, and we have reported it as such (Table 1.14). Choices 5 and 6 represent forms of directiveness, in that options are not openly set forth. Whenever responses differed according to the carrier's sex, we have listed responses for the male carrier in parentheses. There was strong consensus ($\geq 75\%$ in 75% of nations) about nondirective presentation of only one option, adoption. Geneticists in 14 nations would discuss this; exceptions were the German Democratic Republic and Hungary, where respondents said no babies were available, India and Japan, where adoption is socially unacceptable to many people, and Turkey. A. I. D. was widely accepted; 83% would present it as an option, including more than 75% in 11 nations (Australia, Canada, Denmark, France, Israel, Italy, Norway, Sweden, Switzerland, United Kingdom and United States), 3% would advise against it, 3% would advise in favor of it, and the rest would discuss it only if asked. A. I. D. is not socially accepted in Japan.

In all, 75% would describe "taking their chances" of having a normal child as an option, without giving advice, and 25% would advise against it. There was strong consensus in five nations (Canada, Italy, Turkey, United Kingdom, and United States) for nondirective presentation to carriers of both sexes, and in one nation (German Democratic Republic) for nondirective presentation to male carriers only.

Of the total, 74% would present contraception as an option, without giving advice; 15% would advise clients to use it; and 11% would discuss it only if asked. There was strong consensus for nondirective presentation to carriers of both sexes in seven nations (Australia, Canada, Denmark, Italy, Sweden, United Kingdom, and United States), to female carriers in Turkey, and to male carriers in Israel.

In all, 74% would present tubal ligation as an option for female carriers, without giving advice, and 73% would present vasectomy as an option for male carriers. There was strong consensus in five nations (Australia, Canada, Sweden, United Kingdom, and United States) for presenting sterilization nondirectively to both sexes, and strong consensus in one, Hungary, for presenting tubal ligation only. In two nations, German Democratic Republic and Greece, there was strong consensus against presenting vasectomy as an option. In all, 5% would advise sterilization, 4% would advise against it, 15% would discuss it only if asked, and 2–3% would not discuss at all.

In vitro fertilization with a donor egg and surrogate motherhood are two new and controversial options. The first has wider acceptance, in spite of a low success rate. There was strong consensus in six nations (Australia, Denmark, Greece, Israel, Switzerland, and the United States) for presenting in vitro fertilization with donor egg, and strong consensus against in two nations, German Democratic Republic and Japan. Of the total, 66% would present this option without giving advice, 23% would discuss it only if asked, 7% would not discuss, 3% would advise against it, and 1% would advise in favor of it. In their reasoning, respondents saw this as a less harmful option than surrogate motherhood, in spite of its technical difficulty.

There was no consensus about presenting surrogate motherhood as an option; 46% would present it without giving advice, 29% would discuss it only if asked, 18% would not discuss it at all, and 7% would advise against it. There was strong consensus against presenting it in six nations (Federal Republic of Germany,

France, German Democratic Republic, Greece, Japan, and Switzerland). In the United States a majority (67%) would present surrogacy as an option, unasked. Men were 4.63 times more likely than women to present surrogate motherhood as an option, 2.36 times more likely than women to present contraception for female carriers, and 2.25 times more likely than women to present in vitro fertilization with a donor egg. Persons who attended 15–24 religious observances a year (regardless of religious background) were 5.5 times more likely to present taking chances as an option, 1.5 times more likely to present tubal ligation, 1.5 times more likely to present vasectomy, and 1.3 times more likely to present contraception for female carriers than those who attended no religious observances at all. No other background variables were significantly related at the 0.05 level, cross-nationally, to presenting options.

Patient autonomy (right to decide, right to know, making informed decisions) was the reason given by 67%; 14% mentioned preventing birth defects. Four per cent said that they would not discuss an option because it was the province of another medical specialist. Fewer than 1% mentioned benefit or harm to society from any option. In addition to giving reasons for their counseling approach, 28% discussed the specific consequences of using any of the listed options. Those who would give directive advice were more likely to mention consequences ($p < 0.0001$) than those who would be non-directive. Ninety-two per cent saw no conflict between the interests of different persons, or between individuals and society, in the use of any option, including surrogacy.

## 1.3.7 Most and Least Difficult Cases

Of the 14 clinical cases, sex selection and confidentiality of a Huntington disease patient versus duties to relatives at risk were the two that gave the greatest ethical conflict to the greatest number of respondents (25% and 21% respectively, Table 1.15). Confidence intervals (95%) for these two cases overlapped. Geneticists in seven countries (Brazil, Federal Republic of Germany, Israel, Sweden, Switzerland, United Kingdom and United States) ranked sex selection as the case that they found the most difficult to decide. Geneticists in nine countries (Australia, Canada, Denmark, France, German Democratic Republic, Hungary, Italy, Norway, and Turkey) found confidentiality of a Huntington patient most difficult. False paternity was the third most difficult case (13% of respondents), ranked most difficult in Greece, India, Switzerland (tied with sex selection), and Turkey (tied with confidentiality of an HD patient).

The three cases that gave the least ethical conflict (Table 1.16) were prenatal diagnosis for patients who refuse abortion (20%), prenatal diagnosis for sex selection (17%), and prenatal diagnosis in cases of maternal anxiety in the absence of medical indications (13%). Confidence intervals (95%) for the first two cases overlapped. The apparent paradox about sex selection rating as the least and most conflicting situation is explained in part because many respondents had already made up their minds.

**Table 1.15.** Cases Giving Most Ethical Conflict

| Country | Per Cent Selecting Case | | |
|---|---|---|---|
| | Prenatal Diagnosis for Sex Selection | Confidentiality of an HD Patient | False Paternity |
| Australia | 25 | 33 | 8 |
| Brazil | 31 | 19 | 22 |
| Canada | 22 | 26 | 9 |
| Denmark | 7 | 80 | 0 |
| FRG | 23 | 21 | 9 |
| France | 0 | 60 | 0 |
| GDR | 0 | 33 | 0 |
| Greece | 14 | 14 | 29 |
| Hungary | 7 | 20 | 7 |
| India | 16 | 4 | 24 |
| Israel | 29 | 0 | 21 |
| Italy | 9 | 36 | 9 |
| Japan | 20 | 6 | 8 |
| Norway | 17 | 33 | 0 |
| Sweden | 29 | 14 | 14 |
| Switzerland | 40 | 0 | 40 |
| Turkey | 0 | 40 | 40 |
| United Kingdom | 32 | 23 | 10 |
| United States | 30 | 19 | 14 |
| Total | 25 | 21 | 13 |
| (95% Confidence limits) | (20, 30) | (18, 24) | (10, 16) |
| Total, Excluding U.S. | 21 | 22 | 12 |
| (95% Confidence limits) | (15, 27) | (17, 27) | (9, 15) |

## 1.3.8 Counseling Goals and Approaches

In addition to the 14 clinical cases, we included questions about the importance or appropriateness of seven goals and five directive/nondirective approaches to counseling, using the wording of the Sorenson, Swazey, and Scotch survey [20].

There was close to 100% consensus that five of the seven listed goals of counseling were important (Table 1.17). These were 1) "helping individuals/couples understand their options and the present state of knowledge so they can make informed decisions" (99.8%); 2) "helping individuals/couples adjust to and cope with their genetic problems" (99.5%); 3) "the removal or lessening of guilt or anxiety" (99.7%); 4) "helping individuals/couples achieve their parenting goals" (98%); and 5) "the prevention of disease or abnormality" (97%). There was widespread consensus that the first two goals were "absolutely essential" (92% of total, ≥ 75% consensus in 16 nations, and 87% of total, ≥ 75% consensus in 13 nations, respectively). There was less consensus about the importance of the remaining two goals. Of the total, 74% considered "improvement of the general health and vigor of the population" important and 14% considered it absolutely essential. There

**Table 1.16.** Cases Giving Least Conflict % Selecting Case

| Country | Prenatal Diagnosis for Parents Who Refuse Abortion | Prenatal Diagnosis for Sex Selection | Prenatal Diagnosis for Maternal Anxiety |
|---|---|---|---|
| Australia | 8 | 8 | 8 |
| Brazil | 17 | 13 | 13 |
| Canada | 22 | 17 | 4 |
| Denmark | 7 | 21 | 14 |
| FRG | 18 | 30 | 11 |
| France | 0 | 50 | 6 |
| GDR | 0 | 71 | 10 |
| Greece | 29 | 29 | 14 |
| Hungary | 0 | 13 | 20 |
| India | 19 | 35 | 12 |
| Israel | 43 | 7 | 0 |
| Italy | 18 | 27 | 9 |
| Japan | 13 | 21 | 17 |
| Norway | 0 | 33 | 0 |
| Sweden | 10 | 10 | 29 |
| Switzerland | 0 | 40 | 20 |
| Turkey | 0 | 40 | 20 |
| United Kingdom | 21 | 17 | 7 |
| United States | 25 | 11 | 14 |
| Total | 20 | 17 | 13 |
| (95% Confidence limits) | (17, 23) | (14, 20) | (10, 16) |
| Total, Excluding U.S. | 15 | 22 | 12 |
| (95% Confidence limits) | (11, 19) | (17, 27) | (9, 15) |

was $\geq 75\%$ consensus in ten nations (Denmark, France, German Democratic Republic, Greece, Hungary, India, Israel, Japan, Turkey and United States) that this was an important, but not an essential goal. A total of 54% regarded "a reduction of the number of carriers of genetic disorders in the population" as important, but only 5% considered it essential. In three nations, Brazil, India and Turkey, there was $\geq 75\%$ consensus that reducing the number of carriers should be an important goal. The results of the Sorenson, Swazey, and Scotch survey are listed at the bottom of Table 1.17 for comparison. The total per cents in our study considering each goal important or essential are similar to those reported in this 1977–1979 survey of genetic counselors in the United States [20]. In regard to two of the seven goals, responses of geneticists who counseled 10 or more patients per week differed from those who counseled none. Those who did the most counseling were more likely (p < 0.001) to consider it essential to help patients achieve their parenting goals but were less likely (p < 0.04) to consider reducing the number of carriers important.

For two goals (1 and 3), gender emerged as significant cross-nationally. Women were 13.2 times more likely than men to consider "helping individuals/couples understand their options" absolutely essential, and 3.5 times more likely than men

33

**Table 1.17.** Goals of Counseling. Per Cent Believing Important[+] (In parentheses: Absolutely Essential)

| Country | Goal: Helping individuals/couples understand their options and the present state of medical knowledge so they can make informed decisions | Helping individuals/couples adjust to and cope with their genetic problems | The removal or lessening of patient guilt or anxiety | Helping individuals/couples achieve their parenting goals | The prevention of disease or abnormality | Improvement of the general health and vigor of the population | A reduction in the number of carriers of genetic disorders in the population |
|---|---|---|---|---|---|---|---|
| Australia | 100* (100)* | 100* (100)* | 100* (50) | 100* (33) | 92* (17) | 67 (25) | 58 |
| Brazil | 100* (84)* | 100* (81)* | 100* (78) | 97* (41) | 100* (66) | 72 (11) | 81* (6) |
| Canada | 100* (98)* | 100* (87)* | 100* (57) | 98* (41) | 98* (11) | 68 (14) | 51 (2) |
| Denmark | 100* (100)* | 100* (100)* | 100* (60) | 92* (46) | 100* (53) | 86* (4) | 54 |
| Federal Republic of Germany | 98* (89)* | 100* (89)* | 100* (75) | 98* (43) | 91* (23) | 28 | 38 |
| France | 100* (94)* | 100* (88)* | 100* (69) | 94* (63) | 100* (69) | 81* (5) | 50 (6) |
| German Democratic Republic | 100* (57) | 100* (86)* | 100* (38) | 100* (24) | 100* (76)* | 100* | 29 (5) |
| Greece | 100* (100)* | 100* (67) | 100* (33) | 100* (50) | 100* (83)* | 100* (33) | 60 (60) |
| Hungary | 100* (87)* | 100* (67) | 100* (53) | 100* (47) | 100* (93)* | 100* (53) | 73 (7) |
| India | 100* (73) | 100* (76)* | 96* (42) | 96* (35) | 100* (78)* | 88* (35) | 92* (46) |
| Israel | 100* (93)* | 100* (73) | 100* (33) | 100* (40) | 100* (53) | 80* (13) | 73 |
| Italy | 100* (82)* | 100* (73) | 100* (46) | 100* (27) | 91* (36) | 55 | 36 |
| Japan | 100* (76)* | 100* (74) | 100* (53) | 96* (33) | 100* (45) | 88* (20) | 67 (18) |
| Norway | 100* (100)* | 100* (100)* | 100* (67) | 100* (50) | 100* (17) | 50 (33) | 17 |
| Sweden | 100* (90)* | 100* (100)* | 100* (70) | 100* (35) | 100* (25) | 65 (5) | 60 |
| Switzerland | 100+ (100)* | 100* (80)* | 100* (80) | 100* (20) | 100* (40) | 60 (20) | 40 |
| Turkey | 100* (80)* | 100* (50) | 100* (50) | 67 (67) | 100* (100)* | 100* (50) | 100* (100)* |
| United Kingdom | 100* (100)* | 100* (97)* | 100* (71) | 100* (41) | 100* (7) | 71 (3) | 48 |
| United States | 100* (97)* | 100* (90)* | 100* (64) | 99* (43) | 97* (19) | 78* (12) | 47 (2) |
| Total | 99.8* (92)* | 99.5* (87)* | 99.7* (62) | 98* (42) | 97* (31) | 74 (14) | 54 (5) |
| (95% Confidence limits) | | | | (96, 100) | (95, 99) | (69, 79) | (49, 59) |
| Total, Excluding U.S. | 99.7* (89)* | 100* (85)* | 99.7* (61) | 98* (40) | 98* (41) | 70 (15) | 59 (8) |
| (95% Confidence limits) | | | | (96, 100) | (96, 100) | (64, 76) | (53, 65) |
| United States 1979[1] (n = 205) | Not Asked | 100* (83)* | 100* (75) | 99* (44) | 98.5 (52) | 74 (11) | 55 (7) |
| (95% Confidence limits) | | | | | | (66, 82) | (46, 64) |

[+] Includes ratings of Absolutely Essential, Important, and Somewhat Important
[1] Sorenson JR, Swazey JP, Scotch NA (1981) Reproductive Pasts, Reproductive Futures: Genetic Counselling and Its Effectiveness. New York: Alan R. Liss for the March of Dimes, p. 42.

**Table 1.18.** Directive/Nondirective Approaches

| Country | Per Cent Believing Always/Sometimes Appropriate | | | | |
| --- | --- | --- | --- | --- | --- |
| | Suggest that while you will not make decisions for patients you will support any they make | Tell patients that decisions, especially reproductive ones, are theirs alone and refuse to make any for them | Inform patients what most other people in their situation have done | Inform patients what you would do if you were in their situation | Advise patients what they ought to do |
| Australia | 100* | 92* | 92* | 8+ | 8+ |
| Brazil | 84* | 94* | 59 | 13+ | 16+ |
| Canada | 94* | 94* | 83* | 45 | 9+ |
| Denmark | 100* | 100* | 62 | 31 | 8+ |
| Federal Republic of Germany | 91* | 89* | 48 | 30 | 9+ |
| France | 88* | 73 | 31 | 38 | 25+ |
| German Democratic Republic | 90* | 86* | 52 | 10+ | 0+ |
| Greece | 86* | 100* | 57 | 29 | 14+ |
| Hungary | 80* | 53 | 53 | 40 | 40 |
| India | 77* | 89* | 77* | 58 | 56 |
| Israel | 93* | 100* | 67 | 0+ | 20+ |
| Italy | 91* | 82* | 46 | 9+ | 18+ |
| Japan | 90* | 81* | 58 | 45 | 27 |
| Norway | 83* | 83* | 50 | 50 | 0+ |
| Sweden | 90* | 100* | 47 | 11+ | 10+ |
| Switzerland | 100* | 75* | 100* | 50 | 0+ |
| Turkey | 50 | 100* | 75* | 75* | 50 |
| United Kingdom | 100* | 94* | 94* | 30 | 0+ |
| United States | 98* | 97* | 69 | 19+ | 12+ |
| Total | 94* | 92* | 66 | 26 | 15+ |
| (95% Confidence limits) | (91, 97) | (89, 95) | (61, 71) | (22, 30) | (12, 18) |
| Total, Excluding U.S. | 90* | 89* | 64 | 33 | 18+ |
| (95% Confidence limits) | (86, 94) | (85, 93) | (58, 70) | (27, 39) | (14, 22) |
| United States 1979 (n = 205)[1] | 93* | 99* | 66 | 18+ | 13+ |
| (95% Confidence limits) | (88, 98) | (97, 100) | (57, 75) | (12, 24) | (8, 18) |

* Strong (≥ 75%) consensus of appropriateness
+ Strong (≥ 75%) consensus of inappropriateness
[1] Sorensen JR, Swazey JP, Scotch NA (1981) Reproductive Pasts, Reproductive Futures: Genetic Counselling and Its Effectiveness. New York: Alan R. Liss for the March of Dimes, p. 44.

35

to regard "removal of guilt or anxiety" as essential. Length of experience was also related to considering the first goal essential; for each year in genetics, the odds ratio increased by 0.18. No other background variables were significant cross-nationally.

There was very strong consensus about the appropriateness of two of five approaches to counseling (Table 1.18). Both of these stressed nondirectiveness: 1) "suggest that while you will not make decisions for patients you will support any they make" (94%); and 2) "tell patients that decisions, especially reproductive ones, are theirs alone and refuse to make any for them" (92%). There was strong ($\geq 75\%$) consensus in all nations except Turkey on the appropriateness of the first approach, and strong consensus in all but two, France and Hungary, on the second. There was less consensus about the third approach, "inform patients what most other people in their situation have done." Although 66% considered it appropriate, this fell short of our criteria for consensus; there was strong consensus that it was appropriate in six countries (Australia, Canada, India, Switzerland, Turkey, and the United Kingdom). Some geneticists regard this approach as directive, and others do not. The fourth and fifth approaches were directive: "inform patients what you would do if you were in their situation" and "advise patients what they ought to do." Relatively few geneticists (26% and 15% respectively) considered them appropriate. There was a strong ($\geq 75\%$) consensus in seven nations (Australia, Brazil, German Democratic Republic, Israel, Italy, Sweden, and United States) that informing patients what you would do was inappropriate, and a strong consensus in one, Turkey, that it was appropriate. There was a strong consensus in all nations except Hungary, India, Japan and Turkey that advising patients what to do was inappropriate. The results of the Sorenson, Swazey and Scotch survey [2], listed at the bottom of Table 1.18, were in general similar to the worldwide totals.

In regard to two of the five counseling approaches, responses of those who saw 10 or more patients weekly differed from the responses of those who saw none. Geneticists who saw the most patients were less likely to consider it appropriate to inform patients what they themselves would do in the patient's situation ($p < 0.001$) and more likely to consider it appropriate to support patients' decisions ($p < 0.02$).

As with the counseling goals, above, we entered background variables into stepwise logistic regressions. Gender was related to four of the five counseling approaches (Nos. 1, 3, 4, 5) across nationalities. Women were 2.68 times more likely than men to consider it appropriate to "suggest that while you will not make decisions ... you will support any they make." Men were 1.9 times more likely than women to consider it appropriate to "inform patients what most other people have done", 4.6 times more likely than women to consider it appropriate to "inform patients what you would do if in their situation," and 6.9 times more likely than women to consider it appropriate to "advise patients what to do." Clearly, men favored the more directive approaches. Persons who said that they were politically liberal were 3.2 times more likely than conservatives to consider it appropriate to "support any (decisions) patients make." No other background variables remained in the analyses at the 0.05 level.

There was widespread consensus, cross-nationally, about most goals and approaches for counseling. Goals rated most important were those emphasizing the

educational and psychological aspects of counseling, such as providing information as a basis for facilitating informed decisions by clients, helping clients to
cope, or removing clients' guilt or anxiety. The goal rated least important was the
one most closely related to eugenic concerns, "reducing the number of carriers in
the population." Preferred approaches to counseling were also nondirective. There
were some exceptions, notably the two socialist nations, German Democratic Republic and Hungary, where more directive approaches were consistently preferred. Geneticists in these nations see it as their role to give advice, direction, and
guidance [4]. In India, where counseling followed a somewhat directive course in
some situations, some respondents noted that the educational and social distance
between counselor and counselee is likely to be greater in India than in more developed nations; geneticists felt that they had an obligation to give direction to less
educated clients.

The nuances of communication in counseling cannot, of course, be covered in a
questionnaire. Information exchange depends on establishing rapport with patients who may be anxious or unsophisticated, explaining unfamiliar concepts,
and offering reproductive options that may deviate from accepted cultural practices. Non-verbal communication is an inescapable part of counseling. Even cloth-
ing and demeanor may convey the counselor's attitudes, especially to patients
from a different social class or subculture. Further, the perceptions of counselor
and patient may differ markedly about what transpired in a counseling session [24,
25]. Nevertheless, the questionnaire results show that most geneticists at least subscribe to the goal of nondirectiveness.

The relationships between personal background variables, especially gender,
and self-reported counseling approaches were noteworthy. Although we had anticipated that there would be some relationships between background and counseling approach that were cross-national, we expected these to be based on professional factors, such as experience, field, or degree, rather than on personal factors
such as gender, political viewpoint, or religiosity, whose effects are supposedly
eliminated, or at least greatly reduced, by professional training. This was not the
case; most relationships were with personal, not professional, background factors,
notably gender, political preferences, and attendance at religious observances. Our
findings with regard to gender contrasted with those of researchers who compared
views of 47 female and 59 male counselors in the United States and found no differences [27]. Among our respondents, professional training had not erased background differences, at least when morally and socially problematic topics such as
abortion and new reproductive options were concerned.

## 1.3.9 Screening

There were four questions on screening. These concerned: 1) screening in the
workplace for genetic susceptibility to work-related disease, 2) access to results of
screening in the workplace; 3) carrier screening for cystic fibrosis, 4) presymptomatic testing for Huntington disease. At present, none of these is technologically
feasible or accurate on a population-wide basis. Respondents were asked to assume that reliable tests were available.

## 1.3.9.1 Screening in the Workplace

Although no test for genetic susceptibility to occupationally-related disease has yet met the United States Office of Technology Assessment (OTA) criteria for actually predicting disease, an OTA survey of 336 major United States corporations in 1982 showed that 17 had already used genetic tests and 59 anticipated using them within five years [22]. Our question on screening concerned a test already used by some companies:

"Assume that an accurate, simple, and reliable mass screening test has been developed for alpha-1-antitrypsin deficiency. This raises the possibility that factory workers who will be exposed to dust and smoke could be screened. Assume that you are a member of an advisory group that will develop guidelines for mass screening of workers in your country. Do you believe that mass genetic screening of workers and prospective employees in potentially dangerous industries should be mandatory for all would be occupationally exposed, or voluntary?"

Serum alpha-1-antitrypsin (SAT) deficiency is an important biological factor predisposing the occurrence of emphysema. Approximately 80% of homozygous individuals will develop emphysema. The homozygous state occurs in approximately one in 7500 persons in the United States population. Heterozygous individuals have an SAT level about 50% of normal and may be at increased risk for emphysema if they smoke or work in dusty environments. They comprise about 3% of the United States population [22]. At present, the value of SAT tests for predicting the development of emphysema in heterozygous individuals is unknown and unproven.

Geneticists strongly preferred voluntary over mandatory screening, by a 72% majority (Table 1.19). In ten nations (Australia, Denmark, Federal Republic of Germany, Greece, Italy, Norway, Sweden, Switzerland, United Kingdom, and United States) there was a strong ($\geq 75\%$) consensus that screening should be voluntary. In two nations, (German Democratic Republic and Turkey,) there was a strong ($\geq 75\%$) consensus that screening should be mandatory, and in three additional nations (Brazil, Hungary, and India) the majority agreed that it should be mandatory. Those who thought that screening should be voluntary cited the worker's autonomy or right to decide (74%), and the danger of stigmatization, discrimination in employment, or misuse of information by institutional third parties (41%). Advocates of mandatory screening cited protecting the individual worker's health (64%), protecting public health (51%), and efficiency or cost-benefit arguments (22%). Nine per cent of those who advocated voluntary screening and 12% of those who advocated mandatory screening based their choices in part upon concern for the economic interests of employers. Those who believed that screening should be mandatory were significantly more likely ($p < 0.005$) than believers in voluntary screening to cite personal or social consequences of screening; 56% mentioned some specific consequence, as opposed to 40% of those who thought that screening should be voluntary. The two groups also differed significantly ($p < 0.00001$) in whose welfare they placed foremost; 97% who advocated voluntary screening and 58% who advocated mandatory screening ranked the worker's welfare as most important, while 3% who advocated voluntary screening and 37%

**Table 1.19.** Screening for Genetic Susceptibility to Work-Related Disease, and Access to Test Results

| Country | Mass Screening Voluntary | No Access To Results Without Worker's Consent (In Parentheses: No Access At All) | | | | | | | |
|---|---|---|---|---|---|---|---|---|---|
| | | Employer | | Worker's Physician | | Life, Health Worker's Comp. Insurers | | Government Health Dept. | |
| Australia | 92* | 100* | | 67 | | 94* | (47) | 67 | (42) |
| Brazil | 34 | 68 | (10) | 19+ | (3) | 77* | (27) | 39 | (10) |
| Canada | 73 | 91* | (21) | 64 | (2) | 96* | (40) | 81* | (26) |
| Denmark | 86* | 100* | (47) | 60 | (7) | 100* | (59) | 86* | (29) |
| Federal Republic of Germany | 94* | 96* | (64) | 68 | (4) | 95* | (71) | 72 | (44) |
| France | 53 | 100* | (77)* | 29 | | 88* | (56) | 50 | (13) |
| German Democratic Republic | 16+ | 81* | (50) | 22+ | | 90* | (78)* | 38 | (25) |
| Greece | 83* | 50 | | 17+ | | 83* | (17) | 17+ | |
| Hungary | 27 | 79* | (29) | 7+ | | 91* | (29) | 29 | (7) |
| India | 26 | 41 | (14) | 17+ | (4) | 65 | (30) | 32 | (9) |
| Israel | 73 | 100* | (7) | 43 | | 100* | (24) | 71 | (21) |
| Italy | 82* | 100* | (27) | 27 | (9) | 87* | (55) | 36 | (9) |
| Japan | 63 | 77* | (23) | 35 | (5) | 90* | (54) | 44 | (20) |
| Norway | 84* | 100* | (83)* | 100* | | 100* | (83)* | 67 | (33) |
| Sweden | 91* | 100* | (35) | 91* | | 98* | (38) | 79* | (26) |
| Switzerland | 100* | 100* | (60) | 40 | | 100* | (73) | 100* | (60) |
| Turkey | 20+ | 40 | (20) | 0+ | | 50 | (25) | 0+ | |
| United Kingdom | 87* | 84* | (10) | 42 | | 88* | (19) | 81* | (19) |
| United States | 77* | 76* | (12) | 63 | (2) | 88* | (34) | 78* | (27) |
| Total | 72 | 81* | (22) | 53 | (2) | 89* | (40) | 68 | (25) |
| (95% Confidence limits) | (67, 77) | (77, 85) | | (48, 58) | | (85, 93) | | (63, 73) | |
| Total, Excluding U.S. | 68 | 85* | (30) | 46 | (3) | 90* | (44) | 60 | (23) |
| (95% Confidence limits) | (62, 74) | (80, 90) | | (40, 52) | | (86, 94) | | (54, 66) | |

* Strong (≥75%) consensus in favor of voluntary screening or no access to results without consent.
+ Strong (≥75%) consensus for mandatory screening or automatic access to results.

who believed in mandatory screening placed "society's" welfare first. Only one per cent placed the employer's welfare first. Believers in voluntary screening were significantly more likely than others (p < 0.00001) to describe a conflict of interest between worker and employer; 34% described such conflicts, as opposed to 13% who advocated mandatory screening. A majority in both groups, however, described no conflicts.

## 1.3.9.2 Access to Test Results

When asked who should have access to test results for genetic susceptibility to work-related disease, 98% said that the worker should have access; this included 86% who said that the worker should be told the results even if s/he did not ask for them. This view contrasts markedly with the history of concealment of asbestosis test results from workers at some major United States corporations [3].

When asked whether the employer should have access, 81% said that employers should have no access without the worker's consent, including 22% who believed that employers should have no access at all (Table 1.19). There was strong consensus for no access without consent in all nations except Brazil, Greece, India, and Turkey, and strong consensus for no access at all in France and Norway. Thirty per cent believed that it would be to the worker's benefit if the employer had some form of access; employers could shift susceptible workers to less dangerous jobs, though only 6% thought that working conditions in general would be improved. Nineteen per cent described potential economic discrimination, stigmatization, or other misuse of test results by employers. Ten per cent based their responses on the economic interests of the employer.

There was little consensus about whether the worker's physician should have access. There was strong ($\geq 75\%$) consensus in six countries (Brazil, German Democratic Republic, Greece, Hungary, India, and Turkey) that the physician should have automatic access, and in two countries (Norway and Sweden) that the physician should *not* have access without the worker's consent. In all, 61% said that it would be to the worker's benefit for the physician to know; 25%, however, said that the worker had the right to decide. In general, respondents trusted physicians far more than they trusted institutional third parties; only 2% said that the physician should have no access at all.

There was strong consensus in all nations except India and Turkey that insurance companies should have no access to test results without the worker's consent, and strong consensus in two countries (German Democratic Republic and Norway) that they should have no access at all (Table 1.19). Although we asked separate questions about four types of insurers (worker's life insurer, worker's health insurer, employer's worker compensation insurer, employer's health insurer), the responses were so similar that we have averaged them. The distrust of insurance companies was such that 40% of respondents thought that they should have no access at all, even with the worker's consent. Very few (4%) thought that workers would benefit in any way from an insurance company knowing their test results. On the other hand, 30% thought that the information would be misused, to the worker's detriment. Many respondents pointed out that "access with consent" placed the worker in a no-win situation: if the worker denies access, s/he will probably be denied insurance. Some pointed to the need for regulations that would prevent workers from in effect being coerced into giving "voluntary" consent.

When asked whether government health departments should have access, 68% said that there should be no access without worker consent. There was a strong consensus to this effect in six nations (Canada, Denmark, Sweden, Switzerland, United Kingdom and United States). There was strong consensus in two nations (Greece and Turkey) that the government should have automatic access. Fifty per cent thought that it would benefit society if the health department had access, in terms of improved public health, working conditions for all workers, or social planning. In all, 19% (5% in the United States) cited possible misuse of information by the government. One-fourth of respondents, however, believed that governments should have no access to results at all. In general, those who believed that screening should be mandatory were more likely ($p < 0.00001$) to believe that third parties of all kinds should have access without consent.

## 1.3.9.3 Cystic Fibrosis Carrier Screening

Our question was phrased: "Assume that a cheap and accurate test, reliable at all ages, has been developed for cystic fibrosis. It diagnoses both carriers and affected individuals, distinguishes between them, and also separates each of them from non-carriers. The test is now ready for application on a population-wide basis. Also assume that accurate *prenatal diagnosis* has become available for cystic fibrosis. In addition to the relatives of patients with cystic fibrosis, to whom and at what age should the carrier test *first* be given?"

At present, no such test is available on a population-wide basis. Carrier testing and prenatal diagnosis are possible only on a family-specific basis, using DNA probes that require testing of genetic material from a member of the family who has cystic fibrosis, usually a child [2]. Geneticists anticipate that within a few years tests suitable for mass screening will be developed. Cystic fibrosis is the most common autosomal recessive disorder among Caucasians, with an incidence of one in 1600 and a carrier rate of one in 20. The disorder is relatively rare among non-Caucasians. Although treatment is available, it places a high daily burden on the family, and the child undergoes frequent hospitalization. Almost half the children die before the age of 24, and many of the rest before the age of 30. In each subsequent pregnancy, the parents face a one-in-four risk of having another affected child.

Respondents believed that the objectives of mass screening should be 1) informed reproductive planning for carriers; 2) efficiency; 3) preserving patients' (or parents') autonomy; 4) identifying and treating affected children as early in life as possible; 5) preventing births of additional children with cystic fibrosis. There was 75% consensus among total respondents, and a $\geq 75\%$ consensus in each of eight nations (Australia, Canada, Federal Republic of Germany, Greece, Japan, Sweden, Switzerland, and United Kingdom) that cystic fibrosis screening, at whatever age, should be voluntary (Table 1.20). There was strong consensus in three nations, the German Democratic Republic, Hungary, and Turkey, that it be mandatory. Those who believed that workplace screening should be voluntary were more likely to believe that cystic fibrosis screening should be voluntary ($p < 0.00001$). There was no consensus, however, about the optimal age for initial screening in order to achieve program objectives. In all, 20% advocated screening newborns by law, 25% advocated screening newborns with parental consent, 13% would choose screening of children or adolescents under 18, with parental consent, 37% advocated screening adults over 18 by consent, and 5% indicated other ages, by law. Three countries had a strong ($\geq 75\%$) consensus about age: Greece favored adults and Switzerland and Turkey favored newborns. Those who advocated screening newborns by law gave as their reasons the benefits of early treatment (55%), program efficiency (31%), informed reproductive planning for the child's parents (30%), and preventing the births of additional children with cystic fibrosis (22%). Those who preferred newborn screening by consent described benefits of early treatment (47%), preventing births of children with cystic fibrosis (43%), the parents' right to decide (42%), informed reproductive planning (35%), and efficiency (19%). Most advocates of adolescent screening chose the ages between 13 and 17,

41

**Table 1.20.** Group to Receive Mass Carrier Screening for Cystic Fibrosis

| Country | Per cent Responding | | | | |
|---|---|---|---|---|---|
| | Newborns, By Law | Newborns, By Consent | Children <18, By Consent | Adults <18, By Consent | Other Ages, By Law |
| Australia | 0 | 59 | 8 | 25 | 8 |
| Brazil | 25 | 16 | 0 | 53 | 6 |
| Canada | 18 | 27 | 11 | 42 | 2 |
| Denmark | 27 | 20 | 20 | 33 | 0 |
| Federal Republic of Germany | 11 | 30 | 9 | 47 | 3 |
| France | 35 | 12 | 6 | 35 | 12 |
| German Democratic Republic | 67 | 0 | 5 | 10 | 18 |
| Greece | 0 | 0 | 0 | 86* | 14 |
| Hungary | 67 | 7 | 0 | 7 | 19 |
| India | 39 | 31 | 4 | 23 | 3 |
| Israel | 20 | 7 | 7 | 53 | 13 |
| Italy | 18 | 0 | 27 | 46 | 9 |
| Japan | 0 | 51 | 15 | 30 | 4 |
| Norway | 33 | 33 | 0 | 34 | 0 |
| Sweden | 5 | 29 | 0 | 66 | 0 |
| Switzerland | 0 | 80* | 0 | 20 | 0 |
| Turkey | 80* | 0 | 0 | 0 | 20 |
| United Kingdom | 0 | 30 | 27 | 37 | 6 |
| United States | 23 | 22 | 17 | 35 | 3 |
| Total | 20 | 25 | 13 | 37 | 5 |
| Total, Excluding U.S. | 18 | 28 | 10 | 39 | 5 |

* Indicates strong (≥75%) consensus.

arguing that because reproductive activities may begin early, this is the most effective age at which to identify and counsel carriers with regard to family planning. Those who would prefer to screen adults by consent mentioned reproductive planning (74%), program efficiency (46%), and the individual's right to decide (40%). In all, only 4% mentioned the possibility of carrier stigmatization, a figure that seems low in view of past experience with sickle cell and Tay Sachs screening (21, 17). A total of 78% gave priority to the welfare of the person being screened, 10% to the welfare of society, and 9% to the health of future generations. Most (91%) envisaged no conflicts of interest in screening programs for cystic fibrosis. As in the previous question, advocates of mandatory screening were more likely than others ($p < 0.003$) to list and describe the consequences of screening programs.

Most (82%) believed that screening for cystic fibrosis should be applied to the entire population, but 18% believed that it should be applied primarily to Caucasians. In five nations more than 20% said that screening programs should focus on Caucasians. These were Japan (55%), Italy (46%), Canada (27%), Brazil (22%), and Switzerland (20%). Many geneticists in the United States and other nations that favored screening for all said that few persons in their countries were without some Caucasian blood; to restrict screening on the basis of race would be discriminatory.

## 1.3.9.4 Presymptomatic Tests for Huntington Disease

Our third screening situation was phrased: "When a 99% accurate pre-symptomatic test for Huntington disease is developed that applies to all families, who should have access to the results of the test?"

Such tests are not currently available on a population-wide basis. Although DNA testing can be used to detect carriers and for prenatal diagnosis, it is not widely available. Huntington disease is a fatal, non-reversible neurological disorder that first strikes in middle age, and leads to progressive mental and motor deterioration over 10 to 15 years, culminating in death. It is not treatable. It is an autosomal dominant disorder, meaning that each of the patient's children has a 50% chance of developing the disease, without prior warning, in later life. Until then, they live under a cloud of uncertainty. A presymptomatic test, given early enough, would permit potential patients with Huntington's to plan both their lives and their families. Early warning, however, will not lead to better prognosis, and will almost certainly produce depression, stigmatization, and loss of economic benefits for some. Many of those at risk are themselves uncertain about whether or not they would wish to know the results of presymptomatic tests [11].

The question is not whether patients should have access to test results if they ask (98% of our respondents believed that they should), but whether they should be informed of these results even if they do not wish to know. In all, 66% of respondents believed that individuals at risk should be told their test results only if they say that they wish to know (Table 1.21). In other words, persons at risk for Huntington disease should have a "right not to know" whether they will develop the disease in later life. There was strong ($\geq 75\%$) consensus about this right in four nations (Federal Republic of Germany, German Democratic Republic, Switzerland, and United Kingdom).

Access for the individual's spouse, who will face serious emotional and financial burdens if the person is affected, and for relatives at risk of developing Huntington disease, presents serious ethical dilemmas. If the tested individual does not give consent, the geneticist is faced with a conflict between the duty to preserve patient confidentiality and the duty to warn third parties of harm. In all, 62% thought that spouses should have no access to test results without the patient's consent. There was strong ($\geq 75\%$) consensus to this effect in six nations (Australia, Federal Republic of Germany, France, German Democratic Republic, Sweden, and United Kingdom). Twelve per cent, both of the total and in the United States, thought that spouses should have access to test results if they asked, and 26% thought that spouses should be informed of results even if they did not ask. There was strong consensus in three nations, Greece, India, and Turkey, that spouses should be informed. Of those who would inform the spouse, 45% cited reproductive planning, 24% cited preparation for the future, and 19% said that the spouse had a right to know.

There was no consensus about access for relatives at risk of developing Huntington disease. There was strong consensus in Switzerland for no access without the patient's consent and strong consensus in Brazil and Turkey that relatives should have automatic access or be informed. In all, 52% thought that relatives

**Table 1.21.** Access to Results of Presymptomatic Tests for Huntington Disease

| Country | Per Cent Responding No Access to Results Without Patient's Consent (In Parentheses: No Access at All) | | | | | | | |
|---|---|---|---|---|---|---|---|---|
| | Patient[+] | | Spouse | | Relatives at risk for HD | | Employer | Life and medical insurers |
| Australia | 50 | | 75* | (8) | 67 | | 100* (67) | 100* (58) |
| Brazil | 56 | | 44 | (6) | 16[+] | | 94* (31) | 91* (28) |
| Canada | 67 | | 56 | (7) | 65 | (10) | 100* (54) | 100* (46) |
| Denmark | 73 | | 53 | (7) | 27 | | 100* (60) | 100* (67) |
| Federal Republic of Germany | 84* | (4) | 82* | (7) | 69 | (4) | 100* (91)* | 95* (84)* |
| France | 71 | (6) | 77* | (15) | 46 | (8) | 100* (83)* | 100* (67) |
| German Democratic Republic | 75* | | 79* | (16) | 65 | (20) | 100* (89)* | 90* (85)* |
| Greece | 33 | | 17[+] | | 50 | | 100* (17) | 83* (17) |
| Hungary | 53 | (13) | 67 | (20) | 27 | (7) | 93* (60) | 87* (60) |
| India | 30 | (4) | 24[+] | (4) | 27 | (4) | 70 (35) | 60 (40) |
| Israel | 57 | | 50 | | 46 | (8) | 100* (50) | 100* (21) |
| Italy | 67 | | 50 | (10) | 50 | (10) | 100* (60) | 100* (50) |
| Japan | 57 | (8) | 55 | (17) | 37 | (14) | 85* (67) | 88* (70) |
| Norway | 50 | | 67 | | 50 | | 100* (83)* | 100* (83)* |
| Sweden | 71 | | 79* | | 57 | | 100* (62) | 100* (48) |
| Switzerland | 80* | | 60 | | 80* | | 100* (80)* | 100* (60) |
| Turkey | 0[+] | | 0[+] | | 0[+] | | 50 (25) | 75* |
| United Kingdom | 94* | | 77* | | 71 | | 97* (16) | 100* (19) |
| United States | 67 | | 65 | (1) | 57 | (2) | 98* (34) | 94* (36) |
| Total | 66 | (2) | 62 | (5) | 52 | (4) | 96* (46) | 93* (45) |
| (95% Confidence limits) | (61, 71) | | (57, 67) | | (47, 57) | | (94, 98) | (90, 96) |
| Total, Excluding U.S. | 65 | (3) | 61 | (7) | 48 | (5) | 95* (56) | 93* (52) |
| (95% Confidence limits) | (59, 71) | | (55, 67) | | (42, 54) | | (92, 98) | (90, 96) |

[+] Per cents are those who would tell patients only if they want to know, as opposed to informing patients against their will.
* Strong (≥75%) consensus *in favor of* access only with consent.
[+] Strong (≥75%) consensus for access *without* consent.

should have no access without the patient's consent, 24% thought that they should have access, even without the patient's consent, if they wanted the test results, and 24% thought that they should be informed of the results, without the patient's consent, even if they did not ask. Reasons included providing information for relatives' reproductive or future plans (27%), relatives' right to know (25%), and the patient's right to privacy (17%).

When we asked about access for institutional third parties, however, there was overwhelming consensus almost everywhere that employers, life insurers, and health insurers should not have access without consent. Geneticists' distrust of these third parties was such that almost half said that they should have no access of any kind, even if the individual gave consent. Few (5%) saw any benefit for individuals in allowing institutional third parties to know their test results, and 28% believed that institutions would misuse information. Only 4% expressed concern for the economic interests of third parties. A question about access for schools (not reported in Table 1.21) produced responses similar to those for other institutions. Most geneticists thought that schools had no need to know that a student would develop a disorder in middle age.

## 1.3.10 Total Consensus

### 1.3.10.1 International Consensus

There was strong consensus ($\geq 75\%$ in each of 75% of nations) about 3.9 (28%) of the 14 clinical cases, neither (0%) of the two questions on voluntary-mandatory screening, 10 (67%) of 15 questions on access to results of screening, and 8 (67%) of the 12 goals and approaches for counseling. In an additional clinical case, prenatal diagnosis for sex selection, there was strong consensus against actual performance, but willingness to refer to someone who might perform it suggests that there is in fact less than a strong consensus. Areas of strong consensus are summarized in Table 1.22.

In addition, there was a moderate consensus ($\geq 67\%$ in each of 67% of nations) that prenatal diagnosis should not be performed for sex selection (Case 11), that counseling about XO fetuses should be nondirective (1/2 of Case 12), and that A.I.D. should be presented as a reproductive option (1/5 of Case 13). There was also a moderate consensus that "improvement of the general health and vigor of the population" should be an important goal of counseling. In all, there was moderate consensus about 1.7 (12%) of the 14 clinical cases and 8% of goals and approaches of counseling.

The addition of strong and moderate consensus produces a total consensus of 40% for clinical cases, 0% for voluntary-mandatory screening questions, 67% for questions on access to results of screening and 75% for counseling goals and approaches (Table 1.22).

### 1.3.10.2 Internal Consensus

The per cents of consensus within each country are shown in Table 1.23, for both strong and moderate consensus. Strong consensus about clinical cases ranged from 75% (Turkey) down to 18% (India), and strong consensus about screening ranged from 93% (Switzerland) down to 10% (India). There were no clear patterns. Developed nations did not consistently have greater internal consensus than developing nations, nor did the four nations with the longest histories of scientific development in clinical genetics (United Kingdom, United States, Canada, and Denmark) have greater internal consensus than some other nations where genetics has developed more recently. Clearly, there is a lack of internal as well as international consensus.

45

**Table 1.22.** Total Consensus

I. Total Strong Consensus
(≥75% in Each of 75% of Nations)
A. *Clinical Cases*
    1. Protection of mother's confidentiality overrides disclosure of true paternity (Case 1)
    2. Disclose conflicting diagnostic findings, and counsel nondirectively (Case 6)
    3. Disclose new/controversial interpretations (Case 7)
    4. Non-directive counseling about fetuses with XYY, a low burden disorder (1/2 of Case 12)
    5. Present adoption as reproductive option to male and female carriers (1/5 of Case 13, 1/6 of Case 14)
    6. Do not actually perform prenatal diagnosis for sex selection. Willingness to refer, however, gives evidence of compromise and blunts this consensus.
B. *Voluntary - Mandatory Screening*
    None
C. *Access to Results of Screening*
    1. No access for employer, or 4 types of insurers to results of occupational screening without consent; access for patient (6 parts of 8-part question)
    2. No access for school, employer, life, and medical insurers to results of presymptomatic test for HD, without consent (4 of 7 parts)
D. *Counseling*
    5 of 7 goals (Table 1.17)
    3 of 5 approaches (Table 1.18)
II. Total Moderate Consensus
(≥67% in Each of 67% of Nations)
A. *Clinical Cases*
    1. Prenatal diagnosis should not be performed, nor should referrals be given, for sex selection (Case 11)
    2. Nondirective counseling about fetuses with X0, a low burden disorder (1/2 of Case 12)
    3. Present A. I. D. as reproductive option (1/5 of Case 13)
B. *Counseling*
    1 of 7 goals (Table 1.17)

|  | % Consensus | | |
| --- | --- | --- | --- |
|  | Strong | Moderate | Total |
| 14 clinical cases | 28 | 12 | 40 |
| 2 screening questions | 0 | 0 | 0 |
| 15 questions on access to results of screening | 67 | 0 | 67 |
| 12 counseling goals and approaches | 67 | 8 | 75 |

## 1.3.11 Future Priorities

We asked respondents to rank-order, from one to ten, a list of issues that they thought *should be* of most concern to medical geneticists in the next 10 to 15 years. They were asked to rank-order the same list twice, first for their own country and then "around the world." Priorities within each country are summarized in Table 1.24, by country. The rank-ordering for each country was calculated by using the mean score, to four decimal points, for each item. Priorities "around the world" are listed in Table 1.25. The rank-ordering of this table was derived by calculating

**Table 1.23.** Internal Consensus in Each Country*

| Country | % of Clinical Cases | | | % of Screening | | | % of Counseling | | |
|---|---|---|---|---|---|---|---|---|---|
| | Strong ≥75% | Moderate 67–74% | Total | Strong ≥75% | Moderate 67–74% | Total | Strong ≥75% | Moderate 67–74% | Total |
| Australia | 68 | 14 | 82 | 62 | 10 | 72 | 83 | 8 | 91 |
| Brazil | 67 | 17 | 84 | 37 | 3 | 40 | 83 | 8 | 91 |
| Canada | 48 | 14 | 62 | 36 | 29 | 65 | 75 | 8 | 83 |
| Denmark | 65 | 8 | 73 | 61 | 4 | 65 | 75 | 8 | 83 |
| Federal Rep. of Germany | 50 | 27 | 77 | 65 | 10 | 75 | 67 | 16 | 83 |
| France | 35 | 10 | 45 | 35 | 7 | 42 | 67 | 16 | 83 |
| German Dem. Republic | 53 | 5 | 58 | 68 | 25 | 93 | 83 | 8 | 91 |
| Greece | 42 | 16 | 58 | 90 | 0 | 90 | 75 | 8 | 83 |
| Hungary | 36 | 22 | 58 | 30 | 60 | 90 | 58 | 8 | 66 |
| India | 18 | 7 | 25 | 10 | 35 | 45 | 83 | 0 | 83 |
| Israel | 51 | 42 | 93 | 33 | 25 | 58 | 83 | 17 | 100 |
| Italy | 66 | 16 | 82 | 58 | 10 | 68 | 75 | 0 | 75 |
| Japan | 58 | 1 | 59 | 33 | 0 | 33 | 67 | 16 | 83 |
| Norway | 43 | 23 | 66 | 61 | 4 | 65 | 75 | 0 | 75 |
| Sweden | 53 | 10 | 63 | 68 | 4 | 72 | 75 | 0 | 75 |
| Switzerland | 56 | 0 | 56 | 93 | 0 | 93 | 75 | 0 | 75 |
| Turkey | 75 | 0 | 75 | 81 | 0 | 81 | 75 | 8 | 83 |
| United Kingdom | 62 | 1 | 63 | 68 | 4 | 72 | 75 | 16 | 91 |
| United States | 64 | 1 | 65 | 61 | 4 | 65 | 83 | 8 | 91 |

* Consensus is *internal* to each country. A high per cent does not necessarily indicate agreement with other countries or with a worldwide consensus.
Per cents for clinical cases based on 14 cases, including 3 cases with multiple parts (2, 5 and 6 parts, respectively).
Per cents for screening based on 4 questions, including 2 with 7 and 8 parts respectively.
Per cents for counseling based on 12 goals and approaches.

**Table 1.24.** Ranking of Future Priorities in Own Nation

| Nation | Rank-order of Priority | | | | | | | | | |
|---|---|---|---|---|---|---|---|---|---|---|
| | Increased Demand | Allocation Resources | Carrier Screen. | Environ. Damage | New Treatments | Screen. Cancer, Heart Disease | Screen. Workplace | Research Human Embryo | Eugenics | Sex Selection |
| Australia | 1 | 2 | 3 | 4 | 6 | 5 | 7 | 8 | 9 | 10 |
| Brazil | 1 | 2 | 4 | 3 | 5 | 6 | 7 | 8 | 9 | 10 |
| Canada | 1 | 2 | 3 | 5 | 4 | 6 | 8 | 7 | 9 | 10 |
| Denmark | 1 | 2 | 5 | 3 | 4 | 6 | 8 | 7 | 9 | 10 |
| Federal Republic of Germany | 1 | 6 | 3 | 4 | 2 | 5 | 8 | 7 | 9 | 10 |
| France | 1 | 7 | 3 | 4 | 2 | 6 | 8 | 5 | 9 | 10 |
| German Democratic Republic | 1 | 8 | 3 | 5 | 2 | 4 | 6 | 7 | 9 | 10 |
| Greece | 2 | 3 | 1 | 5 | 7* | 7* | 4 | 9 | 6 | 10 |
| Hungary | 3 | 5 | 1 | 2 | 4 | 6 | 8 | 7 | 9 | 10 |
| India | 1 | 4 | 1 | 3 | 7 | 5 | 6 | 8 | 9 | 10 |
| Israel | 2 | 1 | 2 | 5 | 4 | 6 | 8 | 7 | 9 | 10 |
| Italy | 2 | 3 | 1 | 4 | 5 | 6 | 8 | 7 | 9 | 10 |
| Japan | 1 | 8 | 6 | 3 | 2 | 5 | 7 | 4 | 8 | 10 |
| Norway | 1 | 3 | 2 | 7 | 4 | 5 | 8 | 6 | 9 | 10 |
| Sweden | 2 | 6 | 3 | 4 | 1 | 5 | 8 | 7 | 9 | 10 |
| Switzerland | 2 | 7 | 1 | 3* | 5 | 4 | 7 | 6 | 9 | 10 |
| Turkey | 2 | 7 | 1 | 3* | 6 | 3* | 5 | 7 | 10 | 9 |
| United Kingdom | 1 | 3 | 2 | 4 | 6 | 5 | 8 | 7 | 9 | 10 |
| United States | 3 | 6 | 2 | 4 | 1 | 5 | 8 | 7 | 9 | 10 |

* tie

**Table 1.25.** Ranking of Future Priorities Around the World

1. Increased demand for genetic services
2. Carrier screening for common genetic disorders
3. Allocation of limited resources
4. Development of new treatments for genetic disorders, including treatment in utero, organ transplantation, and molecular genetic manipulation
5. Environmental damage to the unborn
6. Screening for genetic susceptibility to cancer, heart disease
7. Research on the human embryo, zygote, and fetus
8. Genetic screening in the workplace
9. Long-range eugenic concerns
10. Sex preselection for sex desired by parents

the rank that each country gave to an item (based on mean score) and then taking the mean of the ranks that each of the 19 countries gave an item.

Geneticists' rankings of future priorities, both at home and abroad, suggest that they put low priority on issues that are of great concern to the public, namely sex selection and genetic screening in the workplace. Future actions on these issues could change the entire structure of society by altering the sex ratio or limiting access to work. If a proposed project to map the human genome within the next ten years is undertaken, eugenic concerns, also given low priority by geneticists, could come quickly to the forefront.

## 1.4 Comparisons Within Cultural/Linguistic Groups

## 1.4.1 Rationale

Two groups of nations had sufficient linguistic similarity and historical/cultural association to warrant special comparisons. These were first, the United Kingdom, Canada, and the United States, and second, the three Scandinavian nations. Norway, with only 6 respondents, was omitted from the statistical comparisons. Cross-tabulations were performed and chi-squares computed for all responses within each group, in order to examine similarities and differences among the nations in each. Readers should interpret the following comparisons with caution, because of the small numbers of practising geneticists in some nations.

## 1.4.2 U.K – U.S. – Canadian Differences

Geneticists in these nations differed at $p < 0.02$ in regard to several background characteristics. These were degree, with fewer Ph.D.'s in the United Kingdom, number of patients per week (more in the United Kingdom), religious background (more Protestants in the United Kingdom), and number of religious observances attended (more in the United States). These differences in background did not remain significant in the regression analyses, and do not explain between-nation differences in choices of action. Doctors in the United Kingdom may still hold a somewhat more dominant position vis-a-vis their patients than doctors in the United States and Canada, although this is rapidly changing. Although doctors in the U.K. are sued with increasing frequency, monetary judgements are smaller than in the other two nations.

These three nations differed among themselves, at the 0.05 level in regard to 5.36 (38%) of the 14 clinical cases, 11% of screening and access questions, and 17% of goals and approaches to counseling. The areas of difference and $p$ values are listed in Table 1.26. In regard to surrogacy, 67% in the United States, 37% in Canada, and 27% in the United Kingdom would discuss this spontaneously, without being asked. More in the United Kingdom (47%) and Canada (42%) said that

**Table 1.26.** Canada – U.K. – U.S.A. Differences

|  | Canada % | U.K. % | U.S. % | p* |
|---|---|---|---|---|
| 1. *Clinical Case* | | | | |
| Present surrogate motherhood as option | 37 | 27 | 67 | 0.00001 |
| Disclose colleague disagreement about ambiguous/ artifactual test results | 66 | 52 | 75 | 0.0001 |
| Perform prenatal diagnosis for sex selection (excludes referrals) | 30 | 9 | 34 | 0.003 |
| Perform prenatal diagnosis for maternal anxiety, in absence of medical indications | 55 | 79 | 78 | 0.01 |
| Disclose XY genotype in a female | 68 | 37 | 64 | 0.01 |
| Disclose new/controversial interpretations of test results | 83 | 78 | 89 | 0.01 |
| Present IVF with donor egg as option | 59 | 63 | 83 | 0.01 |
| 2. *Screening and Counseling Questions* | | | | |
| Access to presymptomatic test results for HD without patient's consent | | | | |
| relatives at risk | 35 | 29 | 43 | 0.01 |
| patient (should be informed, unasked) | 33 | 6 | 33 | 0.02 |
| no access for employer, even with | | | | |
| patient's consent | 54 | 16 | 34 | 0.04 |
| Appropriate to: | | | | |
| Inform patients what you would do | 45 | 30 | 19 | 0.0002 |
| if in their situation | | | | |
| Inform patients what others have done | 83 | 94 | 69 | 0.05 |
| 3. *Other Questions* | | | | |
| Regulations should prohibit commercial laboratories performing prenatal diagnosis for | | | | |
| sex selection | 66 | 83 | 50 | 0.001 |
| maternal anxiety | 37 | 43 | 20 | 0.001 |
| patients who refuse abortion | 21 | 27 | 11 | 0.01 |
| Totals on which approaches differed at p<0.05 level: | | | | |
| 38% of clinical cases | | | | |
| 11% of screening questions | | | | |
| 17% of questions on goals/approaches for counseling | | | | |

* based on chi-square

surrogacy was not accepted than in the United States (22%). Geneticists in the United States were more likely to disclose colleague disagreement about ambiguous/artifactual results (75%) than geneticists in Canada (66%) or the United Kingdom (52%). Geneticists in the United States (34%) and Canada (30%) were more likely to say that they would perform prenatal diagnosis for sex selection than their colleagues in the United Kingdom (9%). Geneticists in the United States (28%) were also more likely to refer clients for sex selection than their colleagues in Canada (17%) or the United Kingdom (15%). Respondents in Canada (18%) and the United Kingdom (17%) were more likely to mention possible harms or benefits to society from sex selection than their colleagues in the United States (6%). More in the United Kingdom (29%) opposed the abortion of a normal fetus than in the United States (18%) or Canada (13%).

Geneticists in both the United Kingdom (79%) and the United States (78%) were more likely to say that they would perform prenatal diagnosis for maternal anxiety (if services were available) than their Canadian colleagues (55%). Reasons for this difference apparently lie in Canadians' greater perceptions of harm to the fetus from the procedure; 28% mentioned harm to the fetus, as opposed to 14% in the United States and 6% in the United Kingdom. Fewer Canadians (14%) mentioned patient autonomy in their reasoning than did their colleagues in the United States (33%) or the United Kingdom (42%). Resources, as expected, entered into reasoning; 39% in the United Kingdom, 28% in Canada, and 20% in the United States mentioned fair and wise use of resources. Nevertheless, as many would like to perform prenatal diagnosis in the United Kingdom, where resources are seen as an important issue, as in the United States, where many regard resources as unlimited. In the United Kingdom and United States, geneticists were more likely to place the mother's welfare first, (87% and 82%) than in Canada (50%). In Canada, 23% put the welfare of the fetus first, as opposed to 9% in the United States and none in the United Kingdom. Geneticists in Canada were more likely to describe a conflict of interest between mother and fetus (23%), geneticists in the United Kingdom were more likely to describe an individual-society conflict over limited resources (19%) and geneticists in the United States were more likely to describe no conflict at all (64%).

Geneticists in Canada (68%) and the United States (64%) were more likely to disclose XY genotype in a female than were their colleagues in the United Kingdom (37%). In their reasoning, geneticists in the United Kingdom (61%) were more likely to regard the truth as a source of harm than their colleagues in Canada (33%) or the United States (32%). More geneticists in the United Kingdom (41%) said that there was "no need for the patient to know" about XY genotype than their colleagues in the United States (19%) and Canada (12%).

More in the United States (89%) and Canada (83%) would not give advice about new or controversial interpretations of test results than in the United Kingdom (78%). (Almost all in all three nations would disclose). More in the United States (83%) would present in vitro fertilization with donor egg as an option than in Canada (59%) or the United Kingdom (63%).

In all, there was a pattern of greater disclosure, both of test results and sensitive information, in the United States and Canada than in the United Kingdom. There was greater willingness to discuss new and controversial reproductive options in the United States than in either Canada or the United Kingdom. With regard to prenatal diagnosis, there was no pattern; more in the United States and United Kingdom said that they would like to perform for maternal anxiety, and more in the United States and Canada would perform for sex selection.

As might be expected, the three nations differed at the 0.001 level with regard to regulating performance of prenatal diagnosis by commercial laboratories, with the United Kingdom more likely to favor regulation than the United States or Canada (see Table 1.12).

Differences on screening questions were in regard to access to results of pre-symptomatic tests for HD. In the United States and Canada, 33% thought that patients should be informed of their test results, even if they did not want to know, as opposed to 6% in the United Kingdom. In the United States, 43% thought that relatives at risk should have access to results, without the patient's consent, as opposed to 35% in Canada and 29% in the United Kingdom. On the other hand, 54% in Canada, 34% in the United States, and 16% in the United Kingdom thought that employers should have no access at all, even with the patient's consent. As with the clinical cases, the pattern is for greater disclosure in the United States and Canada than in the United Kingdom, with the exception of disclosure to institutional third parties.

With regard to counseling approaches, more in the United Kingdom (94%) and Canada (83%) considered it appropriate to inform clients what others have done in the client's situation than in the United States (69%). More in Canada (45%) considered it appropriate to tell clients what they would do if in the client's situation than in the United Kingdom (30%) or United States (19%).

## 1.4.3 Scandinavian Differences

Norway, with only 6 responses, could not be included in the statistical comparisons in Table 1.27. Nevertheless, we mention Norway in the text because there are important cultural differences between Norway and other Scandinavian nations, notably in the persistence of Calvinist influences upon ethics. The reader should keep in mind, however, that the per cents reported from Norway should not be read statistically.

Denmark and Sweden differed at the 0.05 level on 14% of the 14 clinical cases and 8% of counseling goals and approaches. These are listed in Table 1.27. More in Denmark (87%) and Norway (83%) would disclose a diagnosis of HD to relatives at risk, against the patient's wishes, than would disclose in Sweden (48%). Swedes were more likely to mention the patient's right to privacy or the doctor-patient relationship (65%) than their colleagues in Denmark (25%) or Norway (20%). Norwegians were more likely to mention the duty to warn third parties of harm (60%) than their colleagues in Denmark (27%) or Sweden (5%). Danes were more likely to say that relatives had a right to know (71%) than their colleagues in Sweden (48%) or Norway (40%).

More Danes (87%) would disclose a diagnosis of hemophilia A to relatives at risk, against the patient's wishes, than would Norwegians (50%) or Swedes (48%).

52

**Table 1.27.** Danish – Swedish Differences

|  | Denmark % | Sweden % | p* |
|---|---|---|---|
| *Clinical Cases* |  |  |  |
| Disclose a diagnosis of HD to relatives at risk, against patient's wishes | 87 | 48 | 0.03 |
| Disclose a diagnosis of hemophilia A to relatives at risk, against patient's wishes | 87 | 48 | 0.05 |
| *Counseling Questions* |  |  |  |
| Importance of "prevention of disease" as counseling goal | 53 | 25 | 0.01 |
| Total differences at $<0.05$ level: |  |  |  |
| 14% of clinical cases |  |  |  |
| 8% of counseling goals/approaches |  |  |  |

* based on chi-square

In this case, fewer Norwegians would disclose than in the previous case because they said the relatives "had no need to know." This reason was given by 75% of Norwegians, apparently because they considered the disorder treatable. The Danes cited the duty to warn third parties of harm (57%) and the relatives' right to know (39%). Danes and Norwegians were more likely to mention the consequences of their actions than were Swedes, both for this and the previous case.

In general, Danish geneticists were most likely to approve of disclosure to relatives at risk. They felt conflicts about this, however. "Confidentiality of an HD patient" was the case giving greatest ethical conflict in Denmark. The Norwegians, who would also disclose in this case, also rated it as the case that gave most conflict.

In regard to counseling goals, more Danes (53%) saw the "prevention of disease" as absolutely essential than Swedes (25%) or Norwegians (17%).

Although geneticists in Denmark and Sweden differed at the 0.04 level on degree, years in genetics, and age, these characteristics were not significantly related, in the regression analyses, to choices of action.

## 1.5 Developing Nations

Four nations in the survey (Brazil, Greece, India, and Turkey) are classified as developing nations by the World Bank, although, as discussed in 1.2.2.2 above, Brazil and Greece are not poor and may deserve a separate classification by sociologists as "semi-peripheral" economically. In the relative absence of enforceable restrictions on employers, multinational corporations may take advantage of conditions outlawed in their parent countries, especially if a nation does not have a strong workers' movement, as is the case in India and Turkey. Under these conditions, genetic screening for susceptibility to occupationally-related disease takes on new importance. It may be seen both as a viable alternative to cleaning up the workplace and as a means of protecting workers who cannot protect themselves and who must take any work available.

Not surprisingly, these four nations had a distinctive pattern of responses in regard to screening and access to results. In three (Brazil, India, and Turkey) the majority thought that screening in the workplace for susceptibility to occupationally-related disease should be mandatory. These four nations were the only countries without a strong consensus against the employer's having automatic access to the worker's test results. Along with the German Democratic Republic and Hungary, they were the only countries with a strong ($\geq 75\%$) consensus that the worker's physician should have automatic access to the test results. Two (Greece and Turkey) were the only countries with a strong consensus that the government health department should have automatic access to test results. In their reasoning, geneticists from these nations believed that mandatory screening and automatic access for some third parties were beneficial for the worker's health.

Family access to the results of screening tests was also regarded uniquely in these nations. Greece, India, and Turkey were the only nations with a strong consensus that the patient's spouse should be informed, unasked, of the results of a presymptomatic test for Huntington disease. Brazil and Turkey were the only nations with a strong consensus that relatives at risk for Huntington disease should either have automatic access to the patient's test results or be informed, even if they do not ask. In regard to clinical cases, geneticists in these two nations would also disclose diagnoses of HD and hemophilia A to relatives at risk, against the patient's wishes. There was apparently a tendency in these nations to see the patient undergoing screening as part of a family unit rather than as a private, atomized individual. The family unit is seen as having a right to know that transcends individual rights to privacy.

In regard to the goals of genetic counseling, Brazil, India, and Turkey were the only nations with a strong ($\geq 75\%$) consensus that reducing the number of carriers in the population should be an important goal. In view of expanding populations and very limited expenditures on health care in these nations, this view of genetic counseling as "primary prevention" may be a response to demographic realities.

## 1.6 Gender Differences

Some important gender differences emerged across nations. Many of these have already been discussed in previous sections of this chapter. In all, there were significant differences in choice of action at the 0.05 level on 4.17 (30%) of the 14 clinical cases and in moral reasoning in an additional clinical case. The 5.17 clinical cases are listed in Table 1.28. There were no differences on the screening or access questions. There were differences on 6 (50%) of the 12 counseling goals and approaches (Table 1.29).

Crosstabulations, using chi-square as the standard measure of association suitable for nominal-order data, were performed for gender and all responses. For each response where there were significant associations ($p < 0.10$) at the zero-order level between gender and response, stepwise logistic regressions were performed. All personal and professional background variables on which women and men differed significantly were entered into the analyses. These were country, degree

**Table 1.28.** Gender Differences in Responses to Clinical Cases

|  | Case Description | %Women | %Men |
|---|---|---|---|
| Case 1 | False Paternity<br>No differences in choice of action:<br>  Mention marital conflict | 75 | 57 |
| Case 4 | Disclosure which parent carries a translocation<br>causing Down syndrome in the child | | |
| |   Disclose, even if not asked | 63 | 46 |
| |   Tell relatives at risk | 22 | 13 |
| |   See welfare of extended family as most important | 45 | 29 |
| |   Describe consequences of their actions | 57 | 41 |
| Case 6 | Directive/nondirective counseling about conflicting<br>diagnostic findings for NTD | | |
| |   Give directive advice | 5 | 13 |
| |   Patient's autonomy is dominant value | 91 | 82 |
| Case 10 | Perform prenatal diagnosis for an anxious woman,<br>in the absence of medical indications | 76 | 61 |
| |   Patient's autonomy dominant value | 39 | 31 |
| |   Justice is dominant value | 11 | 22 |
| Case 12 | Directive/nondirective counseling about fetuses with<br>low burden disorders | | |
| | X0:    Give directive advice | 6 | 14 |
| | XYY:  Give directive advice | 10 | 17 |
| Case 14<br>(1 of 6<br>parts) | Surrogate motherhood as option for female carrier<br>of tuberous sclerosis | | |
| |   Discuss, unasked | 35 | 52 |
| |   Describe consequences | 34 | 20 |

**Table 1.29.** Gender Differences in Counseling

Goals/Approaches that Women Considered More Essential/Appropriate

|  | p* | Odds ratio* |
|---|---|---|
| 1. Help clients understand options | 0.02 | 13.2 |
| 2. Remove, lessen guilt or anxiety | 0.004 | 3.5 |
| 3. Support any decisions patients make | 0.05 | 2.7 |
| Approaches that Men Considered More Appropriate | | |
| 1. Advise patients what they ought to do | 0.01 | 6.9 |
| 2. Inform patients what you would do if in their situation | 0.002 | 4.6 |
| 3. Advise patients what others have done | 0.02 | 1.9 |

* based on stepwise logistic regression

(M. D. or Ph. D.), number of hours per week in medical genetics, number of years in medical genetics, age, marital status, and number of children (Table 1.30). The purpose of the logistic regressions was to see whether gender was related to responses, over and above nationality, age, and other background variables. Although not reported, logistic regression results support the data in Table 1.28. Gender differences, across nationalities and personal backgrounds, also appeared

**Table 1.30.** Demographics By Gender

|  | Men | Women | p* |
|---|---|---|---|
| Degree, M.D. or equivalent | 86% | 70% | 0.0001 |
| Ph.D. or equivalent | 13% | 24% |  |
| other | 1% | 6% |  |
| Median years in genetics | 14 | 11 | 0.001 |
| Median hours/per week in genetics | 40 | 43 | 0.01 |
| Median age | 47 | 42 | 0.0001 |
| Married | 87% | 70% | 0.0001 |
| Median number children | 2 | 1 | 0.0001 |

* based on chi-square

in the reasoning underlying choices of action (Table 1.28). Cases where differences occurred were Case 1 (false paternity), Case 4 (disclosure of parental translocation), Case 6 (counseling about conflicting diagnostic findings for neural tube defect), Case 10 (prenatal diagnosis for maternal anxiety), and Case 12 (counseling about fetuses with low burden disorders XO and XYY).

Interestingly, there were no gender differences in responses or reasoning with regard to two cases where we most expected them: use of prenatal diagnosis for the purpose of selecting the sex of the child, and disclosure to a woman with XY genotype.

The gender differences in Table 1.28 fall into three types: 1) cases involving marital relationships; 2) directive/ nondirective counseling; 3) a case testing professional response to a woman patient's autonomy (prenatal diagnosis for an anxious woman).

There were gender differences in responses to the two cases in the study that most directly involved the marriage: 1) false paternity; and 2) disclosure of which parent carries a translocation.

In the false paternity case (Case 1), there were no gender differences in choice of action; almost all respondents chose to preserve the mother's confidentiality. Women, however, were more likely than men to mention conflicts between spouses; 75% of women and 57% of men mentioned marital conflicts.

Women were more likely than men to disclose which parent carried the translocation (Case 4) without first asking the parents whether they wished to know; 63% of women and 46% of men would disclose the information, even if parents did not ask for it; 22% of women and 13% of men would also disclose the information to relatives at risk for carrying the translocation. The welfare of the extended family, including relatives at risk and their potential offspring, was the primary consideration for 45% of women and 29% of men in this case; 57% of women and 41% of men mentioned the consequences of their actions.

Men were more likely than women to give directive advice or purposely slanted information in two of the four clinical cases dealing with directive/nondirective counseling. These were 1) advice about aborting or carrying to term when prenatal diagnosis produces conflicting results (Case 6); and 2) advice about carrying to term or aborting fetuses with borderline disorders XO and XYY (Case 12). In both these cases, the overwhelming majority of both men and women (83% and 95%)

would counsel nondirectively. Men were almost twice as likely as women, however, to give directive advice. Although respondents as a whole were more optimistic about XYY than XO, women and men did not exhibit different amounts of optimism. There were gender differences in dominant values underlying the responses to Case 6 (directive/nondirective counseling in cases of conflicting test results). The primary reasons given by 91% of women and 82% of men fell under the heading of patient autonomy.

In the two cases of directive/nondirective counseling of male and female carriers of tuberous sclerosis (Cases 13 and 14), women and men counseled similarly, with one exception: women were less likely than men to describe surrogate motherhood as a possibility, unless the patient asked about it. Of respondents, 35% of women and 52% of men would discuss surrogacy, nondirectively, as a reproductive option, without being asked. An additional 40% of women and 24% of men would discuss surrogacy if the patient specifically asked about it; 34% of women and 20% of men mentioned the possible consequences of surrogacy. Most of the consequences described were negative. There were no gender differences in responses about donor egg and in vitro fertilization as a reproductive option.

Women were more likely than men to perform prenatal diagnosis for maternal anxiety (Case 10), without medical or age indications; 76% of women and 61% of men would perform prenatal diagnosis. (An additional 6% of women and 10% of men would refer the patient elsewhere). Women's reasons for performing prenatal diagnosis were more likely than men's to indicate respect for the patient's autonomy ("she has a right to the service," or "she has a right to decide"). Men's reasons were more likely than women's to reflect the value of justice ("don't waste resources," "equal access to services"). Although women's emphasis on the autonomy of the woman patient appeared cross-nationally, it was most marked within the United States.

Around the world, there were no gender differences in performance of prenatal diagnosis for sex selection. In the United States, however, women were 2.01 times more likely than men to say that they would perform prenatal diagnosis for sex selection, basing their answers on respect for patient autonomy.

In answer to the 12 questions on counseling goals/approaches, women, across nationalities, were more likely than men to consider it important to remove or lessen patient guilt or anxiety and to help clients understand their reproductive options (Table 1.29). They were also more likely to consider it appropriate to support patients' decisions.

Men, across nationalities, were more likely than women to consider it "appropriate" to give directive advice in counseling, such as telling patients what they ought to do, telling patients what the geneticist would do if in their situation, or telling them what others have done (Table 1.29).

Gender differences in moral reasoning are discussed further in 1.7.3 below.

## 1.7 Values and Ethical Reasoning

Although moral reasoning will be discussed at greater length in the concluding chapter, we have described our coding system here and included summary tables for reference.


### 1.7.1 Coding of Qualitative Data

The qualitative portions of the questionnaires, in which respondents described in their own words why they had chosen a course of action, enabled us to compare the reasons given by respondents in different nations. We coded the total number of reasons given for an action, whether the consequences of an action were considered, whose interests were considered most important, and the perception or non-perception of conflicts between the interests of different persons or between moral principles. The first two reasons given were each assigned one of 93 codes.

In addition to coding the first two reasons given for choices of action, we coded four additional aspects of the qualitative responses. These were: 1) total number of reasons given; 2) whether the possible consequences of an action were stated; 3) whose welfare was considered most important when making the decision; and 4) whether a conflict of interest or of principles was perceived when making the decision.


### 1.7.2 Ethical Principles

The 93 codes used to describe respondents' moral reasoning were next organized under six major headings, representing ethical principles commonly discussed in biomedical ethics [1, 6, 8]. These ethical principles are as follows:

1. *Autonomy* (Respect for the Person): the duty to respect the self-determination and choices of autonomous persons, as well as to protect persons with diminished autonomy, e.g., young children, mentally retarded persons, and those with other mental impairments.
2. *Non-maleficence*: the obligation to minimize harm to persons and wherever possible to remove the causes of harm altogether.
3. *Beneficence*: the obligation to secure the well-being of persons by acting positively on their behalf, and moreover, to maximize the benefits that can be attained.
4. *Justice*: the obligation to distribute benefits and burdens fairly, to treat equals equally and to give reasons for differential treatment based upon widely accepted criteria for just ways to distribute benefits and burdens.
5. *Strict Monetary Utilitarianism*: economic interests or material ends have the highest priority in reasoning.

6. *Non-moral reasons* are based on factual claims, scientific, metaphysical, or religious beliefs.

Examples of answers falling under the heading of *Autonomy* are right to decide, right to know, right not to know; optimal decisions are based on the use of medical/scientific information, confidentiality, obligation to tell the truth. Examples of reasons falling under the heading *Non-maleficence* are: do no harm; prevent harm to patient, fetus, child, future children; truth-telling as a source of harm; prevention of guilt or anxiety; preserve the family unit; do not set a precedent that will harm the moral order (the "slippery slope" argument).

*Beneficence* means a positive inclination to do good, as opposed to the mere avoidance of harm. Statements relating to the common good, public health, improvement of life for future generations, of working conditions, or of social equality all fall under the heading "beneficence". So also do the "caring" relationships described by Gilligan [12] as so influential in women's moral thinking. Examples of these are statements of responsibility to family or society, helping to remove guilt or anxiety, providing counseling, telling the truth in such a manner as to maximize good, and helping patients prepare for the future, including preparation for a child with a birth defect or for the stresses of abortion.

*Justice* involves balancing the rights of individuals against the welfare of society. Statements such as "they deserve this (medical) service," or "don't waste resources" fall under the heading of justice, as do statements about equal access, right of all to affordable medical care, or "the interests of the fetus ought to be considered equally with those of living persons."

Examples of *Strict Monetary Utilitarianism* are cost-benefit analyses or protecting the economic interests of third parties. *Non-moral answers* include fear of lawsuit (mentioned by fewer than 1%), my institution or supervisor forbids, I approve/disapprove, or this is technically possible/impossible.

The 93 individual reasons, as organized under these headings, can be found in Table 1.31.

We were interested in whether geneticists in different nations based their actions on different principles. First we summarized the 93 reasons listed in Table 1.31 under the six major principles described: 1) autonomy, 2) non-maleficence, 3) beneficence, 4) justice, 5) strict monetary utilitarianism, and 6) non-moral answers. We summarized the first two reasons given in each of the 14 clinical cases to produce an overall "principles score" for each nation. These are reported in Table 1.32. This table suggests, first, that autonomy is the overwhelming principle in most clinical decision-making, with 59% of the responses falling under this heading. Other principles, such as non-maleficence (20%), beneficence (11%), and justice (5%) pale in comparison. Second, Table 1.32 suggests that there are substantial international differences in the ordering of principles. For example, 64% of responses in the United States, and 63% of responses in Canada, Sweden, and the United Kingdom were based on autonomy, as opposed to 40% in Norway and 36% in Hungary. In contrast, 42% in Hungary and 15% in the United States were based on non-maleficence. Few responses anywhere were based on justice. There were no differences between men and women in overall preferences for the various principles.

**Table 1.31.** Codebook for Moral Reasoning: Principles Approach

---

I. *Autonomy*

   A. The ethical conviction that individuals should be treated as autonomous agents, e.g., unconditional right to self-determination, choice, autonomy, own decision, use of available technical options, right to refuse, full disclosure, right to referral, right to abortion
      patient
      parents
      spouse
      relatives at risk
      geneticist or physician (right to refuse to perform a procedure or to withhold information)
      counselor should be non-directive, support whatever decision clients make
      patient requests should be respected, whether they're right or wrong

   B. Right to know (entitled or deserve to know; reasonable request; includes the right *not* to know)
      patient
      spouse
      parents
      relatives at risk
      geneticist
      professional colleagues or third parties

   C. Optimal choices, or decisions are *based upon use* of medical/genetic information by patient, relatives, geneticist, or referring physician
      Freedom to change mind about abortion

   D. Patient's responsibility
      "duty to know," whether they want to or not, and to use information

   E. Ethical conviction that there is a responsibility or obligation to protect the autonomy of the person even though it may be diminished (*e.g.,* person is vulnerable, incapacitated, has knowledge that is incommensurate with the geneticist's knowledge, or geneticist has knowledge of patient's secrets or diagnosis). Includes anwers mentioning dignity of or respect for other party
      patient
      special mention of position of women in society or family
      child
      relatives at risk
      duty to warn third parties, including relatives, of harm
      duty to warn about new or experimental procedures or interpretations
      explicitly acknowledges that autonomy is diminished

   F. Truthtelling (rule-oriented; use for Kantian arguments)
      honesty, obligation to tell truth
      refusal to lie

   G. Right to privacy or confidentiality
      patient
      parents
      child
      relatives at risk

   H. Doctor-patient relationship
      doctor-patient relationship (trust, confidentiality)
      responsibility to give advice, direction, guidance, education

**Table 1.31.** (continued)

II. *Non-Maleficence (Avoidance of Harm)*

A. Do no harm (include harm to third parties or relatives)
B. Prevent or minimize physical or moral harm or risk of harm (moral harm-deceit)
   to patient (includes burden of disease on parents)
   to fetus or child
   to future children, including prevention of birth defects (includes helping patient have a normal child)

C. Prevent harm to fetus
   oppose abortion
   oppose abortion of normal fetus

D. Preserve family
   preserve family unity

E. Truth-telling to avoid harm

F. Truth-telling as a source of harm
   no benefit gained from truth-telling (no need to know)

   potential misuse of information by third parties
   avoid social stigmatization, discrimination in the workplace

G. Other
   harm through regulations or government intervention
   harm to society if sex ratio upset
   parent's request serves no useful purpose
   don't set a precedent that will harm the moral order ("slippery slope" argument)

III. *Beneficence (Purposeful "Doing Good")*

A. Removal of guilt or anxiety now, help with present problems
   physician's responsibility to provide health care for family, society
   the "Golden Rule" of Christian tradition: Do unto others as you would have others do unto you.

B. Benefits outweigh possible harm

C. Means of truth-telling so as to maximize good (means of telling truth, support, counseling, referrals)

D. Prepare for the future
   family planning, making informed reproductive choices
   prepare patient for the future, including help cope with stresses of disease or abortion
   child will be in normal range, despite genetic diagnosis

E. Improvement of life
   future generations
   health care
   social planning
   insurance coverage
   workers' health (includes responsibility of factory to worker)
   working conditions
   social unity
   protection of persons through regulation or licensing of labs and providers (insure proper level of service, quality control) to prevent misuse

61

**Table 1.31.** (continued)

F. Common good, public health

G. Other
   population limitation
   maintain balanced sex ratio
   eugenic arguments

IV. *Justice*

A. Access
   equal access
   entitlement to full insurance coverage
   right to medical care that is affordable

B. Fairness
   fairness or unfairness; they deserve or don't deserve the service
   interests of the fetus ought to be treated equally with those of living persons

C. Allocation of resources
   use resources wisely, don't waste resources
   appropriate or inappropriate use of technology
   medical indication or no medical indication
   all available services should be provided on request
   gaining acceptance (historical evolution)

V. *Strict Utilitarianism (Monetary)*

   efficiency or utility
   cost-benefit analysis
   protection of economic interests of third parties
   they have a right to whatever service they can pay for out or pocket

VI. *Compromise*

   *Compromise* (stated as such by respondent)
   – includes referral to another center, disclosure to another physician rather than patients

VII. *Non-Moral Answers* (no ethical principles involved)

   fear of lawsuit
   logistically or technically difficult, accurate or inaccurate, correct or incorrect
   law, regulations, supervisor, institution forbids
   not accepted, controversial
   I do not accept or approve of this
   this is not a geneticist's problem; should be dealt with by another professional
   the Bible (or equivalent in my religion) tells me so
   ethics should not be based on regulations or on legislation
   other non-moral reason
   medicine (or genetics) should not be a business
   not applicable in my country
   I approve of this
   mother's anxiety is predictive of fetal health

**Table 1.32**  Major Principles in 14 Clinical Cases*

| Country** | % Responses per Principle | | | | |
|---|---|---|---|---|---|
| | Autonomy | Non-Malef-icence | Beneficence | Justice | Non-Moral Reasons |
| Australia*** | 61 | 17 | 12 | 5 | 4 |
| Brazil | 53 | 25 | 14 | 4 | 4 |
| Canada | 63 | 17 | 10 | 5 | 5 |
| Denmark | 57 | 22 | 11 | 6 | 4 |
| Federal Republic of Germany | 55 | 23 | 13 | 3 | 6 |
| France*** | 45 | 32 | 16 | 4 | 2 |
| Greece | 54 | 29 | 12 | 3 | 3 |
| Hungary | 36 | 42 | 15 | 4 | 3 |
| India | 42 | 39 | 14 | 2 | 3 |
| Israel*** | 55 | 19 | 15 | 4 | 6 |
| Italy | 57 | 21 | 13 | 5 | 4 |
| Japan | 51 | 28 | 10 | 4 | 7 |
| Norway | 40 | 40 | 9 | 6 | 5 |
| Sweden | 63 | 20 | 10 | 2 | 5 |
| Switzerland*** | 53 | 20 | 15 | 5 | 6 |
| Turkey | 58 | 21 | 14 | 3 | 4 |
| United Kingdom*** | 63 | 16 | 8 | 5 | 7 |
| United States | 64 | 15 | 10 | 5 | 6 |
| Total | 59 | 20 | 11 | 5 | 5 |
| Total, Excluding U.S. | 55 | 24 | 12 | 4 | 5 |

Standard measures of association, such as chi-square not applicable because of repeated measurements per respondent.
* Totaled per cents for first and second reasons given for choices of action. Per cents based on responses.
** Data for German Democratic Republic not available.
*** Percents total <100 because 1% gave utilitarian answers.

A similar principle summary for screening and access questions showed greater emphasis on non-maleficence and beneficence, as is appropriate for public health issues (Table 1.33). Here 47% of responses were based on autonomy, 24% on non-maleficence, 22% on beneficence, 2% on justice, and 5% on strict monetary utilitarianism. Again, there were substantial differences in emphasis among nations.

## 1.7.3  The Ethics of Relationships

There are alternative approaches to the analysis of moral reasoning that do not rely on principles. Critics of the principles approach have claimed that in practice it is impossible to make clinical decisions on the basis of moral principles. Instead, clinicians think in terms of relationships, which tend to involve reciprocity [26]. The relationship approach emphasizes "needs" (usually patients') and "responsibilities" (usually clinicians'). In describing responsibilities as a basis of ethical ac-

**Table 1.33.** Major Principles in Screening and Access to Results*

| Country** | % Responses per Principle | | | | |
| --- | --- | --- | --- | --- | --- |
| | Autonomy | Non-Malef-icence | Benef-icence | Justice | Strict Monetary Utilitarianism |
| Australia | 43 | 26 | 24 | 0 | 7 |
| Brazil | 48 | 15 | 27 | 0 | 6 |
| Canada*** | 46 | 27 | 21 | 1 | 5 |
| Denmark | 48 | 31 | 20 | 0 | 4 |
| Federal Republic of Germany*** | 36 | 39 | 22 | 0 | 2 |
| France | 51 | 13 | 25 | 3 | 8 |
| Greece | 49 | 21 | 24 | 0 | 6 |
| Hungary*** | 42 | 27 | 28 | 0 | 3 |
| India | 24 | 26 | 41 | 4 | 5 |
| Israel | 42 | 30 | 23 | 0 | 5 |
| Italy | 44 | 25 | 23 | 4 | 4 |
| Japan*** | 52 | 22 | 22 | 1 | 2 |
| Norway | 31 | 40 | 21 | 8 | 0 |
| Sweden | 55 | 21 | 23 | 0 | 1 |
| Switzerland | 45 | 39 | 16 | 0 | 0 |
| Turkey | 32 | 12 | 49 | 4 | 3 |
| United Kingdom | 51 | 17 | 23 | 1 | 8 |
| United States*** | 51 | 22 | 18 | 2 | 6 |
| Total | 47 | 24 | 22 | 2 | 5 |
| Total, Excluding U.S. | 44 | 26 | 25 | 1 | 4 |

Standard measures of association, such as chi-square, not applicable because of repeated measurements per respondent.
* First and second reasons for choices of action; includes reasons about access to results of screening. Per cents based on responses.
** Data for German Democratic Republic not available.
*** Per cents total <100 because 1% gave non-moral reasons.

tion, this approach incorporates elements of Gilligan's and other feminist theories of moral development [12].

A major appeal of the relationship approach is that it is somewhat closer to the way clinicians think than is the more abstract principles approach. According to the relationship approach, the 93 individual moral reasons coded would fall under five headings:

I.   Rights and Obligations          } – Reciprocals
II.  Needs and Responsibilities      } – Reciprocals
III. Deserts and Justice             } – Reciprocals
IV.  Good of the Health Care System and Other Institutions
V.   Good of Society

**I. Rights and Obligations**
These terms derive from legal concepts and are reciprocals. If the patient has a right, the doctor has an obligation to respect that right, and vice versa. There are

two kinds of rights, both recognized by law: 1) *Rights of noninterference* or freedom from interference (negative rights); and 2) *Rights of entitlement* or access to services even if scarce or expensive (positive rights). Rights of entitlement apply to *all* persons, regardless of deserts or need. For example, a wealthy woman may not *need* to have her abortion paid for by the National Health Service, but she is *entitled* (has a right to) the service without cost. Rights of noninterference are basically the right to be let alone. They include the right to privacy and the right to procreate without government or institutional interference. They do *not* include unlimited visits to government-supported infertility clinics (this would be a right of entitlement if guaranteed by law, or would otherwise be a need).

**A.** Rights of noninterference or freedom from interference (negative rights)
- Right to privacy or confidentiality
- Right to choose or decide, whatever the decision (includes decisions that are *not* based on the use of scientific medical information)
- Right to refuse to perform a procedure or to withhold information (doctor's right)
- Right to refuse a procedure (patient's right)
- Right to elect *available* procedures, such as abortion, prenatal diagnosis
- Right to whatever service they can pay for out of pocket

**B.** Rights of entitlement (positive rights)
- Right to know; right to information
- Right *not* to know
- Right to referral
- Right to procedures that are *not* immediately available (scarce or expensive);
  - includes concepts of *access*
  - Equal access
  - Entitlement to full insurance coverage
  - Right to medical care that is affordable

**C.** Obligations: Acts that are the reciprocals of rights (including both negative and positive rights). Obligations differ from Responsibilities in that they are performances of acts. Responsibilities focus on the promotion of some aspect of the other person's well-being.
- Duty to warn about the dangers of new or experimental procedures
- Duty to warn third parties of harm
- Counselor should be non-directive, support whatever decisions patients make
- Patients' requests should be respected, whether they're right or wrong
- Honesty, obligation to tell the truth
- Refusal to lie
- Patients have a "duty to know", whether they want to or not, and to use the information
- Gaining acceptance (historical evolution)
- All available services should be provided on request
- Law, regulations, supervisor, institution forbids

## II. Needs and Responsibilities

These are reciprocals. Patients need psychological support, comfort, protection from physical or moral harm. Doctors have a responsibility to provide for these needs. One of the major patient needs is *avoidance of harm.* Note that fetuses have needs, but not rights (only *persons* recognized as such by law have rights).

**A.** Needs (Needs focus on some aspect of *well-being*).
- Need for information, need to know, so that optimal choices are made; optimal choices or decisions are based upon use of medical/scientific information
- Truth-telling as a source of harm
- No benefit from truthtelling (no need to know)
- Parents' request serves no useful purpose
- Removal of guilt or anxiety, help with present problems
- Benefits outweigh possible harm
- Special mention of position of women in society or family
- Preserve family unity
- Truthtelling to avoid harm
- Truthtelling as a source of harm
- Prepare for the future
- Family planning, making informed reproductive choices
- Child will be in normal range, despite genetic diagnosis
- Interests of the fetus ought to be treated equally with those of living persons
- Use resources wisely, don't waste resources
- Appropriate or inappropriate use of technology
- Medical indication or no medical indication

**B.** Responsibilities (Responsibilities focus on *promotion* of the other's well-being, as opposed to merely respecting rights).
- includes preservation of moral integrity, relationships
- Protection of persons with diminished capacity, who are vulnerable
- Doctor-patient relationship (trust, confidentiality)
- Responsibility to give advice, direction, guidance, education
- Do no harm
- Prevent or minimize physical or moral harm or risk of harm (Moral harm = deceit)
  - to patient (includes burden of disease on parents)
  - to fetus or child
  - to future children, including prevention of birth defects (includes helping patient have a normal child)
- Prevent harm to fetus
  - oppose abortion
  - oppose abortion of normal fetus
- Avoid potential misuse of information by third parties
- Avoid social discrimination, stigmatization, discrimination in the workplace
- Avoid harm through regulations or government intervention
- Don't set a precedent that will harm the moral order ("slippery slope" argument)
- Physician's responsibility to provide health care for family, society

- The Golden Rule
- Means of truthtelling so as to maximize good (means of telling truth, support, counseling, referrals)
- Prepare patient for the future, including help cope with stresses of disease or abortion

### III. Deserts and Justice

Deserts go beyond rights of entitlement or needs. They are what a particular person or special group deserves because of prior suffering or injustice, or because of prior good works or other special qualities. Hiring policies that attempt to redress previous wrongs by giving special preference to groups that have suffered injustice are based on the concept of deserts. In genetics, examples of deserts would be the family with a Down syndrome child who refuse abortion but ask for prenatal diagnosis in order to prepare themselves for the birth of another Down child. Some geneticists so admired this family and its willingness to bear suffering that they said they *deserve* the service because they are such good parents or because they have suffered so much. Very few reasons given in this survey fall under the concept of deserts. Deserts are something *extra* to be given to people in special circumstances, and are not to be confused with needs.

Justice is the reciprocal of deserts, and includes the concept of fairness and the demand on the doctor to provide what patients deserve.

Fairness or unfairness; they deserve or don't deserve the service

### IV. Good of the Health Care System and other Institutions
- Efficiency or utility
- Cost-benefit analysis
- Protection of economic interests of third parties

### V. Good of Society
- Harm to society if sex ratio upset
- Improvement of life
  - future generations
  - health care
  - social planning
  - insurance coverage
  - workers' health
  - working conditions
  - social unity
  - protection of persons through regulation or licensing of labs and providers
- Common good, public health
- Population limitation
- Maintain balanced sex ratio
- Eugenic arguments

A codebook organized according to ethical relationships can be found in Table 1.34.

A summary of responses, under the different categories of ethical relationships, appears in Table 1.35. Needs was the largest single category, with a total of 32% of

**Table 1.34.** Codebook for Moral Reasoning: The Relationships Approach

I. *Rights of Noninterference (Negative Rights)*

    A. The ethical conviction that individuals should be treated as autonomous agents, e.g., right to self-determination, choice, autonomy, own decision, right to refuse, right to abortion
        patients
        parents
        spouse
        relatives at risk
        geneticist or physician (right to refuse to perform a procedure or to withhold information)

    B. Right to privacy or confidentiality
        patient
        parents
        child
        relatives at risk

    C. Other
        They have a right to whatever service they can pay for out of pocket

II. *Rights of Entitlement (Positive Rights)*

    A. Access
        equal access
        entitlement to full insurance coverage
        right to medical care that is affordable

    B. Right to know (entitled or deserve to know; reasonable request; includes the right *not* to know)
        patient
        spouse
        parents
        relatives at risk
        geneticist
        professional colleagues or third parties

III. *Obligations*

    A. Doctor's obligations
        duty to warn third parties, including relatives, of harm
        duty to warn about new or experimental procedures or interpretations
        truthtelling (rule-oriented; use for Kantian arguments)
        honesty, obligation to tell truth
        refusal to lie
        all available services should be provided on request
        gaining acceptance (historical evolution)
        law, regulations, supervisor, institution forbids
        counselor should be non-directive, support whatever decision clients make
        patient requests should be respected, whether they're right or wrong

    B. Patients' obligations
        "duty to know," whether they want to or not, and to use information

**Table 1.34.** (continued)

IV. *Needs*

A. Needs for information
optimal choices or decisions are *based upon use* of medical/genetic information by patient, relatives, geneticist, or referring physician
they may change their mind about abortion after receiving test results

B. Need to avoid harm
preserve family unity
truth-telling to avoid harm
truth-telling as a source of harm
no benefit gained from truth-telling (no need to know)
benefits outweigh possible harm
parents' request serves no useful purpose

C. Psychosocial Needs
special mention of position of women in society or family
removal of guilt or anxiety now
help with present problem
family planning
making informed reproductive choices
mother's anxiety is predictive of fetal health
(she needs the service)

D. Needs of child/fetus
child will be in normal range, despite genetic diagnosis
interests of the fetus ought to be treated equally with those of living persons

E. Allocation of resources according to patient's needs
use resources wisely, don't waste resources
appropriate or inappropriate use of technology
medical indication or no medical indication

V. *Responsibilities*

A. Ethical conviction that there is a responsibility to protect the autonomy of the person even though it may be diminished (*e.g.,* person is vulnerable, incapacitated, has knowledge that is incommensurate with the geneticist's knowledge, or geneticist has knowledge of patient's secrets or diagnosis)
patient
child
relatives at risk
explicitly acknowledges that autonomy is diminished

B. Doctor-patient relationship
doctor-patient relationship (trust, confidentiality)
responsibility to give advice, direction, guidance, education

C. Avoidance of harm
Do no harm (include harm to third parties or relatives)
Prevent or minimize physical or moral harm or risk of
harm (moral harm = deceit)
to patient (includes burden of disease on parents)
to fetus or child

**Table 1.34.**  (continued)

to future children, including prevention of birth defects (includes helping patient have a normal child)
Prevent harm to fetus
    oppose abortion
    oppose abortion of normal fetus
Potential misuse of information by third parties
    avoid social stigmatization, discrimination in the workplace
    harm through regulations or government intervention
Don't set a precedent that will harm the moral order ("slippery slope" argument)

D. Caring for the Welfare of Others
    physician's responsibility to provide health care for family, society
    the Golden Rule
    means of truth-telling so as to maximize good (means of telling truth, support, counseling, referrals)
    prepare patient for the future, including help cope with stresses of disease or abortion

VI. *Deserts*

Fairness or unfairness; they deserve or don't deserve the service

VII. *Good of Society*

A. Improvement of life
    future generations
    health care
    social planning
    insurance coverage
    workers' health (includes responsibility of factory to worker)
    working conditions
    social unity
    protection of persons through regulation or licensing of labs and providers (insure proper level of service, quality control) to prevent misuse

B. Common good, public health

C. Other
    population limitation
    maintain balanced sex ratio
    eugenic arguments
    harm to society if sex ratio upset

VIII. *Good of the Health Care System*
    efficiency or utility
    cost-benefit analysis
    protection of economic interests of third parties

IX. *Compromise*
    Compromise (stated as such by respondent – includes referral to another center, disclosure to another physician rather than patients)

**Table 1.34.** (continued)

X. *Non-moral Answers* (no ethical principles involved)

fear of lawsuit
logistically or technically difficult, accurate or inaccurate, correct or incorrect
not accepted, controversial
I do not accept or approve of this
this is not a geneticist's problem; should be dealt with by another professional
the Bible (or equivalent in my religion) tells me so
ethics should not be based on regulations or on legislation
other non-moral reason
medicine (or genetics) should not be a business
not applicable in my country
I approve of this

responses. Per cents ranged from 42% in Denmark down to 19% in Turkey. The reciprocal of Needs, which is Responsibilities, accounted for 16% of responses, ranging from 31% in Hungary and India down to 12% in the United Kingdom. Needs and Responsibilities together accounted for 48% of total responses, ranging from 68% in Hungary down to 43% in Turkey. Obligations accounted for 19% of total responses, ranging from 24% in Canada down to 11% in Hungary and India. Rights of noninterference accounted for 15% of responses, ranging from 19% in Japan and Turkey down to 8% in Denmark. Rights of entitlement accounted for 11% of total responses, ranging from 17% in Australia and Brazil down to 3% in France. Together, Rights and Obligations, which are reciprocals, accounted for 45% of total responses, slightly less than Needs and Responsibilities. The total per cents for Rights and Obligations ranged from 54% in Turkey down to 26% in Hungary.

In all, few responses were related to deserts (0.7%, mostly in Canada and Italy), the good of society (0.5%, mostly in Greece, India, and Japan), good of the health care system (0.4%, mostly in the United States and Canada), or compromise (0.1%, mostly in Canada, United Kingdom, and United States). These are not reported in the table. In Greece and India, 4% of responses, the highest per cent of any nation, were for the good of society.

In all, women answered in terms of needs and responsibilities at about the same rates as men (49% vs. 47%). This gives little support to the Gilligan hypothesis that women are more likely than men to structure their moral reasoning in these terms. There were some significant gender differences in reasoning on four of the 14 clinical cases, however. These were 1) confidentiality of an HD patient versus duties to relatives at risk; 2) confidentiality of a hemophilia A patient versus duties to relatives at risk; 3) disclosure which parent carries a balanced translocation; and 4) presenting reproductive options to male carriers of disorders not diagnosable prenatally. In the first two cases, men were more likely to phrase their answers in terms of patients' rights of non-interference or doctors' obligations, while women were more likely to phrase their answers in terms of patients' rights of entitlement or doctors' responsibilities. In the third case, men preferred rights of noninterfer-

**Table 1.35.** Ethical Relationships in 14 Clinical Cases

| Country* | % Responses per Relationship | | | | | | | Non-moral Answers |
|---|---|---|---|---|---|---|---|---|
| | Rights of Noninter-ference | Rights of Entitlement | Obligations | (Total Rights and Obligations) | Needs | Responsi-bilities | (Total Needs and Responsi-bilities) | |
| Australia | 15 | 17 | 18 | (50) | 31 | 13 | (44) | 4 |
| Brazil | 10 | 17 | 13 | (40) | 40 | 17 | (57) | 4 |
| Canada | 14 | 11 | 24 | (49) | 31 | 13 | (44) | 4 |
| Denmark | 8 | 11 | 21 | (40) | 42 | 15 | (57) | 3 |
| Federal Republic of Germany | 17 | 13 | 14 | (44) | 31 | 20 | (51) | 5 |
| France | 12 | 3 | 19 | (34) | 35 | 27 | (62) | 2 |
| Greece** | 15 | 8 | 13 | (36) | 40 | 15 | (55) | 4 |
| Hungary | 10 | 5 | 11 | (26) | 37 | 31 | (68) | 3 |
| India** | 11 | 7 | 11 | (29) | 33 | 31 | (64) | 3 |
| Israel | 13 | 15 | 14 | (42) | 37 | 13 | (50) | 6 |
| Italy | 17 | 13 | 21 | (51) | 31 | 14 | (45) | 2 |
| Japan | 19 | 11 | 17 | (47) | 25 | 20 | (45) | 7 |
| Norway | 13 | 8 | 18 | (39) | 34 | 24 | (58) | 3 |
| Sweden | 18 | 16 | 14 | (48) | 32 | 16 | (48) | 4 |
| Switzerland | 12 | 7 | 20 | (39) | 40 | 15 | (55) | 6 |
| Turkey | 19 | 12 | 23 | (54) | 19 | 24 | (43) | 3 |
| United Kingdom | 15 | 11 | 19 | (45) | 35 | 12 | (47) | 6 |
| United States | 16 | 11 | 22 | (49) | 31 | 13 | (44) | 5 |
| Total*** | 15 | 11 | 19 | (45) | 32 | 16 | (48) | 5 |
| Total, Excluding U.S. | 15 | 12 | 17 | (44) | 33 | 18 | (51) | 4 |

Standard measures of association, such as chi-square, not applicable because of repeated measurements per respondent.
Per cents based on responses, not respondents.
* Data for German Democratic Republic not available
** 4% in Greece and in India listed good of society.
*** Totals are less than 100% because 0.7% were deserts, 0.5% good of society, 0.4% good of health care system, and 0.1% compromise.

72

**Table 1.36.** Ethical Relationships in Screening and Access Questions

| Country* | % Responses per Relationship | | | | | | | | |
|---|---|---|---|---|---|---|---|---|---|
| | Rights of Noninterference | Rights of Entitlement | (Total Rights) | Needs | Responsibilities | (Total Needs and Responsibilities) | Good of Society | Good of Health Care System | Non-moral Answers |
| Australia | 23 | 11 | (34) | 12 | 19 | (31) | 20 | 8 | 3 |
| Brazil | 26 | 13 | (39) | 11 | 19 | (30) | 20 | 5 | 5 |
| Canada | 33 | 7 | (40) | 10 | 23 | (33) | 15 | 5 | 6 |
| Denmark | 33 | 7 | (40) | 15 | 22 | (37) | 13 | 3 | 5 |
| Federal Republic of Germany | 22 | 5 | (27) | 13 | 37 | (50) | 17 | 1 | 4 |
| France | 27 | 6 | (33) | 6 | 19 | (25) | 26 | 7 | 2 |
| Greece | 24 | 11 | (35) | 11 | 19 | (30) | 20 | 4 | 4 |
| Hungary | 22 | 8 | (30) | 16 | 20 | (36) | 28 | 3 | 1 |
| India | 14 | 8 | (22) | 14 | 25 | (39) | 29 | 5 | 4 |
| Israel | 31 | 4 | (35) | 14 | 25 | (39) | 18 | 4 | 3 |
| Italy | 24 | 11 | (35) | 11 | 20 | (31) | 20 | 5 | 5 |
| Japan | 28 | 9 | (37) | 12 | 19 | (31) | 18 | 2 | 9 |
| Norway | 25 | 8 | (33) | 12 | 43 | (55) | 10 | 0 | 0 |
| Sweden | 37 | 8 | (45) | 10 | 24 | (34) | 14 | 1 | 5 |
| Switzerland | 31 | 5 | (36) | 12 | 32 | (44) | 11 | 2 | 7 |
| Turkey | 18 | 11 | (29) | 4 | 15 | (19) | 42 | 3 | 6 |
| United Kingdom | 31 | 10 | (41) | 11 | 16 | (27) | 19 | 7 | 6 |
| United States | 33 | 11 | (44) | 14 | 17 | (31) | 14 | 6 | 4 |
| Total** | 29 | 9 | (38) | 13 | 21 | (34) | 17 | 5 | 4 |
| Total Excluding U.S. | 27 | 8 | (35) | 12 | 23 | (35) | 19 | 4 | 5 |

Standard measures of association such as chi-square are not applicable because of repeated measurements per respondent.
All per cents are based on responses, not respondents.
* Data for German Democratic Republic not available.
** Totals are less than 100 because 2.4% were obligations and 0.2% deserts.

73

ence while women preferred needs. In the fourth case, men preferred obligations while women preferred needs. The first three cases all involved potential conflicts among family members, to a greater degree than most other cases in the study. It is appropriate that if women's and men's moral reasoning is to differ, it should be in regard to these cases. The responses to the four cases where there were significant gender differences lend support to Gilligan's hypothesis that, at least in some cases of family conflict, men think in terms of rights-obligations, while women think in terms of needs-responsibilities.

Ethical relationships in the screening and access questions are summarized in Table 1.36. Here rights outweighed needs and responsibilities. Rights of noninterference accounted for 29% of the responses, ranging from 37% in Sweden down to 14% in India. Rights of entitlement accounted for 9% of responses. Together, rights of noninterference and entitlement totaled 38% of responses, ranging from 45% in Sweden down to 22% in India.

Responsibilities accounted for 21% of responses, ranging from 43% in Norway down to 15% in Turkey. Needs accounted for a total of 13% of responses, ranging from 16% in Hungary down to 4% in Turkey. Together, needs and responsibilities accounted for 34% of responses, just behind 38% for rights. It is appropriate that rights, especially rights of noninterference, should have first place when the bulk of the screening questions involved third party access to patients' test results.

**Table 1.37.** Perception of Consequences of Actions

| Country* | % Responses Describing Consequences |
|---|---|
| Australia | 38 |
| Brazil | 41 |
| Canada | 43 |
| Denmark | 37 |
| Federal Republic of Germany | 37 |
| France | 55 |
| Greece | 45 |
| Hungary | 53 |
| India | 51 |
| Israel | 42 |
| Italy | 43 |
| Japan | 29 |
| Norway | 83 |
| Sweden | 33 |
| Switzerland | 55 |
| Turkey | 31 |
| United Kingdom | 37 |
| United States | 36 |
| Total | 39 |
| Total, Excluding U.S. | 41 |

Per cents based on responses. First and second reasons given in 14 clinical cases and 2 screening questions. Standard measures of association, such as chi-square, not applicable because of repeated measurements per respondent.
* Data for German Democratic Republic not available.

74

**Table 1.38.** Primacy of Welfare.
% Responses Reporting Welfare Most Important*

| Country | Patient*** | Family Unit or Relatives | Child or Fetus | Geneticist | Society |
|---|---|---|---|---|---|
| Australia | 69 | 19 | 4 | 4 | 3 |
| Brazil | 65 | 18 | 9 | 4 | 3 |
| Canada | 71 | 15 | 6 | 4 | 4 |
| Denmark | 67 | 23 | 3 | 4 | 2 |
| Federal Republic of Germany | 68 | 17 | 10 | 3 | 1 |
| France | 54 | 18 | 10 | 8 | 5 |
| Greece | 64 | 18 | 4 | 5 | 9 |
| Hungary | 57 | 15 | 15 | 3 | 4 |
| India | 63 | 15 | 8 | 3 | 9 |
| Israel | 73 | 16 | 4 | 4 | 2 |
| Italy | 69 | 15 | 4 | 2 | 5 |
| Japan | 64 | 13 | 12 | 5 | 3 |
| Norway | 64 | 18 | 9 | 3 | 5 |
| Sweden | 78 | 14 | 4 | 3 | 2 |
| Switzerland | 74 | 18 | 8 | 0 | 0 |
| Turkey+ | 67 | 12 | 7 | 7 | 2 |
| United Kingdom | 78 | 13 | 3 | 3 | 2 |
| United States | 77 | 14 | 5 | 3 | 2 |
| Total | 72 | 15 | 6 | 3 | 3 |
| Total, Excluding U.S. | 68 | 11 | 8 | 4 | 4 |

* Per cents total <100, because 1% saw welfare of "future generations" as most important, and 0.3% the welfare of "institutional third parties."
** Data for German Democratic Republic not available.
*** "Patient" means "parents" if a child or fetus is diagnosed.
+ 5% in Turkey listed "future generations".
Per cents based on responses. Standard measures of association, such as chi-square, not applicable because of repeated measurements per respondent.

The good of society accounted for 17% of responses, ranging from 42% in Turkey down to 10% in Norway. It is appropriate that the good of society be invoked more frequently in screening questions than in clinical cases. In all, 5% of responses involved the good of the health care system and 4% were nonmoral answers. In addition, 2.4% involved obligations, mostly in Australia, Federal Republic of Germany, France, Greece, Hungary, Italy, Japan, and the United States. Only 0.2% involved deserts.

Overall, men's and women's responses were similar. The only area of gender difference was in regard to regulations for commercial laboratories, where men were more likely to give nonmoral answers and women were more likely to respond in terms of the good of society.

**Table 1.39.** Perceptions of Conflict in Clinical and Screening Situations*

| Country*** | No Conflict | Client-Family Conflict | Client-Geneticist Conflict | Parent-Child (or Fetus) Conflict | Individual-Society Conflict |
|---|---|---|---|---|---|
| Australia | 71 | 14 | 5 | 4 | 3 |
| Brazil | 79 | 7 | 6 | 5 | 1 |
| Canada | 67 | 14 | 7 | 5 | 3 |
| Denmark | 78 | 10 | 6 | 1 | 1 |
| Federal Republic of Germany | 72 | 12 | 9 | 3 | 1 |
| France | 73 | 9 | 11 | 3 | 1 |
| Greece | 75 | 8 | 7 | 6 | 4 |
| Hungary | 72 | 10 | 6 | 10 | 2 |
| India | 68 | 12 | 8 | 9 | 3 |
| Israel | 76 | 8 | 7 | 3 | 3 |
| Italy | 74 | 12 | 5 | 2 | 4 |
| Japan | 69 | 10 | 10 | 7 | 3 |
| Norway | 51 | 13 | 9 | 7 | 9 |
| Sweden | 80 | 9 | 7 | 2 | 0 |
| Switzerland | 74 | 8 | 9 | 4 | 1 |
| Turkey | 83 | 5 | 9 | 3 | 0 |
| United Kingdom | 70 | 12 | 7 | 4 | 3 |
| United States | 76 | 9 | 7 | 2 | 2 |
| Total** | 74 | 10 | 7 | 4 | 2 |
| Total, Excluding U.S. | 72 | 11 | 8 | 5 | 2 |

Standard measures of association, such as chi-square, not applicable because of repeated measurements per respondent.
* Totaled for 14 clinical cases and 2 screening questions.
** Per cents total < 100, because 1.7% reported worker-employer conflict, and 1.3% reported conflict between two moral principles.
*** Data for German Democratic Republic not available.

## 1.7.4 Other Aspects of Moral Reasoning

Table 1.37 lists the per cents of responses describing specific consequences of actions. In all, 39% of responses mentioned consequences, ranging from 83% in Norway to 29% in Japan.

Table 1.38 describes the per cents of responses attributing primacy to the welfare of different parties. The welfare of the patient (or the parents if a child was diagnosed) came first in 72% of responses, followed by family unit or relatives in 15%, child or fetus in 6%, geneticist in 3%, and society in 3%. Again, there was considerable variation. Responses putting the patient's welfare first ranged from 54% in France to 78% in Sweden and the United Kingdom and responses placing the child's welfare first ranged from 3% in Denmark and the United Kingdom to 15% in Hungary. In all, however, few (6%) put the welfare of child or fetus first.

Table 1.39 lists the per cents of responses reporting conflicts of interest between different parties. In all, 74% mentioned no conflicts, 10% mentioned conflict between client and relatives, 7% conflict between client and geneticist, 4% conflict between parent and child or fetus, and 2% conflict between individual and society.

## 1.8 Conclusion

We did not find the degree of international consensus that we originally anticipated. There was more variation than consensus about the 14 clinical cases. What conclusions can be drawn?

First, cultural differences in ethics still seem substantial. This finding tends to refute the view that the diffusion of technology carries a Western cultural tradition that resolves ethical disputes in the name of patient autonomy.

Second, some findings were a surprise. Despite the controversies about new reproductive options, most respondents were willing to discuss donor egg and surrogate mothering in a non-directive context. Most will do prenatal diagnosis for maternal anxiety alone, except in some nations that ration prenatal diagnosis through national health insurance. Finally, in some nations we found substantial minorities willing to perform prenatal diagnosis for sex selection unrelated to X-linked disease.

Third, geneticists are almost universally wary of institutional third parties, i.e., insurers and employers, having access to results of genetic screening without the patient's consent. On the other hand, only 10 of 19 nations had strong consensus that genetic screening in the workplace should be voluntary. Obviously, the social and economic structure of each nation will mould ethical views.

Why is there not more consensus about approaches to ethical problems among medical geneticists? Perhaps the reason lies in the recent development of the specialty, which began around 1970. Many respondents had little or no formal instruction in ethics or in formal post-graduate genetics courses in which they might have shared approaches to and standards for such problems. Our respondents probably learned ethics "on the job".

Geneticists' responses suggest that they are not so concerned as the public about such issues as sex selection, genetic screening in the workplace, and long-range eugenic concerns. Certain answers to these theoretical dilemmas would, in practice, gradually alter the sex ratio or birth order in the population, limit access to work, and change society's views about what constitutes a healthy human being. The impact of human genetics on medicine and society can only increase, and will perhaps rekindle concerns about eugenics. If prenatal sex selection unrelated to X-linked disease becomes prevalent, we cannot help but wonder if demands for selection on other non-medical characteristics will follow.

Societal problems tend to sneak up on medicine and catch clinicians unawares. As genetic technology and services become more complex and present more difficult moral dilemmas than in the past, medical geneticists around the world may be drawn together to face these problems. At present, there are impressive cross-cultural differences of opinion.

# References

1. Beauchamp TL, Childress JF (1987) Principles of Biomedical Ethics, 3 rd ed. Oxford University Press, New York
2. Brock JH (1985) Prospective prenatal diagnosis of cystic fibrosis. Lancet i: 1175–1178
3. Brodeur P (1985) Outrageous misconduct: the asbestos industry on trial. Pantheon, New York
4. Czeizel A (1988) The right to be born healthy: The ethical problems of human genetics in Hungary. Alan R Liss, New York
5. Elling RH (1986) Struggle for workers' health. Baywood, Farmingdale, NY, pp 30, 73
6. Englehardt HT (1986) Foundations of Bioethics. Oxford University Press, New York
7. Fletcher JC, Berg K, Tranøy KE (1985) Ethical aspects of medical genetics. Clin Genet 27: 199–205
8. Fletcher JC, Van Eys J, Dorn LD (1989) Ethical considerations in pediatric oncology. In: Pizzo PA, Poplack DG (eds) Principles and practice of pediatric oncology. JB Lippincott, Philadelphia, pp 309–320
9. Fraser FC (1974) Genetic counseling. Am J Hum Genet 26: 636–659
10. Fraser FC and Pressor C (1977) Attitudes of counselors in relation to prenatal sex determination for choice of sex. In: Lubs HA, de la Cruz F (eds) Genetic counseling. Raven, New York, pp 109–120
11. Genetic counseling and the prevention of Huntington's chorea (Editorial, 1982) Lancet i: 147; Perry JL (1981) Some ethical problems in Huntington's chorea. Can Med Assn J 125: 1098
12. Gilligan C (1982) In a different voice: psychological theory and women's development. Harvard University Press, Cambridge, MA and London
13. Hulten M, Needham P, Watt JL, Griffiths M (1987) Preventing feticide. Nature 325: 190
14. McKusick VA (1969) Human genetics. Prentice-Hall, Englewood Cliffs, NJ, p. 181
15. National Foundation-March of Dimes Birth Defects Foundation (1983) International Directory of Genetic Services. National Foundation, White Plains, NY
16. President's Commission for the Study of Ethical Problems in Medicine and Biomedical and Behavioral Research (1983) Genetic screening and counseling. U.S. Government Printing Office, Washington
17. Robach MM and Zeiger RS (1973) The John F. Kennedy Institute Tay-Sachs Program: Practical and ethical issues in an adult genetic screening program. In Hilton B and Callahan D (eds) Ethical issues in human genetics: Genetic counseling and the use of genetic knowledge. Plenum, New York, pp 131–146
18. Sivard RL (1986) World military and social expenditures, 1986. World Priorities, Washington, DC
19. Sorenson JR (1976) From social movement to clinical medicine: the role of law and the medical profession in regulating applied human genetics. In: Milunsky A, Annas GJ (eds) Genetics and the law. Plenum, New York, pp 467–485
20. Sorenson JR, Swazey JP, Scotch NA (1981) Reproductive pasts, reproductive futures: genetic counselling and its effectiveness. Alan R Liss for the March of Dimes-Birth Defects Foundation, New York
21. Stamatoyannopoulos G (1974) Problems of screening and counseling in the hemoglobinopathies. In: Motulsky A and Lenz W (eds) Birth defects: Proceedings of the 4th International Conference, Vienna, 1973. Medica, Amsterdam
22. United States Congress, Office of Technology Assessment (1983) The role of genetic testing in the prevention of occupational disease. U.S. Government Printing Office, Washington, DC pp. 33–61
23. United States Department of Health, Education and Welfare, Public Health Service, National Institutes of Health (1979) Antenatal diagnosis: report of a consensus development conference sponsored by the National Institute of Child Health and Development, assisted by the Office for Medical Applications of Research and the Fogarty International Center, March 5–7, 1979, Bethesda, MD. NIH Publication No. 79-1973, pp I: 201–203
24. Wertz DC, Sorenson JR, Heeren TC (1986) Clients' interpretations of risks provided in genetic counseling. Am J Hum Genet 39: 253–264
25. Wertz DC, Sorenson JR, Heeren TC (1988) Communication in health professional-lay encoun-

ters: How often does each party know what the other wants to discuss? In: Ruben BD (ed), Information and Behavior 2. Transaction Books, New Brunswick, NJ, pp 329–342

26. Whitbeck C (1983) The moral implications of regarding women as people: new perspectives on pregnancy and personhood. In: Bondeson WB, Engelhardt HT, Spicker SF, Winship D (eds), Abortion and the status of the fetus. D. Reidel, Amsterdam

27. Whitbeck C (1987) Fetal imaging and fetal monitoring: finding the ethical issues. Women and Health 13 (1/2): 47–58

28. Zare N, Sorenson JR, Heeren TC (1984) Sex of provider as a variable in effective genetic counseling. Soc Sci Med 19: 671–675

# Preface to Part 2

The nineteen chapters in Part 2 follow a standard outline formulated by the Editors. The outline was given to the co-authors with the invitation to compose their chapters. The choice and ordering of topics was not the responsibility of the authors.

The rationale for a pre-assigned outline for each chapter was based on several reasons. First, we wished to make the information from each nation as inclusive as possible. We wanted each chapter to cover the whole spectrum of social, ethical, and economic problems related to genetic services. In the absence of a formal outline, it is likely that many vital facts and conditions in these nations would have been inadvertently omitted.

Secondly, we hoped that readers would be able to use Part 2 in a systematic and dependable way. An outline provides the means to this end. Readers who wish to scan all nineteen chapters for a particular topic may do so by following the numbered sections in the outline.

Thirdly, we believe that this study is the first international report on the evolution and scope of genetic services in the decade 1975–1985. To achieve uniformity of this empirical task, we felt it necessary to determine, with advice from several experts in medical genetics, how it should be done.

Finally, there are several controversial topics associated with genetic services. These include abortion practices, cost-benefit analyses, social conflicts, and national expenditures for genetic services and health care. We take full responsibility for having invited the discussion of these issues.

The Editors

# Standard Outline for Each Nation (2.1–2.19)

2.1.1    Medical Genetics
2.1.1.1  Scope of the Problem
        Number of Births per year 1975–1985 – Incidence of Genetic Disease – Childhood Mortality and Congenital Malformations
2.1.1.2  Organization of Clinical Genetic Services in _____
        Description of Centers – Services Offered – Number of Postnatal Chromosome Studies – Investigation of Genetic Diseases – Genetic Counseling
2.1.1.3  Prenatal Diagnosis
        Description of Services – Cases by Indication – Policy on Indications
2.1.1.4  Cost-benefit of Early Diagnosis
2.1.1.5  Abortion
        Incidence of Elective Abortion 1975–1985 – Elective Abortion/Live Birth Ratio – Incidence of Abortion After Genetic Diagnosis – Social Abortion/Genetic Abortion Ratio
2.1.2    Ethical Problems
2.1.2.1  Genetic Counseling
2.1.2.2  Prenatal Diagnosis
2.1.2.3  Genetic Screening
2.1.2.4  Other Contexts
2.1.3    Consensus and Variation in _____
2.1.4    Cultural Context of Medical Genetics in _____
2.1.4.1  Sources of Challenge and Support
        Religious – Legal – Political – Parents' Groups – Handicapped Groups – Medical Interest Groups
2.1.4.2  Major Controversies
2.1.4.3  National Expenditures for Medical Genetics
2.1.4.4  Abortion Laws
        Applications to Genetic Indications – Social and Policy Conflicts
2.1.4.5  Studies of Effectiveness of Genetic Services
        Acceptability of Services Among Parents
2.1.4.6  Need for New Laws
2.1.5    Ethical Issues and Future Trends

## 2.1 Ethics and Medical Genetics in Australia

J. G. Rogers and A. M. Taylor

## 2.1.1 The Scope of the Problem

In Australia the number of births per year from 1975–1984 has been relatively stable at approximately 230,000 per year (Table 2.1.1). The figures in Table 2.1.1, which show the childhood mortality rates for the first 12 months of life for the last 10 years, indicate a decline of almost 50% during this period. Whilst the *number* of deaths due to malformation has remained fairly constant, the *proportion* of deaths due to malformation has increased, as other causes of mortality in the first year of life have been reduced. It can be concluded, therefore, that current technology has had minimal impact on the death rate from congenital abnormalities.

Data collection on the incidence of malformations was commenced in 1981, when the National Perinatal Statistic Unit was established under the direction of Dr. Paul Lancaster. Available data showing the incidence of combined and specific malformations and specific disorders are presented in Table 2.1.2. The incidence of major malformations has averaged 1.44% over the last 3 years. This is an underestimate, due to underreporting and late recognition of significant problems, as the data were derived from perinatal data forms, death certificates, autopsy reports, and hospital-generated statistics.

The incidence of some specific malformations is shown in Table 2.1.2 and does not appear to have fluctuated significantly over the last 3 years. The incidence of congenital heart disease is markedly underreported. The incidence of neural tube defects is approximately 0.15%. This figure is lower than that obtained in other surveys (Danks and Halliday 1983; Field 1978) and may reflect either a changing incidence or the impact of prenatal diagnosis.

Table 2.1.2 also includes data generated by Pitt [1962] in a survey of 22,364 births in a major university obstetric hospital. The overall incidence of malformations and clefts is very comparable to the data from the National Perinatal Statistic Unit. Pitt felt that the incidence of congenital heart disease and chromosome disorders were underestimates. Drew [1977], some 15 years later, prospectively studied 10,454 consecutively-born infants in another obstetric hospital that has a special interest in high-risk pregnancies. He found a much higher overall frequency of congenital heart disorders. This is in part explained by the incidence of *patent ductus arteriosus*, but also highlights the underreporting in the other figures presented and the effects of high-risk pregnancies. The frequency of clefts is much higher and reflects the nature of the population sampled.

Table 2.1.3 shows the incidence of a number of birth defects in Australia. The data on PKU, galactosemia (Pitt 1983) and hypothyroidism (personal communication, J. Connelly) were derived from Australian screening programs. The inci-

**Table 2.1.1.** Live Births, Mortality in First Year and Mortality Due to Congenital Malformations, 1975-1984

| Year | Total Live Births | Infant Mortality in First Year | Percentage Due to Congenital Malformations % |
|------|-------------------|-------------------------------|-----------------------------------------------|
| 1975 | 235,426 | 4,744 | 17 |
| 1976 | 227,810 | 4,654 | 20 |
| 1977 | 228,421 | 4,096 | 20 |
| 1978 | 226,301 | 3,954 | 20 |
| 1979 | 233,129 | 2,534 | 28 |
| 1980 | 255,527 | 2,417 | 27 |
| 1981 | 235,842 | 2,482 | 30 |
| 1982 | 238,684 | 2,327 | 30 |
| 1983 | 241,030 | 2,163 | 31 |
| 1984 | 232,425 | 2,452 | 29 |

Data derived from: Congenital Malformations Australia, 1981-1984, National Perinatal Statistic Unit.
Livebirths Australia: Australian Bureau of Statistics, 1975-1984
Causes of Death Australia: Australian Bureau of Statistics, 1975-1984

**Table 2.1.2.** Incidence of Combined and Specific Congenital Malformations (per 10,000 births)

|          | Combined Congenital Malformations | Neural tube Defects | Congenital Heart Disease | Clefts | Chromosomal |
|----------|-----------------------------------|---------------------|--------------------------|--------|-------------|
| 1982[1]  | 146.8 | 15.4 | 38.3 | 14.8 | 16.3 |
| 1983[1]  | 146.9 | 15.4 | 40.2 | 13.9 | 16.4 |
| 1984[1]  | 140.0 | 12.6 | 37.4 | 15.7 | 16.7 |
| 1962[2]  | 151.0 | 16.6 | 21.0 | 16.5 | 9.8 |
| 1977[3]  | 410.0 |      | 97.6 | 25.8 |      |

[1] Source: Congenital Malformations, Australia 1981-1984
[2] Pitt 1962
[3] Drew et al. 1977

**Table 2.1.3.** Estimates of Incidence of Birth Defects in Australia

| Condition | Incidence | Source |
|-----------|-----------|--------|
| Primary Hypothyroidism | 1/4158 | Connelly, personal communication |
| PKU | 0.83/10,000 | Pitt et al. 1983 |
| Galactosemia | 0.45/10,000 | Pitt et al. 1983 |
| Cystic Fibrosis | 1/2556 | Allan et al. 1980 |
| Achondroplasia | 1/26,000 | Oberklaid et al. 1979 |
| All chromosome abnormalities | 1.85/1000 | Bell et al. 1986 |
| Down syndrome | 1.25/1000 | Bell et al. 1986 |
| Spina bifida | 0.99/1000 | Danks and Halliday 1983 |
| Anencephaly | 0.88/1000 | Danks and Halliday 1983 |

dences of neural tube defects (Danks and Halliday 1983), achondroplasia (Ober-klaid et al. 1979) and cystic fibrosis (Allan et al. 1980) were derived from surveys undertaken in Victoria. The incidence of chromosomal abnormalities was derived from Queensland data (Bell et al. 1986).

## 2.1.1.2 Organisation of Clinical Genetic Services

The establishment of genetic services in Australia has been relatively recent and the Government has been slow to recognise community needs. Until recently all medical geneticists needed to go overseas for their training. The organisation of services, sites, and personnel is described in Table 2.1.4 by state. Genetic services are organised on a state-by-state basis, with the exception of Tasmania, which is serviced from Victoria, the Australian Capital Territory, which is serviced from

**Table 2.1.4.** Organisation of Clinical Genetics Services

|  | Queensland | South Australia[1] | Victoria[2] | West Australia | New South Wales[3] |
|---|---|---|---|---|---|
| Qualified Geneticists | 1 | 1 | 4 | 1 | 4 |
| Assistants | 2 | 2 | 3 | 4 | 7 |
| Counselling Clinics per week | 6 | 5.5 | 7[4] | 6 | 3 |
| Clinic Sites | 2 | 5 | 7[5] | 3 | 8 |
| Population (Millions) | 2.6 | 1.4 | 4.2 | 1.4 | 5.6 |

[1] Provides services to Northern Territory
[2] Provides services to Tasmania
[3] Provides services to Australian Capital Territory
[4] Excludes 16 sessions in Tasmania
[5] Includes 4 sites in Tasmania

Sources: Population, Australian Demographic Statistics. Australian Bureau of Statistics, 1986. Personal Communications, Hockey A, Pearn J, Haan E, Sillence D.

**Table 2.1.5.** Chromosome Studies, Victoria, 1977–1986

|  | Blood | Amniotic Fluid | Fibroblast |
|---|---|---|---|
| 1977 | 1,638 | 368 | 71 |
| 1978 | 1,895 | 490 | 73 |
| 1979 | 1,710 | 619 | 77 |
| 1980 | 1,800 | 713 | 66 |
| 1981 | 1,677 | 844 | 180 |
| 1982 | 1,733 | 988 | 209 |
| 1983 | 1,610 | 1,206 | 182 |
| 1984 | 1,897 | 1,402 | 183 |
| 1985 | 2,106 | 1,463 | 243 |
| 1986 | 2,162 | 1,741 | 255 |

Source: Personal Communications, D. Fortune, B. Susil, M. Leversha

New South Wales, and the Northern Territory, which is serviced from South Australia. The number of qualified geneticists is low, and geneticists are assisted by doctors-in-training and other physicians. In all states, clinics are conducted at several different sites, usually general and maternity teaching hospitals. There are several clinics conducted each week.

Table 2.1.5 shows the number of postnatal chromosome studies done in Victoria for the last 10 years. The numbers do not reflect the increasing workload in recent years associated with studies for the fragile X chromosome. The figures for blood chromosome analysis show considerable fluctuation and have increased in recent years as new chromosomal disorders are identified. Amniotic fluid studies have shown a steady increase with increasing utilisation of prenatal diagnosis (Bell et al. 1985). There has been an increase in utilisation for maternal age in recent years, as is reflected in Table 2.1.5. This is in part due to reducing the age at which the test is available and also increased utilisation (Bell 1985). Studies for maternal age in Victoria are still limited to women 37 years and over at the time of birth of their child. There has been a steady increase in the utilisation of fibroblast cultures, which relates to the more intensive study of stillborn infants.

Approximately 2000 samples per year are submitted in Victoria for metabolic screening. Virtually all newborn babies in Australia have a Guthrie test for PKU and hypothyroidism. In Victoria, approximately 800 patients or families are seen each year in a medical genetics clinic. Most of the counselling associated with antenatal diagnosis is undertaken by the obstetricians concerned. Specific disorders such as spina bifida, cystic fibrosis and muscular dystrophy are counselled by the specialists concerned with their care. Joint clinics have been established for genetic ophthalmology and genetic dermatology.

## 2.1.1.3 Prenatal Diagnosis

Genetic services for prenatal diagnosis are offered in all states of Australia. In most states, prenatal diagnosis can either be obtained in the public sector via government-funded hospitals, or in the private sector. There has been a strong move to have amniocentesis performed by a small number of highly-experienced operators, and this has been achieved in most states. In Victoria, many patients are referred directly to obstetricians who specialise in antenatal diagnosis and only a small proportion of the patients are seen by a medical geneticist. The antenatal diagnostic services are based in obstetric teaching hospitals. Services such as fetoscopy and fetal blood sampling are undertaken only in Victoria and New South Wales. Most cytogenetics laboratories are based within the major teaching hospitals, although private laboratories operate in Queensland.

Unfortunately data are not available on an Australia-wide basis and data presented in Table 2.1.6 are for Victoria and Tasmania. This shows the total number of tests done from 1976–1985, according to indications. A total of 8,228 women out of a total of 670,196 who have had liveborn or stillborn infants have utilised prenatal diagnostic services. This table indicates the number of expected abnormalities, such as Down syndrome in advanced maternal age, and unexpected abnormalities, such as neural tube defects in advanced maternal age. The total number of terminations for each category is shown.

The policy on indications for prenatal diagnosis is made on a state-by-state basis. Some states allow amniocentesis for all women 35 and over, whilst other states allow it only for women 37 and over, due to limited availability of resources. The initial policy in Victoria and New South Wales was to allow amniocentesis only for women 40 and over. With increasing availability of facilities, this age limit has been lowered. The policy is to lower the age limit even further in Victoria, to 35, when facilities become available. Most states would only undertake amniocentesis for women who accept termination of pregnancy following a positive diagnosis of genetic disorder.

Australia has attempted to centralise testing for lysosomal enzyme disorders. These tests are undertaken in the laboratory of Dr. Tony Pollard at the Adelaide Children's Hospital. Some testing for inborn errors of metabolism is undertaken in the Murdoch Research Institute in Melbourne. A number of laboratories currently undertake intrauterine diagnosis of thalassaemia by globin chain synthesis. Laboratories for DNA diagnostic studies are currently under development in a number of centres.

Amniocentesis is readily available in Australia for maternal age, neural tube defects, previous chromosomal disorders, inborn errors of metabolism, haemoglobinopathies and haemophilia. DNA techniques are being developed or are available for haemoglobinopathies, haemophilia, Huntington disease, adult polycystic kidney disease, Duchenne muscular dystrophy, myotonic dystrophy and alpha-1-antitrypsin deficiency. Samples are sent to other centres in the world for specific indications. Diagnostic samples are also received by laboratories in Australia from other countries.

## 2.1.1.4  Cost-Benefit of Early Diagnosis

No formal analysis of the cost-benefits of counselling is available for Australia. Table 2.1.6 shows the number of terminations performed on the basis of intrauterine diagnosis in Victoria and Tasmania. This shows an overall incidence of expected abnormalities of 3.2%. The vast majority of patients elected to terminate babies who were found to have major abnormalities. Estimates prepared by Jane Halliday and David Danks (personal communication), suggest that in Victoria 40% of women 37–39 years and 50% of women 40 years and over present for testing. Halliday and Danks estimate that this would lead to the detection of approximately 9 Down syndrome children at a cost of U.S.$24,850 per child. This is approximately one-twelfth of the lifetime cost of care, which has been estimated at U.S.$189,000 per affected child. The same group, in looking at spina bifida, estimated the cost of detecting one spina bifida child to be U.S.$9,450 which is one-seventeenth of the cost of care of an affected child for 20 years, estimated at U.S.$165,550. These figures are comparable with Hayes and Hayes' [1982] estimate of the cost of intrauterine diagnosis at one-twelfth of the cost of maintaining an affected child in an institution for 10 years (conversion rate A$1 = U.S.$0.70).

**Table 2.1.6.** Prenatal Diagnosis (Victoria and Tasmania) 1976-1985[1]

| Indication | Number of Tests done | Expected Abnormalities (%)[2] | Unexpected Abnormalities | Total Termina-tions |
|---|---|---|---|---|
| Maternal age | | | | |
| 35–36 | 753 | 4 (0.5%) | 1 | |
| 37–39 | 3,008 | 43 (1.4%) | 15 | |
| 40+ | 1,582 | 43 (2.7%) | 3 | |
| | 5,343 | 100 (1.9%) | 19 | 97 |
| Previous neural tube defect | 1,201 | 21 (1.7%) | 9 | 24 |
| Previous chromosome anomaly | 625 | 5 (0.8%) | – | 4 |
| Parental translocation carrier | 101 | 11 (10.9%) | – | 11 |
| X–linked disorders | 73 | 21 (28.8%) | 1 | 13 |
| Thalassaemia | 133 | 38 (28.6%) | 1 | 36 |
| Metabolic disorders | 103 | 23 (22.3%) | 1 | 23 |
| Anxiety | 249 | – | 3 | 3 |
| Other(inside guidelines) | 290 | 2 | – | 2 |
| Sonar abnormalities | 110 | 62 | – | 58 |
| Total | 8,228 | 268 (3.2%) | 35 | 271 (3.3%) |

Total pregnancies (livebirths and stillbirths) for Victoria and Tasmania 1976-1985: 670, 196
Source: Perinatal Deaths, Australia. Australian Bureau of Statistics.
[1] Data provided by Jane Halliday, Murdoch Institute
[2] Expected abnormalities are the type of abnormality being sought on the basis of indications.


## 2.1.1.5 Abortion

Table 2.1.6 shows the total number of abortions undertaken when major defects were detected by prenatal diagnosis in Victoria from 1976-1985.

Table 2.1.7 shows the reported incidence of elective abortion and the abortion/pregnancy ratio for South Australia from 1975-1984. It indicates an increase in the incidence of abortion from 0.13 in 1975 to 0.17 in 1979, where it has remained up to 1984.

Table 2.1.8 gives a breakdown of terminations by indication in South Australia. The extraordinarily high percentage of abortions for mental disorder (96%) is a result of the abortion law in Australia, which permits that abortions be performed

**Table 2.1.7.** Abortion/Livebirth Ratio in South Australia 1975–1984

| Year | Abortions | Abortion Rate* | Registered Livebirths | Abortion Ratio++ |
|---|---|---|---|---|
| 1975 | 2,996 | 11.3 | 19,986 | 0.13 |
| 1976 | 3,289 | 12.0 | 18,947 | 0.15 |
| 1977 | 3,499 | 12.6 | 19,260 | 0.15 |
| 1978 | 3,793 | 13.4 | 18,558 | 0.17 |
| 1979 | 3,880 | 13.5 | 18,413 | 0.17 |
| 1980 | 4,081 | 14.0 | 18,430 | 0.18 |
| 1981 | 4,095 | 13.8 | 19,271 | 0.17 |
| 1982 | 4,047 | 13.5 | 19,199 | 0.17 |
| 1983 | 4,033 | 13.3 | 19,830 | 0.17 |
| 1984 | 4,091 | 12.2 | 20,052 | 0.17 |

* Rate per 1000 for women 15–44 (excludes abortions in women under 15 and over 44 but includes abortions to women of unknown age)
++ Abortions divided by (abortions + livebirths)
Source: Hart G, Medical Termination of Pregnancy in South Australia, 1970–1984, Technical Report number 1, Pregnancy Outcome Unit, South Australian Health Commission.

**Table 2.1.8.** Indications for Abortion, South Australia

| Diagnosis | 1975–1979 | | 1980–1984 | |
|---|---|---|---|---|
| | No | % | No | % |
| Mental disorder (290–319) | 16,795 | 96.3 | 19,159 | 94.2 |
| Obstetric conditions (630–676) | 142 | 0.3 | 11 | 0.1 |
| Anencephaly (740) | 4 | – | 34 | 0.2 |
| Other brain/spinal anomalies (741,742) | 3 | – | 28 | 0.1 |
| Other congenital anomalies (743–759) | 231 | 1.3 | 147 | 0.7 |
| Rubella exposure (647.5) | 68 | 0.4 | 28 | 0.1 |
| Other perinatal conditions (760–779) | 41 | 0.2 | 10 | 0.1 |
| Other conditions | 162 | 0.9 | 920 | 4.5 |
| Total | 17,446 | 100.0 | 20,337 | 100.0 |

Source: Hart G, Medical Termination of Pregnancy in South Australia, 1970–1984

*only if* the physical or *mental* welfare of the mother is endangered. This has been liberally interpreted by medical practitioners. Approximately 1% of the reported terminations in South Australia, 1980–1984, were for birth defects.

## 2.1.2 Ethical Problems Faced by Medical Geneticists in Australia

Of the 14 geneticists practising in Australia, 12 replied to the questionnaire. Whilst the response rate was high, it is difficult to draw firm conclusions from such a small sample. From the responses, there appears to be a reasonably strong consensus concerning such issues as patient autonomy, confidentiality of genetic data, intrauterine diagnosis, genetic screening, and the right to abortion and contraception. In the day-to-day practise of genetic counselling, ethical problems do not at present appear to play a major role. The apparent lack of explicit ethical problems confronted in the course of practical counselling in Australia may in part relate to the relatively low frequency of occurrence of situations such as those presented in the questionnaire and also the relatively small community of genetic counsellors.

## 2.1.3 Consensus and Variation on Approaches to Ethical Problems in Australia: Responses to the Questionnaire

### Confidentiality vs. Duties to Third Parties

There was strong consensus that information about affected individuals with Huntington disease and haemophilia A should be given to relatives if they ask, even without the patient's consent. Australia differed from other Anglo-Saxon countries, such as the United Kingdom, Canada, and the United States, where there was no consensus on duties to third parties. Australian geneticists appear to believe that the obligation to respect the individual's autonomy can be overridden by their obligation to avoid the harm that may come from not informing relatives.

Australian geneticists would appear to have a primary commitment to the presenting client, rather than to the family or community. Confidentiality would be overridden only when a relative presents for counselling.

There was strong consensus, as there was in all countries, about protecting the mother's confidentiality in the disclosure of paternity. The principle operating here is presumably that nondisclosure would cause less harm to the husband than it would to the third parties in the two previous cases.

### Full Disclosure

There was strong consensus amongst Australian geneticists, as there was in most other countries, about full disclosure of ambiguous, uncertain or conflicting laboratory results. This is consistent with a non-directive approach to counselling. Fewer Australian geneticists (50%) said that they would disclose disagreement between colleagues than in the United States and Canada, where there was strong ($\geq 75\%$) or moderate (67–74%) consensus about disclosing disagreement. This may relate to the likelihood of medico-legal action in North America.

There was moderate consensus (67%), compared with no consensus in the other Anglo-Saxon countries, about disclosing which parent carried the balanced translocation. Four would only disclose information to parents with their consent, indicating recognition of the possible conflict between truth-telling (autonomy) and causing unnecessary harm. Two would override patient confidentiality and tell relatives even without consent. It is interesting to speculate why there was not wider agreement on duties to third parties in this case, as there was in the case of Huntington disease and haemophilia A.

This lack of agreement is a surprising result. Disclosure may temporarily disturb a family's equilibrium. A well-trained counsellor, however, would be able to handle the emotions that arise. In addition, there are important counselling implications, such as the variable risk, dependent on which parent carries the translocation, and the use of A.I.D. or IVF with a donor egg, which cannot logically be discussed without disclosure. Chromosome studies on other family members should be strongly encouraged for the appropriate relatives of a translocation carrier. This cannot be done without identifying the carrier.

There was no consensus about disclosing XY genotype in a female in Australia, nor in the UK and USA. Seven would disclose the information and five would give other reasons for the infertility. If full disclosure is equivalent to truth-telling and is supported by the principle of autonomy, then for Australian geneticists, autonomy was constrained by considerations of avoiding harm to the individuals concerned.

### Directive/Non-directive Counselling
Australian geneticists clearly favoured a non-directive approach to counselling, both in terms of their responses to moral dilemmas and preferred approaches. This applied to decisions about fetuses with a possible neural tube defect, with Turner syndrome, or with XYY genotype, and in general to discussing options available to both male and female carriers of tuberous sclerosis. For fetuses with XO or XYY genotype, three and two geneticists respectively would try to counsel so as to avoid termination. Somewhat disturbingly, it appears that not all geneticists would describe fully the risks and problems associated with each of the options.

There were some interesting qualifications to the non-directive approach. There was no consensus on counselling for carriers of tuberous sclerosis about taking their chances, with five out of 12 and four out of 11 respectively either avoiding discussion or advising against this option. There was no consensus on counselling about surrogate motherhood, with six (46%) avoiding discussion of this option. This may indicate the sensitivity that exists about this issue in Australia, where it has been a matter of considerable controversy.

### Indications for Prenatal Diagnosis
There was strong consensus, as in ten other countries, that if a family with a Down syndrome child requested prenatal diagnosis it should be performed, even if the parents opposed abortion. There was strong consensus (83%) that prenatal diagnosis should not be performed for sex selection.

In general, geneticists were agreed that one of the important goals for genetic counsellors was lessening patients' guilt and anxiety. However, they would not pursue this goal in an unqualified way. According to the data, there was no consensus that prenatal diagnosis should be performed for maternal anxiety alone. Six (50%) would perform the procedure. Four would refuse, with or without discussion, and two would refer the patient to someone else. Limited resources do not seem sufficient to explain this reservation, because five (42%) believed that regulations should prohibit commercial laboratories from performing prenatal diagnosis for this purpose. As with other medical investigations, geneticists felt that prenatal diagnosis should be performed only for specific indications.

90

## Screening

There was strong consensus in Australia (92%) and strong ($\geq 75\%$) to moderate (67–74%) consensus in 11 other countries that screening should be voluntary. Australian geneticists, like geneticists in all other countries, agreed that the individual should have access to the results of screening. Australian geneticists also agreed that employers and insurance companies should not have access to results without the individual's consent. There was moderate consensus (67%) that the worker's doctor and the Health Department should not have access to results of screening without consent. Four out of twelve geneticists felt that the Health Department and worker's doctor *should* have automatic access.

There was moderate consensus (67%) that relatives should not have access to results of presymptomatic tests for Huntington disease without patient consent. Four geneticists felt that relatives should have access irrespective of the patient's wishes. These reservations may reflect perceived conflict between the interests of the individual and those of third parties and/or the wider community. It is interesting to compare this response with the case of diagnosed Huntington disease, where there was strong consensus in favour of revealing information to relatives without patient consent. If a presymptomatic test is 99% accurate, relatives need only the results of their own screening tests, without disclosure of the results of other family members. Thus confidentiality need not be overridden.

There was no consensus in Australia, nor in 15 other countries, about the best age to begin carrier screening for cystic fibrosis, though 59% preferred newborns, with parental permission.

## Problems Causing Greatest and Least Conflict

Disclosing the results of a positive diagnosis of Huntington disease to relatives at risk caused the greatest conflict for Australian geneticists. This case was selected by four out of 12. The second-greatest conflict, selected by three out of 12, concerned the use of prenatal diagnosis for sex selection. The main reason offered was the conflict between responsibilities to different parties. Other reasons offered were the high risk of harm whatever you do and there being no clear course of action leading to the best outcome.

Geneticists reported the least conflict about disclosing which parent carried a balanced translocation (four out of 12) and the second least conflict about disclosure of new/controversial interpretations of low AFP results (two out of 12).

## Counselling

Geneticists throughout the world were agreed that the most important goals were preventing disease; lessening patient guilt and anxiety; and helping patients to understand options, to cope with genetic disorders, and to achieve their parenting goals. There was moderate consensus (67%) amongst Australian geneticists that improving the health and vigor of the population was also an important goal, but there was no consensus about the importance of reducing the number of carriers of genetic disorders in the population, though 58% considered this important. This seems to reflect a primary concern among Australian geneticists for their clients and lesser concern for the health of the community at large. This may also represent an avoidance or unwillingness to get involved in eugenic issues. There was strong agreement amongst Australian geneticists that the basic approach to counselling should be non-directive and that it is not appropriate to give advice or to state what the geneticist would do.

### Future Priorities

High future priorities for Australia were the increased demand for genetic services and allocation of limited resources. Given the small proportion of gross national product devoted to health and the even smaller proportion devoted to genetic services, this is not surprising. High priority was given to carrier screening and to preventing environmental damage to the unborn.

Goals in counselling concern the individuals and their families, whereas future priorities are community-oriented. This explains the apparent discrepancy between the relatively low importance attached to the counselling goals of reducing the number of carriers and increasing the health and vigor of the population and the *high future priorities* assigned to carrier screening and preventing environmental damage to the unborn. Presumably, a future high priority for carrier screening reflects hopes of reducing the number of affected individuals in the community. This priority, together with the priority of avoiding environmental damage to the unborn, can be seen as ways of preventing the occurrence of birth defects and increasing the health and vigor of the population. The discrepancy in weighting between related counselling goals and future community priorities may also reflect geneticists' reluctance to confront positive eugenic concerns (Smith 1984).

In Australia, there was strong or moderate consensus on 82% of clinical cases, on 72% of screening questions and on 91% of goals and approaches for counselling. Australian geneticists appear to agree upon approaches to ethical problems. This may reflect their common heritage in training, as well as the relatively small medical community involved. Australian geneticists have respect for parental autonomy, accept the importance of full disclosure, and in general prefer non-directive approaches to counselling. All of these are underpinned by the principle of autonomy. As reflected in decisions about cases, however the principle of autonomy can be overridden by the obligation to avoid harm. Australian geneticists not only take responsibility for avoiding harm to their patients, but also to third parties.

Concern for the wider community was not so clearly demonstrated, either in support for mandatory screening or in goals such as reducing the number of carriers or improving the health and vigor of the population. This was, however, balanced by assigning high future priorities to carrier screening and to prevention of environmental damage to the unborn. This may reflect the recognition by geneticists of the increasing need to broaden their responsibilities, not only to third parties, but to the wider community.

## 2.1.4 The Cultural Context of Medical Genetics in Australia

### 2.1.4.1 Sources of Challenge and Support

Australia has a large and varied immigrant population which includes Greek, Italian, South-East Asian, Turkish, Yugoslav, Lebanese and other Middle Eastern peoples with divergent views and attitudes towards disease, birth defects, and the sex of the child. For example, lethal metabolic disease is better accepted by some groups in a female child than in a male child. These differences have a considerable impact on the practise of medical genetics and on genetic counselling. Problems include counselling via interpreters and the occasional need to use a telephone interpreter service for a rare language, communicating "alien" concepts of birth defects and genetics, and dealing with the social and psychological approaches taken by different groups (Cox 1975). A consequence of this immigrant population is a widespread thalassaemic screening program. Whilst cousin marriages are common amongst the Turkish and Arab immigrants, Australians regard this practise with suspicion. Some members of the Turkish community call marriages between the offspring of brothers first cousin marriages, whereas the offspring of sisters are second cousin marriages. One difficulty that has become apparent in counselling Cambodian and Vietnamese refugees is the conflict between our scientific understanding of genetics and their alternative understanding of diseases as results of spirits or karma.

Since the liberalisation of attitudes to abortion in law and in practise, the Right to Life organisation, backed by the Catholic Church, has constituted a strong organised opposition to abortion. This does not appear to have affected delivery of genetic services directly, apart from an occasional demonstration outside a clinic or a hospital where such services are offered. Differing social, religious and cultural views about abortion can affect clients and may contribute to the chronic grief or guilt that occasionally follows termination. By the same token, ready availability of abortion may lead to failure to appreciate the emotional and other difficulties that may follow termination. These problems may be ameliorated by adequate counselling and support.

Religious views have an impact on the practise of medical genetics; for example, we have found in practise that there are differences between Irish and other European Catholics in regard to their views on abortion. Utilisation of genetic services, including intrauterine diagnosis, by the Catholic community seems proportional to their numbers in the population (26%). Many members of the Moslem community oppose prenatal diagnosis, termination of pregnancy, and post-mortem examination.

Political parties appear to have no systematic attitudes toward medical/genetic issues and offer limited active support. There have been no formal studies regarding general acceptability of genetic services.

## 2.1.4.2  Major Controversies

Controversy has arisen in Australia as the result of limited resources being available for antenatal diagnosis. Guidelines have been introduced in some states so that limited laboratory facilities can cope with the workload. In some states of Australia amniocentesis is offered to all women 35 years and over and in other states only to those age 37 years and over. Sharp controversy arose in Victoria in the early days of amniocentesis when an attempt was made to limit amniocenteses to a small group of experienced operators. In 1984, of a total of 1402 amniocenteses performed, 71% were by seven operators, the remaining 29% by 66 operators. Increased technical problems were encountered amongst less experienced operators (Prenatal Diagnosis Report for Victoria and Tasmania 1984, Department of Genetics, Royal Children's Hospital).

Some controversy has arisen over attempts to rationalise services. For example, in Victoria, with a population of 4.2 million in 1986, there were two laboratories that undertook globin chain synthesis and two units that undertook fetoscopy or other methods of fetal blood sampling. Rationalisation has occurred in most states of Australia for the study of lysosomal disease, which is undertaken in Adelaide.

There has been controversy, as yet unresolved, over the role of non-medical persons in the counselling of patients (Kenan 1986). Very limited use has been made of genetic associates comparable to those in the United States. With increasing demand for screening and intrauterine diagnosis, Australia will need to establish programs and positions for non-physician genetic counsellors. In Australia, specialist paediatricians appropriately undertake counselling of many families within their own area of expertise.

## 2.1.4.3  National Expenditures for Medical Genetics

Australia has been slow to develop genetic services. Table 2.1.9 shows the proportion of the total budget allocated to health care between 1980 and 1985. As can be seen from Table 2.1.4, the small number of medical geneticists providing services is indicative of the small proportion of the health care budget allocated to genetic services. No further data are available.

**Table 2.1.9.**  Budget Allocations for Health Care in Australia 1980–1985*

| Year | Total Current Outlay $US (in millions) | Health Outlay $US | Health as Percentage of Government Expenditures % |
|------|------|------|------|
| 1980 – 1981 | 23,433 | 2,526 | 10.8 |
| 1981 – 1982 | 26,810 | 2,019 | 7.5 |
| 1982 – 1983 | 31,492 | 2,375 | 7.5 |
| 1983 – 1984 | 36,661 | 3,035 | 8.3 |
| 1984 – 1985 | 41,563 | 4,238 | 10.2 |

* From Commonwealth Government Finance – Australia, Australian Bureau of Statistics

## 2.1.4.4 Abortion Laws in Australia

The Davidson case was a famous test case concerning abortion in Australia in 1969. Section 65 of the Abortion Provision of the Crimes Act states that it is an offence to *unlawfully* procure an abortion. Justice Menhennitt interpreted this to imply that some abortions could be lawful. In particular, the principle of duress or necessity was taken to justify abortions, and the circumstances in which this principle could be applied were defined as:

i.   a person must believe on reasonable grounds that abortion was necessary to preserve the woman from a serious danger to her physical or mental health.
ii.  the dangers of performing an abortion were not out of proportion to the danger of continuing the pregnancy.

Most Australian jurisdictions now have similar provisions. In practise, this interpretation of the law has led to the ready availability of safe abortions at a reasonable cost.

## 2.1.4.5 Studies of the Effectiveness of Genetic Services

There have been three studies evaluating the effectiveness of genetic services: by Bell et al. [1986], Rosshandler et al. [1981], and a report entitled "Prenatal Diagnosis Report for Victoria and Tasmania, 1983," produced by the Department of Genetics, Royal Children's Hospital, Melbourne. It appears that a relatively narrow segment of the population utilises genetic services, those who are more highly educated and have a higher income (Rosshandler et al. 1981). The studies all show the limited penetration of genetic services into the marketplace and the need for greater community awareness and education about them. In Western Australia, there appears to be a greater utilisation of genetic services than in any other state. This may be due to the ease of educating such a small medical community.

## 2.1.4.6 Need for New Laws

Laws in anticipation of technical change are difficult to frame. There is a need for closer alignment between the law and medical practise involving non-treatment of severely disabled infants, as demonstrated by a 1985 case. The grandfather of a baby born with spina bifida took out affidavits alleging that the child was being neglected and starved by the hospital with the mother's consent, though this was denied by the mother. The case came before Judge Vincent, who made it clear that under no circumstances was the adoption of a deliberate course of action to terminate life warranted by the law. The child was taken into the temporary care of the court, which did not deprive the mother of custody or of parental rights. Justice

Vincent wrote an order directing the hospital that necessary and reasonable steps be taken "....in accordance with good medical practise and in consultation with the mother" in regard to the care of the child (Transcript 1986, p. 21). Judge Vincent would not rule on what he deemed a further question raised on behalf of the child by the grandfather. This was whether the hospital should perform an operation on the child that might save its life. The case highlighted the pressing need to bring the law into line with medical decisions not to treat, which would be regarded as acceptable medical practise.

The Victorian Infertility (Medical Procedures) Act of 1984 was partially proclaimed in 1986, being the first legislation introduced anywhere in the world aimed at regulating IVF and embryo research. Section 6.3 of the Act defines what constitutes experimental procedures and requires all experimental procedures to be approved by the Standing Review and Advisory Committee. The more controversial part of the Act, not yet proclaimed, would prohibit the use of fertilised ova for any purpose other than implantation. This legislation, however, is already creating difficulties. The Standing Committee is evaluating proposals for experimentation with fertilised ova as if the unproclaimed provisions of the Act were already in force. This has directly affected IVF research and the procedures of egg freezing, micro-injection of sperm and embryo-biopsy (Dawson 1987). The controversy already generated by this legislation makes clear that the ethical, legal, social, and scientific problems surrounding embryo research are not going to be easily resolved, deriving as they do from fundamental conflicts between the requirements of experimental research and social and ethical mores.

## 2.1.5 Ethical Issues and Future Trends

Trends that are likely to raise ethical problems in the future include easy methods of analysis of DNA for the presence of Down syndrome or other major chromosomal errors, allowing an increased utilisation of DNA screening techniques. The risk of miscarriage with chorion villus sampling will need to be balanced against the likely gain from widespread use of screening.

The possibility of mass screening for carrier status, for example of cystic fibrosis, raises ethical issues such as the appropriate age for screening, necessary resources for counselling, and confidentiality of the results. Identifying carriers of a disorder where there is no prospect of intrauterine diagnosis or treatment can be socially damaging (Stamatoyannopoulos 1973).

Persons with disorders that may not produce symptoms until later in life, such as Huntington disease, will need to face the issue of diagnosis without treatment. Identifying carriers will, however, allow them to utilise intrauterine diagnosis. This could eliminate Huntington disease in one generation.

The appropriate utilisation of gene transfer as a means of treatment will have to be addressed. Criteria for patient selection and information about the likely risks and benefits will need to be developed. Whilst there are good arguments for gene transfer in somatic cells, it is unlikely that gene transfer could be sensibly applied to germ cells. Having identified normal and abnormal germ cells, there is no logic in selecting and treating the latter. The same argument applies to the feasibility of utilising in vitro fertilisation and the testing of a single cell to recognise a genetic disorder. This may eventually coincide with the ability to transplant a gene into such an embryo to correct the disorder. The question of whether such a gene transplant is warranted when utilising in vitro techniques would have to be carefully examined. A non-affected embryo could just as easily be selected, and the cost of such choices will need to be considered, including the substantial additional cost of using IVF as opposed to diagnosis in utero. The allocation of scarce resources in the total field of health care may well limit the appeal of genetic technologies. Cost-benefit of the technologies and the overall ethics of allocation of resources will need to be carefully considered.

There is an increasing personal awareness on the part of medical geneticists stimulated by controversies that have arisen amongst geneticists and in the community. There has been a broadening of membership of ethics committees to include laypersons and non-medical professionals. At present these committees are primarily concerned with evaluation of research projects. There are two bioethics centres in Victoria. The centre for Human Bioethics at Monash University is run by a multi-disciplinary Council composed of scientists, philosophers, jurists, physicians and a community worker. The Bioethics Centre at St. Vincent's is located in a major Catholic teaching hospital. There are currently a small number of professional ethicists. The medical, financial and academic climate in Australia makes it unlikely that there will be a significant increase in the number of professional ethicists. There is a gradual acceptance of the view that medical ethicists can make a significant contribution to debate, thinking and teaching about ethical issues. It is likely that in a few major centres ethicists will become important resource persons. There appears to be a developing awareness of ethical issues due to increased publications in the medical literature, community awareness and debate, and increased patient involvement in decision-making. There have also been Government-sponsored Commissions of Inquiry into issues such as in vitro fertilisation and euthanasia in Victoria.

Increased diversity in the Australian population will lead to medical practitioners and medical geneticists who have more diverse value systems. Hence there may be greater variation in approaches to ethical decision-making in the future. Australia's multi-racial society with its many different sets of values makes the achievement of consensus within the wider community difficult. The setting up of Commissions of Inquiry, and the National Health and Medical Research Council's Ethics Committee may provide specific guidelines. Increased ethical awareness through community education will enhance the quality of ethical debate.

The growing community awareness of genetic issues and a greater awareness of the need for an ethically informed approach amongst geneticists will ensure development along ethically acceptable paths. The relatively small size of Australia's core group of geneticists will facilitate development of an ethical approach. The limited economic appeal of genetic technologies will further constrain unethical practises. If new technologies become lucrative and their utilisation spreads beyond the core group of geneticists, the value placed on economic gain may influence the development of genetics in less ethically-acceptable directions.

97

# References

Allan JL, Robbie M, Phelan PD, Danks DM [1980] The incidence and presentation of cystic fibrosis in Victoria 1955-1978. Aust Paediatr J 16: 270-273

Bell JA, Pearn JH [1985] Prenatal cytogenetic diagnosis: medical and social implications. Indications, acceptance by doctors and patients, impact and cost: a 10-year review. Med J Aust 142: 80-83

Bell JA, Pearn J, Cohen G, Ford J, Halliday J, Martin N, Mulcahy M, Purvis-Smith S, Sutherland G [1985] Utilization of prenatal cytogenetic diagnosis in women of advanced maternal age in Australia, 1979-1982. Prenat Diag 5: 53-58

Bell J, Hilden J, Bowling F, Pearn J, Brownlea A, Martin N [1986] The impact of prenatal diagnosis on the occurrence of chromosome abnormalities. Prenat Diag 6: 1-11

Cox D [1975] "Welfare of Migrants". Australian Commission of Inquiry into Poverty. Australian Government Publishing Service, Canberra

Danks DM, Halliday JL [1983] Incidence of neural tube defects in Victoria, Australia. Lancet i: 65

Dawson K [1987] *In vitro* fertilisation: Legislation and problems of research. British Medical Journal 295: 1184-1186

Drew JH, Parkinson P, Walstab JE, Beischer NA [1977] Incidences and types of malformations in newborn infants. Med J Aust 1: 945-949

Field B [1978] Neural tube defects in New South Wales, Australia. J Med Genet 15: 329-338

Fletcher JC, Berg K, Tranøy K [1985] Ethical aspects of medical genetics. A proposal for guidelines in genetic counseling, prenatal diagnosis and screening. Clin Genet 27: 199-205

Fletcher JC, Wertz DC, Sorenson JR, Berg K [1987] Ethics and human genetics: a cross-cultural study in 17 nations. In: Vogel F, Sperling K (eds) Human genetics: proceedings of the 7th International Congress of Human Genetics. Springer-Verlag, Heidelberg, pp 657-672

Hayes SY, Hayes R [1982] Mental Retardation Law Policy and Administration. New South Wales Health Commission, Sydney, Australia

Kenan RH [1986] Growing pains of a new health care field: Genetic counseling in Australia and the United States. Aust J Soc 21: 172-182

Oberklaid F, Danks DM, Jensen F, Stace L, Rosshandler S [1979] Achondroplasia and hypochondroplasia. Comments on frequency, mutation rate, and radiological features in skull and spine. J Med Genet 16: 140-146

Pitt DB [1962] A study of congenital malformations, Part 1. Major malformations in single births. Aust N.Z. J Obs & Gynaecol 2: 23

Pitt DB [1963] Major malformations and multiple births. Aust N.Z. J Obs & Gynaecol 3: 40-43

Pitt D, Connelly J, Francis I, Wilcken B, Brown DA, Robertson E, Hill G, Masters P, Raby J, McFarlance J, Bowling F, Hancock J [1983] Genetic screening of newborn Australia. Results for 1981. Med J Aust 1: 333-335

Rosshandler S, Danks DM, Rogers JG [1981] An economic survey of genetic clinic clients. Med J Aust 2: 641

Smith GP [1984] Eugenics and family planning. Exploring the Yin and the Yang. Univ Tas Law Rev 6: 4-24

Stamatoyannopoulos G [1973] Problems of screening and counselling in the haemoglobinopathies. Proceedings of the IVth International Conference on Birth Defects, Vienna, p 268

Transcript [1987] of hearing before the Honourable Mr. Justice Vincent in the Supreme Court of Victoria. July 2. Re F; F against F Ref. No. PD 2/7. Melbourne, Victoria

# A Selected Bibliography of Bioethics in Australia: IVF and Human Embryo Research

Brumby M, Kasimba P [1987] When is cloning lawful? Journal of In Vitro Fertilization and Embryo Transfer, 4: 198-204

Committee to consider the social, ethical, and legal issues arising from in vitro fertilization [1984]

Report on the disposition of embryos produced by in vitro fertilization. Victorian Government Publishing Service, Melbourne

Dawson K [1987] In vitro fertilisation: Legislation and problems of research. British Medical Journal, 295: 1184–1186

Dawson K [1987] Fertilisation and moral status: A scientific perspective. Journal of Medical Ethics, 13: 173–178

Dawson K, Hudson J (eds) [1987] IVF: The current debate. Centre for Human Bieothics, Clayton, Victoria

Senate Select Committee on the Human Embryo Experimentation Bill 1985 [1986] Human embryo experimentation in Australia. Australian Government Publishing Service, Canberra

Singer P, Kuhse H [1986] The ethics of embryo research. Law, Medicine and Health Care, 14: 133–137

Singer P, Wells D [1984] The reproductive revolution. Oxford University Press, Oxford

Unlacke S [1987] In vitro fertilization and the right to reproduce. Bioethics 1: 240–254

## 2.2 Ethics and Medical Genetics in Brazil

F. M. Salzano and S. D. J. Pena

### 2.2.1 *Medical Genetics in Brazil*

### 2.2.1.1 *Scope of the Problem*

**The Country and the People**

Brazil is a country of continental size. Distances to be traveled between its most extreme North-South or East-West points reach 4,300 km, while its total area is 8.5 million km². The country is divided into five large regions (North, Northeast, Southeast, South and Center-West), which display a vast array of climates and ecological characteristics. The socioeconomic conditions of these regions are also very different, the most developed being the Southeast and South.

Distributed over this vast territory are 125 million persons, placing Brazil as the sixth country in the world in terms of population. There is wide variation in the number of persons living in the different regions, the lowest demographic density occurring in the North and the highest in the Southeast. The population as a whole is increasing at an average annual rate of 2.5%; life expectancy at birth is only 55 years for males and 59 for females with, however, much regional diversity.

The racial background of this population is highly heterogeneous, with European, Black and Amerindian contributions. The Caucasoid component derives mainly from Portugal, but in the South and Southeast especially the Italian, Spanish, Japanese and German nationalities are also represented. The Amerindian population is now estimated at only 220,000 individuals and has not been included in the 1980 census, which yielded the following percentages in relation to race: whites, 54; mixed, 39; black, 6; Asian, 1.

A clear geographic pattern can be observed in Brazil's ethnic distribution: trihybrid (white/Indian/black) persons predominate in the Northeast, dihybrid (white/Indian) in the North and Center-West, while European descendants relatively free from admixture are largely found in the Southeast and South. This statement, however, is valid only in general terms. The process of race admixture was widespread, with the formation almost everywhere of complex arrangements (for more details see Salzano and Freire-Maia 1970; Salzano 1987).

Brazil, with its US$150.00 of annual per capita income, is very far away from the levels of developed nations. In addition, this income is very unevenly distributed. Considering the 40.3 million workers that constitute the economically active portion of the population, we will see that the poorest 50% receive only 12.6% of this income, while the wealthiest 1% receive 16.9%. The consequences of this underdevelopment and unfair social conditions are manifold. In the large cities, 24% of the houses do not have a water supply, 11% do not have electricity, and 62% do not have adequate water closets. In the rural areas the situation is even worse. The high mortality rate (9%!) in the first year of life, high levels of undernutrition (calculated as 67%), and the high prevalences of infectious diseases (malaria afflicts 1.5 million Brazilians) should be considered in any discussion related to government support for genetic counseling or prenatal diagnosis, although, as indicated above, these conditions vary regionally (Salzano 1979a; Sanford 1985).

## 2.2.1.2  Organization of Clinical Genetic Services in Brazil

### History: The Early Days
The first genetic studies in Brazil date back to the beginning of the 1930s. Three persons were catalysts for progress: C. A. Krug, F. G. Brieger and A. Dreyfus. Krug and Brieger were plant geneticists, while Dreyfus worked mainly with insects. Dreyfus and the Rockefeller Foundation, through its Director, Harry M. Miller Jr., were responsible for the first stay of Theodosius Dobzhansky in Brazil in 1943. The association between this distinguished geneticist and the Brazilian researchers lasted for three decades, and especially in the first half of this period his influence was marked. As a result, most Brazilian geneticists of this period started their work as *Drosophila* investigators. This was true of three of the four persons who were first responsible for developing the field and who had a formative influence upon a large number of specialists in human genetics: N. Freire-Maia, O. Frota-Pessoa and one of us (FMS). The fourth was P. H. Saldanha, who worked with humans from the very beginning. In the early 1960s, however, other key persons for the development of Brazilian human genetics began their investigations. Mention can be made especially of B. Beiguelman, W. Beçak, A. Freire-Maia, H. Krieger and E. S. Azevêdo. Influence from the outside occurred especially through the association with two well-known U.S. population geneticists, J. V. Neel and N. E. Morton. More details about these events and the people who participated in them can be found in da Cunha et al. [1961], Salzano (1979b) and Beiguelman [1981].

### Recent Developments in Brazilian Medical Genetics
Although some of the researchers indicated above had published papers on medical genetics earlier, the boom in this area really occurred after the establishment, in Brazil, of techniques for the study of human chromosomes. This happened during the 1960s, and involved the work of W. Beçak, mentioned above, plus that of C. Bottura, I. Ferrari; J. C. Cabral de Almeida, M. S. Mattevi, W. Pinto Jr., and H. R. S. Nazareth. It was at that time also that I. Roisenberg started his work on the inherited defects of coagulation, which is still being continued (Beiguelman 1981).

In the last two-and-a-half decades the number of centers and people involved with medical genetics in Brazil increased markedly. A list of the main groups is presented in Table 2.2.1.

As can be seen, their distribution is quite uneven, with most of them being located in the Southeast region, and more specifically in São Paulo. Eighteen (56%) of the institutions listed are from this region, while none is found in the Northern re-

**Table 2.2.1.**  Information about Centers of Medical Genetics in Brazil

| Geographical location (region, city, State) | Institution | Main investigators |
|---|---|---|
| *Northeast Region* | | |
| Natal, RN | Federal University of Rio Grande do Norte | T. J. A. Moura, L. L. A. Sena |
| João Pessoa, PB | Federal University of Paraíba | H. G. Nunesmaia |
| Recife, PE | Federal University of Pernambuco Secretary of Health, State of Pernambuco | E. O. Silva D. A. Sampaio |
| Salvador, BA | Federal University of Bahia | E. S. Azevêdo, M. R. P. Bueno, L. M. A. Moreira |
| *Center-West Region* | | |
| Brasília, DF | University of Brasília | A. R. T. Gagliardi, H. L. Ferreira, R. S. Mello |
| Cuiabá, MT | Federal University of Mato Grosso | T. J. Lister |
| Goiânia, GO | Federal University of Goiás | V. Toledo |
| *Southeast Region* | | |
| Vitória, ES | Federal University of Espírito Santo | D. M. Silva |
| Uberlândia, MG | Federal University of Uberlândia | M. A. Spanó |
| Belo Horizonte, MG | Federal University of Minas Gerais | S. D. J. Pena, M. N. T. Marques |
| Rio de Janeiro, RJ | Federal University of Rio de Janeiro  Oswaldo Cruz Institute | J. C. Cabral de Almeida, I. M. Orioli, D. N. F. Conceição, G. Carakushansky, H. Krieger |
| São José do Rio Preto, SP | Paulista State University | M. Varella-Garcia, P. C. Naoum |
| Ribeirão Preto, SP | University of São Paulo | I. Ferrari, M. A. Zago, J. M. Pina Neto, C. Casartelli |
| São Carlos, SP | Federal University of São Paulo | C. A. A. Barbosa |
| Botucatu, SP | Paulista State University | D. V. Freire-Maia, A. R. Costa |
| Campinas, SP | State University of Campinas | B. Beiguelman, W. Pinto Jr., A. S. Ramalho, L. A. Magna, C. Hackel, J. F. P. Arena |
| Sorocaba, SP | Pontifical Catholic University | I. Armando |
| São Paulo, SP | University of São Paulo | O. Frota-Pessoa, P. H. Saldanha, M. Zatz, A. M. Viana-Morgante, A. Wajntal, P. A. Otto, R. B. Levisky, P. G. Otto, C. H. Gonzales, O. C. O. Barreto |

**Table 2.2.1.** (continued)

| Geographical location (region, city, State) | Institution | Main investigators |
|---|---|---|
| | Paulista School of Medicine | R. Monteleone Neto, J. A. D. Andrade, M. E. S. Fernandes, A. J. B. Cunha, M. G. Lima |
| | Research Center on Oncology | L. Mori, G. M. Machado-Santelli |
| | Butantan Institute | W. Beçak, M. L. Beçak, R. C. S. Santos |
| | Association of São Paulo Maternity | T. R. Gollop |
| | Institute of Medical Assistance to Public Servants | C. L. Borovik, D. Brunoni |
| | Bioscience/Lavoisier Laboratory | B. J. Schmidt |
| *South Region* Londrina, PR | Londrina University | E. M. P. L. C. Marchese |
| Curitiba, PR | Federal University of Paraná | N. Freire-Maia, M. Pinheiro, F. A. Marçallo, R. F. Pilotto, B. Arce-Gomez, I. J. Cavalli |
| Florianópolis, SC | Federal University of Santa Catarina | N. Ferrari, E. T. Pereira, M. D. Muniz, C. E. A. Pinheiro |
| Santa Maria, RS | Federal University of Santa Maria | R. Z. Flores |
| Porto Alegre, RS | Federal University of Rio Grande do Sul | F. M. Salzano, I. Roisenberg, M. S. Mattevi, B. Erdtmann, R. R. Fischer, C. J. Geiger |
| | Porto Alegre Clinical Hospital | R. Giugliani, L. Schüler, M. R. S. Carvalho |
| | Porto Alegre School of Medical Sciences | H. M. M. Mendez, G. A. Paskulin |

gion. The listing of main investigators presented in Table 2.2.1 is somewhat arbitrary, but 72 (85%) live in the Southeast or South regions.

**Genetic Counseling**

Only about 30 of the centers listed in Table 2.2.1 provide genetic counseling, and the number of groups that furnish regular counseling to a relatively large number of persons is even smaller.

Who seeks genetic counseling and why? What kind of behavior do these counselees present in this type of situation? These questions have been considered, in relation to the Porto Alegre center at the Federal University of Rio

103

**Table 2.2.2.** Patients Seen at the Genetics Service of the Instituto Hilton Rocha in Belo Horizonte in the Period July 1982–June 1986, Classified by Type of Referral

| Type of referral | Number |
|---|---|
| 1. Genetic counseling | 1,049 |
|    1.1. Genic disorders | 522 |
|    1.2. Elevated maternal age | 219 |
|    1.3. History of fetal losses | 217 |
|    1.4. Exposure to teratogens | 27 |
|    1.5. Consanguinity | 26 |
|    1.6. Miscellaneous | 38 |
| 2. Diagnostic evaluation | 324 |
| 3. Chromosome studies | 289 |
| 4. Miscellaneous | 81 |
| Total | 1,743 |

Grande do Sul, by Kanan [1981], Witt and da Rocha [1982], Mattevi and Salzano [1982] and Geiger et al. [1985]. Reports by Castilla et al. [1977] and Gonçalves [1981] examined some of them at two centers in the State of São Paulo. As was shown by Geiger et al [1985], in the period between November, 1978 and July, 1982 three types of patients were found to be the most common in Porto Alegre: (a) those with chromosome aberrations (24%); (b) chromosomally normal, with several malformations (21%); and (c) with genic diseases (12%). (Genic diseases refer to those conditions that are caused by point mutations, as opposed to those caused by chromosome aberrations). The figures for Belo Horizonte are different, reflecting the peculiarities of the genetics unit located there, which serves a high-income population and, although having a general scope with special interest in reproductive genetics, is located on the premises of the Instituto Hilton Rocha, a majòr ophthalmological hospital. In the four-year period July 1982 – June 1986, 1743 families were referred to this genetics service for consultation. The indications for referral were varied and can be divided into four large groups (Table 2.2.2). Most of the families (1049 cases, 60%) were seen for genetic counseling *sensu strictu*, and the reasons are given in detail in the Table. It is important to note that 310 families (30% of those counseled) received *prospective* genetic counseling, the most common indication being advanced maternal age, with most cases proceeding to undergo amniocentesis. The second group was composed of patients referred for diagnostic evaluation of neurological problems (including mental retardation), dysmorphism or growth problems. Many of these patients received chromosome or metabolic investigations. The third group consisted of patients referred for chromosome studies on the basis of a specific clinical hypothesis: 134 for Down syndrome, 76 for Turner syndrome, 34 for ambiguous genitalia, 20 for Klinefelter syndrome and 25 for various other conditions.

Several authors (e. g. Simpson 1975; Harris and Begleiter 1976; Magnelli 1977; Castilla et al. 1977; Klein and Wyss 1977; Bochkov 1979; Czeizel et al. 1980; Gonçalves 1981) have described the types of patients referred to their services and discussed the distributions observed. In these series the prevalence of patients with chromosome aberrations varied from 7% (Czeizel et al. 1980) to 48% (Magnelli

1977). The values for Porto Alegre (24%) and Belo Horizonte (17%) are in the middle of this range. On the other hand, the percentage of genic diseases found in Porto Alegre (13%, of which 10% are monogenic and 2% polygenic) is lower than those presented in these eight investigations. This finding may reflect (a) difficulties of identification; (b) lack of interest in referring genetically affected patients to that service; or (c) unawareness of the existence of the service on the part of practicing physicians. The figure for genic diseases for Belo Horizonte is higher (30%).

A detailed description of the types of chromosome aberrations found in Porto Alegre in the period 1965-1979 was given by Mattevi and Salzano [1982], and a report for 1980-1985 is currently in preparation. Types of ascertainment varied, but in the present discussion we will concentrate on the chromosome abnormalities observed in patients referred by physicians. As expected, most of these abnormalities were those related to Down syndrome; however, there was a large difference in the prevalence of this syndrome in the two periods (57% among 235 patients with aberrations in the first vs. 71% among 169 in the other; chi-square: 8.4, 1 d.f., $p < 0.01$). The difference cannot be explained by dissimilarities in the mean ages of the patients' mothers, which were almost identical (28.5 and 28.8, respectively). It should be mentioned that, due to the high costs of the reagents and the amount of work involved, in Porto Alegre no chromosome studies are performed in women over 35 years of age whose children show the typical signs of the syndrome. Another difference observed was in the frequencies of autosome translocations and inversions. In the second period, a large number of translocations was found (21 vs. 9), which was partially compensated by a smaller number of inversions in these chromosomes (1 vs. 10; chi square: 12.6; 1 d.f.; $p < 0.001$). All these findings indicate the subtle ways in which these populations of patients change, since our policy regarding the cases that should be accepted for genetic counseling was not altered during these years.

In the 1978-1982 period in Porto Alegre, Down syndrome was responsible for 17% of all cases that came to the Federal University of Rio Grande do Sul Service (Geiger et al. 1985). A similar frequency was obtained by Castilla et al. [1977] in Ribeirão Preto, and by Gonçalves [1981] in another Brazilian center (14% in both studies); but the numbers found in Europe (Klein and Wyss 1977, 9%; Czeizel et al. 1980, 4%) were much lower. The percentage found in Belo Horizonte (8%) is similar to the European figures. This may indicate a tighter selection for access to chromosome studies and/or a more diversified source of subjects in the latter centers.

Most of the genetic counseling centers are located in universities or State institutions and provide free services, or ask only for payment for the reagents used. Therefore, the results described above can be taken as representative of the populations from which they were derived. Private services for karyotype determinations also exist in some cities.

**Genetic Screening**

Presently the most important monogenic disease in Brazil is undoubtedly sickle cell anemia. As was indicated above, 45% of our population has varying degrees of Black admixture, and of these, 5-6% are heterozygotes $Hb^A/Hb^S$. But even in persons classified as white this genotype is present in about 1%. The estimated total number of people with sickle cell disease among Blacks and mixed is estimated as 45,000 (Salzano 1985).

Considering this large number of people, it is surprising to see how few systematic investigations on this condition have been performed in Brazil. Moreover, many of the earlier studies could have confounded sickle cell anemia with other entities, such as sickle cell beta-thalassemia. This situation is rapidly changing now, with the establishment of a Cooperative Group for Research in Hemoglobinopathy that includes 77 researchers, coordinated by the Center of Reference for Hemoglobins, headed by P.C. Naoum, who works in São José do Rio Preto. Other strong centers studying this subject are located in Campinas (A.S. Ramalho, F.F. Costa), São Paulo (J.T. Araujo), Ribeirão Preto (M.A. Zago) and Porto Alegre (M.H. Hutz, F.M. Salzano). Systematic screening of populations for the purpose of genetic counseling, however, is being performed at São José do Rio Preto and Campinas only (for details see Zago et al.1983; Naoum et al.1984; Naoum 1985; Zago and Costa 1985; Ramalho 1986).

Heterozygotes for beta-thalassemia can occur in about 1% of the Caucasoid fraction in the Brazilian South and Southeast, and higher prevalences may exist in unmixed descendants of Italians. Ramalho et al [1985] described the program they have for detecting such individuals and giving them appropriate information. An association (Associação Brasileira dos Talassêmicos) for the help of thalassemia homozygotes and their relatives exists in São Paulo, which has connections with the Thalassemia International Federation.

A program for carrier detection and prevention of Tay-Sachs disease was established in the Jewish community of Porto Alegre. After one year of an extensive public education program, 298 young volunteers of reproductive age were screened for the responsible gene by the tear test. Possible carriers were further submitted to the leukocyte hexosaminidase A assay to confirm the diagnosis. Seven heterozygotes were detected and received genetic counseling (Buchalter et al.1983).

Screening for phenylketonuria (PKU) and hyperphenylalaninemia was carried out both among 4,914 normal and 86 mentally retarded children of the southern city of Rio Grande by Esperon [1978]. Of the six phenylketonurics discovered two could be treated with the low phenylalanine diet. In Porto Alegre the study of the prevalence of metabolic disorders concentrated mostly on high-risk patients (those with developmental, visual or auditory deficiencies, other diseases, or who were in pediatric intensive care units). Highest frequencies were encountered among patients with osteoarticular disorders or renal-ureteral lithiasis. Due to their relatively high prevalences, the organic acidurias seem to constitute a good target for the investigation of inborn errors of metabolism in severely ill children (Wannmacher et al. 1982; Wajner et al. 1986).

A large and relatively comprehensive screening program for phenylketonuria and congenital hypothyroidism has been under way in the city of São Paulo for the past five years. This program is voluntary and sponsored by an association of parents and friends of mentally deficient persons (APAE – Associação de Pais e Amigos do Excepcional). So far, over 500,000 newborn children have been screened, the general incidence being 1/15,760 for phenylketonuria and 1/3,100 for congenital hypothyroidism (B.Schmidt, personal communication, 1986). These figures are similar to those reported for other countries (Collaborative Study 1975; Medeiros-Neto et al. 1986).

The pioneer program in São Paulo has triggered a large national discussion as to whether newborn screening for PKU and congenital hypothyroidism should become mandatory in Brazil. Some argue that since the major health priorities in Brazil are malnutrition and infectious diseases, it would make no sense to invest precious funds in the screening of rare congenital diseases. Others point out that the program in São Paulo has been shown to be cost-effective and that the growing middle class in Brazil can pay for the costs and has the right to have access to such programs. Three states (São Paulo, Rio de Janeiro and Minas Gerais) have already passed legislation in this direction, but only São Paulo has a large-scale operative program. The Ministry of Health has set up a committee to study the possible implementation of a federally-funded country-wide newborn screening program, but it seems unlikely that such a program will be launched in the very near future. Meanwhile, it is probable that several smaller programs will be organized by private laboratories to operate on a voluntary basis.

## 2.2.1.3 *Prenatal Diagnosis*

Prenatal diagnosis by second trimester amniocentesis was introduced in Brazil only in the 1970s by the late Heleneide Nazareth at the Escola Paulista de Medicina in São Paulo (Nazareth et al. 1981). Since then expansion has been slow: only five laboratories offer routine amniotic fluid prenatal cytogenetics in Brazil, and all of them are concentrated in the Southeast region (four in the State of São Paulo and one in Minas Gerais).

To collect some data about prenatal services in Brazil, a short questionnaire was sent to the heads of the five laboratories mentioned above, and all answered. The data show that to date a total of 1891 genetic amniocenteses have been performed in Brazil. Most were done for cytogenetic studies, 63% of the total being performed for advanced maternal age and 16% because of a previous child with a chromosome disorder. The figures are similar to those reported from Toronto in the period 1971-1978 (Rudd and Doran 1980), but more recent North American data show higher percentages of cases done for maternal age, such as the 89% from New York City in the period 1979-1983 (Benn et al, 1985). The complications of amniocentesis in Brazil were relatively few: there were a total of 22 fetal losses after the procedure (1%, only 0.3% occurring in the week following the amniocentesis). This figure is lower than the fetal loss rate reported in the control group for the large collaborative studies in the USA and England (Rodeck 1984). On the other hand, the overall number of cases in which the amniocentesis had to be repeated for culture failure or slow culture growth was relatively high (141, 7.5%) when compared with recent North American figures (2%, Benn et al. 1985) but comparable to older figures, such as the 6% repeats in Winnipeg from 1973 to 1978 (Greenberg and Hamerton 1980) and 8% from Vancouver in the same period (Baird 1980). It should be noted that the Brazilian laboratories were very heterogeneous in their need to repeat amniocenteses, the proportion varying from a reported low of 3% to a high of 35%. In the 1891 cases studied there were two errors of diagnosis (0.1%) and in 27 cases (1%) a diagnosis could not be reached.

The questionnaires also included questions about chorionic villus sampling, which has been recently introduced in Brazil (Gollop et al. 1986). All five laboratories involved in prenatal diagnosis by amniocentesis had some experience with chorion biopsy. In all, approximately 90 such procedures have been done in the country as a whole, with an 81% success rate. In 15% of the cases a diagnosis could not be made and in 3% there was fetal loss before term.

Considering the size of the Brazilian population, this experience with prenatal diagnosis is very limited. The total number of prenatal diagnoses done in the period 1975–1986 in the whole country is smaller than the number of genetic amniocenteses done in metropolitan New York in one year (Benn et al. 1985). In our view, two major interrelated causes contribute to this limitation: cultural-religious-legal factors and economic ones.

Brazil is largely a Roman Catholic country, and the Catholic Church's ban on abortion certainly limits the acceptance of prenatal diagnosis. This is reinforced by the Brazilian Penal Code, which considers therapeutic abortion a crime with heavy penalties (see Section 2.2.4.4 below). Cultural factors are also very relevant: for instance, it is our experience that women in the 35–40 age group (generally representing professional women who marry late or women initiating a second marriage) are much more receptive to genetic amniocentesis than those in the 40–45 age group, who are generally multiparae having an unplanned pregnancy.

Economic factors influence not only the demand but also the supply of prenatal genetic services. In this respect we have to analyze the considerable costs involved in setting up and maintaining the tissue culture and cytogenetical facilities which are indispensable for the operation of a prenatal diagnosis laboratory. One of the major problems is the legal and bureaucratic impediments to the importation of scientific equipment and supplies. For instance, Brazil does not produce $CO^2$ incubators of reasonable quality and it is almost impossible to obtain the licence to import one from outside. Foreign scientific equipment available in Brazil, such as microscopes etc., will cost 3 to 5 times its price abroad. Tissue culture plasticware, culture media and other supplies have practically to be smuggled into the country, after being purchased with expensive dollars bought in the black market.

Considering all these major difficulties, it is not surprising that few centers have ventured into prenatal diagnosis. Interestingly, all laboratories offering prenatal services in Brazil are private profit-oriented services, in contrast to the predominantly university-based laboratories in North America and Europe. A large number of the universities in Brazil are owned by the federal government and are plagued by restrictive legislation and bureaucratic inertia that limit the collection of fees from patients. The universities also lack the accounting flexibility necessary to run a prenatal diagnosis laboratory. This situation is worrisome, since it entails a lack of peer review and other regulatory activities of the academic environment. Efforts are being made to organize a Brazilian Society of Medical Genetics, which will assume this regulatory role by setting standards of genetic practice, establishing also quality control procedures and laboratory certification.

## 2.2.2 Ethical Problems Faced by Brazilian Medical Geneticists

### Previous Discussions

Humans are moral animals. All of us feel a certain degree of compulsion to favor what we consider to be good, as well as to condemn and to eliminate what is evil. But the systems of moral norms vary from one individual to the other, and from one culture to the other, despite the existence of some universal principles.

The sets of written and unwritten codes of conduct that exist in Brazil are the result of a complex interrelationship between our culture and the people who interpret it. A historical review and discussion of medical ethics in our country has been provided by Landmann [1985]. But the sets of regulations that exist are not unconditionally accepted. Those aspects related to genetics have been recently discussed at three meetings: (a) VI Latin American Congress of Genetics, held in Maracaibo, Venezuela, 1983 (Lemoine 1984); (b) the National Forum of Medical Genetics, organized by the Brazilian National Academy of Medicine and held in Rio de Janeiro, 1985 (Rocha 1985); and (c) the 32nd Brazilian Congress of Genetics, held in Curitiba, 1986. In the first meeting the Brazilian legislation was compared with legislation from other Latin American countries, and in the other two the dilemmas faced by our medical geneticists due to obsolete and sometimes inappropriate laws were stressed. In the last meeting, the present survey was explicitly discussed, with results that will be detailed in section 2.2.3.

### Brazilian Legislation

To understand the situation in Brazil the following aspects of its legislation should be mentioned: (a) *Contraception*: There is no legal prohibition of this type of birth control, and the present code of medical ethics (enacted by the Federal Council of Medicine and officially published in the Federal Register of May 25, 1984) ignores it. But there is prohibition of the public dissemination of anticonceptional methods (Article 20, Law of Penal Contraventions; Decree-Law no. 4,113 of February 14, 1942); (b) *Sterilization*: The new code of medical ethics simply indicates that the specific legislation on this matter should be followed. In relation to the Penal Code, Prof. Benjamin Morais (cited in Landmann 1985) asserts that tubal sterilization performed in accordance with the woman's wish constitutes no crime. A vasectomy program functions openly in São Paulo, and 4,169 men were sterilized, at their request, in a 32-month period between 1981 and 1983 (Castro et al. 1984). In Teresina, Piaui, 63% of the women desiring contraception had chosen sterilization as their preferred method (Merrick 1983); (c) *Artificial insemination by donor*: No mention of it appears in the new code of medical ethics, but the procedure was formally prohibited in the previous code (officially published in the Federal Register of January 11, 1965); (d) *Abortion*: Abortion is prohibited by law, except when the mother's life is in danger or in cases of rape. See section 2.2.4.4 below; (e) *Workers' health protection*: The labor legislation has no provisions regarding predisposing genetic characteristics, although it has many rules with reference to workers' health protection in general.

**Health for a Few or Health for All?**

The World Health Organization's established target for year 2000 is that of health for all. This, of course, can be viewed more as a slogan than as an attainable objective. There are formidable problems among the underdeveloped nations, and even among those of the First World. In some cases, the quality of life may be deteriorating due to the industrial or nuclear pollution.

In Brazil the situation is complex, due to the coexistence of developed and underdeveloped areas. While in the Southeast and South some of the conditions approach those of the most advanced nations, in the other regions the situation is similar to those seen in other poor countries. Our health policy, therefore, has to be flexible. While high priority should be given to the most prevalent endemic diseases, it would be erroneous not to consider also the needs of the industrialized areas. This has already been recognized through the mass vaccination campaigns against poliomyelitis, which is very rare here, in the importation of sophisticated equipment for heart transplantation, as well as in the emphasis given to the Acquired Immunodeficiency Syndrome (AIDS), which affects only a few hundred Brazilians.

There is a case, therefore, for much more involvement of the Brazilian public health system with genetic diseases, which it has practically ignored until now. Areas in which this interaction could be especially profitable are those related to chromosome aberrations, and, in general, those concerned with the etiology and prevention of mental deficiency.

## 2.2.3  Consensus and Variation in Approaches to Ethical Problems

### 2.2.3.1  The Present Survey

**Nature of the Sample**

How representative is the sample of 32 medical geneticists? The following points should be kept in mind: Researchers living in eight Brazilian States (two in the South, three in the Southeast, and three in the Northeast regions) have been included; their mean age was 42 years, and sexes were about equally distributed (18 males, 14 females); most of them (69%) were married, having an average of two children; half had been raised in Catholic families, but seldom attended church services; more tended to view themselves as liberal (56%) than as conservative (13%); professionally, 18 had a medical degree, and the fact that 14 had Ph.D.s instead of M.D.s can be explained by the fact that Brazilian human genetics traditionally developed from animal genetics; the majority had a lengthy experience in medical genetics (average: 14 years of practice), with work about evenly distributed between the clinic and the laboratory; the average number of patients counseled per week was six.

We therefore can view this sample as mostly representative of Brazilian medical geneticists, especially of those with more seniority.

110

## 2.2.3.2 Pattern of the Answers

The majority of the investigators sampled would choose the following alternatives: (a) full disclosure to parents who carry a balanced translocation; (b) providing information to relatives at risk, if asked, if Huntington disease or hemophilia A patients refuse to permit disclosure; (c) disclosure, in cases of ambiguous prenatal test results, that there *may be* an abnormality; (d) disclosure of false paternity to the mother alone; (e) providing complete information about XO and XYY fetuses, and letting the couple decide what to do; (f) explanation of all reproductive possibilities to carriers of a tuberous sclerosis gene.

In their responses to the second part of the questionnaire, the majority of geneticists (a) would try to dissuade a woman from having prenatal diagnosis for anxiety alone (but a significant number would perform prenatal diagnosis); (b) would not tell a woman with testicular feminization syndrome that she is chromosomally male; (c) would grant a request for prenatal diagnosis in a woman of 42, even if she would oppose abortion; (d) would refuse to do prenatal diagnosis for sex preselection; (e) would disclose conflicting laboratory results, refusing to give advice about what to do.

The question that evoked the greatest ethical conflict was prenatal diagnosis for sex selection alone. The testicular feminization case gave the least ethical conflict.

Turning now to questions of more social concern, the majority would favor a mandatory law for mass screening of industrial workers for alpha-1-antitrypsin, as well as screening for cystic fibrosis for all persons over 18 years of age. Access to the screening results should only be given (with the patient's approval) to persons who could not interfere with his/her career or rights.

In the questions of priorities in Brazil and the rest of the world, understandably, increased demand for genetic services and allocation of limited resources were items indicated as very important for Brazilians, but not necessarily for geneticists around the world. It was also felt that research on human embryos or fetuses, as well as treatment in utero and molecular genetic manipulation, should probably be given more emphasis outside than inside Brazil.

Prevention of disease, removal of patients' guilt or anxiety, helping patients to cope with genetic problems and to understand the present state of medical knowledge should be the main goals in genetic counseling. Counseling *should not* be much concerned with eugenics or other problems at the population level. In general, the counselor's attitude should be non-directive and supportive.

In giving explanations for their choices, Brazilians valued especially (at the ratio of 2:1:1) the ethical principle of autonomy, followed by that of beneficence and that of non-maleficence.

This was the dominant pattern; but for each question a varied array of items was selected; as impressive as the pattern just described was the polymorphic nature of the answers, pointing to the multivalent aspect of the human personality.

## 2.2.3.3  Comparison with Data from other Countries

In terms of the sample, Brazilians were somewhat younger, had fewer males, fewer married persons, and fewer offspring than most other groups. They had more Ph. D.s and fewer pediatricians than the others, less experience in medical genetics, worked more hours in the laboratory and fewer hours at administrative tasks. Although they were predominantly of Catholic background, they were less likely to attend religious ceremonies than researchers of other nationalities. They were similar to geneticists in other countries in hours per week seeing patients, total hours worked per week, number of patients per week and self-reported liberal or conservative political persuasion.

As a whole, Brazilian answers to the questionnaire were similar to those of geneticists from other countries. There were some differences, however: (a) in the case of prenatal diagnosis for an anxious woman without medical indications, most Brazilians would refuse to do the test. The reasoning here involved placing the principle of non-maleficence over that of autonomy; (b) most Brazilians would not tell the woman with testicular feminization that she was XY (non-maleficence over autonomy); and (c) Brazilians would give somewhat more emphasis to mandatory than to voluntary screening tests.

In terms of research priorities, Brazilians stressed, in contrast to people of most other nations, that more investigations on environmental damage to the unborn, as well as on genetic screening in the workplace, should be performed.

Other differences, in relation to the goals of genetic counseling, were more emphasis on the prevention of disease, reduction in the number of carriers, improvement of the population's health, and on helping patients achieve their parenting objectives; Brazilians would also be less willing than others to indicate what they would do in the counselee's situation. While their main emphases were on the individual or family, they were still more "populationists" than their fellows in other countries.

## 2.2.3.4  Discussion at the 32nd Brazilian Congress of Genetics

The organization of a roundtable at the 1986 Brazilian Congress of Genetics, mentioned previously, had two main objectives: (a) to inform Brazilian geneticists about this project and the main tendencies observed in the studied sample; and (b) to discuss the ethical issues involved and obtain further opinions about them. A simplified questionnaire was handed to the audience and those that wanted to give their opinion in writing were encouraged to do so.

The results are summarized in Table 2.2.3. Nine males and 20 females answered the questionnaire, out of a total of about 150; they were much younger (average: 34 years) than the sample included in the survey and a sizeable number (34%) were students. Their general opinion can be summarized as follows: (a) *In favor* of abortion of a genetically malformed fetus, of adoption of children when there is risk of genetically malformed offspring, of legislation regulating the practice of ge-

**Table 2.2.3.** Results of a Survey Conducted at a Session of the 1986 National Meeting of the Brazilian Society of Genetics in which Questions of Bioethics had been Discussed[a] (n = 29)

| Problem | In favor | Against | No Opinion |
|---|---|---|---|
| 1. Abortion of a fetus malformed due to genetic reasons | 26 | 2 | 1 |
| 2. Adoption of children when there is risk of genetically malformed offspring | 24 | 4 | 1 |
| 3. *In vitro* fertilization (in general) | 16 | 12 | 1 |
| 4. Surrogate motherhood (in general) | 11 | 18 | 0 |
| 5. Prenatal diagnosis for sex preselection | 2 | 27 | 0 |
| 6. Prenatal diagnosis in the absence of any medical or genetic indication | 15 | 14 | 0 |
| 7. Legislation regulating the practice of genetic counseling and prenatal diagnosis | 26 | 1 | 2 |
| 8. Genetic screening (either mandatory or voluntary) in the workplace | 27 | 1 | 1 |
| 9. Disclosure of genetic risk to relatives of patients even if patients oppose it | 18 | 8 | 3 |
| 10. Disclosure to the couple of accidentally discovered nonpaternity | 5 | 22 | 0 |

[a] Nine males and 20 females answered a short questionnaire with the indicated questions. Their average age was 34 years (range: 18–61), and in relation to professional experience they could be classified as follows: (a) Undergraduate students: 3; (b) Graduate students: 7; (c) University professors or professionals: 17; (d) No information: 2.

netic counseling and prenatal diagnosis, of genetic screening (either mandatory or voluntary) in the workplace, and of providing information on genetic risk to relatives of patients even if patients are against disclosure: (b) *Against* prenatal diagnosis for sex preselection and disclosure of accidentally discovered non-paternity; (c) *Undecided* about *in vitro* fertilization, surrogate motherhood, and prenatal diagnosis in the absence of any medical or genetic indication.

At the business meeting of the Society a motion was approved for the legalization of abortion when there are clear indications that the fetus is severely malformed.

## 2.2.4 Cultural Context of Medical Genetics in Brazil

### 2.2.4.1 Sources of Challenge and Support

**Brazilian Culture**
As can be surmised from the previous paragraphs, the two samples studied, despite differences in composition, were basically in agreement in relation to the questions at issue. Why? To interpret these results we have to consider the Brazil-

ian cultural heritage. The mixing of cultures occurred simultaneously with the mixture of races, and a good outline concerning these processes can be found in Ribeiro [1977]; but the dominant influence came from Portugal. It is impossible, in the space available to us, to characterize even the main outlines of this culture (see, for instance, chapter 5 of Figueiredo 1977). Some of its features, however, are important in the present context. These are: (a) a generally peaceful, non-belligerent nature; (b) an emphasis on the family as the basic social unit; (c) the marked influence of the Church in all aspects of personal relationships; and (d) the tendency to favor tradition over innovation, knowledge acquired in books over experimentation, and a general lack of interest in science.

In contact with the Indian and African cultures, the Portuguese descendants have changed. The Black influence especially served to strengthen the mystical component of our personality. In the South and Southeast, European immigrants from other countries (especially Italy, Germany, and Spain) have left their mark; their influence in regard to the four features described above, however, has been small. To these ethnic influences we should add the constancy of authoritarian governments that, with rare exceptions, have exerted power in Brazil. The tendency among the questionnaire respondents, even if not marked, to favor the implementation of compulsory measures may stem from this historical fact.

**The Church**
While most Brazilians, especially those engaged in science, seldom attend church services, the influence of the Catholic religion in shaping the personalities of the questionnaire respondents cannot be overemphasized. The early contact with religious practices of varied nature, the type of teaching that they have received at the schools, and the political importance of church officials, all contribute to this influence. The laws prohibiting abortion and the restrictions on information about contraceptive practices are therefore not surprising. The position of this religion on questions of mating and reproduction was always heavily biased towards non-interventionism in natural processes.

## 2.2.4.2 Major Controversies

See 2.2.4.6 below.

## 2.2.4.3 National Expenditures for Medical Genetics

See 2.2.2 above.

## 2.2.4.4 Abortion Laws in Brazil

Abortion is prohibited by law, except in two situations, when the mother's life is in danger or in case of rape (article 128 of the Penal Code). There are heavy penalties for the woman who seeks abortion, as well as for the physician or midwife who performs it (one to three and one to four years in prison, respectively, articles 124 and 126 of the Penal Code). If the woman suffers injury or death, the penalties are increased by one-third and one-half, respectively (article 127 of the Penal Code). It should be mentioned, however, that illegal abortion clinics exist almost every-where.

## 2.2.4.5 Studies of Effectiveness of Genetic Services

See 2.2.1 above.

## 2.2.4.6 Need for New Laws

Most of the Brazilian legislation related to biological problems is out-of-date (review in Salzano 1983). At the moment the main discussion centers on the legalization of the abortion of malformed fetuses, but other questions also merit examination. Resistance against change, however, is strong, and we should remember that the Brazilian law permitting divorce was probably only approved because the president at that time was Protestant. But winds of change are blowing in our country now, with the elaboration of an entirely new Constitution; it is possible that in the wake of these changes important aspects of this obsolete legislation may be altered.

## 2.2.5 Ethical Issues and Future Trends

**The World**
The fantastic technical development of our time is freeing our species from the vagaries of the environment and creating the possibility of direct manipulation of our genetic material. The perspectives opened by this technical progress are enormous, but at the same time our responsibility is greatly increased, raising ethical problems that are the very subject of this book. This trend towards control of our reproduction will certainly continue, as well as an increased interdependence among nations in terms of economic resources. Together with these positive tendencies, however, negative ones exist, the most threatening for our genetic material being the increased exposure to nuclear and other types of industrial waste. We are therefore facing a future dominated by machines and technocrats, and it is important that we do not lose sight of the strictly human aspects of our existence.

**Brazil**

We can confidently expect that the benefits that come with industrialization will be extended to the underdeveloped areas of the North, Northeast, and Center-West regions, and an effort should be made to prevent its negative aspects from spreading to these areas. Progress in biotechnology may be important for the eventual control of the large number of endemic infectious diseases that still plague these places. With this control, attention could then be focused, with added emphasis, on the most prevalent hereditary diseases and congenital malformations, with the implementation of programs of prevention and treatment both *in utero* and after birth.

In cultural terms, everything should be done to avoid a reversal of the current trend towards a liberalization of our society, and to avoid a return of authoritarianism. Appropriate changes in the legislation and proper public education may help to avoid much suffering and unhappiness. Care should be taken, however, to prevent the new technological devices from being used in unethical ways. The words liberty and responsibility are closely interconnected, and advances towards more freedom should be paralleled by a corresponding sense of respect towards self and others. We close on an optimistic tone, hoping for a country in which the conditions for welfare will be more evenly distributed, irrespective of the sex, race, religion, or social class of its citizens.

# References

Azevêdo JL [1986] Desempenho e rumos da Genética no Brasil. Sociedade Brasileira de Genética, Ribeirão Preto

Baird PA [1980] La pratique de diagnostic prénatal à Vancouver. In: Le Diagnostic prénatal – Cahiers de Bioéthique 2. Les Presses de L'Université Laval, Québec, p 54

Beiguelman B [1981] A Genética Humana no Brasil. In: Ferri MG, Motoyama S (eds) História das Ciências no Brasil, Vol 2. Editora Pedagógica e Universitária e Editora da Universidade de São Paulo, p 273

Benn PA, Hsu LYF, Carlson A, Tannenbaum HL [1985] The centralized prenatal genetics screening program of New York City. III: The first 7,000 cases. Am J Med Genet 20:369-384

Bochkov NP [1979] Genetic counseling in the USSR. Progr Clin Biol Res 34: 31-40

Buchalter MS, Wannmacher CMD, Wajner M [1983] Tay-Sachs disease: screening and prevention program in Porto Alegre. Rev Bras Genet 6: 539-547

Castilla EE, Ferrari I, Monteleone Neto R, Parreiras IMO, Paz J, Pina Neto JM, Simões AL [1977] Levantamento dos casos atendidos no ambulatório de Genética Médica (HC-FMRPUSP) no período de 1974 a 1976. Cienc Cult (Suppl) 29: 717

Castro MPP, Mastrorocco DA, Castro BM, Mumford SD [1984] An innovative vasectomy program in São Paulo, Brazil. Intern Fam Plan Persp 10: 125-130

Collaborative Study [1975] Frequency of inborn errors of metabolism, especially PKU, in some representative newborn screening centers around the world. Humangenetik 30: 273-286

Czeizel A, Métneki J, Osztovicz M [1980] Cases of a genetic counselling clinic. Acta Paediatr Acad Sci Hung 21: 33-54

Da Cunha AB, Frota Pessoa O, Blumenschein A [1961] Atas do Primeiro Simpósio Sul-Americano de Genética. Faculdade de Filosofia, Ciências e Letras da Universidade de São Paulo, São Paulo

Duarte FAM [1984] Cadastro de geneticistas brasileiros. Sociedade Brasileira de Genética, Ribeirão Preto

Esperon LCM [1978] Erros inatos do metabolismo dos aminoácidos. Fundação Universidade do Rio Grande, Rio Grande

Figueiredo N [1977] Amazônia: tempo e gente. Prefeitura Municipal de Belém, Belém

Geiger CJ, Salzano FM, da Rocha FJ [1985] Who seeks genetic counseling and why - a Brazilian evaluation. Rev Bras Genet 8: 395-403

Gollop TR, Eigier A, Vianna-Morgante AM, Naccache N [1986] Chorionic villi sampling for early prenatal genetic diagnosis. Rev Bras Genet 9: 381-385

Gonçalves A [1981] Avaliação do desempenho de um ambulatório de genética em nosso meio. Rev Bras Clin Terap 10: 593-596

Greenberg CR, Hamerton JL [1980] Profil du diagnostic prénatal à Winnipeg. In: Le Diagnostic prénatal - Cahiers de Bioéthique 2. Les Presses de L'Université Laval, Québec, p 47

Harris DJ, Begleiter ML [1976] First year's experience in a new genetics clinic. Missouri Med 73: 271-274

Kanan JHC [1981] Comparação de diversas características biológicas entre duas amostras de malformados portadores de cariótipos normais e anormais e de seus familiares. Bachelor's Thesis, Universidade Federal do Rio Grande do Sul, Porto Alegre

Klein D, Wyss D [1977] Retrospective and follow-up study of approximately 1,000 genetic consultations. J Génét Hum 25: 47-57

Landmann J [1985] A ética médica sem máscara. Editora Guanabara, Rio de Janeiro

Lemoine VR [1984] Genética. VI Congreso Latinoamericano de Genética y I Congreso Venezolano de Genética. Asociación Venezolana de Genética, Maracaibo

Magnelli NC [1977] Evaluation of seven years of activity at a genetic counselling clinic. Proc III Latin American Congr Genet : 153-159

Mattevi MS, Salzano FM [1982] Effect of chromosome changes on body and mind development. Adv St Birth Defects 5:67-87

Medeiros-Neto G, Maciel RMB, Halpern A [1986] Iodine deficiency and congenital hypothyroidism. Aché, São Paulo

Merrick TW [1983] Fertility and family planning in Brazil. Intern Fam Plan Persp 9: 110-119

Naoum PC [1985] Grupo cooperativo em hemoglobinopatias. Hemo Antropo 11: 1-20

Naoum PC, Mattos LC, Curi PR [1984] Prevalence and geographic distribution of abnormal hemoglobins in the State of São Paulo, Brazil. Bull Pan Am Health Organ 18: 127-138

Nazareth HRS, Pinto W Jr, Andrade JAD [1981] Diagnóstico prénatal de aberrações cromossômicas. Primeira experiência brasileira. Rev Bras Genet 4: 459-470

Ramalho AS [1986] As hemoglobinopatias hereditárias. Um problema de saúde pública no Brasil. Sociedade Brasileira de Genética, Ribeirão Preto

Ramalho AS, Magna LA, Costa FF, Grotto HZW [1985] Talassemia menor: um problema de saúde pública no Brasil? Rev Bras Genet 8: 747-754

Ribeiro D [1977] As Américas e a civilização. Vozes, Petrópolis

Rocha E Jr [1985] Ética médica. Fórum nacional. Academia Nacional de Medicina, Rio de Janeiro

Rodeck CH [1984] Obstetric techniques in prenatal diagnosis. In: Rodeck CH, Nicolaides KH (eds) Prenatal diagnosis. John Wiley & Sons, Chichester, p 15

Rudd N, Doran T [1980] Le programme de diagnostic génétique prénatal de Toronto. In: Le Diagnostic prénatal - Cahiers de Bioétique 2. Les Presses de L'Université Laval, Québec, p 40

Salzano FM (1979a) Abnormal hemoglobin studies and counseling in Brasil. Proc First Intern Conf Sickle Cell Disease: a World Health Problem: 67-69

Salzano FM (1979b) Estudo sobre a evolução biológica no Brasil. In: Ferri MG, Motoyama S (eds) História das ciências no Brasil, Vol 1. Editora Pedagógica e Universitária e Editora da Universidade de São Paulo, São Paulo, p 241

Salzano FM [1983] A Genética e a lei. Aplicações à Medicina Legal e à Biologia Social. TA Queiroz, Editor e Editora da Universidade de São Paulo, São Paulo

Salzano FM [1985] Incidence, effects, and management of sickle cell disease in Brazil. Am J Ped Hematol/Oncol 7: 240-244

Salzano FM [1987] Brazil. In: Schwidetzky I (ed) Rassengeschichte der Menschheit. Vol. 12, R Oldenbourg, München, p 137

Salzano FM, Freire-Maia N [1970] Problems in human biology. A study of Brazilian populations. Wayne State University Press, Detroit.

Sanford H [1985] Demografia e saúde - aspectos políticos. In: Fonseca AS (ed) Demografia e saúde. Forum nacional. Academia Nacional de Medicina, Rio de Janeiro, p 18

Simpson NE [1975] Experiences of a genetic counselling clinic in Kingston, Ontario. Can J Publ Health 66: 375–378

Wajner M, Wannmacher CMD, Gaidzinski D, Dutra-Filho CS, Buchalter MS, Giugliani R [1986] Detection of inborn errors of metabolism in patients of pediatric intensive care units of Porto Alegre, Brazil: comparison of the prevalence of such disturbances in a selected and an unselected sample. Rev Bras Genet 9: 331–340

Wannmacher CMD, Wajner M, Giugliani R, Giugliani ERJ, Costa MG, Giugliani MCK [1982] Detection of metabolic disorders among high risk patients. Rev Bras Genet 5: 187–194

Witt RR, da Rocha FJ [1982] Aspectos do comportamento dos pacientes submetidos a aconselhamento genético entre 1980 e 1981. Rev Gaúcha Enf 3: 185–195

Zago MA, Costa FF [1985] Hereditary haemoglobin disorders in Brazil. Trans Royal Soc Trop Med Hyg 79: 385–388

Zago MA, Costa FF, Tone LG, Bottura C [1983] Hereditary hemoglobin disorders in a Brazilian population. Hum Hered 33: 125–129

# Books on Ethics and Medical Genetics Published in Brazil

Fernandes PSL [1972] Aborto e infanticídio. Sugestões literárias, São Paulo

Landmann J [1985] A ética médica sem máscara. Editora Guanabara, Rio de Janeiro

Opitz, JM [1984] Tópicos recentes de Genética Clínica. Sociedade Brasileira de Genética, Ribeirão Preto

Rocha E Jr [1985] Ética médica. Fórum nacional. Academia Nacional de Medicina, Rio de Janeiro

Salzano FM [1979] Você e sua herança. Civilização Brasileira, Rio de Janeiro

Salzano FM [1983] A Genética e a Lei. Aplicações à Medicina Legal e à Biologia Social. TA Queiroz, Editor e Editora da Universidade de São Paulo, São Paulo

Vieira S, Hossne WS [1987] Experimentação com seres humanos. Editora Moderna, São Paulo

## 2.3 Ethics and Medical Genetics in Canada

D.J.Roy and J.G.Hall

## 2.3.1 Medical Genetics in Canada

Medical genetics services in Canada are part of the Universal Health Care System, which provides hospital and physician insurance to all citizens. Health care funding is administered provincially, with each province having a slightly different system. Each province contributes funding, and in addition Federal funds are distributed to each of Canada's ten provinces, that is, British Columbia, Alberta, Saskatchewan, Manitoba, Ontario, Québec, New Brunswick, Nova Scotia, Prince Edward Island, and Newfoundland. The two Canadian territories of Yukon and North West Territories also receive federal funding and provide most medical care locally, but refer patients to the other provinces for specialized care, such as genetic services.

Even though Canada is the world's second largest country in area, there are only 25.5 million inhabitants, with most of the population living in towns and cities close to the US-Canadian border. Much of Canada is very sparsely populated. Seventy-six percent live in urban areas [10]. Thus one of the real challenges for the Canadian health care system is to provide equivalent services to all citizens.

### 2.3.1.1 Scope of the Problem

**Number of Births Per Year**
In 1985, there were 379,480 births, only a small increase from ten years previously, when there were 359,328 births. The standard of health appears to have improved in the last 10 years, since life expectancy has risen from 69 to 70 years for Canadian men and 76 to 77 years for Canadian women, and infant mortality has decreased from 17.5 deaths per thousand live births in 1971 to 9.6 deaths per thousand live births in 1981. The neonatal mortality rate, which was 12.4 deaths per thousand live births in 1971, declined to 6.2 deaths per thousand in 1981.

**Incidence of Genetic Diseases and Congenital Malformations**
There is a birth defects reporting system, run by the Federal government. The information is sketchy, however, since it is largely dependent on birth and death certificates. From that system, congenital anomalies are estimated to occur in 2% of births. In British Columbia there is a population registry of birth defects, genetic diseases, and chronic handicapping conditions. It has over 60 sources of ascertainment, so that an individual may be ascertained at any time after birth. This provides much more accurate data, which indicate that 5% of the population have a congenital anomaly or genetic disease [2].

## 2.3.1.2  Organization of Clinical Genetics Services

### Description of Centers

Each province provides medical genetics services through designated centers. New Brunswick, Nova Scotia and Prince Edward Island share a single center. All medical genetic centers or clinical genetic units are in tertiary care facilities. There are from one to eight centers per province (except as mentioned in the Maritime provinces). The organization of clinical genetics services is slightly different from province to province. The Canadian College of Medical Geneticists (CCMG) has exerted a major influence on the standards of care, training, and quality of services. Centers may apply to the College for evaluation of training and service programs. Cytogenetic laboratories are tested for proficiency by a program established in Ontario. Genetics centers exist in British Columbia at Vancouver and Victoria; in Alberta at Calgary and Edmonton; in Saskatchewan at Saskatoon; in Manitoba at Winnipeg; in Ontario at Hamilton, Kingston, London, Ottawa, Toronto (Hospital for Sick Children, Toronto General Hospital, Surrey Place), Credit Valley in Mississauga, Oshawa, and North York; in Québec at McGill University, Université de Montréal, Université Laval and Université de Sherbrooke); in Newfoundland at St. John, and in Nova Scotia at Halifax.

### Services Offered

All centers provide general genetic counseling and some prenatal diagnostic services. The extent of other services, however, varies a great deal. For instance, in the area of prenatal diagnosis, all centers provide amniocentesis. Some have very sophisticated ultrasound prenatal diagnosis. Two centers have fetoscopy available. Eight centers can provide chorionic villus sampling and are taking part in the Canadian collaborative study to assess the relative risks of CVS as compared to amniocentesis.

### Investigation of Genetic Disorders

All provinces have newborn screening programs, but again there is variation in terms of the tests that are routinely performed. PKU and hypothyroid screening are performed in all provinces. Maternal serum alpha-fetoprotein (MSAFP) evaluation is available upon request in all provinces, but general population screening programs of MSAFP for all pregnancies are present only in Manitoba and Ontario. There is some concern that proper funding for the whole program be developed before it is begun in other provinces. In 1983, the Society of Obstetricians and Gynecologists of Canada (SOGC), the Canadian Pediatric Society (CPS), and the Canadian College of Medical Geneticists (CCMG) made joint recommendations and guidelines for indications for prenatal diagnosis and recommendations for those individuals who should provide prenatal diagnostic services [21].

### Genetic Counseling

Genetic health care services vary from province to province. As mentioned previously, counseling services are primarily available for the pediatric age group and pregnant women. Many centers, however, are beginning to develop adult genetic services. Most are considered regional service centers. Three provinces have active outreach programs with clinics around the province and another has a network for treatment of metabolic disorders. Most hospital-based clinical services provide ward consultations. Many centers work with specialty clinics such as cystic fibrosis, neural tube defects, lipid disease, etc. Most tertiary care centers provide teratogen information, although only several centers have specifically organized a teratogen information service.

### The Québec Network of Genetic Medicine

Four regional centers, each affiliated with a medical faculty of a Québec university, make up the Québec Network of Genetic Medicine, established in October 1969 by a group of researchers [5, 6, 19]. These centers are Hôpital Sainte-Justine, affiliated with Université de Montréal, Montreal Children's Hospital, affiliated with McGill University, the Centre Hospitalier de l'Université Laval (CHUL), and Centre Hospitalier Universitaire de Sherbrooke (CHUS).

The Network offers blood neonatal screening for congenital hypothyroidism, hereditary tyrosinemia and phenylketonuria, urinary screening for enzymatic disorders and abnormalities of membrane transport, prenatal diagnosis, and carrier screening in high risk populations.

Up to the beginning of April 1983, the blood neonatal screening program had found 48 cases of PKU and 67 cases of tyrosinemia in 1,054,950 newborns screened, and 197 cases of congenital hypothyroidism in 915,112 screened newborns. In the prenatal diagnosis program, 150 chromosomal abnormalities, 230 neural tube defects, and 96 other abnormalities were detected in 9,188 amniocenteses performed up to March 31, 1983 [5].

The program for carrier screening in high-risk populations is centralized at Montreal Children's Hospital. The program covers Tay-Sachs and thalassemia, is focused on high schools, and offers opportunities for geneticists to participate in the continuing education of teachers [5, 20]. From July 1972 to April of 1983, 913 Tay-Sachs carriers were found as a result of 17,575 tests performed. From 1979 to April 1983, 7,252 thalassemia carrier tests led to the detection 430 beta-thalassemia carriers, 25 alpha-thalassemia carriers, and 9 other variants [5].

### Laboratories

In general, laboratory services related to medical genetics are provided through the departments of pathology or laboratory medicine in Canada. A few chromosome laboratories are in departments of pediatrics and genetics or in research laboratories. In general, as a new technique develops, it is first developed as a research technique within a department or division of Human or Medical Genetics and then it is transferred to a service laboratory.

There are now four kinds of laboratory functions available and associated with genetic services in Canada: metabolic laboratories, cytogenetic laboratories, embryopathology laboratories, and DNA service laboratories. All tertiary care centers now have both metabolic and cytogenetic laboratories available to them. There has been an attempt to network between laboratories so there is less duplication of specialized techniques requiring special expertise.

The volume of various laboratory services provided varies greatly from center to center. Two centers have an embryopathology service. Six centers now provide

DNA linkage studies as a service item. At this time, most DNA studies are done in research labs or sent to large service labs in the United States. Appropriate mechanisms for funding of this new service are not yet in place.

**Volume of Service**
A survey of numbers of families seen and laboratory tests provided to medical genetic patients has not been done since 1979. An informal survey, however, revealed that all centers are active and growing. The growth rate has been quite different between centers, with some centers having grown approximately 50% in the last seven years while other centers have grown up to 500%. The patient-family load also varies between centers, from 100 families to 7,000 families per center per year. For instance, very rough estimates of the number of patients (families) seen from all the genetic centers in Ontario for 1985–1986 indicate that 3,000 families were seen as outpatients for genetic counseling, 700 were seen in outreach clinics, 600 were seen as ward consults, and 4,600 were seen for prenatal diagnosis. From British Columbia for 1985–1986, 1,200 families were seen as outpatients for genetic counseling, 160 in outreach clinics, 300 as ward consults, 2,600 for prenatal diagnosis and 500 in special-disease oriented clinics.

## 2.3.1.3 Prenatal Diagnosis

**Description of Services**
The indications for prenatal diagnosis developed by the SOGC, CPS and CCMG in 1983 have been followed almost completely in all centers since that time. The CCMG has also developed a Code of Ethics (Appendix) for its members in the practice of medical genetics [4]. This provides for exchanges of information under appropriate confidentiality guidelines, among medical geneticists from Canadian centers, in order to provide appropriate care to family members who have come to a particular center.

**CVS**
With regard to provision of CVS: five centers in Canada are actively involved in the collaborative study to determine the relative risk of CVS versus amniocentesis for prenatal diagnosis. Three other centers have just joined the trial. In Canada, CVS is only offered to women with appropriate indications for prenatal diagnosis (primarily advanced maternal age, i.e., maternal age 35 at the time of delivery), who are willing to take part in a randomized trial. It is anticipated that this study will be finished in early 1988. At that time the role of CVS will be assessed as a service option for prenatal diagnosis in Canadian centers that have gone through the appropriate preparatory processes. There have been established strict obstetric and laboratory guidelines for developing expertise in order to provide CVS as a service.

### 2.3.1.4  Cost-Benefit of Early Diagnosis and Genetic Counseling

Cost-benefit studies have been done on programs for prenatal detection of Down syndrome, neural tube defects, and for alpha-fetoprotein screening [16, 17, 18]. This has allowed more rational planning of service programs in these areas. These studies have been possible because of the availability of data from the British Columbia Health Surveillance Registry, which means the number of affected individuals born can be determined.

A cost-benefit analysis of the Québec Network's thalassemia carrier screening program demonstrated that the total direct cost per case prevented is less than the cost of a single year of treatment for an affected individual [6]. A cost-benefit analysis of the Québec Network of Genetic Medicine as a whole concluded that the cumulative net economic benefit derived from the Network's implementation was $29.8 million for the period 1969–1985 [13].

The Québec Network of Genetic Medicine has demonstrated that its services are both socially advantageous and financially profitable. A cost-benefit analysis concluded that the Network yielded net benefits worth at least $30 million.

This cost-benefit study merits special attention. It was after the introduction of screening and treatment programs for hypothyroidism in 1974 that the Network's computed annual benefits exceeded its costs. The study, then, indicates that forecasts about the profitability of a service are likely to be erroneous if they do not include potential benefits that may accrue from innovative screening programs for other congenital disorders. The study also suggests that administration of the Network by active researchers may favor timely introduction of new screening and treatment programs, and cut the losses in net benefits that would result from unnecessary delay in implementing innovations [6].

### 2.3.1.5  Therapeutic Abortion

Statistics on therapeutic abortions performed are available from Statistics Canada. In 1975 there were 359,323 births and 49,399 abortions, giving a rate of 13.7 abortions per 100 live births. In 1984, there were 377,031 births and 62,291 abortions, giving a rate of 16.5 abortions per 100 live births. Between 1978 and 1981 the ratio of abortions/live births was consistently above 17.5. Thus currently the ratio may be increasing.

There are no exact or accurate figures for the number of "genetic" abortions for all of Canada. They are available, however, for some years in some provinces. In British Columbia (which has the highest abortion rate in Canada), for instance, during the year 1984, there were approximately 43,911 live births and 11,449 abortions, of which 35 terminations of pregnancy were related to known genetic problems diagnosed in the fetus. Thus less than 0.3% of terminations of pregnancies in British Columbia in 1984 were related to genetic indications. During that year there had been almost 2,000 genetic prenatal evaluations or diagnostic studies done as service in British Columbia, 2.5% of which were positive or showed abnormalities present.

Over a period of three years, 1983–1985, 116 pregnancies were terminated after 8,876 prenatal diagnoses performed in four of the centers in the province of Ontario. This number does not account for all terminations of pregnancy following prenatal diagnosis in the province during this period, but does indicate the order of magnitude of therapeutic abortions performed for genetic reasons [Hutton EM, Neidhardt A, Simpson N, Uchida I 1986, personal communication].

## 2.3.2 Ethical Problems: Results of the Survey

### 2.3.2.1 Genetic Counseling: The Ethics of Communication

Genetic counseling, though based upon methods and procedures designed to deliver a correct diagnosis, is essentially a process of communication about the occurrence or risk of occurrence of a genetic disorder in a family [1]. The survey questionnaire reflected the importance of this definition. In at least 12 instances, the primary ethical issues presented in the survey's 14 cases and 11 questions about screening and counseling focused on the disclosure of information about genetic disorders. The content, confidentiality, or mode of communication in genetic counseling was the core of the ethical problem posed in these instances. We have formulated three general questions to organize our presentation of the Canadian responses to the survey questions dealing with the ethics of communication in genetic counseling.

**Should medical genetics tell the whole truth, and nothing but the truth, to those who have a right to information about a genetic disorder in a family?**

The CCMG instructs its fellows that they should "not withhold information from patients unless this can be fully justified as being in the best interests of the patient [4]." The 47 Canadian medical geneticists responding to the survey questionnaire exhibited varying strengths of consensus about how this guideline should be interpreted and implemented in practical situations.

The respondents' strongest consensus was in favor of giving parents a thorough explanation when the results of prenatal testing indicate the possibility, but fail to offer a confirmed diagnosis, that a fetal anomaly is present. Three of the survey's cases raised this issue. When elevated maternal serum alpha-fetoprotein values indicated the possibility of a small neural tube defect, 94% of Canadian geneticists agreed that parents should be told that the test results conflict and that no directive advice should be given about termination or carrying to term. In the two other cases, one dealing with colleague disagreement about the possibility of trisomy 13 mosaicism, the other with new and controversial interpretations suggesting the possibility of Down syndrome, the consensus in favor of full disclosure of colleague disagreement was 66% and the consensus in favor of full disclosure of new interpretations, without giving advice, was 83%. Canadian respondents universally rejected communication options that amounted to lying or concealing the truth. Honesty, respect for the parents' right and responsibility to make their own reproductive decisions, and the ethos, or fundamental assumption, of non-directive counseling were the reasons cited most frequently in support of full disclosure in these three cases.

There was a considerable measure of hesitancy to take the initiative in giving complete information to parents of a Down syndrome child, when one parent has been identified as the carrier of a balanced translocation. Nearly 40% of Canadian medical geneticists would rather invite or allow parents to indicate whether they want to know who the carrier is. One statement of reasons in support of this approach characterized the relationship of the genetic counselor to parents as "I am, in a sense, their servant."

The parents' need for complete information in order to plan their own families, and to help potentially affected relatives to plan theirs, was prominent among the reasons put forth by the 60% of the respondents who would take the lead in disclosing full information to parents without being asked. One observation emphasized the generally poor quality of genetics education in this country. For this reason, counselors should not be overly confident that parents understand the genetic and reproductive implications of balanced translocation sufficiently to take the lead in asking the appropriate questions.

One respondent who chose the option of discussing disclosure options with the couple before drawing blood samples for karyotyping emphasized the importance of preparatory counseling. The counseling conversation is much more complex in reality than the survey's brief wording of the answer options would indicate. The important notion is that the genetic counselor often has to help the couple go through a lot of thinking before eliciting their choice of disclosure options.

The principle of full disclosure meets a challenge when the truth may psychologically disturb or confuse the person seeking counsel, or even disrupt this person's self-image and life. Slightly less than a third of Canadian respondents (32%) turned to the exception clause of the CCMG guidelines on full disclosure when presented with the case of a woman found to be chromosomally male (46, XY) after tests to diagnose the causes of her infertility. Though all these respondents would offer the woman an explanation of her infertility and would avoid using the term "chromosomally male," some would ease her gently into an understanding that a person can be a woman even if she does not have the usual 46, XX karyotype. These respondents were primarily concerned to reassure the woman about her femaleness and to prevent psychological disruption. There was a moderate consensus (68%) in favor of full disclosure. This approach was motivated, in part, by the fear that the woman would suffer greater harm were she later to learn the truth from others, possibly in circumstances less protective of her feelings than the counseling context. Several respondents observed that the decision on full or partial disclosure in such a case is contingent upon how well the counselor knows the patient. Others qualified their choice of the full disclosure option as valid only for an educated, intelligent woman. They would otherwise tailor the information to fit the woman's capacity to understand.

Nearly all the respondents, whichever option they chose, emphasized the need to prepare the woman adequately for reception of the doubly painful information about her inability to have a child and her chromosomal anomaly. None of the respondents chose the untruthful option of saying the cause of infertility was unknown.

## Are genetic counselors ever justified in disclosing confidential patient information to third parties?

The CCMG guidelines enjoin College fellows to "keep information obtained from patients in confidence unless written permission for release has been given, or unless it can be shown this is likely to produce significant detrimental effects to the health of other individuals, currently or in the future [4]."

Canadian respondents were strongly in agreement (87%) that they would tell only the mother what laboratory tests reveal about a child's parentage when the child has an autosomal recessive disorder and the father has been found not to be a carrier. One respondent justified this approach as "likely to be least harmful and disruptive and does not involve false statements." Many believed it to be the mother's responsibility, not the genetic counselor's, to inform the husband, if necessary, that he is not the child's biological father. Avoiding a possible marriage break-up ranked very prominently among the reasons given to justify this approach. One respondent questioned the realism of the case presented. How likely is it that half the siblings would be illegitimate?

Would Canadian geneticists divulge information either to siblings of a person with Huntington disease, or to relatives of a woman with a child having hemophilia A, if these persons refuse permission for disclosure? Canadian respondents presented a wide divergence of views on the proper approach to take in each of these situations. Over a fourth (28%) of the respondents would protect confidentiality in the Huntington disease case, and nearly as many (26%) would do so in the hemophilia A case. Seven (15%) and 8 (17%), respectively, would send the information, and transfer the disclosure decision, to the referring physician. In each of the two cases, 32% would disclose the information to siblings or relatives, even if they did not ask. An additional 25% of respondents in each case would inform siblings or relatives *only* if these persons requested the information. In each case, 24 respondents (not the same persons) were prepared, with varied qualifications of approach, to utilize the exception clause of the CCMG guideline for confidentiality (see opening paragraph of this section).

## Should genetic counselors be directive or supportive when communicating with patients?

The CCMG advises its fellows to "provide supportive rather than directive advice to patients in regard to reproductive decisions [4]." Canadian respondents demonstrated moderate to strong consensus in support of non-directive counseling regarding the various options open to maternal and paternal carriers of the tuberous sclerosis gene. One respondent's rationale for this non-directive approach was the succinct statement: "Families require information, not advice, regarding family planning. They should feel that the choice is theirs." The strongest consensus, 86% for both male and female carriers, was for explaining risks and problems associated with the option of simply taking one's chances. Two innovative options available to a woman with tuberous sclerosis, however, appeared to be problematic to a number of Canadian respondents. Slightly more than half (51%) the responding geneticists would discuss the option of surrogate motherhood only if asked to do so; 37% would present it as a possibility, and 12% would not discuss it at all. Though 59% would take the lead in raising the option of in vitro fertilization with a donated ovum, 38% would discuss this option only if the parents indicated an interest.

Almost all Canadian medical geneticists would be non-directive in telling parents about a diagnosis that the fetus has either Turner syndrome (45, X) or a 47, XYY chromosome anomaly. They would give parents complete information about the disorder, its prognosis, and the likely future state of the child, and about problems and decisions the parents may have to confront in the future. Slightly more than 25% of respondents, 12 in the 47, XYY case and 13 in the 45, X case, indicated that they would give complete information and also describe the emotional difficulties that may be associated with a choice of abortion. One respondent believed that these possible difficulties associated with termination are an integral part of the complete information that genetic counselors owe parents in these cases. One geneticist supported the more strictly non-directive approach because parents should bring "their own biases, not the counselor's" into their reproductive decision.

Canadian medical geneticists were generally very reluctant to advise parents about the reproductive decisions they should make. Over 94% of respondents believed that the appropriate professional behavior in genetic counseling was to provide information concerning available options and support parents in their reproductive decisions, but not to advise them about what these decisions should be. The strong consensus in support of this concept correlates positively with the very strong Canadian views on the absolutely essential character of two counseling goals. Helping clients to understand options, then helping them to cope with their decisions, were judged as absolutely essential goals by 98% and 87% of respondents respectively.

## 2.3.2.2  Prenatal Diagnosis: Ethics of Access

The SOGC recommendations present a detailed indications policy for prenatal diagnosis. The recommendations do have a bearing on three cases in the survey questionnaire, since they specifically stipulate that maternal anxiety and prenatal determination of fetal sex for non-medical reasons are conditions for which genetic amniocentesis is not indicated; and prior commitment to termination of pregnancy following the diagnosis of fetal abnormality should *not* be a prerequisite for prenatal diagnosis [21].

### Refusal to Terminate Pregnancy

Access to prenatal diagnosis in Canada is generally not contingent upon a woman's prior agreement to utilize termination of pregnancy if tests indicate that a fetal anomaly is present. Eighty-nine percent of Canadian respondents indicated that they would perform the diagnosis or provide a referral in the case of a 42-year-old pregnant woman, already mother of a Down syndrome child, who is opposed to abortion. Respect for parental autonomy was most prominent among the reasons given to support this approach. However, 16 of the 40 respondents agreeing to perform the diagnosis also mentioned that the parents might change their minds about abortion when confronted with the reality of a Down syndrome diagnosis. They should have this opportunity to change their minds.

### Maternal Anxiety as Indication

There was neither strong nor moderate consensus among the Canadian respondents about performing prenatal diagnostic testing when maternal anxiety is the only indication. Over half (55%) would accept the woman's request, and an additional 15% would give a referral, though most would do so only after first attempting to dissuade her. The reasons given to justify this departure from the CCMG guidelines include the "greatest happiness" principle, respect for autonomy, and reduction of anxiety. One respondent considered irrational anxiety to be "a medical condition that justifies a remedy – even though potentially harmful." Another respondent was "glad to some extent no regulations preclude offering her the test."

### Sex Selection

Almost a third (30%) of Canadian respondents would perform prenatal diagnosis, and 53% would refuse, when the parents' sole objective, selecting the sex of the child, is unrelated to medical conditions in the fetus. Another 17% would refer the couple to another unit prepared to offer prenatal diagnosis for sex selection.

Reasons cited to justify accepting the couple's request clustered around two poles: first, an emphasis on the duty to be non-directive, captured in the phrase, "The ethical position of an information provider does not justify refusal"; second, the chance to save a life the parents seem determined to destroy if they do not receive information as to the fetal sex. One expression of this view stated: "It is better on balance to take the chance that the fetus will be male and be allowed to survive than the loss of fetuses of both sexes if the test is refused."

Refusals to perform prenatal diagnosis for sex were generally based on professional considerations. The central view was: sex, as such, is not an abnormality and its diagnosis for reasons totally unrelated to medical indication does not fall within the mandate and scope of genetic counseling and prenatal diagnosis. A consequentialist consideration was also cited to stress that granting such requests in a society that does not accept abortion on demand could "create a public outcry which may result in withdrawal of services for families at genetic risk."

This issue is obviously controversial. There was a strong consensus among Canadian medical geneticists, however, that this issue should not be a focus of major concern in Canada over the next decade. Nearly 55% of Canadian respondents ranked this issue in tenth place, and 32% ranked it ninth on a 1 to 10 order of priority concerns for the future.

### Commercial Laboratory Involvement in Prenatal Diagnosis

Canadian medical geneticists were strongly (77%) in favor of regulations to prohibit a commercial laboratory from performing prenatal diagnosis routinely if the laboratory was not associated with a medical genetics unit to interpret results. Seventy-nine percent of Canadian respondents were against regulations governing the access of parents who will not terminate pregnancy to the prenatal diagnostic services of such a laboratory; 63% were against regulations when maternal anxiety alone is the indication and 34% were against regulations when sex choice is the couple's reason for seeking prenatal testing.

## 2.3.2.3 Screening: Ethical Issues

The guidelines of the CCMG advise its fellows that one of their responsibilities to society is to "encourage the establishment of screening programs for the detection of specific genetic disorders in population groups." The guidelines also specify three conditions. Such screening programs should be "justified by the frequency of the disorder, as well as the availability of a management approach and the related economic resources [4]." The guidelines offer no specific counsel on the four issues raised in the survey questionnaire.

### Genetic Screening for Occupational Susceptibility

There was moderate agreement (73%) that screening of workers for alpha-1-anti-trypsin deficiency should be voluntary. Over a fourth of the respondents, however, (27%) were in favor of mandatory screening.

Protection of the individual from avoidable serious illness, and of industry and society from avoidable health care costs were the principal reasons offered in support of mandatory testing. Two of the eleven respondents in favor of mandatory screening, and one in favor of voluntary screening, emphasized the industry's responsibility to offer all workers a clean and safe environment.

Respect for worker autonomy and freedom of choice, and the fear of discrimination based on genotype, were the main reasons given to support voluntary screening. One respondent argued: "This case carries with it the possibility of much more than worker protection. It may obstruct employment, deny health and life insurance and socially stigmatize 'deficient' subjects." Another respondent believed that most workers, if properly educated, would want to be tested.

The Canadian respondents varied considerably in their views about who should have access to information obtained from genetic screening for occupational susceptibility to health hazards in the working environment. All supported worker access, and 71% were in favor of employer access if workers consent. Only one of the 47 Canadian medical geneticists would refuse access of a worker's physician to screening results, but 62% would permit the physician to receive this information only if the worker consents. A five to four ratio, approximately, characterized the respondents' views about whether a worker's life insurer or health insurer should have access with the worker's consent or no access at all. For every four respondents who were against any access at all, five were in favor, provided that the worker approved. Over half of the Canadian geneticists, 56%, would permit health department access if the worker approved; 26% thought that the government should have no access at all, and 18% thought that the government should have automatic access.

### Pre-symptomatic Testing for Huntington Disease

The survey focussed attention on the scope of access to results of an accurate pre-symptomatic test for Huntington disease, a test hypothetically applicable to all families.

The Canadian medical geneticists exhibited neither strong nor moderate consensus on any of the response options. The strongest Canadian consensus centered on the person at risk for Huntington disease. This person may not want to know the test results or may want to determine the moment for being informed. Sixty-seven percent of Canadian respondents expressed the need to respect this preference. The request (53%) or approval (14%) of such persons should be a condition of their being told about the results.

Schools should not have access to test results, according to 60% of respondents. The other 40% would grant access only if the person at risk approved. There was no consensus, but rather a near 50–50 split in each instance, among Canadian respondents as to whether medical insurers, life insurers, and employers should have no access at all or access only with approval of the person tested.

About half of the respondents would grant access to a spouse or to relatives only on the condition that the person tested approved this (49% for the spouse, 55% in the case of relatives). Forty-four percent thought that a spouse, and 35% thought that relatives should be informed independently of the tested person's approval. Seven and 10% respectively thought that spouse or relatives should have no access at all, even with patient approval. One should mention that the reasons respondents gave to justify their choice of answers suggest considerable agreement among Canadians on the ethical need of a spouse, as bearing co-responsibility for reproduction, to know about such test results.

### Screening for Cystic Fibrosis Carriers

Canadian responses ranged across 9 of the 12 available questionnaire answers to the question, to whom in the population, and at what age, should the carrier test for cystic fibrosis *first* be given. However, 87% of the responses split in nearly 50–50 clusters at both ends of the proposed age spectrum. Forty-five percent thought that the test should be given to all newborns, either by law (18%) or only with parental consent (27%). Administering the test to persons over 18 years of age, by consent, was favored by 42% of Canadian respondents, including 16% choosing the restriction "of Caucasian descent who request it."

Most Canadian medical geneticists (80%) supported the view that participation in carrier screening for cystic fibrosis should be voluntary, not imposed by law. While some cited cost-effectiveness to justify the restriction to Caucasians, others referred to possible discrimination, or the semblance of discrimination and possible resulting political controversy, as reasons for rejecting this restriction. Differing views about the benefits of early treatment also influenced the respondent's choice of age group for the test.

It is perhaps worthwhile to emphasize that these answers were given before cystic fibrosis DNA linkage had been established, making it possible for some families with an affected child to predict which individuals in the family are likely to be carriers. It would be interesting to see whether the same questions would now evoke different responses from the same geneticists.

## 2.3.3 Consensus and Variation in Canada

See 2.3.2 above.


## 2.3.4 Cultural Context of Medical Genetics in Canada

Canada is a country in which consensus is difficult to achieve and is not always desired. A wide spectrum of ethnic, cultural, and religious diversity, and notable regional and provincial differences set the context for reproductive ethics. The province of Québec, for instance, possesses a system of law and a culture quite different from those of the other provinces. Some provinces, such as Newfoundland and Prince Edward Island, have small populations and tend to be culturally and morally more homogeneous than the larger, more cosmopolitan provinces. As a general rule, Canada takes pride in respecting these differences, and in preserving diversity of custom and thought. This is reflected by a strong desire on the part of medical geneticists to provide information to families and allow them to make their own decisions.

With the exception of quite general guidelines (see the Appendix), centralized and uniform policies do not characterize the Canadian approach to the ethical issues of medical genetics. Moreover, an important number of medical geneticists appear quite reluctant to be categorized.

Although a neighbor, Canada is quite different culturally from the United States. The strong emphasis in Canada on multiculturalism (versus a melting pot) and the existence of universal health care reflect fundamental differences in the values of the society. Canada is often slower to implement new developments, but usually provides service to all in a cost-effective and rational way.


### 2.3.4.1 Sources of Challenge and Support

In general, there has been reasonable support from various provincial health ministries for genetic services, particularly prenatal diagnostic services and outreach clinic programs. However, the cost of these services may provide an obstacle in the future to their provision, since in the present climate of economic constraint, it is difficult to put in place new services. Sometimes private foundations have stepped in. For instance, the Huntington Disease Foundation has developed a DNA bank for their members and has two centers across Canada to provide service for Huntington families. In reality, however, it is appropriate that such services should be developed and provided by health care ministry funds.

The groups in support of mentally retarded individuals in Canada have recently been successful in preserving various rights of retarded individuals, particularly with regard to sterilization procedures. In this regard it is important to note that the Supreme Court of Canada declared in its judgment of October 23, 1986, in Re: "Eve," that sterilization for non-therapeutic purposes of persons unable to consent is not covered by the *parens patriae* jurisdiction of the courts in Canada.

## 2.3.4.2  Major Controversies

Perhaps the sharpest controversy in Canadian medical genetics has to do with lack of financial support to provide care to all individuals. At this time medical genetics care is provided in larger tertiary care centers, in urban areas, and service is not easily accessible for rural segments of the population. With the increasing numbers of people seeking genetics services, a significant increase in funding will be necessary. On the other hand, most provinces are developing comprehensive outreach programs.

## 2.3.4.3  National Expenditures

In 1984, 8.5% of Canada's national product, or $1,450 per capita ($US1,115), was spent on health care [10]. This is a grand total of $36.3 billion ($US27.9 billion) spent in 1984 on health care in Canada. A very small fraction of this amount was spent on medical genetic services. Accurate information on the exact national expenditure is not available, but a fairly accurate estimate can be made for some provinces. In British Columbia in 1984, less than $1 million was spent on genetic evaluation, diagnostic and counseling services. This figure does not include laboratory costs and procedure costs. In a province of 2.8 million people, however, it means that less than $0.35 per person was spent on provision of medical genetic professional services.

## 2.3.4.4  Abortion Laws

Until recently, abortion was legally approved in Canada under conditions defined in the 1969 amendment to the Criminal Code. On indication that continuance of pregnancy would likely endanger a woman's health or life, Section 251 of the Code recognized abortion as legally permitted, provided it were done in an accredited hospital. The Code also required prior approval of the abortion by majority vote of a therapeutic abortion committee composed of not less than three physicians, exclusive of the physician who conducts the termination of pregnancy. However, Canadian abortion law did not require hospitals to establish therapeutic abortion committees; it did not recognize fetal abnormality as an acceptable indication for abortion, nor did it set any gestational limits for a legally permitted abortion.

   In practice, the possibility of abortion provided for in the Canadian Criminal Code was quite illusory for many women [7]. The law faced numerous challenges over the years, particularly from Dr. Henry Morgentaler, who set up abortion clinics outside of accredited hospitals. Dr. Morgentaler was indicted several times and several times acquitted in trials by jury. A recent indictment was appealed to the Supreme Court of Canada. After a year and a half of deliberation, the Supreme

Court, in its decision of January 28, 1988, struck down Section 251 of the Criminal Code as violating Section 7 of the Canadian Charter of Rights and Freedoms. This section of the Charter prohibits infringements of an individual's right to life, liberty and security of the person. The Supreme Court found that:

"State interference with bodily integrity and serious state-imposed psychological stress, at least in the criminal law context, constitutes a breach of security of the person. Section 251 clearly interferes with a woman's physical and bodily integrity. Forcing a woman, by threat of criminal sanction, to carry a foetus to term unless she meets certain criteria unrelated to her own priorities and aspirations, is a profound interference with a woman's body and thus an infringement of security of the person. A second breach of the right to security of the person occurs independently as a result of the delay in obtaining therapeutic abortions caused by the mandatory procedures of s.251 which results in a higher probability of complications and greater risk. The harm to the psychological integrity of women seeking abortions was also clearly established [11]."

Theoretically, this decision means that any doctor can now perform abortions in any hospital, clinic, or doctor's office. However, doctors or hospitals are not obligated by this decision to perform abortions, and it remains to be seen how the various provinces of Canada will attempt to regulate abortion practice as related to prenatal diagnosis of genetic disease. It is difficult to predict how new abortion legislation, now in preparation, will regulate abortion practice in Canada.

## 2.3.4.5 Studies of Effectiveness of Genetic Services

There have not been any studies in Canada looking at the effectiveness of genetic services. However, Québec has been exemplary in doing a number of studies evaluating the effectiveness of various programs relating to specific genetic disorders. Studies from Québec on screening have clearly shown that public education is the key to the acceptance of any program. With proper education, screening programs have been readily accepted and utilized in Québec [18].

## 2.3.4.6 Need for New Laws

Historically, each province has developed its own clinical genetic services. To date, it has not seemed necessary to develop laws to prevent abuses of the new developments in biology and human genetics. In most centers the provision of new and unique types of service or care are discussed thoroughly at a local level as well as at the CCMG meetings, and a consensus is achieved on the way technology should be used.

## 2.3.5 Ethical Issues and Future Trends

Canadian medical geneticists approach ethical issues in a non-analytical, non-directive, and non-judgmental way. They certainly do not pontificate on matters of reproductive right and wrong, nor, for that matter do they seem to consider the analysis of ethical issues associated with their practice to be one of their prime responsibilities. They rather respond to these issues in a practical way, largely by honoring the maxims deriving from their roles and their goals.

Medical geneticists in Canada see themselves primarily as information-providers and support-givers. Responses to this study's questionnaire emphasized two goals as being absolutely essential: helping prospective parents to understand their reproductive options, and then helping them to live in peace with their reproductive choices.

Physicians and surgeons normally would fall short of fulfilling their responsibilities were they systematically to avoid forming clinical and clinical-ethical judgments about what is best for their patients, even if it remains ethically necessary to negotiate treatment plans with patients in the light of what patients judge their own best interests to be. Medical geneticists work quite differently. By professional conviction, they do not claim to possess, and generally refuse to exercise Aesculapian authority. They believe it would be meddlesome and ethically inappropriate to intervene directively in the reproductive lives of people coming to them for information and support. Medical geneticists in Canada do not seek patient compliance with their proffered advice about optimal reproductive choices. Indeed, they generally refuse to offer such advice.

Medical geneticists in Canada are also non-judgmental. They do not see it as their responsibility to help parents to evaluate ethically their reproductive choices, nor would they ethically question the reproductive decisions of the parents they counsel. The maxims supporting these governing assumptions are: inform accurately and honestly, support sensitively, but do not advise, dictate, or criticize parents' reproductive decisions.

The focus of medical geneticists' professional attention to ethical issues is on individual patients, parents, and families, not on society or the population at large. They consequently tend to shy away from designing or adopting uniform solutions to ethical issues. Such solutions might constrain them to subordinate parental choices, however eccentric these might be, to some overarching policy. Respecting and promoting the autonomy of individual parents seems to be the dominant value professed by the majority of medical geneticists in this country.

One medical geneticist, as mentioned earlier in this chapter, characterized the relationship of the genetic counselor to parents as: "I am, in a sense, their servant." Though a fair number of medical geneticists might subscribe to this summary description, few would accept an interpretation that would make them slaves of a client's demands. The medical ethos implied in the adjective, *medical* genetics, seems to motivate geneticists occasionally to refuse their services to persons who would demand and use these for purposes that have nothing to do with medicine. There is little indication, however, that medical geneticists in Canada have systematically reflected on the extent to which the ethos of medicine could conceivably motivate them to modulate their commitment to the principle of non-directiveness.

134

## A Need for More Systematic Reflection?

There is little evidence or reason to believe that medical geneticists in Canada are likely to abandon or dramatically modify their current approach to ethical issues. They may, though, find it opportune over the next decade to initiate a more explicit program of professional reflection on the societal and ethical impact of advances and applications of developments in genetics.

Promoting the value of parental autonomy may increasingly require more than information alone. A Belgian geneticist, Herman Van Den Berghe, has expressed the view that, while genetic knowledge and technology are growing with astonishing speed, society is not prepared to receive this information, let alone to do something with this information that has a sound ethical basis. Even geneticists who find this view to be somewhat alarmist may share Van Den Berghe's concern that geneticists are taking on an enormous responsibility simply by offering this technology to the population at large. It may well become increasingly necessary for geneticists explicitly to study the question as to whether "with only a handful of people we are very deeply influencing an unprepared society [22]."

When consumers who demand a technology, and policy makers who regulate its introduction into society, fail to achieve more than a superficial understanding of scientific technology, they invite potential social disequilibrium. While innovations abound, resources are limited. Societies today can ill afford the need to backtrack on decisions, taken years earlier, to introduce costly and competing technologies that later prove to be ineffective or only marginally beneficial.

The possibility of social conflict also has to be recognized. Scientists and professionals may espouse priorities very different from the values that rule, and the anxieties that perturb, other people. If long-term anxieties are successfully classified and brushed aside as merely "popular," "unscientific," and, therefore, "insignificant," a needed check and balance on the short-term goals of scientists and professionals, passionately interested in the recognition and advancement of their own work, may be seriously weakened and lost. Conversely, if long-term anxieties and images of potential distant mischief are collapsed into immediate threats, the risks of heavy, uninformed constraints on science and new technologies run high.

These considerations bear directly upon the way Canadian medical geneticists have ranked the foci of future ethical concern. Increased demand for genetic services and allocation of scarce resources were identified as the issues of greatest concern for medical geneticists over the next decade or so. Eugenics and sex preselection were ranked lowest in the order of future concerns.

## The Allocation of Limited Resources

Canadian medical geneticists are making important contributions to discourse in Canada about how scarce resources should be distributed. The Canadian multicenter randomized trial of CVS and amniocentesis is an effort rigorously to assess the relative safety and accuracy of CVS for fetal diagnosis. The decision to mount this trial had to confront the view that first trimester diagnosis cannot ethically be withheld from women who present early enough in pregnancy to take advantage of it. The Canadian trial gives greater weight to the view that validated knowledge about safety, accuracy, and efficacy comes before patient acceptance or demand in the order of conditions that must be fulfilled before a procedure is justifiably proposed as a standard of clinical practice [15]. The protection of patients and the just distribution of limited resources are strong ethical indications in Canada for the need of suitably controlled trials of diagnostic and therapeutic innovations.

The allocation of limited resources may raise questions in Canada that are even more difficult to handle than those we already face. Those who plan health care budgets may display increasing interest in studies demonstrating that the costs of screening and birth-prevention programs compare very favorably with the costs normally involved in treating and caring for babies born with genetic disorders and congenital abnormalities. Canadians may have to decide how committed they are to the goal of developing therapies and cures for the devastating conditions resulting from chromosomal abnormalities, genetic disorders, and multifactorial congenital abnormalities. Will Canadians likely judge, in the years to come, that selective abortion of defective fetuses is the socially and economically preferred route to follow?

Choices have been described as tragic when they reveal a determination has been made that some people are not equal to others; or when these choices imply that life, the basis for the enjoyment and achievement of all other goods, is not valued as priceless in a society [3]. Tragic choices are already being made in Canada, but we may have to make them more explicitly in the future.

Cost-benefit studies of screening programs for genetic disorders may close with reminders that information should be given and used in ways that respect the human dignity of those born with defects that are prenatally detectable. We may have to ponder more carefully over the next decade whether such reminders will retain anything greater than the force of humanitarian platitude if societies, in fact, adopt cost-benefit conclusions as the foundation for social policies on genetic disease.

### Eugenics

Canadian medical geneticists have given low ranking to eugenics as a future ethical concern. That merits a pause for thought. It is probably true that medical geneticists in the majority are not motivated by any eugenic intention in their daily work, particularly if eugenics is taken to mean efforts to improve the human species. Geneticists in Canada have clearly manifested an individual-family perspective on ethical issues and are not professionally concerned in any programmatic way with the impact of parental reproductive choices on society, much less on the human species. Moreover, prospective parents are primarily concerned about themselves, their children, and their families, not about improving the genetic stock of humanity.

Discussions about eugenics are semantically trying because the term has several quite different meanings. Such discussion also frequently becomes emotionally charged because the term is laden with depressing historical associations that medical geneticists do not, rightly so, want to see linked to their practice and to the services they offer.

It is, however, difficult to avoid recognizing that the cumulative effect of individual parental decisions for selective abortion on the basis of fetal indications amounts to a eugenic trend in modern societies. "Eugenics," as E. A. Murphy has written, seems to be used more and more to refer to short-term gains, namely, avoidance of genetic disease in the current generation [13].

This recognition does not *per se* entail an accusation of moral reprehensibility, but may signal the emergent need for reasoned argument about eugenics. Though it is perhaps too early to know whether we will witness an intense debate about eugenics over the next decade, two prominent persons have recently raised the issue in relation to medical genetics. Ruth Hubbard, while not questioning a woman's right to have an abortion, detects an important difference between decisions about what *kind* of baby to bear and decisions about *whether* to bear a baby at all. The former decisions, in her view, are bedeviled by overt and unspoken judgments about which lives "are worth living" and about "who should and who should not inhabit the world [9]." Benno Müller-Hill has advanced the thesis that the rise of genetics is marked by a gigantic repression of its history. His charge is disturbing:

> The recognition of one of many genetic defects in the human embryo allows or warrants – these are the words scientists like to use – its destruction. The killing of deficient newborn babies as practised in Germany between 1939 and 1945 has simply become anachronistic. Most geneticists sincerely believe that here they have created new values. They do not see that they appeal to the forces of the market which state that cost-efficiency considerations make it advisable, for both parents and state, to destroy the cost-intensive embryo [12].

Medical geneticists in Canada and in other countries may vehemently, and correctly reject any such link between their work and reprehensible eugenic programs of the 1930's and 1940's. The point to be made here, though, is somewhat different. Vehement rejection of eugenic charges may not suffice over the next decade as the power of diagnostic technology increases. Medical geneticists and others may well have to engage themselves more explicitly than ever before in methodological and interdisciplinary reflection on the history of genetics and on the future course of genetics in an evolving society. More attention may have to be given, as Loren Graham has advised, to the second-order links between science and values, those links, namely, "which are contingent on existing political and social situations, current technological capabilities, and the persuasiveness of current ideologies, flawed in an intellectual sense as they may be [8]."

# Acknowledgements

The authors wish to acknowledge the help and suggestions of Drs. A. Hunter, N. Simpson, B. McGillivray, C. Scriver, C. Laberge, A. Neidhardt, L. Dalaire, E. Hutton, and P. MacLeod. D.J. Roy's work was supported in part by a grant from Imperial Oil Limited.

# References

1. Ad Hoc Committee on Genetic Counseling [1985] Genetic counseling, Am J Hum Genet 27: 240–242
2. Baird PA [1987] Measuring birth defects and handicapping disorders in the population: the British Columbia Health Surveillance Registry, CMAJ 136: 109–111
3. Calabresi G, Bobbitt P [1978] Tragic choices. W.W. Norton, New York
4. Canadian College of Medical Geneticists [1986] Professional and ethical guidelines. CCMG, Ottawa
5. Charbonneau M, Laberge C, Scriver CR, Dussault JH , Lemieux B, Melançon S [1986] The Quebec network of Genetic Medicine. In Press
6. Dagenais DL, Courville L, Dagenais MG [1985] A Cost-benefit analysis of the Quebec network of genetic medicine. Soc Sci Med 20: 601–607
7. Dickens BM, Cook R [1979] The development of commonwealth abortion laws. International Comparative Law Quarterly 28: 424–457
8. Graham LR [1977] Political ideology and genetic theory: Russia and Germany in the 1920's. Hastings Center Rep 7: 30–39
9. Hubbard R [1985] Prenatal diagnosis and eugenic ideology. Women's Studies Int Forum 8: 567–576
10. Iglehard JK [1986] Canada's health care system. N Engl J Med 315: 202–208
11. Morgentaler v. The Queen, Supreme Court of Canada, January 28, 1988 (unreported)
12. Müller-Hill B [1987] Genetics after Auschwitz. Holocaust and Genocide Studies 2: 3–20
13. Murphy EA [1978] Eugenics: An ethical analysis. Mayo Clin Proc 53: 655–664
14. Ostrowsky JT, Lippman A, Scriver CR [1985] Cost-benefit analysis of a thalassemia disease prevention program. Am J Publ Hlth 75: 732–736
15. Roy DJ [1986] First-trimester fetal diagnosis: prudential ethics. CMAJ 135: 737–739
16. Sadovnik AD, Baird PA [1981] A Cost-benefit analysis of prenatal detection of Down syndrome and NTDs in older mothers. Am J Med Genet 10: 367–378
17. Sadovnik AD, Baird PA [1982] A Cost-benefit analysis of prenatal diagnosis for NTD selectively offered to relatives of index case. Am J Med Genet 12: 63–73
18. Sadovnik AD, Baird PA [1983] A Cost-benefit analysis of population screening for NTD by measurement of maternal alpha-fetoprotein levels. Prenatal Diagnosis 3: 117–126
19. Scriver CR, Laberge C, Clow CL, Fraser FC [1975] Genetics and medicine: an evolving relationship. Science 200: 946–951
20. Scriver CR, Scriver DE, Clow CL, Schok M [1978] The education of citizens: human genetics. Amer Biol Teacher 40: 280–284
21. Society of Obstetricians and Gynecologists of Canada [1983] Canadian recommendations for prenatal diagnosis of genetic disorders. Bulletin 5: 1–10
22. Van Den Berghe H (198a) Impact of genetics on society. Birth Defects: Original Article Series. Alan R Liss, New York 23: 1–5

# Appendix

## Code of Ethics for the Canadian College of Medical Geneticists

The C.C.M.G. was established to ensure adherence to acceptable standards in delivery of medical genetics services in Canada. This includes standards for the training and competence of those delivering these services.

Fellows of the C.C.M.G. are commonly physicians or members of other professional bodies who have their own established codes of practice. However, in addition to these different professional skills, the practice of medical genetics requires a specialized understanding of genetic mechanisms in basic biology and the impact of these not only on individual recipients of medical genetics services but also on their offspring and the present and future population groups to which they belong. An appreciation of the limitations of this knowledge at any particular point in time is especially important.

In view of these considerations, the C.C.M.G. has approved the following guidelines for fellows in relation to their responsibilities not only to patients and to society as a whole but, also, to one another as members of this professional body.

### Responsibilities to Patients
Fellows of the C.C.M.G. should:

1) Provide genetic services to individuals without regard for race, sex, or religious beliefs.
2) Take all reasonable measures to establish or ensure accuracy of diagnosis in patient or family.
3) When indicated, seek appropriate expertise in interpreting results of specialized genetic and other investigations.
4) Be able to justify risk figures provided to the patient and other members of the family.
5) In conveying information to patients, should have the patients' best interests in mind and should attempt to ensure an appropriate level of understanding of this information.
6) Avoid withholding information from patients unless this can be fully justified as being the most reasonable course to take in a specific situation.
7) Discuss with the family all reasonable alternatives for handling their risk situation.
8) Provide supportive rather than directive advice to patients in regard to reproductive decisions.
9) Appreciate when patients and families need special support services and should take the initiative in acquainting patients with the availability of these or in directing patients to them.
10) Keep in confidence information obtained from patients unless it can be shown that this is likely to produce significant detrimental effects to the health of other individuals, currently or in the future.
11) Follow generally accepted guidelines in obtaining informed consent from patients prior to their inclusion in research studies.

### Responsibilities to Society
Fellows of the C.C.M.G. should:

1) Take the initiative in pursing family members at significant risk of high burden genetic disorders in the most appropriate manner.
2) Encourage the establishment of screening programs for the detection of particular genetically determined disorders and risk states when the frequency of these in specific population groups and the availability of appropriate techniques and economic resources justifies this.

3) Endeavor to improve the distribution and quality of medical genetic services so that no segment of society is deprived of such services.
4) Encourage any reasonable effort to extend and improve the education of the public on medical genetic matters.

**Responsibilities to the Profession**
A fellow of the C.C.M.G.:

1) As an individual, will conduct himself (herself) beyond reproach and will act within his (her) area of competence. He (she) will report to the appropriate body of his (her) peers, conduct by a confrere, which is considered unbecoming to the profession.
2) Will first communicate to confreres, through recognized scientific channels, the results of any medical genetic research, to allow confreres to establish an opinion of its merits or validation of results before presenting to the public or using in service clinical applications.
3) Will recognize his (her) responsibility to give the generally held opinions of the profession when interpreting scientific knowledge to the public; and in presenting any personal opinion which is contrary to the generally held opinion of the profession, he (she) will indicate he (she) is doing so, and will avoid any attempt to enhance his (her) own personal reputation.
4) Will request the opinion of an appropriate confrere acceptable to the patient when diagnosis or treatment is difficult, or when the patient requests it. Having requested the opinion of a confrere, he (she) will make available all relevant information.
5) Will, when his (her) opinion has been requested by a confrere, report in detail his (her) findings and recommendations to the attending physicians, and may outline his (her) opinion to the patient. He (she) will continue with the care of the patient only at the specific request of the attending physician, and with the consent of the patient.
6) Will cooperate with those individuals who, in the opinion of the geneticist, may assist in the care of the patient.
7) Will make available to a confrere, on the request of a patient, a report of his (her) findings and counselling of that patient.
8) Will avoid any personal profit motive for diagnostic procedures or treatments from any facility in which he (she) has a financial interest.

## 2.4 Ethics and Medical Genetics in Denmark

A.J. Therkelsen, L. Bolund, and V. Mortensen

## 2.4.1 Medical Genetics in Denmark

### 2.4.1.1 Scope of the Problem

With a population of around 5.1 million, Denmark has around 50,000 births per year. The birth rate has been declining steadily from 14.3 per 1000 inhabitants in 1975 to 10.0 per 1000 in 1983, increasing slightly again in 1984 and 1985 to 10.1 and 10.5 respectively. The total number of births in 1985 was 53,989, with 240 still-borns. The total number of births in 1986 will be approximately 57,000. Childhood mortality is low, being around 8 per 1000 below 1 year of age and 9 per 1000 below 14 years of age.

The total incidence of genetic diseases and malformations is only approximately known, but a survey (part of the EUROCAT project [3]) is underway in the county of Funen, which will supply us with a fairly precise estimate of the total frequency of congenital malformations. The frequencies of some of the most common malformations are given in Table 2.4.1, together with corresponding frequencies in Sweden, Norway, and Finland. The total rate of congenital malformations in Denmark is estimated at 14–15 per 1000 liveborn.

The frequency of chromosome abnormalities is estimated fairly precisely by the work of Johannes Nielsen et al. [10] and appears in Table 2.4.2. With respect to monogenic inherited diseases, the frequency is known for only a few conditions

**Table 2.4.1.** Frequency of selected congenital malformations among children born in 1983 registered in the county of Funen (EUROCAT), Sweden, Norway, and Finland respectively

|  | County of Funen (DK) | Sweden | Norway | Finland |
|---|---|---|---|---|
| Anencephalus | 4.1 | 1.5 | 2.9 | 2.6 |
| Spina bifida (open) | 6.7 | 4.5 | 6.4 | 1.8 |
| Hydrocephalus | 3.6 | 3.2 | 2.9 | 1.4 |
| Cleft palate, isolated | 7.2 | 5.7 | 5.4 | 10.5 |
| Cleft lip, with/without cleft palate | 14.4 | 14.1 | 12.4 | 8.9 |
| Atresia/stenosis oesophagi | 4.1 | 2.7 | 1.7 | 1.4 |
| Atresia/stenosis anorectalis | 3.6 | 2.0 | 1.5 | 0.5 |
| Hypospadias | 12.3 | 15.0 | 13.5 | 6.3 |
| Reduction deformity of limbs | 7.2 | 5.3 | 5.4 | 4.7 |
| Omphalocele/gastroschisis | 5.1 | 1.2 | 4.8 | 1.1 |
| Down syndrome | 6.2 | 12.5 | 9.9 | 8.3 |

**Table 2.4.2.** Incidence of autosomal abnormalities in 20,222 newborn children

| Karyotype | Total | Rate/1,000 Newborn | |
|---|---|---|---|
| +21 | 25 | 1.23 | |
| +13 | | | |
| +18 | 5 | 0.25 | |
| +8 and ring | 3 | 0.15 | 0.60 |
| Unbalanced abnormalities | 4 | 0.20 | |
| +Mar | 11 | 0.54 | |
| 13/14 translocation | 22 | 1.09 | |
| 14/21 and 15/21 | 7 | 0.35 | |
| Reciprocal translocations | 27 | 1.34 | 3.91 |
| Inversions* | 5 | 0.25 | |
| Others | 7 | 0.35 | |
| Autosomal Abnormalities | 116 | 5.74 | |

* Cases of inversion 9, 14.32/1,000, are not included

**Table 2.4.3.** Types and frequencies of genetic disease in a pediatric department in Denmark

| | | Total | % of total no of patients | | |
|---|---|---|---|---|---|
| Monogenic | Autosomal Dominant | 12 | | | |
| | Autosomal Recessive | 34 | 55 | (10.3%) | 2.7% |
| | Sex-linked | 9 | | | |
| Chromosomal Aberrations | Numerical | 11 | | | |
| | Structural | 3 | 14 | (2.6%) | 0.7% |
| Multifactorial | | | 463 | (87.0%) | 22.5% |

but the total frequency is estimated at about 1%, as in other Western countries. The frequency of genetic disease in a representative pediatric department is known to be around 25% [5] and is distributed as shown in Table 2.4.3.

## 2.4.1.2 Organization of Clinical Genetic Services in Denmark

The best organized part of the genetic service in Denmark is prenatal diagnostic work. Prenatal diagnosis was started in Denmark in 1970, and the number of investigations rose rapidly, as appears in Fig. 1. In 1978, it was formalized by the Ministry of Internal Affairs and three centers were equipped to do the work [2]. The three centers and their activities appear in Table 2.4.4. In 1986, a fourth laboratory was established.

The results of all prenatal investigations are listed in the Danish Cytogenetic Central register, together with all postnatal chromosome investigations performed since 1961.

With respect to genetic counseling, the picture is more difficult to evaluate. Counseling related to pre- and postnatally diagnosed chromosome abnormalities and monogenic diseases is given by the scientific staff in the laboratories perform-

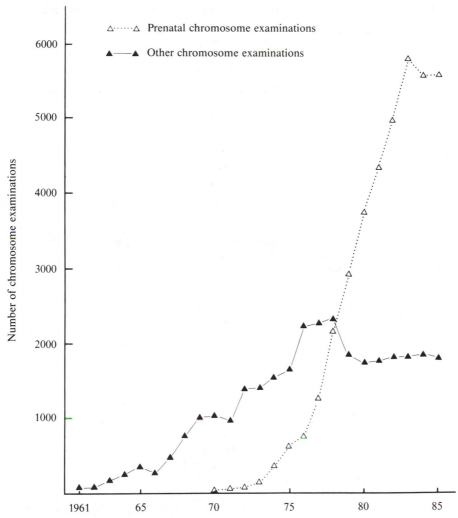

**Fig. 1.** Prenatal chromosome examinations and other chromosome examinations in Denmark from 1961–1985

ing the diagnostic work. Genetic counseling in other cases is only partly performed by these people. Genetic counseling is also performed at the University Institutes in Copenhagen and Aarhus (Table 2.4.6) and genetic counseling covering Funen is given by the head of the Institute of Medical Genetics at the University of Odense, with assistance from one co-worker. The counseling is undoubtedly very inefficient for many of the genetic diseases, as only about four person-years at most is used for diseases unrelated to prenatal diagnosis. It has been estimated that around 15 person-years are necessary for full coverage.

No formalized education or specialist status of clinical geneticists exists in Denmark, but a committee has recently been set up by the National Board of Health for the purpose of solving this problem.

**Table 2.4.4.** Number of amniotic fluid examinations in Denmark by laboratory/genetic center 1970-1985

| Year | John F. Kennedy Institute Glostrup 1 | Rigshospitalet Copenhagen 2 | Institute of Human Genetics Aarhus 3 | Total 4 |
|------|------|------|------|------|
| 1970 | 1 | 1 | 6 | 8 |
| 1971 | 7 | 9 | 18 | 34 |
| 1972 | 12 | 30 | 26 | 68 |
| 1973 | 42 | 57 | 42 | 141 |
| 1974 | 109 | 183 | 55 | 347 |
| 1975 | 124 | 343 | 147 | 614 |
| 1976 | 181 | 407 | 194 | 782 |
| 1977 | 221 | 688 | 372 | 1,281 |
| 1978 | 438 | 1,038 | 684 | 2,160 |
| 1979 | 725 | 1,424 | 765 | 2,914 |
| 1980 | 840 | 2,067 | 840 | 3,747 |
| 1981 | 1,068 | 2,267 | 1,007 | 4,342 |
| 1982 | 1,072 | 2,788 | 1,096 | 4,956 |
| 1983 | 1,161 | 3,264 | 1,420 | 5,845 |
| 1984 | 890 | 3,252 | 1,454 | 5,596 |
| 1985 | 982 | 3,167 | 1,478 | 5,627 |

## 2.4.1.3 Prenatal Diagnosis

As it appears in Fig. 1, the number of postnatal investigations seems to be rather stable, around 1800 per year. The number of prenatal investigations was around 5600 per year in 1984 and 1985. Prenatal investigation is performed in 10-11% of all pregnancies. The indications for offering prenatal diagnosis are laid down by the National Board of Health [12] and appear in Table 2.4.5. The diagnostic service is an offer to pregnant women, and acceptance should be voluntary. As an indication of the extent to which the offer is accepted, it is worth mentioning that 68.4% of all pregnant women $\geq$ 35 years of age had prenatal diagnosis performed in 1985. In some counties, the acceptance rate was very high - in one county 84.3% - whereas the lowest acceptance rate in a county was 53.2%.

The variation is very large and should be attributed to three main factors:

1. The distance from patient to genetic center is negatively correlated with the acceptance rate.
2. The degree of patient information varies geographically and from center to center, and with distance from a center.
3. Patients' religion. The most religious people are found in rural areas, and they are often opposed to prenatal investigation.

The indication "anxietas" is used fairly commonly in Denmark. In 1985, 11.4% of the investigations were made on this indication. The frequency with which the indication is used varies from center to center and especially between the hospitals

144

**Table 2.4.5.** Indications for prenatal diagnosis (Danish National Board of Health 1981) and number and frequency of investigations during the three-year period 1980-1982

| Indications | Total number of prenatal investigations 1980-1982 | |
|---|---|---|
| 1. Maternal age ≥ 35 | 7,268 | (61.4%) |
| 2. Paternal age ≥ 50 | 128 | (1.1%) |
| 3. Previous child with chromosome abnormality | 215 | (2.1%) |
| 4. Chromosome abnormality in parent | 57 | (0.5%) |
| 5. Chromosome abnormality in sibs and/or children of sibs | 1,443 | (12.2%) |
| 6. Previous spontaneous abortion (≥ 3) | 96 | (0.8%) |
| 7. Previous child with mental defect or malformations of unknown etiology | 413 | (3.5%) |
| 8. Previous child with inborn errors or X-linked disease | 184 | (1.6%) |
| 9. Previous child with neural tube defect or neural tube defect in family | 496 | (4.2%) |
| 10. Miscellaneous (Anxietas, mental retardation in family, exposure to toxic substances)* | 1,495 | (12.6%) |
| Total | 11,831 | |

* Outside the indications given by the National Board of Health

**Table 2.4.6.** Genetic laboratories in Denmark

| Name of laboratory | Investigations performed | | | Number of staff members | |
|---|---|---|---|---|---|
| | Prenatal karyotyping | Postnatal karyotyping | Inborn errors (including DNA-diagnostics) | Academics | Technicians and Secretaries |
| Chromosome laboratory Rigshospitalet, Copenhagen | + | + | – | 4.5 | 18.5 |
| Metabolic Laboratory Rigshospitalet, Copenhagen | – | – | + | 4 | 8.5 |
| Institute of Medical Genetics University of Copenhagen | – | + | + | 1.5 (0.5) | 3.5 (1) |
| Chromosome Laboratory John F. Kennedy Institute Glostrup | + | + | – | 3 | 14 |
| Metabolic Laboratory John F. Kennedy Institute Glostrup | – | – | + | 4 | 5.5 |
| Dept. of Clinical Genetics Institute of Human Genetics University of Aarhus | + | + | + | 4 (0.5) | 14.5 (2) |
| Chromosome Laboratory Aarhus Psychiatric Hospital Arhus | – | + | – | 2 | 6.5 |
| Dept. of Clinical Genetics County of Vejle, Brejning 7080 Børkop | + | + | – | 1 | 5 |
| Nos. in parentheses: staff for inborn errors | | Total | | 24 | 76 |

doing the sampling (highest frequency 26.6% and lowest 3.1%). The main reason for the variation is the difference of opinion between amniocentesis centers. In our area, for instance, the chief of staff of the center at Aarhus is opposed to amniocentesis with this indication, whereas the chief of staff in Aalborg is very liberal.

The amnion fluid investigations are gradually being replaced by chorion villus investigations, and by the end of 1986 a total of 1095 investigations of this type had been performed, of which 695 were made in 1986. The total number of prenatal genetic investigations in 1986 was 6701, as against 5627 in 1985.

Prenatal diagnosis of monogenic diseases is done partly through international collaboration, whether the diagnosis is obtained by enzymatic methods or by DNA technology. The total diagnostic capacity in Denmark is illustrated in Table 2.4.6, giving the number of staff available in the different laboratories.

## 2.4.1.4  Cost-benefit of Early Diagnosis and Genetic Counseling

Unfortunately, no cost-benefit analysis of genetic counseling has been made in Denmark, whereas it has been made with respect to prenatal diagnosis of Down syndrome [9]. In this investigation, it was shown that prenatal chromosome investigation of women $\geq$ 35 years of age for Down syndrome alone would give a benefit of around Dkr.4 million ($555,000) per year. Adding the benefit caused by the concomitant diagnosis of other chromosome abnormalities and neural tube defects, prenatal investigations are very attractive from an economic point of view. A sizeable benefit has also been shown for neonatal screening for PKU [9], and preliminary investigations seem to show a benefit from screening of all pregnant women for alphafetoprotein in serum [4], although this screening program is so far used in only part of the country.

## 2.4.1.5  Abortion

The number of elective abortions based on prenatal diagnosis is shown for the period from 1975-1985, together with the total number of elective abortions, in Table 2.4.7. The number of abortions induced for genetic reasons is small compared to the total number of legally-induced abortions.

**Table 2.4.7.**  Legally induced abortions in Denmark from 1975-1985

Number of abortions induced

| Year | Genetic reasons | Total | Total number of liveborns |
|---|---|---|---|
| 1975 | 14 | 27,884 | 72,071 |
| 1976 | 15 | 26,842 | 65,267 |
| 1977 | 35 | 25,662 | 61,878 |
| 1978 | 42 | 23,699 | 62,036 |
| 1979 | 56 | 23,193 | 59,464 |
| 1980 | 68 | 23,334 | 57,293 |
| 1981 | 83 | 22,779 | 53,083 |
| 1982 | 79 | 21,462 | 52,658 |
| 1983 | 92 | 20,791 | 50,821 |
| 1984 | 85 | 20,742 | 51,800 |
| 1985 | 65 | 19,919 | 53,749 |

## 2.4.2 Ethical Problems Faced by Medical Geneticists in Denmark

### 2.4.2.1 Genetic Counseling

When idealizing the principles of genetic counseling, it is often claimed that the counselor should be completely open and objectively inform the patient and his or her relatives of the latest knowledge and all possible means of action available, giving the patient the best possible background for a decision, without giving direct advice. In practice, ethical conflicts arise in many situations, such as:

When the patient is unable to digest the information intellectually and/or emotionally, and simply asks the counselor what to do; when the diagnosis is uncertain or based on estimates of likelihood; when statistical information needs to be interpreted; when the consequences of carrier status are discussed; when it comes to approaching related individuals at risk who have not asked for counseling – especially when the patient does not agree to disclose information about his or her situation. The conflicts often involve objective versus directive, passive versus active, and individual versus social approaches to counseling.

### 2.4.2.2 Prenatal Diagnosis

These ethical problems often become emphasized when prenatal diagnosis is considered. Although abortion is "free" in Denmark (see section 2.4.4.4 below) until the twelfth week of pregnancy (and much of the prenatal diagnostics can now be performed before this time), selective abortion on the basis of a *genetic* diagnosis is generally considered an emergency measure which is only reluctantly chosen. It may be noted that abortion due to viral infection during early pregnancy is more easily accepted than abortion for genetic reasons, probably due to the fact that the nature of genetic disease is not properly understood, but is experienced as clearly different from other types of disease.

There is a very strong consensus that if prenatal diagnosis is offered, it should clearly be an offer and the possibility of saying no to genetically selective abortion should be guaranteed. The individual should be protected from pressures from the society. The right to be different should be guarded. However, the right of self-determination can come into conflict with the interests of the child to be and with the interests of society. In some cases, the interests of society might have to be protected from the demands of the individual. Not all requests for prenatal diagnosis can be granted. Although difficult to define, there is a common code of ethics in the society that must not be neglected, and the acute need to make priorities for expenditures within the health system also sets limits on the prenatal diagnostic efforts offered.

## 2.4.2.3  Genetic Screening

The range of ethical problems encountered in relation to specific genetic diagnostic tests widens when it comes to screening for a spectrum of conditions, as in prenatal chromosome and alphafetoprotein screening. In this case, the parents cannot possibly take all the different possible outcomes into account before they decide whether or not to accept the offer of prenatal screening tests. They might end up in unexpected or awkward situations that require a choice.

Another form of screening is population screening for particular genetic defects or predispositions to disease. Here the ethical dilemma is between the desire of the individual to receive information and the interests of employers, insurance companies and other agencies of the society. The problem is aggravated by the possibilities and needs for comprehensive registration in modern society.

## 2.4.2.4  Other Contexts

There is a general feeling of insecurity in the population with respect to recent developments in the field of genetics. Scientific progress has been too rapid to allow the general public to achieve a balanced view of the situation. The emotionally most central aspects of human existence are involved, and the glory of nature is seen as being threatened. Geneticists often feel inadequate in their attempts to inform the public and to participate in the open debate and political counseling that is required. The risk of crude conflicts and bans is imminent, whereas consensus based on informed public debate and respect for individual differences seems difficult to achieve. The introduction of *in vitro* fertilization as a treatment for infertility has roused a debate concerning the starting point of human life. The development of the *in vitro* fertilization technique, experimentation on human fertilized eggs and pre-embryos, the use of intra-uterine devices for contraception, and the right to free abortion are different aspects of this ethical debate. In this context, the ethical problems related to future possibilities of somatic gene therapy, germ line genetic intervention, and genetic manipulation are often brought up.

## 2.4.3  Consensus and Variation in Approaches to Ethical Problems Among Danish Medical Geneticists

If one is to describe a dominant approach to the ethical problems facing medical geneticists in Denmark, it is fair to say that they take – as in many other countries – their starting point in the interpersonal situation between doctor and patient, where the patient is in the center and the patient's needs decide the course of action proposed. The ethical demand rises out of this situation. Only secondly are consideration for third parties and wider social circumstances, such as family planning and eugenic considerations, taken into account. Therefore, autonomy is

148

the ethical value most often put forward to justify a given action, and it is only natural that the clinical case that caused Danish geneticists the greatest trouble should be the question regarding Huntington disease (Case 2). This is so because there is a conflict between confidentiality towards the patient and responsibility towards different parties, and there is a high risk of causing harm. Ultimately, consideration for siblings and relatives at risk overrides confidentiality. When there is strong consensus that one should provide information to relatives, it comes out of a wish to help.

When there is a strong consensus to inform, as in the case of disclosure of professional disagreement about interpreting findings (Case 7), it is not necessarily out of respect for the rule always to tell the truth, but rather as a means to relieve the professional conscience. This is not always in the interest of the patient. It is not for fear of legal consequences, because lawsuits against physicians are very rare in Denmark.

Against this background, it might seem a bit astonishing that three out of 14 persons would prefer to lie in the case of false paternity, although the majority of Danish geneticists would choose to tell the mother alone. Again, the protection of the mother's confidentiality was not due to an abstract principle, but was here enforced because all other kinds of action would harm the family unit and would not make anybody happier.

When it comes to directive counseling, Danish geneticists are very reserved. They think that the ideal situation is for the patient to reach his or her own decision on the basis of complete information. It is the patient's possibility of making an informed decision that determines the kind of answers and advice doctors give, for instance in the tuberous sclerosis case (Cases 13 and 14), where the consensus to inform about insemination, vasectomy, adoption, and contraception was overwhelming. Danish geneticists want only to inform and try not to give advice.

Also, in regard to the actions suggested in the tuberous sclerosis case with a female carrier, there was a large degree of consensus, except when it comes to surrogate motherhood. This might be due to the fact that, at the time the survey was taken, this problem was heavily debated, and it is now legally prohibited to make contracts concerning surrogate motherhood. In this case, there was no consensus on the ethical reasons given, however. The right to know for parents and the motive of preventing birth defects were cited almost as often as the patient's right to make an informed decision.

The Scandinavian countries are often looked upon as very closely related, mostly with good reason. Therefore, it was expected that a Scandinavian consensus would emerge. This was the case, but interesting variations also appeared. For instance, in Denmark and Sweden there was a strong consensus on the question of performing prenatal diagnosis when the indication was maternal anxiety (Case 10). In Norway, there was no consensus on this point. Norway seemed to have a stronger tendency towards directional counseling.

The difference between Norway and Denmark also appears in the case of prenatal diagnosis for parents who are opposed to induced abortion (Case 9). In Denmark, there was a strong consensus (13 out of 15) in favor of performing prenatal diagnosis, on the grounds of the parents' right to decide, while three out of six Norwegian geneticists would not do so.

When it comes to performing prenatal diagnosis for sex selection (Case 11), there was a difference between Sweden and Denmark. In Denmark, the overwhelming majority of geneticists (13 out of 15) would not do so, obviously because they did not consider the question of sex selection a medical problem. Thus, it would be a waste of medical resources. In Sweden, as in the USA, prenatal sex selection was the problem that caused the greatest conflict; 6 out of 19 would perform prenatal diagnosis with this indication. On the questions about screening there was a higher degree of consensus. All Scandinavian countries stressed that mass screening should be voluntary, based on the worker's right to decide. While some East European countries propose to make it mandatory, it is supposedly due to a different tradition concerning workers' rights.

It is questionable to comment on these geographical differences, because the material is very sparse. But it seems that in many ways Sweden resembles the USA more closely than do Norway and Denmark. This also shows in the questions about patient's confidentiality versus duties to third parties. Respect for confidentiality was more pronounced in Sweden and the USA than in Denmark. In Norway, a stronger religious influence may sometimes lead to a more restrictive attitude, as is seen, for instance, in not performing prenatal diagnosis for maternal anxiety.

On the whole, one must say that there is a high degree of consensus concerning the actions proposed by Danish geneticists. With medical professionalism come certain standards and guidelines, which geneticists want to impose on others as well. For instance, 12 out of 14 Danish geneticists felt that sex preselection should be prohibited in private clinics. Although there was consensus about courses of action in many situations, ethical reasons given to justify the proposed actions differed considerably. The reason most often given was the patient's right to make an informed decision. The principle of autonomy was maintained. This was also the case in the answers to the question of who should have access to the results of genetic screening. The most common opinion was *not* to give access to third parties (or to give it only with the worker's approval), with reference to the right to privacy; secondly, there was a wish to exclude the possibility of misuse. When 6 out of 15 responded that the worker's doctor should have access without the approval of the worker, the interpretation might be that concern for the worker's health can override the principle of autonomy. As a whole, respondents seemed to want as few regulations as possible, assuming that the problems were best solved in an immediate contact between the medical geneticist and patient. That is probably also the reason for the lack of consensus on the question of carrier testing for cystic fibrosis.

The great variation in ethical reasons cited might be due to the fact that doctors are given practically no formal training in ethical reasoning. They are not accustomed to relating their ethical judgments to philosophical traditions, and they often give "non-moral" answers. They rely on the professional standards and their ethical intuitions, handed down through the ordinary medical training and not taught in special courses. In recent years, however, there has been a growing interest in ethical issues that has resulted in some publications [1, 8]. Legislation concerning an ethical council has recently been passed [6].

150

## 2.4.4 Cultural Context of Medical Genetics in Denmark

### 2.4.4.1 Sources of Challenge and Support

The Danish welfare society regards itself as an open democratic society; but it is seldom challenged to specify the values which are supposed to form the basis of our culture.

The Danish Evangelical Lutheran church comprises 90% of the population, but, organized as a folkchurch, it does not constitute a pressure group. Nobody can speak in the name of the church.

The advances of medical genetics have stirred up some public debate, and religious leaders, bishops and theologians have taken an active part and called attention to the ethical issues inherent in medical genetics.

During the first ten years of prenatal diagnostic work, very little public debate took place in Denmark concerning its use. The 1980's have seen some, but it has not influenced the use of prenatal diagnosis to any significant extent. A small political party is against its use for religious reasons, but on the whole, religious motives play an insignificant role. Patient organizations, of which Denmark has a total of 52, have taken little part in the debate, and of those related to genetic diseases only an association of Turner-patient contact groups has expressed strong opposition to prenatal diagnosis.

### 2.4.4.2 Major Controversies

In recent years, there has been a tendency towards reevaluating the arguments in favor of abortion. In the light of the advances in gene technology, in the methods of artificial reproduction, and the consequent possibilities for gene manipulation, concerns have been raised. Among other things, the argument about the woman's right to decide in matters concerning her own body without considering the rights of the fetus has been questioned. However, there are no signs of any altering of the legal status of the abortion act. A growing awareness of the moral dilemmas inherent in the abortion issue may lead to an increased responsibility in family planning, and, for some groups of people, a renunciation of artificial means in regard to reproduction.

In a recent change in the adoption law, it has become legally prohibited to help establish contact between one woman and another who wants to bear her child [7]. Remarks on the legislation said that "agreements on delivery of a baby for compensation are at odds with quite basic principles in our society. Children ought not to be bought and sold, and this also applies to unborn children."

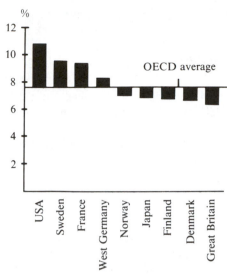

**Fig. 2.** Fraction of gross national product used on health care in 1983

## 2.4.4.3 National Expenditures for Medical Genetics

As mentioned above, the efficiency of genetic counseling is relatively low. At the moment, we are trying to intensify it by introducing a formal training program for medical geneticists. Although Denmark is usually considered a country with very intensive health care, it is astonishing, as shown in Fig. 2, that among the OECD countries [11] Denmark devotes the second lowest fraction of the gross national product to health care, 31.7 billion kroner (US$4.4 billion) out of a gross national product of 613.3 billion kroner (US$85.2 billion). Calculated per inhabitant, Denmark is the fourth lowest of the countries described in Fig. 2 – still below the OECD average and lower than Federal Republic of Germany, Norway, France, Sweden, and the U. S. A. The total cost of clinical genetics for laboratory diagnostic work and genetic counseling is estimated to be around 30 million kroner (US$4.17 million) – a small fraction of the total expenditure on health care (0.1%).

## 2.4.4.4 The Law of "Free" Abortion

According to the 1973 law on "free" abortion, every woman living in Denmark has – if she so wishes – the right to induced abortion before the twelfth week of pregnancy. The law is decisive that it is the woman's right (a possible husband is not even mentioned). It is determined that the woman shall be given information about the auxiliary services provided, if she wants to carry the pregnancy to term. She is also to be informed of the character, consequences, and risks of the abortive operations, but the woman does not have to give reasons for wanting an abortion.

It is entirely her own decision. The 12-week limit was established out of concern for the safety of the woman against complications. After the twelfth week, the woman can get an abortion by permission, according to indications. These indications are medical (health of the woman or the child), ethical (rape, incest), or social. The permission is relatively easy to obtain and is always given in the case of abnormal findings in connection with prenatal diagnosis. So legal regulations do not put obstacles in the way of induced abortion for genetic reasons.

When the "free" abortion act was passed in 1973, it was regarded as an act of justice by the majority of the population. The ethical motives behind the legislation were to stamp out illegal abortions and to give women equal opportunities. As it were, women who could pay, could always get an abortion; to remove this inequality and give equal access to abortion, to facilitate the administrative procedure, and to contribute to women's liberation, the abortion law was passed. This in fact meant that the legal system adapted to the actual behavior of the population.

Since 1973, there has not been much public discussion on the abortion issue. The number of legal abortions went up almost 200% and has now stabilized at around 20,000 abortions per year, compared to some 50,000 births (Table 2.4.7). Opposition to the legislation has come from some religious groups. One political party, the Christian Democratic party, which was founded mainly in opposition to the legislation on pornography and abortion, has approximately 2.5% of the voters as supporters. This party has twice – unsuccessfully – proposed changes in the free abortion act. Some of the bishops of the Danish Evangelical Lutheran Church, of which 90% of the population are members, have, together with the Catholic bishop, also protested against the law. They have thus aroused an awareness of the ethical dilemma inherent in the abortion issue, but it has not had any direct influence on the legislation or the actual practice of medical genetics.

## 2.4.4.6 The Need for Laws in the Future

There are many demands for, but also strong opposition to, new laws in this field. The opposition has mainly warned against the idea that one can solve ethical problems with bans and absolutely rigid rules and regulations. In spite of this opposition, a law was recently passed [6] which completely prohibits experiments with fertilized human eggs *in vitro* except in the established process of *in vitro* fertilization to achieve pregnancy. Thus a form of medical treatment is accepted, but any attempts to improve the methods are prohibited. The law also prohibits attempts to develop human clones, chimeras, or interspecies hybrids. The latter bans are obviously not controversial. Neither is the establishment of an ethical council that should stimulate an informed public debate and suggest a law on the handling of fertilized eggs and gametes to be used for fertilization. The ethical council should also guide the authorities in their attempts to create rules and recommendations for the registration and use of genetic information and the introduction of new methods of diagnosis and treatment. The need for new laws in this field should be satisfied by this development.

153

## 2.4.5 Ethical Issues and Trends in Medical Genetics

The development of medical genetics is likely to continue unabated for the next decade. A more or less complete human gene map will soon be achieved. This will open up the possibility of following the inheritance of any clearly definable genetic defects (or traits). Most relevant human genes will soon be cloned. The techniques of transfer and controlled expression of such genes in cells of the human body will open up the possibility of gene therapy (or genetic manipulation). The ethical issues involved are already being debated, but one can foresee that the questions will become more and more subtle. Unless the techniques are banned altogether, which seems unlikely, the necessity of taking a differentiated ethical standpoint in individual cases, on the basis of general recommendations reached by open debate, will become more and more obvious.

It is therefore obvious that there will be an increasing demand for ethical guidance in the future. Newly-developed institutional settings for doing applied ethics might provide important ethical resources. The ethical council will hopefully play an important role by interacting with existing local and national ethics committees, as well as with the authorities. At the same time it will stimulate and participate in the public debate. The establishment of a clinical specialty in medical genetics should also be helpful. It would define a group of physicians that can be held responsible and that can aid in the enormous educational work necessary.

The survey as a whole seems to demonstrate that with a given technology and professional standard comes a relatively high degree of consensus concerning the actual course of action proposed or taken. The variation is mainly in the ethical justification of courses of action. It is to be expected that this variation will diminish. With the internationalization of technology comes the internationalization of ethics. But as a fringe phenomenon, a counter movement might develop, based on an abandoning of the use of artificial means and an increased personal responsibility for life-style and health. The ability of society to guide medical genetics on ethical paths is questionable. The best hope is that medical geneticists themselves show a kind of ethical awareness by consciously choosing ethically justified solutions. This is best achieved when they can work in an environment where a free debate and public opinion can meet with and influence or illuminate professional standards. To further this goal, it is worth trying to strengthen the ethical council and committees in their double task of serving as resource organs both for the legislative and administrative authorities and for public opinion.

## References

1. Andersen D, Mabeck CE, Riis P (eds) [1986] Medicinsk etik. FADL's forlag, København
2. Betænkning om om prænatal genetisk diagnostik. Betænkning nr.803 København 1977. In Danish
3. De Walls P, Lechat MF [1986] Eurocat report 1. Surveillance of congenital anomalies years 1980-1983. Department of Epidemiology, Catholic University of Louvain, Bruxelles
4. Goldstein HG [1987] Report from 2nd economic office, Ministry of Internal Affairs, May 18th

5. Jensen PKA, Rasmussen K, Bro P [1982] Belastningen af genetiske sygdomme blandt indlagte på en regional børneafdeling. Ugeskrift for Læger 144: 2489–2492. In Danish

6. Law of the Establishment of an Ethical Council and the Regulation of Certain Biomedical Experiments. Law no. 353, Ministry of Internal Affairs, June 3rd, 1987. In Danish

7. Law no. 326, June 4th 1986. Ministry of Justice. In Danish

8. Munck E, Bjerg S [1986] Ansvarlighed. Medicinsk etik, Gyldendal, København. In Danish

9. Nielsen G, Mikkelsen M, Wamberg E [1974] Cost-benefit analyse af forebyggende åndssvageforsorg. Socialt tidsskrift 9: 147–167. In Danish

10. Nielsen J, Sillesen I [1975] Incidence of chromosome aberrations among 11,148 newborn children. Humangenetik 30: 1–12

11. OECD rapport [1985] Measuring health care 1960–1983, Paris

12. Sørensen SK [1981] Meddelelse til læger, jordremødre og sygehuse om forebygende undersøgelser for kromosomsygdomme, medfødte stofskiftesygdomme, neuralrørsdefekter m. v. hos fostre. Sundhedsstyrelsen 21st April, 1–7. In Danish

## 2.5 Ethics and Medical Genetics in the Federal Republic of Germany (FRG)

T.M. Schroeder-Kurth and J. Huebner

### 2.5.1 Medical Genetics in the FRG

#### 2.5.1.1 Scope of the Problem

According to the Statistical Year Book of 1985, the population of the FRG on December 31, 1983 was 61,306,700, of whom 56,732,500 were Germans and 4,574,200 were foreigners. Forty-nine percent belonged to the Protestant church, 44.6% to the Catholic Church, 1.1% to other Christian confessions, 1.3% to other religious groups, 0.1% were Jews, and 3.9% indicated no religious preference.

Table 2.5.1 describes the numbers of live births, stillbirths, and early childhood deaths from 1975 to 1985. The rate of early childhood deaths has decreased. The numbers of live births to mothers 35 years of age and over are included in the table to show the changes in the percents of pregnant women who could have requested prenatal diagnosis. The percentage of births to mothers older than 35 decreased from 10.05% in 1975 to a low of 7.11% in 1982 and slowly increased again to 8.19% in 1984. The percentage of foreign mothers of advanced age is higher than the percentage of German mothers of advanced age. In 1982, 11.33% of foreign mothers and 6.55% of German mothers were 35 or over; in 1983, these percents were 12.14% and 7.78% respectively (Statistische Jahrbücher 1976–1986). Births to women aged 37 and over have decreased in recent years. The increase in births to women 35 and over between 1982 and 1984 was due to an increase in births to those aged 35 and 36.

**Table 2.5.1.** Live Births, Stillbirths, Infant and Child Deaths, 1975–1986

| Year | Total Live Births | Live births to mothers ≥ 35 years | Total Still-Births | Total Early Childhood Deaths | | | |
|------|------|------|------|------|------|------|------|
| | | | | 1st week | 1st year | 1–5 years | 5–10 years |
| 1975 | 600,512 | 63,679 | 4,689 | 6,967 | 11,875 | 2,197 | 1,959 |
| 1976 | 602,851 | 60,069 | 4,444 | 5,936 | 10,506 | 1,866 | 1,749 |
| 1977 | 582,344 | 53,363 | 3,794 | 4,916 | 9,022 | 1,668 | 1,628 |
| 1978 | 576,468 | 51,405 | 3,650 | 4,314 | 8,482 | 1,662 | 1,436 |
| 1979 | 581,984 | 49,400 | 3,325 | 4,026 | 7,855 | 1,524 | 1,255 |
| 1980 | 620,657 | 48,482 | 3,308 | 3,904 | 7,821 | 1,448 | 1,081 |
| 1981 | 624,557 | 47,485 | 3,204 | 3,401 | 7,257 | 1,361 | 946 |
| 1982 | 621,173 | 44,152 | 2,996 | 3,000 | 6,782 | 1,318 | 859 |
| 1983 | 594,177 | 46,315 | 2,790 | 2,748 | 6,099 | 1,268 | 989 |
| 1984 | 584,157 | 47,838 | 2,567 | 2,474 | 5,633 | | |
| 1985 | 586,155 | 50,465 | 2,414 | 2,217 | | | |
| 1986 | ~626,000 | | | | | | |

**Table 2.5.2.** Gross estimate of genetic counseling sessions and chromosome diagnoses needed (1984): 56 million Germans, 44 million foreigners; 580,000 newborns, including 44,000 mothers ≥ 35 years

| Conditions | Frequency in risk–groups (RG) or population (P) | % of analyses with positive results | Expected abnormalities in population | *Estimated Needs* Chromosome diagnoses postnatal | prenatal | Genetic counseling sessions |
|---|---|---|---|---|---|---|
| *embryos/fetuses[1]* trisomies (due to advanced maternal age ≥ 35 years) | 0.02/RG | 2% | 880 | | 44,000 | 44,000 |
| other chromosome aberrations (recurrence, translocations) | 0.0001/P | 10% | 600 | | 6,000 | 6,000 |
| other diseases (recurrence, screening) | ? | – | | | 4,000 | > 5,000 |
| *newborns[2]* chromosome aberrations severe malformations monogenic diseases | 0.005/P 0.02/P 0.01/P | 5–20% | 2,900 11,600 5,800 | ~20,000 | | ~25,000 |
| *other populations[3]* monogenic and multifactorial diseases and anomalies repeated abortions sterility problems | ? ? ? | 5–20% 1–5% | | ~30,000 | | ~50,000 |
| consanguinity | rare/P | | | | | |
| exposure to mutagens or teratogens during pregnancy | frequent in pregnancies | | | | | |
| **Total** | | | | 50,000 | 54,000 | 130,000 |

1. If all mothers ≥ 35 years would accept prenatal chromosome diagnosis, the same number of counseling sessions would be needed. The actual finding of chromosomal abnormalities in this group is about 2%, which leads to 880 aborted fetuses. The incidence of structural rearrangements in the general population is about 1:10,000; however, not all carriers reproduce. Thus numbers given are rough estimates.
2. Emery and Rimoin (1983)
3. Includes older children and adults. The estimated number of genetic and non-genetic diseases and anomalies (Vogel and Motulsky 1979) may not be directly related to the actual need for chromosome analyses or genetic counseling, because not all individuals ask for clarification of diagnosis or counseling (personal estimation).

Table 2.5.2 shows expected numbers of children with severe genetic and non-genetic birth defects, using an estimate of 3% of live births. There is no registry in the FRG for congenital malformations or genetic diseases, because of intensive protection of the individual's privacy. The calculation of a 3% risk for newborns is based in part upon a prospective study of 14,000 pregnancies (Deutsche Forschungsgemeinschaft 1977). It includes 1% for dominant new mutations, 0.3% for X-chromosomal and autosomal recessive disorders, 0.2% for severe malformations and 0.5% for chromosome abnormalities (Vogel and Motulsky 1979).

## 2.5.1.2 Organization of Clinical Genetic Services in the FRG

Since 1970, compulsory national health insurance has covered genetic diagnostic services, mainly chromosome analyses and counseling. Since 1977, the costs of genetic counseling have also been reimbursed by most private health insurers. There are difficulties in reimbursement for newer and more complicated diagnostic techniques. However, the compulsory health insurance now covers DNA analysis, and private health insurers are expected to follow. In general, preventive measures such as counseling or prenatal diagnosis are not included in the original charter of a health insurance company. In practice, such expenses are paid and the fees are fair.

In 1986, there were 27 units at universities for genetic counseling and human genetic diagnostics (chromosome analysis and/or biochemical investigations), 8 units for counseling and diagnostics at larger hospitals or State Health Offices, and 9 private commercial enterprises that offered counseling and/or chromosome analysis (one center per $1.7 \times 10^6$ inhabitants and one laboratory for prenatal diagnosis for $1.36 \times 10^6$ inhabitants).

If all families accepted prenatal diagnosis, an estimated 54,000 prenatal chromosome analyses would be needed every year (Table 2.5.2). Of these, 44,000 would be for advanced maternal age. Each prenatal diagnosis should be preceded by a counseling session. In addition, an estimated 20,000 newborns will have genetically-caused birth defects, including 2,900 with chromosome aberrations and 11,600 with severe malformations, some of which are of chromosomal origin. Far more newborns are suspected of having chromosomal abnormalities than will have positive laboratory results. In order to identify all newborns with chromosome aberrations or malformations of genetic origin, an estimated 20,000 postnatal chromosome analyses would be needed annually. Each of these analyses should be preceded by a counseling session. In addition, the parents of newborns with monogenic diseases should receive counseling, making a total of approximately 25,000 counseling sessions needed for parents of newborns every year.

An estimated total of 130,000 counseling sessions are needed per year (Table 2.5.2). Approximately 49,000 sessions, or 38% of those needed, actually take place, an estimate based on the services provided by nine of the larger units. Genetic counseling, however, is not restricted to counseling units. Many pediatricians and doctors with other specialties counsel patients in hospitals and in office practice. Also, genetic diagnosis of metabolic diseases is mainly done in hospitals, universities, and foundations specializing in these diseases.

In most genetic counseling units, the counselor depends on investigations that have already been done at larger clinics. Sometimes, after reviewing the patient's file, the counselor has to refine the genetic diagnosis through more specific investigations. There is no central laboratory for human genetic diagnostic techniques, but some Institutes of Human Genetics offer their services for specific diagnoses.

## 2.5.1.3 Prenatal Diagnosis

### Description of Services

Prenatal diagnosis of genetic diseases by amniocentesis is presently offered by 44 laboratories capable of tissue culturing and chromosome analysis. Many more centers for prenatal care and private gynecologists practice amniocentesis. Thus, it proved impossible to count all who do amniocentesis.

In recent years, prenatal diagnosis by amniocentesis has increased rapidly, as shown in Table 2.5.3. The percent of mothers age 35 or over who received amniocentesis rose from an estimated 29% in 1982 to an estimated 47% in 1986. If chorion biopsies are included, the percent receiving prenatal diagnosis may exceed 50% in 1986.

Table 2.5.4 shows the numbers of amniocenteses performed in each state, the percent of the total FRG population and the number of labs in each state, and the estimated percent of women aged 35 years and over who received amniocentesis in the years 1982, 1984, 1985, and 1986. The uptake of prenatal diagnosis has been slow in some states, such as Niedersachsen, Saarland, Nordrhein-Westfalen, and Bayern. On the other hand, the City-States of Hamburg and Bremen, which serve women from surrounding states, reported numbers out of proportion to their populations.

CVS began in 19 university laboratories in 1985; four additional centers planned to introduce it in 1986. A total of 924 chromosome analyses from CVS were reported in 1985, which included about 30 biopsies primarily done for other diagnostic reasons. The expected number of CVS investigations for 1986 in 23 laboratories totaled 3,355, which meant a 3.6-fold increase. Our own laboratory expected to perform about 250 CVS procedures in 1986. By September 1986, about 82 had been done, due to a shortage in personnel in the gynecology depart-

**Table 2.5.3.** Development of Prenatal Diagnosis in the FRG

|  | Livebirths | Mothers ≥ 35 Years | Total Prenatal Chromosome Diagnoses | Total Performed for Advanced Maternal Age | % of Mothers ≥ 35 served |
|---|---|---|---|---|---|
| 1982 | 621,173 | 44,152 | 15,838 | ~12,670 | 28.6 |
| 1983 | 594,177 | 46,315 | | | |
| 1984 | 584,157 | 47,838 | 22,506 | 16,628 | 34.8 |
| 1985 | 586,155 | ~48,000 | 26,130 | ~19,310 | 40.0 |
| 1986 | 586–590,000 | ~49,000 | ~31,180 | ~23,042 | ~47.0 |

Expected/Estimate

159

**Table 2.5.4.** Amniocenteses by State

| | 1984 % of FRG Population | 1986 No. of Labs# | 1982 Total Amniocenteses | 1982 % Mothers ≥35 served* | 1984 Total Amniocenteses | 1984 % Mothers ≥35 served* | 1985 Total Amniocenteses | 1985 % Mothers ≥35 served* | 1986 Total Amniocenteses | 1986 % Mothers ≥35 served* |
|---|---|---|---|---|---|---|---|---|---|---|
| Schleswig-Holstein | 4.27 | 2 | 847 | 36 | 1,025 | 36 | 1,116 | 40 | 1,160 | 41 |
| Hamburg | 2.63 | 5 | 1,216 | 96 | 1,606 | 89 | 1,704 | 99 | 1,770 | 101** |
| Niedersachsen | 11.82 | 2 | 674 | 10 | 817 | 11 | 1,032 | 14 | 1,150 | 15 |
| Bremen | 1.10 | 1 | 640 | 114** | 754 | 104** | 638 | 87 | 650 | 89 |
| Nordrhein-Westfalen | 27.46 | 9 | 3,929 | 24 | 4,877 | 28 | 5,290 | 30 | 6,340 | 35 |
| Hessen | 9.08 | 5 | 1,263 | 24 | 2,172 | 35 | 2,749 | 47 | 3,280 | 55 |
| Rheinland-Pfalz | 5.93 | 3 | 792 | 22 | 1,416 | 37 | 1,960 | 51 | 1,980 | 50 |
| Baden-Württemberg | 15.08 | 8 | 3,452 | 36 | 5,412 | 56 | 6,541 | 66 | 7,360 | 74 |
| Bayern | 17.89 | 5 | 1,892 | 17 | 2,939 | 25 | 3,446 | 30 | 5,500 | 46 |
| Saarland | 1.71 | 1 | 182 | 19 | 244 | 23 | 316 | 28 | 500 | 44 |
| Berlin (West) | 3.02 | 2 | 952 | 53 | 1,267 | 63 | 1,433 | 73 | 1,500 | 75 |
| Total# | 100.0 | 43 | 15,838 | 29 | 22,506 | 35 | 26,130 | 40 | 31,180 | 47 |

* percents estimated
# an additional laboratory did not participate
** percents are > 100 because the numbers reported include women from other states.

**Table 2.5.5.** Breakdown of Indications for Prenatal Chromosome Diagnostics from 42 Laboratories, 1984

| Total Prenatal Chromosome Diagnoses | Indication: Maternal Age ≥35 | Advanced Paternal Age ≥40 | Other Medical Indications | | | Maternal Anxiety (No Medical Indication) |
|---|---|---|---|---|---|---|
| | | | Recurrence Risks | X-linked Diseases | Other Inherited Disorders | |
| 22,506 | 16,628 | 1,220 | 1,655 | 71 | 526 | 2,406 |
| 100% | 73.9% | 5.4% | 7.4% | 0.3% | 2.3% | 10.7% |
| Range: | 63–87% | 0–15% | 2–17% | 0–3.7% | 0.3–11% | 0–29% |

ment and in the cytogenetic laboratory. Other units may encounter the same problem.

**Breakdown of Cases by Indication**

Colleagues in 38 prenatal diagnostic laboratories answered a special questionnaire in early 1985 about indications for prenatal diagnosis in their units. This questionnaire was separate from the Ethics and Human Genetics survey. Data from an additional four private laboratories, which could not provide a breakdown of indications, were treated as comparable to data from University laboratories in compiling Table 2.5.5. Results of the survey showed that 73.9% of all diagnoses were done for advanced maternal age. Percents ranged from 63% to 87% in individual laboratories. Paternal age of 40 years or over was the indication in 5.4% of all cases, with a range of 0–15% (Table 2.5.5). Other medical indications accounted for 10% of prenatal diagnoses, with a range of 0–17%. Maternal anxiety or need for reassurance of the fetus's genetic "normalcy" accounted for 10.7% of prenatal diagnoses, with a range of 0–29%, indicating that there was considerable variation in the acceptability of this non-medical indication.

Maternal and paternal age limits accepted as indications for amniocentesis are shown in Table 2.5.6. As a result of difficulties in establishing counseling units and laboratories in some states, such as Niedersachsen and Saarland (Table 2.5.4) and the small numbers of laboratories in relation to the size of population in some states, age limitations are necessary in most units. Thirty units were in line with recommendations in national and international publications, i.e., 35 years and above. Six units, however, declared lower or higher limits.

The controversy over whether or not there is a paternal age effect is reflected in Table 2.5.6. Ten units did not accept amniocentesis for paternal age alone. Some of the others reported somewhat curious regulations. Cut-off lines at 50–60 years mean that they at least offered amniocentesis to extremely rare father-mother age combinations, thus not overburdening the laboratories' capacities.

Fifteen units answered questions about regulations for CVS (Table 2.5.6). One of 15 units would provide CVS at age 33 years, nine units at 35 years, and five at

**Table 2.5.6.** Arbitrary Limits of Maternal and Paternal Age for Acceptance of Amniocentesis or CVS, 1985 (n = 36 laboratories)

| Amniocentesis | | | | CVS | |
|---|---|---|---|---|---|
| Maternal age limits | No. of labs | Paternal age limits | No. of labs | Maternal age limits | No. of labs |
| ≥ 33 | 1 | ≥ 40 | 6 | ≥ 33 | 1 |
| ≥ 34 | 3 | ≥ 41 | 3 | ≥ 35 | 9 |
| ≥ 35 | 30 | ≥ 45 | 4 | ≥ 38 | 4 |
| ≥ 36 | 1 | ≥ 48 | 1 | ≥ 40 | 1 |
| ≥ 37 | 1 | ≥ 50 | 8 | no response | 11 |
| | | ≥ 55 | 3 | | |
| | | ≥ 60 | 1 | | |
| | | not accepted as an indication | 10 | | |

more advanced ages. The situation is similar to the earlier development of amnio-centesis, when doctors had to learn the procedure. However, as frequently stated in the literature, the problems with CVS are many and are not restricted to the bi-opsy itself. For CVS there is a minimal consensus among gynecologists, counsel-ors, and cytogeneticists about the services offered, about informed consent of the mother/parents, about care for the puncture/biopsy, and about minimum stan-dards of cytogenetic quality. Usually 12–15 cells are evaluated. Broad variations exist in tissue culture methods and in time intervals until the result is given to the mother-in-waiting. CVS by mail will soon become possible when laboratories have enough capacity and personnel available. Today CVS is done in centers, but not in doctors' practices, while amniocentesis is increasingly transferred to commercial laboratories outside the centers.

Table 2.5.7 gives more information about laboratories' restrictions on capacity and indications for amniocentesis. Nineteen of 37 units were already working at full capacity. Surprisingly, 18 units reported that they were not yet working at full capacity. About 20% more amniocenteses were expected in 1986 than in 1985 (Table 2.5.4).

The conditions for prenatal diagnosis seemed to follow a generally accepted concept. Private patients, who pay about two to three times the fee paid by com-pulsory national health insurance for the same investigation, had no advantage. In most units, the indication could be given by the gynecologist who did the amnio-centesis. Only five units required a full genetic counseling session prior to amnio-centesis. All units, without exception, accepted indications given by medical genet-icists, and 34 of 37 units accepted maternal anxiety as a reason for amniocentesis.

Whether counseling services were offered prior to prenatal diagnosis depended on the unit's philosophy of genetic counseling and human genetic diagnostics, availability of personnel, and the cooperation of gynecologists and cytogeneticists. Some centers offered prenatal diagnosis only after thorough genetic counseling. Others accepted patients for amniocentesis from gynecologists without knowledge of the woman's personality, genetic background, or conflicts involved. Many col-leagues in clinical genetics considered counseling for prenatal diagnosis in the ad-vanced age group less important than counseling for hereditary disorders. Other colleagues regretted that they could not offer counseling because of shortages of personnel. Even a training program for medical geneticists supported since 1980 by the benevolent society "Aktion Sorgenkind" (Action for the Child with Special Needs) barely accepted the need for counseling before prenatal diagnosis.

**Table 2.5.7.** Center Policies on Amniocentesis (n = 37 genetics units)

| Regulations and Conditions for Amniocentesis | Yes | No |
|---|---|---|
| Unit currently working at full capacity | 19 | 18 |
| Favors private patients | 0 | 37 |
| Genetic counseling prior to amniocentesis | 5 | 32 |
| Indication by: | | |
| 1. Gynecologist | 32 | 5 |
| 2. Medical geneticist | 37 | 0 |
| 3. Maternal anxiety or other psychosocial reason acceptable | 34 | 3 |

## 2.5.1.4  Cost-benefit Analysis

A short comment will suffice. It is not our purpose to add anything to the calculations that have been done by others and we will not give figures here. It is ethically objectionable to describe the life of a handicapped human being in economic terms per year, although such calculations must be made by politicians to coordinate social and medical programs. In this context, medical doctors must use their experience to help promote these programs. However, we strongly oppose a cost-benefit approach to the lives of handicapped persons. Also, we strongly oppose any development of an economically-driven preventive protocol for pregnancies and any pressure to abort when a genetic marker is found in a fetus.

## 2.5.1.5  Abortion

The abortion law (§218 in the Penalty Law) was changed in May 1976. Induced abortion was exempted from penalty under certain conditions:

1. The pregnant woman has to declare that it is her free will to abort;
2. A physician has to confirm the indication;
3. A social counselor or physician has to advise the pregnant woman about social support for continuation of the pregnancy; and
4. The abortion has to be done by another gynecologist independent of the doctor who confirmed the indication.

Indications are the following: Psychosocial reasons, ethical or criminal reasons (rape or incest), both indications exempted until the twelfth week of pregnancy; the so-called eugenic reason (abnormal child, high risk for a severe genetic or non-genetic disease), which exempts abortion until the twenty-second gestational week; and medical reasons (saving the mother's life), without time limits. The law requires that all induced abortions be reported anonymously. Table 2.5.8 reports the statistics on abortions since the law was changed. The numbers in the first column represent the officially registered cases reimbursed by health insurance and include out-patients. They have been broken down according to the legally-recognized indications. There is, of course, much concern about the unknown additional number of unregistered abortions done during short-term clinical stays, done for private patients, or done outside the FRG. The estimated total number of fetuses aborted in the FRG has been included in Table 2.5.8 because of serious concerns among the public and the Board of Medical Associations (Bundesärztekammer). Because of these differences between numbers of officially-reported abortions and estimates of actual numbers, it is difficult to make any comparisons between the numbers of abortions for psychosocial indications and the numbers of abortions for the so-called eugenic reason. Such ratios have been included, but should be interpreted with caution.

163

**Table 2.5.8.** Induced Abortions in the FRG, 1975–1985

| Year | Officially Registered | Estimated No. "Suspected Reality" | % Indications for Registered Abortions | | | | | Psychosocial/ Genetic Abortion Ratio | Induced Abortion/Live Birth Ratio No. of Abortions per 100 Live Births | |
|---|---|---|---|---|---|---|---|---|---|---|
| | | | Psycho-Social | Medical | Fetal Abnormality | Ethical (Rape, Incest) | Not Stated, other Reasons | | Officially Registered | Estimated "Reality" |
| 1975 | | 80,000–350,000 illegal abortions suspected | | | | | | | | |
| 1976 | (13,044)[+] | | 45.0 | | | | | | | |
| 1977 | 54,309 | ~140,000 | 57.7 | 29.0 | 4.3 | ±0.1 | 8.9 | 19.0 | 9.3 | 24.0 |
| 1978 | 73,548 | | 67.0 | 22.9 | 3.7 | ±0.1 | 6.3 | 18.0 | 12.8 | |
| 1979 | 82,788 | ~325,000 | 70.6 | 20.8 | 3.8 | ±0.1 | 4.7 | 20.0 | 14.2 | 55.8 |
| 1980 | 87,702 | | 72.1 | 20.1 | 3.5 | ±0.1 | 4.2 | 20.6 | 14.1 | |
| 1981 | 87,535 | ~212,000 | 74.8 | 17.6 | 3.2 | ±0.1 | 4.3 | 23.4 | 14.0 | 33.9 |
| 1982 | 91,064 | ~220,000 | 76.9 | 16.7 | 2.5 | ±0.1 | 3.8 | 27.6 | 14.7 | 35.4 |
| 1983 | 86,529 | | 80.2 | 14.3 | 2.1 | ±0.1 | 3.3 | 38.2 | 14.6 | |
| 1984 | 86,298 | ~230,000 | 83.8 | 12.0 | 1.9 | ±0.1 | 2.7 | 44.1 | 14.8 | 39.4 |
| 1985 | 83,538 | ~260,000 | 84.3 | 11.1 | 1.3 | ±0.1 | 1.7 | 64.8 | 14.3 | 44.3 |

[+] Changes in the Abortion Law, May 18, 1976, allowed exemptions from penalty. Anonymous registration is required, but not regularly carried out; No. of abortions in 1976 reflects second half-year registration (Bräutigam and Grimes 1984; Goebel 1984; Kuhn 1986; Statistical Year Book 1985).

In 1985, for every abortion done for fetal abnormality, there were an estimated 64.8 abortions for psycho-social reasons. There were 14.3 officially registered abortions and an estimated 44.3 actual abortions for every 100 livebirths.

## 2.5.2 Ethical Problems Faced by Medical Geneticists in the FRG

### 2.5.2.1 Genetic Counseling

The basic ethical problem is the question of how to deal with knowledge. Is there a right not to know, for those who do not want to know? A general renunciation of access to knowledge would not do justice to the structure of our scientific-technical civilization. On the other hand, every human being must have the right to refuse medical investigations. Despite possible risks, it is a human right to forego prenatal diagnosis, and this must be granted. Refusal, however, should only be the decision of a mature citizen after thorough counseling. Use or refusal of modern diagnostics must be based on a responsible and fully-informed decision.

An additional ethical consideration in providing genetic knowledge is how much time a counselor should take to counsel each patient and how much time the organization should allow the counselor to take. On this depends how much detailed information, with its consequences and ethical implications, the counselor can bring forward. Short-cutting counseling certainly curtails the ethical consideration of a problem. This becomes particularly visible in cases where prenatal diagnosis is routinely done without counseling. Too little time leaves counselor and counselee too far apart. The counselor delivers his or her personal scientific knowledge, without ethical reflections, to the counselee, without further discussion. The counselee is left alone with her or his decision and receives no help. But even worse would be directive counseling.

Setting standards for successful outcomes of counseling poses another ethical problem. If the counselee follows the advice of the counselor, it might be counted as successful counseling. But if the counseling was a true mutual discussion about pending decisions, someone should ask afterwards how the patient acted on the basis of the advice s/he received.

### 2.5.2.2 Prenatal Diagnosis

In prenatal diagnosis ethical problems include options for abortion and questions of acceptable medical indications (Schroeder-Kurth 1985b). In many laboratories, prenatal diagnosis by amniocentesis is done without counseling the pregnant women, simply as a service on request. Risk of fetal loss is no longer a medical argument against amniocentesis on request, but limited resources reinforce the responsibility for a just allocation of services to those at higher risk for a diseased child.

165

In specific genetic diseases prenatal diagnosis can help to verify the state of health of the expected child. If there is a pathological result, the parents either prepare themselves for a retarded child and look for therapy or they decide to terminate the pregnancy. This is not therapy but killing. Even in ethical discussions, this fact will be camouflaged by choice of words, e.g., "interruption of pregnancy," "genetic prevention," or "avoidance of genetic diseases." What is involved is a selective killing of genetically abnormal beings. The ethical status and right to life of a fetus, as compared with a newborn, remains controversial. This question also extends to human zygotes and embryos; in the FRG legal protection of embryos begins 14 days after fertilization.

Any decision about the above-mentioned problems is complicated by the risk of prenatal diagnosis. If termination of pregnancy is out of the question, should an amniocentesis or CVS be performed? The answers will differ, depending on the ethical convictions of the patient and the genetic defect under investigation (Schroeder-Kurth 1985b, 1982b).

The possibility of identifying certain defects by prenatal diagnosis or at least of ascertaining a high probability of defect opens another perspective: a trial pregnancy. Pregnancy can be risked on condition that in case of a pathological result the fetus will be aborted. Such a "decision of the second degree" for a pregnancy creates an "artificial situation" (Huebner 1981), in which the mother's relation to the child and its acceptance – depending on its still uncertain state of health – will be postponed into the second trimester.

To some commentators trials of pregnancy are no longer an ethical problem. "With further improvement of prenatal diagnosis it will soon be possible to help a couple that today still has to forego children of their own on account of a high genetic risk" (Genetische Beratung 1979, p. 53). Ethically, however, a trial pregnancy is still a dubious consideration, because the price may be abortion of a fetus considered abnormal.

For further discussion of ethical problems in prenatal diagnosis, see 2.5.4 (Cultural Context of Medical Genetics) below.

## 2.5.2.3 Genetic Screening

Screening of newborns is widely used in the FRG for diseases that are treatable. Screening for CF falls into this category. However, CF heterozygote screening poses ethical problems. In the opinion of medical geneticists in the FRG, screening should only be done with consent.

## 2.5.2.4 Other Contexts:

For a discussion of the future of the handicapped in an age of prenatal testing, see 2.5.4 (Cultural Context of Medical Genetics) below.

## 2.5.3 Consensus and Variation: Survey Results

The results of the study showed that medical geneticists in the FRG paid great attention to the autonomy of the patient and respected the free decisions of counselees. A consensus in approach emerged from all answers: The counselor was more concerned about the parents' welfare than about protection of the unborn. Parental protection overruled the protection of the fetus, with one exception: sex choice of an otherwise normal baby. In all, 94% would refuse to perform prenatal diagnosis. The welfare of the child and the conflict between client and geneticist was well recognized. In the international comparison, the reasons given against sex selection fell into the most-used categories and represented a strong defense against misuse of methods, resources and goals of medical genetics.

Although there was consensus against CVS or amniocentesis for sex selection, the discussion is still open. The arguments concentrate on various types of feminist views, and on present laws and their sloppy interpretation by doctors and patients, as well as on individualistic grounds. A doctor's decision may also rest on the desperate principle of saving half of the children, the wanted ones, in situations where parents threaten to abort. The majority of counselors, however, oppose accepting CVS for sex selection, probably because the Ethical Committee of the Society of Anthropology and Human Genetics recommended opposition. This guideline agrees with the position of geneticists around the world. Sex selection has the lowest priority today and in the future for medical geneticists in the FRG.

Options that respondents would present in counseling were limited to those options with the greatest support from the majority in this society. For example, the option of "taking chances" for a person at risk for tuberous sclerosis posed severe problems for several counselors. Patient autonomy was respected, but it was clearly limited by guidelines, principles, or professional duties of medical doctors to weigh their responsibilities against the individual desires of patients.

Discussions on presenting reproductive options must take into account current legal restrictions. Donor egg, IVF and surrogate motherhood are regulated by the Medical Board and medical law. Thus these methods can be discussed only theoretically, since no actual option exists within the FRG.

A sizeable number of counselors (28%) would describe the emotional difficulties associated with terminating a pregnancy when counseling the parents of XO or XYY fetuses. The percent describing difficulties of termination exceeded the percent in all other countries except Hungary and Japan. None in the FRG would advise abortion for these conditions.

Respondents reported that the questions that gave them the greatest ethical conflict were sex selection, confidentiality of a Huntington disease patient versus duties to relatives at risk, and disclosure of new/controversial test results.

Geneticists experienced the least ethical conflict about prenatal diagnosis for sex selection, for parents who refuse abortion, and for maternal anxiety.

Perceptions about the sex selection case were interesting: 23% said that this problem gave them the greatest ethical conflict, and 30% said it gave them the least conflict. The latter had apparently already made up their minds before seeing the question.

The request for prenatal diagnosis in Case 9 (parents who refuse abortion) aims to prepare the parents for a retarded child, while in Case 10 (maternal anxiety) prenatal diagnosis could serve to prevent the birth of a child with retardation. In view of this contradiction, prenatal diagnosis seemed to be accepted as a good diagnostic tool; its practicability justified its use for both purposes.

In genetic screening there was a strong consensus that programs should be discussed first with the persons who are at risk. Screening projects should only be done on a voluntary basis with full disclosure of results to the persons screened, but with no access for third parties. The fear of third-party misuse of occupational screening results was greater among medical geneticists in the FRG than in most other countries. Unfortunately, the decision for or against screening programs at commercial and industrial enterprises is not under the control of persons who participated in the study. Fear of misuse also strongly influenced answers to questions such as "Who should have access to results of presymptomatic tests for Huntington disease?"

It is interesting how frequently specific reasons for choice of action were given in responses to the questionnaires. Most frequent reasons given were the right of the patient to privacy and the possible misuse of information by third parties. Emphasis was also given to the autonomy of the patient, scientific information as the basis for the best decisions, the patient's right to know or not to know, and honesty and the duty to speak the truth. On the other side, the possible suffering of future children and the refusal to abort a normal fetus appear relatively seldom. Family planning was the most frequently given second reason, followed by the intention to safeguard the unity of the family. It was argued repeatedly that guilt and fear should be reduced and also that limited resources should be used wisely.

In describing the reasons for their choices of action, many did not mention the consequences of their choices. For example, 79% did not describe the possible consequences of disclosing or not disclosing colleague disagreement about test results, and 60% did not mention the consequences of screening for susceptibility to occupationally-related disease. This seems to indicate a deficit in reflection on sociological and social-ethical questions.

## 2.5.4 The Cultural Context of Medical Genetics in the FRG

In view of the steadily increasing number and range of decisions in medical practice, ethical considerations are necessary in new situations. Increasingly, we begin to have life and death at our disposal, which forces us to decide about the value of human life. If, in addition, the possibilities of gene technology are considered, some talk of a "leap of quality" in human evolution, which would necessarily require a "new ethic."

More and more genetic disorders can be identified by prenatal diagnosis. The methods of gene technology allow more exact analyses, which can be used for screening programs. Interpreting the test results requires an ever-increasing ethical demand: Which deviations from the genetic norm justify a termination of pregnancy? Which abnormalities should be declared acceptable? What burden can be carried by the child, the mother, the family, the society? Who makes the decision? What kind of life can consequently be considered "worthwhile living" and what not? The last question was recently discussed in a very pragmatic way by the philosophers Kuhse and Singer [1985].

In Germany, the misuse of genetics by the Nazis for eugenic programs suppressed these issues, and eugenic considerations have been avoided in genetic counseling in the FRG. Recently many discussions have recalled these problems.

A basic problem is what kind of mentality the growing possibilities of genetic counseling and prenatal diagnosis are creating among the public. There is the danger that a "biological norm" may be created, which classifies genetically burdened human beings as "avoidable" and consequently unacceptable by society. This would create a "duty to have a normal (nonhandicapped) child." This position no longer recognizes the "diakonic" task of the handicapped in society. By "diakonic task" we mean that the handicapped, by their presence, perform a real social service. Diakonic comes from the Greek word for servant, and is used in the New Testament to describe the Order of Deacons who cared for the poor, sick, and elderly in the early Christian Church. The handicapped are deacons in a symbolic sense. Their presence serves to make us reflect on what it means to be human. Their presence also serves to draw communities together in making sacrifices to provide for their well-being, and thereby enriches the fabric of human relationships. A society without the handicapped would lose its sense of community and its willingness to care for others. The ideal of perfect health sacrifices the reality and complexity of life and human relations, which do not exist without suffering. At risk is humane solidarity with the sick and handicapped and their families.

## 2.5.4.1  Sources of Challenge and Support

There are four influences on ethical reflection:

**a)** The individual counselor depends upon his or her own ethical convictions and expects concrete help from professional and theological ethics. Counselors' expectations are based mostly upon traditional ethics; they look for critical assistance with their own tasks and expect hints at the ethical borderlines. They await ethical guidelines that regulate further developments and draw a line between "can-still-be-done" and "not-allowed-anymore." In line with this expectation appears an ethical casuistry that creates a "prescription-for-action." The development of medicine and genetics requires continuous revision of guidelines, but this does not negate their usefulness. Roman Catholic moral theologians, in particular, fill this demand for guidelines (Boeckle and von Eiff 1982; Gruendel 1984; Reiter 1985) but Protestant theologians do so as well (Eibach 1983, 1986; Thielicke 1986).

**b)** The questionnaire results suggested that only a small number of participants were oriented and motivated towards religion. In all, 38% of participants did not attend any personal religious observances in the past year, 40% attended 1 to 4 times a year, 11% attended 5 to 14 times a year, and 11% attended 15 or more times a year. Accordingly, far-reaching reservations exist toward metaphysical reasons for ethics and rules on which traditional ethics are mostly based. There follows a certain ethical positivism and pragmatism, which does not reflect fundamental and basic arguments, but refers to personal convictions about the problem. General acceptance and enforceability are the criteria; yardsticks are legal judgments, normative rules of professional societies, and laws of the State. Within this framework the personal conscience may act (van den Daele 1985; Sass 1985).

c) Protestant theologians, in particular, pose the fundamental question of resubstantiation of ethics. This question cannot be pursued except in human situations where advice and help are requested. Christian love must accompany the fate of every human being. This requires detailed and extended dialogues and discourse, in which, in companionship with all affected persons, decisions are made (Huebner 1981, 1986; Honecker 1985, 1986; Link 1981). In consequence, an "ethic of genetic counseling" will include reflections on different situations without neglecting the truthfulness of more general ethical concepts; general principles and results will be integrated into specific considerations. Based on their pastoral experiences, Catholic moralists are arguing in the same way (Sporken 1981).

d) To complete the picture, so-called "alternative groups" should be mentioned. They are basically opposed to any kind of genetic counseling and prenatal diagnosis and point to bad experiences during the Nazi regime. As part of their general criticism of society, they are afraid of manipulation by the upper classes (Sierck and Radtke 1984), while feminists fear domination by the patriarchate (Hansen and Kollek 1985). Such views are represented by the political party "Die Grünen" (The Green Party) and also by groups of the handicapped.

These questions and problems have been discussed among geneticists themselves, in interdisciplinary symposia (Wendt 1970; Boland et al. 1981; Kuhn 1983; Engert and Quakernack 1985), and also in meetings for various types of participants (e.g. Schloot 1984). In the meantime, the subject "Ethics" has become firmly established in professional congresses. Human geneticists inform the public and teach medical colleagues and interested laypeople about the possibilities of genetic counseling and diagnostic techniques. Each counseling unit has developed its own instructive pamphlet. In the FRG the Bundesärztekammer (German Medical Association) has published recommendations for IVF and prenatal diagnosis, which will be integrated into the medical laws.

No professional chair of Medical Ethics exists yet at a university in the FRG. On their own initiative, some lecturers teach about relevant questions and problems. For instance, docents at the Institutes for Medical History at Freiburg, Heidelberg, and Frankfurt offer courses about Medical Ethics. Sometimes problems are treated in public lectures at universities, so-called "Studium generale" (Vogel 1982), and other lectures and in seminars offered at the theological faculties of some universities, for instance in Heidelberg and at the Kirchliche Hochschule in Berlin.

The Protestant and Catholic Academies in the FRG and in the GDR are in the forefront of the discussion of genetic and medical-ethical problems. They have organized meetings, symposia and working groups (e.g. Strauss 1971; Ritschl 1981). Since 1976, a group of researchers from various disciplines has existed at the Institute for Interdisciplinary Research of the Evangelische Studiengemeinschaft (FEST) in Heidelberg, which discusses ethical problems in genetic counseling. In the meantime, several books with interdisciplinary articles have been published (von Troschke and Schmidt 1983; Reiter and Theile 1985; Wehowsky 1985). Catholic moral theologians, evangelical ethicists, and practical philosophers have given their contributions on this subject. Some have written publications of their own (Altner, 1980; Eibach, 1983, 1986; Huebner, 1986; Ritschl, 1986; Loew, 1985).

The Evangelical Church in Germany published a leaflet on ethical considerations about the embryo and fetus with the title "Von der Würde werdenden Lebens" ("On the Dignity of Developing Lives") in 1985. The Synod of the Evangelical Church in Germany edited a declaration in 1987 entitled "On Respect for Life" (Evangelische Kirche in Deutschland, Kirchenamt 1987; Das Leben achten, 1988). The "Diakonisches Werk" of the Evangelical Church in Germany has paid as much attention to genetic counseling (Schober 1983) as the "Deutscher Evangelischer Krankenhausverband" (Association of German Protestant Hospitals) (Schenk 1984). There are similar activities in the Roman Catholic Church and Associations. The regional Protestant Churches and their synods are concerned about ethical problems of biotechnology. Local parishes and religious communities are also interested; the theme has been presented in religious lectures in schools and has been widely discussed at popular meetings of the "Deutscher Evangelischer Kirchentag," which take place every two years.

The German government has created an interdisciplinary working group on "in-vitro fertilization, genome analysis and gene therapy." The results will be used for future legislation. The Parliament of the FRG initiated an "enquête" commission that dealt with gene technology and related problems (Catenhusen and Neumeister 1987). The Churches have also been contacted. Political parties support foundations dealing with these problems, mostly in the form of public meetings, the proceedings of which are published (e.g., in a series about "Gene Technology, Chances and Risks," 1985, 1986). Although emphasis is given to the steadily progressing gene technology, the questions of genetic counseling and prenatal diagnosis are being dealt with publicly at the same time.

## 2.5.4.2 Major Controversies

The most controversial ethical problem concerns the termination of pregnancy. Although prenatal diagnosis followed by abortion, subject to medical indication, is accepted by society in the FRG, the Churches in particular point to the ethical problem – the killing of human life. On the question of whether prenatal diagnosis should be offered if the patient refuses an abortion *a priori*, 15% of participants in the survey answered in the negative. The Bodelschwingh'schen Anstalten in Bethel near Bielefeld, which cares for many severely handicapped human beings, has decided not to introduce prenatal diagnosis (Peters 1983). The nurses as well as the patients would not understand the rationale for such a procedure. The critical ar-

171

gument is the practical experience that prenatal diagnosis may be followed automatically by abortion if the fetus is abnormal. This would make personal decisions and responsibility for abortion impossible.

Another controversy concentrates on genetic counseling. Should counseling only provide information, should there be directive or non-directive advice, should psychological and social aspects be included, or should it be a discussion between partners that also includes some pastoral care? How a counselor deals with the patient's wish for prenatal diagnosis without medical indication depends on the philosophy of counseling and on whether the counselee can be followed beyond the one-time consultation. The basic concept of genetic counseling determines its efficiency, which will in turn determine its financial support. Counseling philosophies in different regions conflict with each other – for instance Marburg and Frankfurt versus Freiburg and Ulm. New gene technologies (DNA analysis and synthesis) and chorion villus sampling have created the most severe controversies, since consequences cannot be foreseen. Situations like disclosure to relatives at genetic risk of Huntington disease, against the patient's wishes, are presently the most discussed dilemmas.

## 2.5.4.4 Abortion Laws

See 2.5.1.5 above.

## 2.5.5 Ethical Trends in Medical Genetics

There are two basic trends that will affect future ethical discussions.

1. The possibilities of prenatal diagnosis will continue to expand. More and more irregularities in the genome will be identifiable. The significance of such irregularities must be evaluated: Simple genetic variants must be separated from real sickness and retardation, and the latter must be evaluated for severity and possible therapy. There are many borderline cases. Steadily expanding knowledge will eventually require redefinitions of indications justifying the termination of pregnancy. Prenatal diagnosis could be extended to every pregnancy, if the risk for the mother is further minimized. Such genetic screening or a "genetic passport to life" also increases problems in the protection of personal data.
2. The danger is that an individual human being will be judged more and more on the basis of biological interpretations; it follows that he or she will no longer be recognized without prejudice as a human partner. The consequence would be an adversarial attitude towards medical institutions, which does not accept and recognize the medical doctor as a helping and responsible human being, but faces him or her as an employee of a service institution that can be sued in case of displeasure. Doctors, on the other hand, will try to safeguard themselves against this possibility. Such a "juridification of the medical art" contradicts the

traditional ethos of medicine and stymies personal engagement. The same goes for the increasing commercialization of medical praxis, in view of calculated considerations of profit, e.g., by purchase and financing of expensive technical installations. The tight technical control of pregnancy and the fetus may blunt the mother's emotional experience of the fetus as a developing human being and the growing intimacy of the parent-child relationship.

In sum, the development of human love between parents and child does not permit the reduction of "health" to an abstract value, in particular if a child is accepted as a gift from God's hand. Health care *per se* should not become an end in itself, but only a means to serve the afflicted person.

# References

Altner G [1980] Leidenschaft für das Ganze. Zwischen Weltflucht und Machbarkeitswahn. Kreuzverlag, Stuttgart

Boeckle F, von Eiff WA [1982] Wissenschaft und Ethik. Christlicher Glaube in moderner Gesellschaft XX. Freiburg, pp 119-147

Boland P, Krone HA, Pfeiffer RA (eds) [1981] Kindliche Indikation zum Schwangerschaftsabbruch. Bamberger Symposion. Wissenschaftliche Information VII: 7. Milupa-AG, Friedrichsdorf/Ts

Bräutigam HH, Grimes DA [1984] Ärztliche Aspekte des legalen Schwangerschaftsabbruchs in der Bundesrepublik Deutschland und in den USA. Bücherei des Frauenarztes, Band 14. Enke Verlag, Stuttgart

Catenhusen WM, Neumeister H (eds) [1987] Chancen und Risiken der Gentechnologie. Enquete-Kommission des Deutschen Bundestages. Dokumentation des Berichts an den Deutschen Bundestag. Gentechnologie - Chancen und Risiken 12. Schweitzer-Verlag, München

van den Daele W [1985] Mensch nach Maß? Ethische Probleme der Genmanipulation und Gentherapie. Beck'sche Schwarze Reihe 299. München

Das Leben achten [1988] Maßstäbe für Gentechnik und Fortpflanzungsmedizin. Gütersloher Verlagshaus Gerd Mohn, Gütersloh

Deutsche Forschungsgemeinschaft [1977] DFG Forschungsbericht: Schwangerschaftsverlauf und Kindesentwicklung. Harald Boldt Verlag, Boppard

Eibach U [1983] Experimentierfeld: Werdendes leben. Eine ethische Orientierung. Vandenhoeck & Ruprecht Verlag, Göttingen

Eibach U [1986] Gentechnik - der Griff nach dem Leben. Eine ethische und theologische Beurteilung. Brockhausverlag, Wuppertal

Emery AEH, Rimoin D [1983] Nature and incidence of genetic diseases. In: Emery AEH, Rimoin D (eds) Principles and practice of medical genetics. Ch. Livingstone, Edinburgh, pp 1-3

Engert J, Quakernack K (eds) [1985] Pränatale Diagnostik. Zweites Bochumer Symposion. Wissenschaftliche Information XI, 3. Milupa-AG, Friedrichsdorf/Ts

Erhard B [1985] Verdunkelung, wo Klarheit erforderlich ist. In: Hoffacker P, Steinschulte B, Fietz PJ (eds) Auf Leben und Tod. Abtreibung in der Diskussion. Gustav Lübbe Verlag, Bergisch Gladbach, pp 159-170

Evangelische Kirche in Deutschland, Kirchenamt (ed) [1985] Von der Würde werdenden Lebens. Extrakorporale Befruchtung, Fremdschwangerschaft und genetische Beratung. Eine Handreichung der Evangelischen Kirche in Deutschland zur ethischen Urteilsbildung. Hannover

Evangelische Kirche in Deutschland, Kirchenamt (ed) [1987] Zur Achtung vor dem Leben. Maßstäbe für Gentechnik und Fortpflanzungsmedizin. Kundgebung der Synode der Evangelischen Kirche in Deutschland (Berlin 1987). Hannover

Floehl R (ed) [1985] Genforschung - Fluch oder Segen? Gentechnologie - Chancen und Risiken 3. J. Schweitzer Verlag, München

Fuhrmann W, Vogel F [1982] Genetische Familienberatung. Ein Leitfaden für Studenten und Ärzte. Heidelberger Taschenbücher 42. Springer-Verlag, Berlin, Heidelberg

Genetische Beratung [1979] Ein Modellversuch der Bundesregierung in Frankfurt und Marburg. Bundesministerium für Jugend, Familie und Gesundheit. Bonn-Bad Godesberg, p 53

Gentechnologie – Chancen und Risiken. (1985–1988) Vol 1–16. J. Schweitzer Verlag, München

Gentechnologie und Recht. Symposium des Justizministeriums Baden-Württemberg [1984] Triberg

Goebel P [1984] Abbruch der ungewollten Schwangerschaft. Ein Konfliktlösungsversuch? Springer-Verlag, Berlin, Heidelberg

Gruendel J [1984] Ethik und Humangenetik. In: Schloot W (ed) Möglichkeiten und Grenzen der Humangenetik. Campus Forschung 408, pp 219–247

Hansen F, Kollek R (eds) [1985] Gen-Technologie – Die neue soziale Waffe. Konkret Verlag, Hamburg

Hartung K, Wendt GG (eds) [1986] Praxis der genetischen Beratung. Möglichkeiten und Ergebnisse. Ein Leitfaden der Stiftung für das behinderte Kind zur Förderung von Vorsorge und Früherkennung. Umwelt & Medizin Verlagsgesellschaft, Frankfurt/M

Honecker M [1985] Verantwortung am Lebensbeginn. In: Flöhl R (ed) Genforschung – Fluch oder Segen? Interdisziplinäre Stellungnahmen. Gentechnologie – Chancen und Risiken 3. München, pp 144–160

Honecker M [1986] Humangenetik und Menschenwürde. Gen-Technik aus der Sicht der evangelischen Ethik. Lutherische Monatshefte, pp 75–79

Huebner J [1981] Zur Ethik genetischer Beratung. Theologisch-ethische Aspekte technischer Möglichkeiten in der modernen Medizin. Ztsch f Evangelische Ethik 25: 102–108

Huebner J [1982] Die Welt als Gottes Schöpfung ehren. Zum Verhältnis von Theologie und Naturwissenschaft heute. Chr. Kaiser Verlag, München

Huebner J [1986] Die neue Verantwortung für das Leben. Ethik im Zeitalter von Gentechnologie und Umweltkrise. Chr. Kaiser Verlag, München

Illhardt FJ [1985] Medizinische Ethik. Springer-Verlag, Heidelberg

In-vitro-Fertilisation, Genomanalyse und Gentherapie. Bericht der gemeinsamen Arbeitsgruppe des Bundesministers für Forschung und Technologie und des Bundesministers der Justiz [1985] In: Gentechnologie – Chancen und Risiken, Vol. 6. J. Schweitzer Verlag, München

Jonas H [1984] Das Prinzip Verantwortung. Versuch einer Ethik für die technologische Zivilisation. Suhrkamp Taschenbuch 1085

Kuhn W (ed) [1983] 92. Tagung der Nordwestdeutschen Gesellschaft für Gynäkologie und Geburtshilfe. Zusammenfassender Bericht. Bad Pyrmont, Alete Wissenschaftlicher Dienst 1/83

Kuhn W [1986] Schwangerschaftsabbrüche. Dtsch Ärzteblatt 83: 1604–1606

Kuhse H, Singer P [1985] Should the baby live? The problem of handicapped infants. Oxford University Press, London

Link Ch [1981] Die Herausforderung der Ethik durch die Humangenetik. Ztsch f Evangelische Ethik 25: 84–101

Löw R [1985] Leben aus dem Labor. Gentechnologie und Verantwortung Biologie und Moral. C Bertelsmann Verlag, München

Müller H, Olbing H (eds) [1982] Ethische Probleme in der Pädiatrie und ihren Grenzgebieten. Urban & Schwarzenberg, München

Perger C [1985] Genetische Beratung in Würzburg. Eine Analyse von 456 Beratungssituationen und 1655 zytogenetischen Untersuchungen aus den Jahren 1980–1983. Diss. Würzburg

Peters A [1983] Pränatale Diagnostik. Stand einer Diskussion. Diakonie 9: 125–131

Reif M, Baitsch H [1986] Genetische Beratung. Hilfestellung für eine selbstverantwortliche Entscheidung? Springer-Verlag, Berlin, Heidelberg

Reiter J, Theile U (eds) [1985] Genetik und Moral. Beiträge zu einer Ethik des Ungeborenen. Grünewald Verlag, Mainz

Ritschl D (ed) [1981] Medizinische Ethik. Evangelische Theologie 41 [6]: 481–606

Ritschl D [1982] Das "story" – Konzept in der medizinischen Ethik. Ztsch f Allgemein Medizin 3: 121–126

Ritschl D [1986] Konzepte, Ökumene, Medizin, Ethik. Gesammelte Aufsätze. Chr. Kaiser Verlag, München

Sass HM [1985] Extrakorporale Fertilisation und Embryotransfer. Zukünftige Möglichkeiten und ihre ethische Bewertung. In: Flöhl R (ed) Genforschung – Fluch oder Segen? Gentechnologie – Chancen und Risiken 3. München, pp 30–58

Schenk W (ed) [1984] Helfen und Heilen. Auftrag und Angebot. Bericht zum Evangelischen Krankenhauskongreß 1983. Deutscher Evangelischer Krankenhausverband e. V., Stuttgart

Schloot W (ed) [1984] Möglichkeiten und Grenzen der Humangenetik. Campus Verlag, Frankfurt

Schober T [1983] Auch vorgeburtliches Leben steht nicht einfach zur Disposition. Diakonie 9: 78–81

Schroeder-Kurth TM [1982a] Ethische Probleme bei genetischer Beratung in der Schwangerschaft. Monatssch. f. Kinderheilkunde 130: 71–74

Schroeder-Kurth TM [1982b] Schwangerschaftsabbruch – Ethische Probleme bei der genetischen Beratung. Geistige Behinderung VI: 224–236

Schroeder-Kurth TM [1985a] Indikationen zur Pränatalen Diagnostik. Grundsätze und Konflikte. Zeitsch f Evangelische Ethik 29: 30–49

Schroeder-Kurth TM [1985b] Die Bedeutung von Methoden, Risikoabwägung und Indikationsstellung für die Pränatale Diagnostik. In: Reiter J, Theile U (eds) Genetik und Moral. Grünewald Verlag, Mainz

Schroeder-Kurth TM [1985c] Humangenetische Beratung. Evangelische Kommentare 18: 392–394

Sierck U, Radtke N (eds) [1984] Die Wohltäter-Mafia. Vom Erbgesundheitsgericht zur Humangenetischen Beratung. Hamburg

Sporken P [1981] Die Sorge um den kranken Menschen. Grundlagen einer neuen medizinischen Ethik. Patmos Verlag, Düsseldorf

Statistische Jahrbücher der Bundesrepublik Deutschland [1976–1986] Kohlhammer Verlag, Stuttgart

Strauss J (ed) [1971] Biologisches Erbe und menschliche Zukunft. Tutzinger Texte 9. Claudius Verlag, München

Thielicke H [1986] Theologische Ethik II/1. J.C.B. Mohr/Paul Siebeck Verlag, Tübingen

von Troschke J, Schmidt H (eds) [1983] Ärztliche Entscheidungskonflikte. Falldiskussionen aus rechtlicher, ethischer und medizinischer Sicht. Medizin in Recht und Ethik 12. Enke Verlag, Stuttgart

Vogel F [1982] Die Zukunft des Menschen aus dem Blickwinkel der Humangenetik. In: Kontroversen der Zukunft. Studium generale an der Universität Heidelberg, Heidelberg, pp 16–23

Vogel F, Motulsky A [1979] Human genetics. Approaches and problems. Springer-Verlag, Heidelberg

Wehowsky St (ed) [1985] Schöpfer Mensch? Gen-Technik, Verantwortung und unsere Zukunft. Gütersloher Taschenbücher/Siebenstern 574, Gütersloh

Wendt GG (ed) [1970] Genetik und Gesellschaft. Marburger Forum Philippinum. Wissenschaftliche Verlagsgesellschaft, Stuttgart

Wendt GG, Theile U (eds) [1975] Genetische Beratung für die Praxis. Enke Verlag, Stuttgart

## 2.6 Ethics and Medical Genetics in France

J. F. Mattei and M. Gamerre

### 2.6.1 Medical Genetics in France

Ethical questions in medicine, as a research worker once said in jest, only interest retired scientists and gossips. Indeed, science possesses its own ethics – those of its use and effectiveness – and the risks it entails are too often exaggerated. In addition, public opinion always tends to confuse fiction with reality, as if it cannot dispense with a shudder of fear in imagining mass production of small docile monsters. The reality this time is a little bit different, as it is doctors themselves who are questioning the deeper implications of their work, and who are worried about the increasing powers given them by recent developments in medical genetics. Which path should be chosen between innocent complacency and die-hard conservatism expressing refusal? Our aim is first of all to describe the situation of medical genetics, then to analyze the ethical problems experienced by geneticists and to clarify present thought on these questions in France.

#### 2.6.1.1 Scope of the problem

In the period from 1975 to 1985, the number of births was between 805,000 and 720,000 a year, which corresponds to a fertility rate that has declined, with a few fluctuations, from 1.92 to 1.82. The population is therefore not renewing itself, since this fertility rate is less than 2.1. At the same time, the infant mortality rate has declined from 13.6 to 8.3 per 1,000 live births, reflecting the considerable improvement in the quality of care and the effectiveness of preventive medicine (Table 2.6.1). Between 1976 and 1981, the rates for congenital malformations were close to 2.6%. Taking into account the difficulties in monitoring, an estimation closer to the reality can be derived using the data from a systematic investigation carried out in Paris (Goujard et al. 1984). (See Table 2.6.2). Precise recording of malformations is now systematically organized in four regions of France (Paris, Lyons, Strasbourg, and Marseilles) within the framework of the International Clearinghouse for Birth Defects Monitoring Systems (1984, Annual Report) and of an E. E. C. Concerted Action Project (Registration of Congenital Anomalies in Eurocat Centers 1979–1983).

"Congenital anomalies" represent the second cause of death in the first year, after "lesions of obstetrical origin and diseases of the newborn" (WHO nomenclature). These data are not shown in national investigations. They must therefore be studied in the mortality statistics in registry offices. Infant mortality rates from

176

**Table 2.6.1.** Population, Births, Birth Rate, Fertility Rate

| Year | Population on January 1 (in millions) | Births (in thousands) | Birth rate (per 1,000) | Fertility rate | Infant mortality rate (per 1,000 births) |
|------|------|------|------|------|------|
| 1975 | 52,600 | 745 | 14.1 | 1.92 | 13.6 |
| 1976 | 52,810 | 720 | 13.6 | 1.83 | 12.6 |
| 1977 | 52,973 | 745 | 14.0 | 1.88 | 11.5 |
| 1978 | 53,182 | 737 | 13.8 | 1.83 | 10.6 |
| 1979 | 53,372 | 757 | 14.1 | 1.87 | 10.1 |
| 1980 | 53,587 | 800 | 14.9 | 1.96 | 10.0 |
| 1981 | 53,840 | 805 | 14.9 | 1.97 | 9.7 |
| 1982 | 54,091 | 797 | 14.7 | 1.94 | 9.5 |
| 1983 | 54,556 | 749 | 13.7 | 1.82 | 9.1 |
| 1984 | 55,064 | 760 | 13.8 | 1.81 | 8.2 |
| 1985 | 55,282 | 768 | 13.9 | 1.82 | 8.3 |

**Table 2.6.2.** Frequency of Malformations in the Paris Region in 1982[a] (per 100 live births)

| Malformations | | Paris 1981 |
|------|------|------|
| Central nervous system | | 0.17 |
| Cardiovascular system | | 0.42 |
| Respiratory system | | 0.03 |
| Hairlip and/or cleft palate | | 0.10 |
| Digestive system | | 0.13 |
| Genito-urinary system | | 0.30 |
| Osteomuscular system | | 0.93 |
|    Club foot | (0.20) | |
|    Congenital dislocation of the hip | (0.23) | |
| Trisomy 21 | | 0.12 |
| Other malformations | | 0.34 |
| Malformed children | | |
|    Single malformation | | 1.56 |
|    Malformation syndrome | | 0.13 |
|    Multiple malformations | | 0.39 |
| Total | | 2.08 |

[a] Goujard J, Gracco de Lay MO, Crost M, Maillard F (1984)

congenital anomalies have decreased during the last twenty years throughout the European Community, from 4% in 1960 to 2.5% in 1980, with rates always being higher for boys than for girls. For example, the average for the years 1965, 1966, and 1967 gives 3.82% for boys and 3.19% for girls (INSERM, 1978). This decrease in infant mortality from congenital anomalies has, however, been less than the decrease in total infant mortality, so that the proportion of deaths from congenital anomalies has increased from 20% to 40% of deaths in the first year. Mortality from cardiac anomalies alone represents 35% to 50% of infant mortality from congenital anomalies. As a guide, INSERM 1978 statistics give the percentage of deaths due to various malformations with respect to the total due to malformations: spina bifida: 4.9%; hydrocephaly: 6.4%; cardiovascular: 52.8%; digestive system: 10.1%. Taking into account the stability observed in the frequency of malformations, the results can be considered as corresponding to an improvement in the survival of malformed children.

## 2.6.1.2  Organization of Clinical Genetic Services in France

Medical genetics has developed steadily and become organized in France during the last 40 years. Observation of hereditary diseases and congenital malformations first of all led a certain number of physicians, mainly pediatricians, to give genetic counseling, using basic data from formal genetics and the study of genealogies of hereditary diseases. Fairly quickly, progress in biology made possible more accurate diagnoses and more logical classifications of these illnesses. So as to offer families all the necessary guarantees of reliability and seriousness, Medical Genetics Centers have been organized in the university hospitals, uniting specialists in medical genetics and biologists. For a population of about 55 million, there now exist 25 Medical Genetics Centers, structured according to local particularities. The ideal would be to unite in the same place the different departments necessary to ensure high quality genetic counseling: genetic counselors, a hospital section, cytogenetic and molecular biology laboratories, prenatal diagnosis consultation with the help of obstetricians and echographists, data processing for epidemiological studies and computerized diagnosis, and finally a library and a teaching and research structure (Giraud 1979). As an example, the Medical Genetics Center at Marseilles, developed through the efforts of Professor F. Giraud and located in a children's hospital of 500 beds, is aimed at a population of three million and receives about 2,500 new families for genetic counseling and/or prenatal diagnosis each year (Giraud 1986).

It is difficult to estimate with precision the number of chromosome studies carried out in France each year for postnatal diagnoses. For example, for a regional population of three million the two cytogenetic laboratories at Marseilles carry out about 1,600 chromosome analyses each year within the framework of check-ups for malformations, mental retardation, repeated miscarriages or sterility. The Center has one academic and five technical/administrative staff per 1,000 investigations/year (Table 2.6.3).

Investigations for genetic diseases are conducted by specialized services, according to the nature of the disease. For metabolic disorders, national and international collaboration exists between medical genetics centers and some laboratories interested in particular enzymatic determinations. At present the exploration of certain diseases, using recent recombinant DNA techniques, is being organized. Five laboratories in France have been certified for the diagnosis of hemoglobinopathies, hemophilia, Duchenne muscular dystrophy and mental retardation linked to X chromosome fragility. It is clear, nonetheless, that such organization will evolve as a function of needs and techniques.

178

**Table 2.6.3.**   Facilities for Clinical Genetics in France[a]

| 25 | Medical Genetics centers (one per 2.2 $\times$ $10^6$ inhabitants) for: | |
|---|---|---|
| | Postnatal chromosome analysis | 1 academic + 5 tech/admin. staff per 1,000 investigations/year |
| | Prenatal chromosome analysis | 1 academic + 6 tech/admin. staff per 1,000 investigations/year |
| | Genetic counseling | 3 clinical geneticists + 1 admin. for about 1,000 counselings/year |

[a] Data estimated on the basis of the Medical Genetics Center at Marseilles.

## 2.6.1.3  Prenatal Diagnosis

In France, prenatal diagnosis, particularly for the detection of chromosome and metabolic anomalies, is thoroughly tried and tested. This is due to the close collaboration between the Caisse Nationale d'Assurance Maladie (Social Security or CNAM), a non-profit association for the detection and prevention of metabolic illnesses and child handicaps (called Association Francaise or AF and chaired by Prof. Frézal), and specialized teams. According to the case, the different specialties (genetics, obstetrics, echography, cytogenetics and biochemistry) make up a coordinated network, as at Marseilles in the Prenatal Diagnosis Center. Such an organization, besides centralizing medical care for the patients, enables the different specialists to meet each other and discuss problems. Whatever the type of organization, prenatal diagnosis fits into the framework of a convention signed by the partners CNAM and AF. This convention determines the indications for prenatal diagnosis, fixes the examination charge reimbursed (1,000 FF or $170, in 1985, for a chromosome study) and decides which laboratories to certify (in 1985 there were 30 laboratories in 23 different towns, covering the entire country).

The convention provides that the indication for prenatal diagnosis must be provided by a medical geneticist, the obstetrical procedure carried out by a trained team, and the study conducted in a certified laboratory. Only the indications recognized by the convention and the studies carried out under these conditions are reimbursed. Prenatal diagnosis centers must send the AF a precise statement of the examinations each month and a follow-up of the pregnancies terminated in the last year each year. In addition to the recognized and indisputable indications, experimental work is financed by the CNAM on new techniques. Thus in 1986 a national program was organized for cystic fibrosis using DNA probes and enzymatic determinations; in 1987 a program started for the diagnosis of disorders linked to the X chromosome, using recombinant DNA techniques.

At present, the CNAM convention contains three indications: maternal age of 38 years or more, the birth of a previous child affected with a chromosome anomaly, or the existence of a balanced parental chromosome translocation. Between 1980 and 1985, 32,990 chromosome studies were carried out for these reasons (Table 2.6.4). In 1985, the 30 certified laboratories conducted 9,301 prenatal diagnoses in search of chromosome anomalies as specified by the convention. This is

**Table 2.6.4.** Prenatal Chromosome Diagnosis by Indications[a]

| Year | Total | Maternal age ≥ 38 years | Previous child with chromosome anomaly | Parental transloca-tion |
|------|-------|-------------------------|----------------------------------------|-------------------------|
|      | (n)   | (%)                     | (%)                                    | (%)                     |
| 1980 | 2,759 | 74.7 | 16.7 | 8.6 |
| 1981 | 3,912 | 76.3 | 16.0 | 7.7 |
| 1982 | 4,440 | 79.5 | 13.8 | 6.7 |
| 1983 | 5,454 | 80.7 | 14.0 | 5.3 |
| 1984 | 7,124 | 82.8 | 12.2 | 5.0 |
| 1985 | 9,301 | 84.7 | 10.9 | 4.3 |
| Total | 32,990 | | | |

[a] These data are regularly updated by Doctor M.L. Briard for the A.F. and published in an internal bulletin called "La Dépêche".

**Table 2.6.5.** Percent of Women ≥ 38 Years Receiving Prenatal Diagnosis

| Year | 1980 | 1981 | 1982 | 1983 | 1984 | 1985 |
|------|------|------|------|------|------|------|
| %    | 13.8 | 19.0 | 21.7 | 28.1 | 34.2 | 41.0 |

an increase of more than 30.6% compared with 1984, twice that in 1983 and three times more than in 1980. For 84.7%, the indication was maternal age (≥ 38). The proportion of women 38 years and over who are benefitting from prenatal diagnosis is now over 40%. This rate is still insufficient, but it is nevertheless a remarkable advance, since it increased from 13.8% to 41% between 1980 and 1985 (Table 2.6.5). A glaring inequality must be noted in access to prenatal diagnosis. The greater the geographical distance from the centre and the lower the socioprofessional level, the less likely the woman is to receive the service. Since 1980, the anomaly rate observed has been 3.17% of the total number of examinations carried out. In 2.64% there has been an abortion upon request of the couple, since it concerned unbalanced autosomal, and more rarely gonosomal, anomalies. In 0.52% of total cases the pregnancy was continued in agreement with the parents; most often it was a question of balanced translocations (Robertsonian or reciprocal translocations and pericentric inversions) or gonosomal anomalies (such as 47, XYY).

For two years now, the question of possible indications for chorionic villus biopsies has been posed. All the arguments in favor of this sampling method are known, and it is useless to reconsider them. It must be noted that the method has progressively gained ground and it is difficult to see what recommendation or what regulations could oppose it. However, it does not seem desirable that chorionic villus sampling be purely and simply substituted for amniocentesis, since the risk of miscarriage remains significantly greater than that from amniocentesis. The discussion is thus not over in France, and the AF has undertaken a survey to gather data.

The convention signed between the CNAM and the AF was completed by another convention dated July 1, 1982 for prenatal diagnosis of metabolic diseases. Two clauses have already been signed, one for prenatal diagnosis of hemoglobino-pathies and the other for hemophilias; both came into effect on July 1, 1984. Between July 1, 1982 and December 31, 1985, 443 metabolic diagnoses were carried out, enabling detection of 85 affected fetuses; between July 1, 1984 and December 31, 1985, 109 diagnoses for hemoglobinopathies were carried out.

As can be seen, the organization of prenatal diagnosis in France is particularly rigorous. This is due both to the interest shown by the public authorities and the will of the AF. The public authorities have found it necessary to delineate a prenatal diagnosis policy because prenatal diagnosis is an individual decision having a long-term impact, and because the demographic structure of the French female population clearly shows that the demand for prenatal diagnosis will grow in the next ten years. In this context, what criteria does the CNAM use for reimbursement? Social, psychological, and economic factors, without doubt, are considered, but the decisions of the CNAM are not made on the basis of cost-benefit analyses alone. Consideration of the effectiveness, risk, other possible side effects, and ethical problems are also taken into account. The decision to insure the neonatal screening of phenylketonuria and hypothyroidism (786,000 examinations paid for in 1984, for example, at 20 FF or $3 per double test) was not difficult; the test was simple, reliable, not very expensive, and covered almost all the newborn (99.53%). The decision to insure was more difficult for prenatal diagnosis, even for chromosomal anomalies. Not only is prenatal diagnosis more expensive than neonatal screening, but it must be reserved for women at risk, and so some, perhaps arbitrary, criteria must be defined. For other diagnoses, in a difficult economic period, there must be criteria for selection. The frequency with which the disease occurs, the absence or presence of benefit for the patient, the therapeutic possibilities, and the quality and accuracy of the diagnosis must all be taken into consideration. It is because the CNAM was able to depend on an organization like the AF that it decided to set up screening strategies.

The AF started by defining accurately the mission of clinical genetics departments and their connection with the laboratories. The specific role of clinical genetics departments is to give genetic counseling. This is a new field and requires an everyday familiarity with the problems it raises. Furthermore, genetic counseling cannot be limited to the estimation of a risk. It occurs in a psychological climate that contributes to making it a medical act. The medical geneticist appears as a natural intermediary between the clinical departments, which are responsible for the diagnosis and treatment of the patients, and the laboratories. The suggested organization is thus in conformity with the French medical tradition and gives the best chances of success to the French program.

## 2.6.1.4 Cost-benefit of Early Diagnosis and Genetic Counseling

The aims of a public health program cannot be defined independently of the elements of cost. Evaluation in monetary terms of cost and benefit in the prevention of handicaps is often arbitrary or unacceptable, since it is not possible to calculate

**Table 2.6.6.**  Estimated Costs of Prenatal Diagnosis (French Francs)

| Procedure | Cost (estimated 1985) |
|---|---|
| Genetic consultation | 110 |
| Obstetrics consultation | 110 |
| Echography | 250 |
| Amniocentesis | 109 |
| Alpha-fetoprotein test | 205 |
| | 784 |
| Laboratory analysis for amniotic karyotype (CNAM) | 1,010 |
| Total | 1,794 FF |

the "cost of suffering". Thus it is not so much a question of finding a cost-benefit balance point as of determining whether this program is financially possible and whether it contributes to the collective well-being.

To give an order of magnitude, we have taken as reference the noteworthy work conducted by Fardeau [1983], which we have updated. We have thus deliberately limited ourselves to the comparison of the costs assumed by the State, i.e., the cost of a prenatal diagnosis versus the cost of caring for a trisomic patient in a specialized institution.

Analysis of the reimbursed costs of the different counseling, obstetrical, and laboratory procedures involved in prenatal diagnosis works out on average to about 1,800 FF ($300) (Table 2.6.6). In fact, the real costs are higher because of the underestimation of the reimbursed costs, the hospitalization necessary in some cases, and the information provided to the doctors and target population. Information includes all activities undertaken to inform physicians and the public of the existence of prenatal diagnosis, of its consequences, of its medico-legal implications, of its evolution, of the ever-changing new possibilities, and the conditions of application. This implies conferences, newspaper and audio-visual campaigns, and post-graduate training for physicians. This cost should decrease with time when all physicians have received training in genetics during their studies. Finally, a unitary cost for a prenatal chromosome diagnosis comes on average to 3,500 FF (about $600). Cost analysis of institutional care for a trisomy 21 is particularly difficult, since it varies according to type of institution. Despite the artificial character of such an analysis, the approximate average annual cost of a trisomy 21 can be calculated by multiplying the average daily cost in a medico-educative institution established by the Minister of Health. This comes to around 130,000 FF (about $22,000). Taking into account a life expectancy on the order of 30 years, this corresponds to a total of 3,900,000 FF ($660,000).

On the basis of utilization of prenatal diagnosis in 1985 (7,880 women 38 or more years old, or 41% of this population; 124 trisomy 21 detected, or 1.7% of examinations carried out), a rate of service which is, as we have seen, far from being satisfactory, the "benefit" of prenatal diagnosis can already be appreciated, since it would mean a saving on the order of 500 million francs (83 million dollars). This "benefit" appears even greater if the extra medical cost of severely polyhandicapped trisomies, the supplementary material charges for the families, and the discovery of chromosomal anomalies other than trisomy 21 are taken into account.

In the organizational conditions in France (which has reliable technique, and all prenatal diagnostic activity kept in the public sector and off the market), a cost-benefit balance point cannot be defined scientifically as a function of maternal age. Elements of program cost have no use except for decision-making, which can only be the domain of Public Welfare. The most rational decision seems to be to specify a capacity likely to bring the incidence in women of 35 and over down to the level of younger women and to inform completely the doctors and women concerned. It is thus essential, first, to assess the knowledge and behavior of doctors in the field of genetic risk and genetic counseling, and then to determine the channels of communication to be used. In a survey carried out in the group of Ayme concerning the "Circulation and adoption of new knowledge in medical genetics: a regional study of genetic counseling and prenatal diagnosis", Julian [1986] emphasizes some very interesting points. The first point is that doctors lack information. In fact, 22% of general practitioners (G. P.'s) did not know that prenatal diagnosis must be proposed to a mother of 38 and over, and 26.5% of obstetricians and 51% of G. P.'s did not seem to know of the medico-legal obligation in France to inform the parents of the possibility of having a prenatal diagnosis! (The inquiry concerned 819 doctors in all, of whom 54 were obstetricians, 35 gynecologists, 103 pediatricians, and 627 G. P.'s). The extension of prenatal diagnosis to an increasing number of disorders creates more and more ethical problems, into which the doctor is called personally, with all his or her cultural and social experience, beyond the role of technical expert. It is remarkable to note that fewer than half the doctors taking part in the survey were in favor of an abortion of the six malformations proposed. It is no less remarkable that a third of the doctors "did not know" which attitude to adopt (Table 2.6.7). The percent undecided may be explained by: reluctance or refusal to give a personal opinion, lack of real knowledge of the pathology or seriousness, or variable expression of the disorder. In fact, when reservations about termination existed, in 20% of cases these were moral, in 11% religious, and in 39% of professional origin. (Professional reservations

**Table 2.6.7.** Views of Doctors Concerning Termination of Pregnancy[a]
(n = 819)

| Disorder | Termination of Pregnancy | | |
|---|---|---|---|
| | Yes % | No % | Do Not Know % |
| Trisomy 21 | 78 | 3 | 19 |
| Hemophilia | 22 | 42 | 37 |
| Turner syndrome | 47 | 15 | 37 |
| Klinefelter syndrome | 44 | 17 | 39 |
| Spina bifida | 52 | 17 | 31 |
| Cystic fibrosis | 46 | 18 | 35 |
| Total | 48 | 19 | 33 |

[a] Julian C (1986)

are different from moral or religious reservations in that they only concern the physician's conception of his/her profession: "to care for and not eliminate the patients who cannot be cured!" This concept is not directly linked to religion or individual morals even if there could be certain superpositions.) There are other reasons for reservations, for example the maternal risk and psychological trauma of an abortion in the fifth month. Such a reservation would disappear in 32% of cases if the abortion could take place before the tenth week, as is now possible with chorionic villus biopsy. There are, however, often very significant differences in the attitudes of doctors according to their age, sex, number of children, and specialty (it appears that male pediatricians more than 50 years old with several children are in general more conservative than the younger, mainly female obstetricians), which emphasizes the amount of subjectivity and the difficulty in defining "ideal" conduct.

## 2.6.1.5 Abortion

In Table 2.6.8 we have compiled the figures for births, social abortions, prenatal diagnoses, and abortions for genetic indications. It is difficult to know accurately the number of abortions not reported and impossible to estimate the number of abortions motivated by "risk of malformation" or "echographic anomalies," since genetics centers are unfortunately not consulted systematically in such cases.

It can, however, be noted that abortions for chromosome abnormalities occur in the ratio of 1.5 per 10,000 births, and 5.9 per 10,000 social abortions. The phenomenon is thus negligible quantitatively and it could be asked – the couples themselves to not hesitate to ask – whether it is reasonable to equivocate on "limiting" medical indications for termination of pregnancy at 20 weeks of gestation in cases of a potentially curable disease, whereas "all" seems legally allowed up to 12 weeks. At this point it is suitable to ask ourselves about the ethical problems for medical geneticists.

## 2.6.2 Ethical Problems Faced by Geneticists in France

**Definition**

Without wishing to lose ourselves in meddlesome semantic considerations, we must nevertheless remark that "ethics" is defined in the Larousse dictionary (which is an authority in France) as "the Science of Morals". The way in which the problem is tackled today almost everywhere inverses this definition by conveying "ethics" as "the morals of Science." In fact, to be clear, realistic and frank, it is a question of defining situations in which the doctor engages in a dialogue with his or her conscience to try and determine a behavior which best respects the idea we have of the "human person" and human dignity. In such naturally conflicted situations, the conscience of the doctor as man of science, the same conscience of the same doctor quite simply as a human in his/her social-cultural-educational

**Table 2.6.8.** Comparison of Live Births, Social Abortions and Genetic Abortions

| Period | Births | Social abortions[a] | Prenatal chromosome diagnoses | Genetic abortions |
|--------|--------|---------------------|-------------------------------|-------------------|
| 1980/1985 | 4,679,000 | 1,200,000 | 32,990 | 706 |

[a] In France abortion is legal upon request by the woman in the first 12 weeks of amenorrhea.

and religious context, the objective circumstances which present both beneficial possibilities and risks, legal conditions, subjective interpretations involving the potential severity of the handicap, and the perception the doctor has of the present and future reactions of the couple, all mingle and oppose each other.

In such circumstances one must know how to remain humble. For us it does not seem possible to define the limit between good and evil, between normal and abnormal, between acceptable and unacceptable, between the potential human being and the real human being, and even between life and death with certainty, since for some, death is only a passage. It does not seem possible for us to fathom the processes of consciences and their internal debates. It is clear that no one can presume to possess divine truth in a society where the decision of each individual engages the community, and inversely where the decisions of the community cause repercussions for everyone. It is thus a good thing that medical geneticists question themselves when faced with new problems that arise; it would, however, be bad if it filled them, *a priori*, with a masochistic guilt.

What are these new problems? They result, first, from the distinctiveness of medical genetics. This discipline diverges fundamentally from traditional individual medicine to address itself to a couple and more generally to two extended families, with all the underlying psychological difficulties that we can imagine. This discipline is above all directed towards prevention and rarely proposes therapeutic solutions. This discipline leads the doctor to give a prognosis for a "being" who does not exist yet ("what would be the risk in case of a new pregnancy"?) and to give this prognosis in terms of probability. This discipline is ambiguous, since it rests upon "genetic counseling". "Counseling" is not necessarily the best term, since it conveys the subjective involvement of the medical geneticist in what should be objective "genetic information" provided to a couple in a given situation. In this general context, recent technical advances in biology, in particular, have given rise to new problems. These can be arranged schematically into three different groups. 1) It is now known how to conceive life outside naturally occurring or traditionally accepted processes (all the so-called medically assisted procreation techniques, such as artificial insemination, in vitro fertilization and "surrogate mothers"); 2) The quality of this life can be forecast (above all through prenatal diagnosis, but also through screening and possibly through the development of predictive medicine); 3) Modification of the nature of life itself is foreseeable (this is the aim of genetic engineering and recombinant DNA techniques).

## 2.6.3  Consensus and Variation in Approaches to These Problems

The selection and description of the sample deserve a few words. In fact, 35 questionnaires were sent to those responsible for genetic counseling. Knowing that important decisions are usually discussed within the team, it did not appear necessary to ask all the doctors in a particular team, which would have biased the results of the inquiry, since large teams would have had a much greater weight in the statistical analysis of the data. This deliberate choice of the doctor in charge of each team is probably not the optimal approach. It is possible that the results convey the reality of the situation but eliminate individual opinions. The age of the respondents was between 31 and 64, with an average of 48. This results from the method of sample selection, and could give a false impression that medical genetics is a discipline that does not attract the young in France. This interpretation would be wrong. In Marseilles, for example, three doctors were questioned (54, 43, 31 years old) but six other doctors are also involved in genetic counseling (53, 39, 35, 34, 31, 27 years old). This selection method is also responsible for the fact that only 17 replies were obtained from the 35 persons asked to respond. It is clear that many department heads had reactions of rejection or mistrust, confusedly conveying their fear, their refusal to be contested, and their consciousness of holding a pragmatic attitude without a well-thought-out basis. These problems, added to the French highly individualistic and insubordinate spirit, explain at least in part, the unreturned questionnaires. France ranked 16th of the 19 nations in participation rate. On the other hand, it is interesting to observe that those who replied had an average of 18 years experience, and devoted about 30 hours a week to medical genetics, seeing an average of 13 patients a week. Thirteen amongst them had had supplementary training in genetics and 15 were pediatricians who had developed medical and genetic counseling activities. Only 2 of 17 did not belong to any professional organization, and more than half were men (11 of 17), but this proportion was different among the youngest. Fifteen were married and had an average 3.73 children each, which is significantly more than the average French family. (It is difficult to know whether this peculiarity results from the orientation of "pediatrics", or "genetics", or both.) Of the 15 who called themselves Catholics, three were non-practicing, whereas nine practiced regularly. Finally, three claimed to be rather conservative and five liberal. In all, it was a very biased sample with disadvantages (young geneticists under-represented), advantages (geneticists having many years of practical experience and thus a sound reference to fact), and peculiarities (almost all pediatricians, Catholics, and with many children).

**Medical Confidentiality**
Concerning Huntington disease and the revelation of the diagnosis with its genetic consequences for the relatives, there was no consensus amongst the doctors of our country. Six would respect the desire of the patient not to reveal anything; two would warn the family, whereas five would wait to be questioned; three, finally, would transfer the problem onto the referring doctor, which can obviously be a solution. In this particularly difficult case, there was no consensus in 12 other countries (Canada, FRG, GDR, Greece, Hungary, India, Israel, Japan, Sweden, Swit-

zerland, U.K., U.S.A.). The same lack of consensus in France was found in the analog situation concerning hemophilia A; for some, "confidentiality is the first right of the patient"; for the others, "it is a duty to inform the subjects concerned when a prenatal diagnosis is possible". On the other hand, in France, as in all the countries, medical confidentiality was the rule when analyses carried out revealed that the putative father was not the biological father: only the mother was informed of the conclusions and the possible genetic consequences.

### Medical Truth: the Whole Truth or Not?

An example concerned the discovery of a balanced translocation in a parent of a trisomy 21 child. In France there was no real consensus on the attitude to be adopted. For example, if the parents did not wish to know, six doctors would not tell them; seven, on the contrary, would tell all, whether the couple asked or not, and four would tell all also to the relatives concerned. In general, there was a strong consensus for the pursuit of openness and objectivity, notably when making known ambiguous or contradictory laboratory results. Telling the truth was rejected with a strong consensus when it was a question of revealing to a woman that her karyotype was 46, XY. It is thus not the pursuit of truth in itself that was the motivating force. The truth was itself appreciated as a function of numerous other considerations, such as medical responsibility or the consequences of the revelation of the diagnosis on the psychological and/or therapeutic level.

### Is genetic counseling to be directive or not?

Logically, genetic information given to couples should be perfectly objective. In fact, this is an unrealistic ideal, since everyone, and particularly the geneticist, appreciates the facts differently according to his or her own experience and adjusts his or her behavior according to the way the interlocutor reacts. Who amongst us has not tended to minimize negative aspects when faced with a pessimistic couple, and vice versa? It is utopian to imagine that doctors can be perfectly objective and non-directive even if they wish to remain so. This internal conflict is resolved differently in different circumstances. For example, in France everybody responding to the questionnaire agreed not to be directive when a 45, X fetus was discovered after prenatal diagnosis. On the other hand, when it concerned a 47, XYY fetus there was no longer any consensus and some advocated not saying anything or minimizing the facts. When one parent was affected with tuberous sclerosis, there was no agreement about the advisability of sterilization or contraception. These disagreements were observed in many other countries, and it is bewildering to realize that completely different reproductive conduct can be "counseled" in the same situation, according to the doctor and the country.

### Indications for Prenatal Diagnosis

It was difficult to interpret results for these questions, since some replies may have been influenced by laboratories' difficulties in coping with demand and some replies may have been formulated by geneticists whose main activity was not prenatal diagnosis. How can the importance of maternal anxiety be determined? How can prenatal diagnosis be refused categorically for this motive alone? Is it logical to carry out a prenatal diagnosis for a couple who will refuse an abortion? So many sources of internal conflict resulted in a total lack of consensus in our country. The French were, however, agreed about refusing prenatal diagnosis for choosing sex in the absence of any genetic indication. This was not, however, the case in the U.S.A., Hungary, India, Canada, and Sweden!

## Screening

New screening strategies, the development of preventive medicine, and economic considerations pose new problems. For risk factors linked with a work-related disease, the choice between mandatory screening (recommended in the GDR, Hungary and Turkey) and voluntary screening (Australia, Denmark, FRG, Greece, Italy, Norway, Sweden, Switzerland, U.K., U.S.A.) was not clear for the French who replied. There was, on the other hand, an almost complete consensus that screening results should be made available to the worker alone and not communicated either to the employer, the life insurer, or the health insurer, except with the consent of the worker. It seemed difficult to specify the "rights" and "place" of the Minister of Health, and in this regard there was no consensus about access for the government health department. As for the screening of cystic fibrosis carriers when a reliable test is developed, the French were undecided about whether it should be voluntary or about the age group to which it should first be given. With respect to a presymptomatic screening test for Huntington's chorea, everyone agreed that the patient should be the only one to have automatic access to the results, except for relatives at risk.

All things considered, the five main problems experienced by the French can be summarized as:

## Medical Confidentiality

It is still a fundamental tradition of medicine, but is more and more questioned according to the case, with regard for family consequences and taking into account possible preventive measures.

## Medical Truth

It imposes itself more and more often, on account of medico-legal liability and possibilities of prevention, but because of individual subjectivity, the doctor sometimes continues to view cases differently according to the context.

## Genetic Counseling

Should it be directive? ... no, but ...

## Prenatal Diagnosis Indications

Are there non-indications?

## Screening

It would be better only to consider volunteers and to give them the results individually. But is it certain that the necessary measures will be taken, and what will be the effectiveness from the point of view of public health?

Detailed comparison with other countries is presented in the synthesis in Section 2.6.4 and the complete Tables in Part I of this book.

## 2.6.4 Cultural Context of Medical Genetics in France

There is no organized teaching of medical ethics in France. In the last few years, however, due to progress in genetics, numerous problems have appeared and have led to the creation of organized structures for reflection and for development of recommendations. It is thus that the National Consultative Committee on Ethics (CCNE) was created, that many local committees have been organized in the university faculties and research organizations and that the religious authorities have contributed to the debate. There is no month without a large circulation magazine, a successful book, or a television program dealing with the problems of medically assisted procreation, prenatal diagnosis, or genetic engineering. In the last five years, the staff of our Medical Genetics Center have been regularly asked to take part in debates on the subject before doctors, non-doctors, the religious or the non-religious, associations, or political personalities.

Founded by decree on February 25, 1983, the CCNE for the natural sciences and medicine is chaired by Professor Jean Bernard. It includes 36 appointed members, chosen either because of "their connection with the main philosophical or cultural groupings" (nominated by the President of the Republic), because of "their competence and their interest in ethical problems", or because they "belong to the sector of research" (nominated by various institutions or ministries). The mission of the CCNE, according to the decree that gave birth to it, consists in giving an opinion "on the moral problems raised by research in the fields of biology, medicine, or health," whether these problems concern the individual, social groups, or the whole of society.

In 1985, the CCNE for the first time gave precise recommendations concerning the organization of prenatal diagnosis:

"To maintain the indispensable rigorous quality in biological and echographical diagnoses, it is recommended that certified prenatal diagnosis centers be established, and that no medical decision concerning an abortion be taken without a previous consultation at such a center. These centers should be multidisciplinary, including at least one medical geneticist, a biological geneticist, and a specialist obstetrician in fetal echography. They should be linked with one or several biological laboratories capable of carrying out the necessary studies. Practically, it is a matter of urgency to train doctors and technical staff in these disciplines. In the legal field, according to the terms of the law of January 17, 1975, a legally recognized motive for abortion is the existence of a strong probability that the child to be born will have a particularly severe disease recognized as incurable, which must be appraised by combining four elements: the degree of certainty of the diagnosis, the severity of the disease, age of onset of the disorder, and effectiveness of treatment. The consent to the abortion must be signed by two doctors, at least one of whom is competent in genetics and belongs to a certified center. Finally, the decision to continue or terminate the pregnancy belongs in the last resort to the parents, duly informed of the results of the examinations. It is essential to take care that the information cannot be understood as exerting pressure on them. The parents should never be resented for opposing prenatal diagnosis or abortion".

In December 1986, the CCNE expressed propositions and recommendations in the field of "medically assisted procreation". Since 1984, the CCNE has affirmed that the human embryo must be "recognized as a potential person". This qualification constitutes "the fundament of the respect which it is owed". Two years later, taking account of the present uncertainty about the status of the embryo as to the "threshold of emergence of the human being", the CCNE maintained in a quite coherent manner that the principle of respect for the forthcoming human being must be recognized from conception.

The CCNE, while recognizing that in vitro fertilization with transfer of the embryo is an acceptable procreation technique, considers it desirable to avoid increases in an uncertain, difficult and costly technique, which is not without physical and especially psychological risk for the couples. The CCNE furthermore directs the attention of the medical body and potential patients to the dangers of procreative desperation. The medical indications for in vitro fertilization must be limited to couples suffering from sterility or an established hypofertility and driven by a common parental project within a stable and effective relationship between man and woman. No other medical indication for in vitro fertilization can now be proposed. Concerning "supernumerary embryos", the CCNE considers that their destruction can only be envisaged in the search for the least evil and that destruction is inevitable when conservation is not possible. This destruction offends all those for whom the life of the embryo must be protected from the moment of fertilization. Conservation of these human embryos by deepfreezing must be carried out in certified centers and must be limited to twelve months maximum following fertilization. The medical motives for a possible extension of this time must be examined by the CCNE. Concerning the donation of embryos, the CCNE would like the legal aspects to be elaborated before embryo donation to other couples can be envisaged. Since the embryo is a potential person, research on embryos must be subjected to regulations and must be controlled by an authority whose composition reflects different currents of thought. For the moment, the CCNE has declared itself in favor of a moratorium of three years, during which time all research aimed at the realization of a genetic or gene diagnosis before transplantation would be suspended, due to the risks that methods of a eugenic character will develop. The CCNE also lists research work which should be forbidden by law, notably all research that seeks to modify the human genome. The CCNE emphasizes the urgent need to regulate all these activities by law and to certify centers that will be empowered to use techniques of medically assisted procreation.

Concerning the problem of surrogate mothers, there have already been about twenty births in France following a "uterus loan". In fact, the transfer of a child before its birth is forbidden and contracts exchanged between the mother and the parents are valueless (Article 1128 of the Common Law). The CCNE and the Council of the Order of Doctors have been very reserved about these practices. The CCNE would like to persuade everyone who has shown an interest in this method not to resort to it. In all humility, faced with a problem still poorly grasped by science, it seems clear that the central question, that of the interest of the future child, is not yet resolved. Nobody can sufficiently ensure that the arrangement of a birth with the intention of separating the child from the mother who has carried it serves the interest of the child. This way of responding to infer-

190

tility contains potential insecurity for the child, for the parents who want a child, for the woman who brings the child into the world, and for the third parties who intervene in all this. The satisfaction of a legitimate desire of some persons risks producing the suffering and contempt of others.

The opinion of the CCNE was received in various ways. It was approved by the Minister of Health and the Family. It met, on the other hand, the disapproval of the French Episcopate concerning certain recommendations that do not correspond to the most fundamental demands of respect for the person in all human beings, no matter how small or how fragile, such as destruction of the embryo or its use for scientific ends. It is in fact the status of the human embryo that is at stake; when does the embryo become a "person"? To say that the embryo must be respected cannot depend on a scientific observation, since the progression of knowledge risks modifying the definitions with each new discovery.

The problem has appeared sufficiently serious for Cardinal Lustiger to recall officially the great fundamental principles that inspire the moral judgement of the Church in these matters. These principles are: 1) Respect for the human being and a personal right to life, from conception and at every stage in the development of existence; 2) Respect for the marriage unit; it requires the fidelity of the married couple and their commitment to become mother and father only by each other; 3) Respect for human paternity and maternity in the integration of their physical, psychological, social, moral and spiritual dimensions; 4) Respect of the right of the child to be conceived, carried, brought into the world and educated by its own parents. It is true that in our country the liberalization of the legislation on abortion allows, under certain conditions, acts directly opposing respect for the human being and human beginnings. These legal or statutory provisions have sometimes placed doctors in intolerable situations. In effect, abortion is now allowed for reasons ranging from real distress to simple convenience in the name of a pseudo-right. It is advisable to make sure that this drift does not deform moral judgement, including that of the medical world, to the point of creating an implicit consensus based on the practical, with little ethical conflict. Cardinal Lustiger reaffirms "that for the Catholic Church each human life is infinitely precious, even when it does not appear as much, in the fragility, sometimes already tainted, of its beginnings." This is why the practice of prenatal diagnosis requires a precise moral judgement. In the case of malformations, often arising from chromosomal diseases that cannot, for the moment, be cured, the fetus must be granted the prerogatives proper to a human being and the respect to which all patients have a right. However, for very severe, and, as yet, incurable diseases, we now find ourselves obligated to enter into the alternative of life or death. The significant proportion of normal diagnoses that result constitute an argument in favor of prenatal diagnosis, since worried mothers who would otherwise be tempted to resort to abortion will be happy, be reassured and have their child saved. As for abnormal diagnoses, they create tragic and unbearable situations for the doctors and parents, since the commandment of God is to respect the human being and a personal right to life from conception. This means that a diagnosis of an anomaly entails a gesture of death. This also means that doctors should consider these moral demands seriously when evaluating the reasons for or against a prenatal diagnosis. The State and all civil, scientific or medical authorities must at all events be denied the right to link prenatal diagnosis to abortion in the case of malformations or chromosomal diseases. This still means the capacity to appraise the reasons for decisions and actions as a team. Cardinal Lustiger concludes by saying, "The Christian way of life does not allow any of us to escape difficult and painful tensions, sometimes going as far as contradiction."

## 2.6.5 Future Trends

After having summarized the opinions of the moral (CCNE) and religious (Cardinal Lustiger) authorities of our country, all supplementary commentary seems absurd. It must nevertheless be emphasized that the debate concerning ethics and genetics is well under way in France. It has, unfortunately, not provided any solutions, but can it be otherwise? In any case, it has the merits of existing, and of perhaps announcing a profound change in our society, and it is necessary. As a result of the striking progress realized by medicine and biology in the matter of reproduction, the moral fundamentals have been called into question by breaking the links between sexuality and reproduction, and between procreation and transfer of the genetic inheritance. It is thus indispensable that at the start of a veritable biological revolution, our societies specify the nature of their views on the embryo, since in 20 or 30 years the most far-reaching science fiction scenarios will already be outdated. For French geneticists the most important problems that will be posed in the coming years are, in rank order, the increase in demand, new genetic treatments, screening of healthy carriers, teratogenic agents, and research on the human embryo. On account of these new possibilities, we are now in a position to make new choices, and thus to assume new liberties and new responsibilities. Our idea is surely not to renounce this liberty; we must therefore take up the challenge that has been presented.

## References

Fardeau M, Garden H, Crost M, Derleau M, Goujard J [1983] Les aspects économiques du diagnostic prénatal par amniocentèse précoce. Rapport INSERM-CNAMTS, Laboratoire d'Economie Sociale

Giraud F [1979] Les Centres de Génétique Médicale. Organisation et fonctionnement. Arch Franç Pédiat 36: 221–224

Giraud F [1986] La consultation de génétique en 1986. In: Journées Parisiennes de Pédiatrie. Flammarion éditeur, Paris, pp 1–6

Goujard J, Gracco de Lay MO, Crost M, Maillard F [1984] Malformations congénitales et pathologie néonatale. In: Rumeau-Rouquette C, du Mazaubrun C, Rabarison Y (eds) Naître ené France, 10 ans d'évolution, vol. I. INSERM-DOIN édit, Paris, pp 45–53

INSERM [1978] Malformations congénitales, Risques périnatals, Enquête prospective, vol. 1. Editions INSERM, Paris

International Clearinghouse for Birth Defects Monitoring Systems [1986] Annual Report, 1984. Government Printer, Wellington, New Zealand

Julian C [1986] Diffusion et adoption de nouvelles connaissances en matière de génétique médicale: une étude régionale du conseil génétique et du diagnostic prénatal. Mémoire DEA en Economie de Santé, Marseille

Mattei JF [1984] Expérience du diagnostic prénatal des anomalies chromosomiques et des maladies du métabolisme. In: Journées Parisiennes de Pédiatrie. Flammarion éditeur, Paris, pp 43–51

Pfeiffer RA, Frézal J, Giraud F, Anders G, Robert JM [1982] Le généticien confronté aux problèmes d'éthique médicale. IXéme Journées Européennes de Conseil Génétique, Erlangen, September 1982. J Genet Hum 30 suppl: 447–466

## 2.7 Ethics and Medical Genetics in the German Democratic Republic (GDR)

R. Witkowski, H. Körner, and H. Metzke

### 2.7.1.1–2 Scope and Organization of Clinical Genetic Services

The state of the art in the GDR has been summarized as follows by Prof. Dr. H. Bach [1], Director of the GDR Genetic Counseling Center (Friedrich-Schiller-Universität Jena):

"Palpable problems faced human genetics in the GDR after the Second World War, in the aftermath of the abuse of that discipline in favor of National-Socialist racist ideologies and the resulting 'measures of racial hygiene' which had caused tremendous suffering to people. A plausible suspicion was not the only obstacle which inhibited progress in human genetics. There were also unscientific, questionable ideas on mechanisms of inheritance (Lysenko) and on the biological future of man (CIBA Symposium in London, 1963). It was not until the late sixties that a justified prejudice against human genetics was greatly reduced and action was taken and supported by the GDR Ministry of Health to give this medical specialty a sound footing for development. A Human Genetics Research Project was launched in 1971 for the purpose of coordinating all current activities, primarily those in cytogenetics and biochemistry, and of providing the hardware and software necessary for adequate undergraduate and postgraduate education. Within this Project, in the seventies, emphasis was placed on providing effective future-oriented resources in research and practice, including methods for diagnosis of chromosomal abnormalities and inborn errors of metabolism, prenatal diagnosis, mass screening for phenylketonuria and cystic fibrosis, and screening of high-risk groups for Wilson's syndrome and other ailments. At the same time, a mutagenicity test system was established to identify and eliminate mutagenic factors in the environment. The GDR Society of Human Genetics was founded in 1978. Its standing working committee on "Human Genetic Counseling" undertook to coordinate all activities of counseling services throughout the GDR.

"The GDR's first two model counseling centers were opened in 1971. The experience they had gained by 1975 was evaluated by the GDR Ministry of Health and used as a basis on which to set up a GDR-wide system of counseling services on human genetics. Against the background of the existence of a high-density network of health services in the GDR and because of relatively short travelling distances in this small country, the idea of setting up a great number of small centers was abandoned. Instead, only 20 centers were established, but these were efficiently staffed and properly equipped.

"Hence, at least one counseling center, in charge of roughly one million peo-

194

ple, is at present available in each of the 15 administrative regions of the GDR. A counseling service, as a rule, is attached to a department of medical genetics at a school of medicine or is located on the premises of another larger state-run health institution. There is no privately-run financing. A counseling service is headed by a medical geneticist (medical specialist in human genetics) or by a biological geneticist with complementary medical specialization.

"A counseling service has its own laboratories for cytogenetic and prenatal diagnosis and is in a position of resorting to other methods of genetic diagnosis, either on its own or in cooperation with other centers.

"Specialization in methods and diseases has been introduced in the GDR for optimum utilization and concentration of experience and equipment. Counseling services are differentiated into those for neuromuscular diseases, ophthalmology, ENT, metabolic disorders, and other fields. These specializations, as well as evaluation of achievements and experience, including data processing, are under the umbrella of the GDR Counseling Center on Human Genetics. Postgraduate education programs, regular exchanges of experience among genetic counseling personnel, standardized documentation of findings, expert opinion services at a national level, and no-delay access to literature are additional responsibilities of the GDR Center, which is also in charge of centralized recording of cases for the purpose of providing helpful information to regional services that may find themselves in difficult situations.

"When the development of medical genetics and counseling began, emphasis, right from the beginning, was placed on close cooperation and dialogue, not only with medical professionals and other scientists but also with philosophers, sociologists, and lawyers, with a view to creating the broadest possible basis on which to draft ethical principles of counseling. Prevention of any kind of misuse of findings and possibilities resulting from research and clinical practice in human genetics is considered a permanent obligation of crucial importance. Any interference with individual freedom of decision is considered a violation of human dignity. Yet, any properly perceived free decision does necessarily depend on sound information about all facts involved, since these usually have repercussions not only for the individual directly concerned, but for society and unborn life. That is why we believe in the need for thorough enlightenment of the people concerned as an indispensable condition for any aid offered for decision-making in the context of genetic counseling.

"The system of counseling services, as it stands with all its accompanying and complementary facilities, is good enough to satisfy present demands of the general public in all parts of this country, and it is expected also to meet growing demands in the future. All persons who need advice do not yet take advantage of the genetic counseling offered. That is primarily attributable to persistent ignorance about possibilities among potential patients and even among many physicians. It is, however, a duty of a medical professional in our time to brief high-risk persons on the possibilities implied in human genetics and to help them in making appropriate contacts. Knowledge of human genetics is expanding at a high rate, and it cannot be expected that every medical practitioner will be capable of offering counsel. Trusting cooperation is, therefore, desirable with the established counseling services [1]."

The 20 centers of genetic counseling in the GDR serve a population of 15 million, with about 230,000 births annually. There are 5,800 counseling cases annually, most of them requiring several sessions. In 1985, postnatal cytogenetic examinations were applied to 2,600 probands.

### 2.7.1.3  Prenatal Diagnosis

There were nearly 1,000 prenatal chromosomal analyses after amniocentesis (chorionic villus sampling was just beginning), including all pregnant women over 38 years of age who asked for prenatal diagnosis (80%), 25% of pregnant women between 35 and 38 years of age, and all pregnancies at risk for a familial structural chromosome aberration. There is an agreement among the cytogeneticists in the GDR that a maternal age of 37 years or more is a strong indication for prenatal diagnosis, whereas between 35 and 37 years amniocentesis or chorionic villus sampling are not offered in every case. Advanced paternal age is not regarded as an indication.

In 1985, about 3,000 AFP tests were applied to maternal serum or amniotic fluid for prenatal diagnosis of neural tube defects. About 200 postnatal and 20 prenatal examinations were made for genetic defects of metabolism.

### 2.7.1.5  Abortion

On the average, 30 induced abortions a year were recommended based on genetic diagnoses, mainly of trisomies, male fetuses at risk for X-linked defects, and neural tube defects. Most severely defective fetuses, however, were found ultrasonographically by gynecologists without contact with a geneticist. Consequently, geneticists have no exact knowledge of the number of induced abortions of genetically defective fetuses.

Abortion has been legalized in the GDR and is performed at a pregnant woman's request up to the twelfth week of pregnancy. Advanced pregnancy will generally not be prematurely terminated unless the mother's life would be physically or psychologically endangered by delivery of an infant that is nonviable (e.g., anencephaly, multiple severe defects) or severely disabled (Down syndrome, neural tube defect). Although no legal limit for the latter exists and borderline cases occur, including gonosomal aberrations, the consensus among genetic centers about indications for prenatal diagnosis and induced abortions is quite strong.

## 2.7.2  Ethical Problems

Severe conflict situations and intricate ethical problems arise concerning the valuation of human life, dignity, individuality, and integrity. The medical geneticist, first of all, has to elucidate causative factors underlying pathogenesis of a disease

196

or malformation and has to see if preventive action can be taken. Prevention in all spheres of medical genetics must be primarily oriented to the needs and wishes of individuals and families.

## 2.7.2.1  Genetic Counseling

The person seeking medico-genetic counsel usually is a clinically intact individual rather than a suffering patient in need of curative treatment. Such persons ought to be told, if they are carriers of pathogenetic genes that might lead to the development of disease in themselves or their descendants or relatives. The counseling session is a confrontation affecting not only the individual concerned, but partners, family and wider kinship group. The session is of acute relevance, not merely to one moment in time, but possibly to the whole life span.

People coming for counseling are usually open-minded and have an interest in having their relatives counseled as well. However, there may be situations in which it is absolutely intolerable for the person concerned to know that he or she is the carrier of abnormal genes and has transmitted them. The carrier may be a loving grandparent grieving the ailment of a desperately longed-for grandchild. The carrier may be the mother or father of an affected child. In this case, knowing which one is the carrier may increase already existing tensions in the family or tensions resulting from the burden of a sick child, and may entail mutual accusations.

Enforcement of "the truth" can have disastrous consequences. Feelings and attributions of guilt must be ameliorated by counseling, and nothing must be done that might be conducive to the buildup of a guilt complex.

If an affected person or carrier has clearly expressed disinterest in information or if the counselor knows from earlier consultations that the person concerned would not understand the information, that attitude should be respected. Nevertheless, everything possible should be done to promote necessary preventive action. Prenatal diagnosis should be offered in the case of another pregnancy and should be made acceptable to the potential recipient.

Counsel-seeking persons are normally sympathetic to the idea of prophylaxis for the entire family. Affected persons quite often inform their own siblings and other relatives about the possibility of genetic counseling or ask the counselor to get in touch with the family. This will depend on the family situation, social environment, and on how the individual has "digested" the counseling session. In rare cases, people find themselves unwilling to put other family members in touch with genetic counseling, in spite of appeals to their responsibility and offers to find ways and means not to penetrate and violate privacy and to maintain the confidentiality of the person. No one should have the right to interfere in such cases in favor of a "higher interest." The counselor is then plunged into severe conflict. The patient's trust and the impermissibility of violating individual dignity stand against the chance of preventing the birth of a severely ill child to other relatives. Yet, there is also a risk in confronting a family with problems that would otherwise have been left unknown and that they may not even consider relevant.

Every person in need of genetic counseling should be aware that confidence will be reciprocated, that aid can be expected, that personal dignity and integrity will be protected, and that no one will make any decision without consulting the patient. Genetic counseling is intended to enable the client to make voluntary informed decisions, and these must never result from coercion.

Counseling of a potential carrier of Huntington disease on risks to self, children or other relatives is a rare but extremely complicated situation. Knowledge of possible disease may be such a burden that life no longer seems worthwhile. However, awareness can just as well mobilize the carrier to activity and to determination not to pass on the disease to his or her children. If a client asks for an assessment of risk, geneticists agree that it should be provided. Whether unaware relatives may or should be informed is a difficult question depending on the situation in each family.

Similar problems are related to revelation of gonosomal chromosome aberrations, such as 46, XY in women or 46, XX, 47, XXY, and 47, XYY in men. Revelation of chromosomally inversed sex findings may cause loss of identity to the person concerned. Given the absence of enlightenment among the general public, the resulting burden would be hard to bear. Here, findings should be so explained that the recipient of information should not receive the impression that "actually I should be male" or "actually I should be female." Mere presentation of the chromosomal formula, so called "pure information," can cause extreme damage. Referring physicians should be aware of this, and should be adequately informed by the geneticists.

## 2.7.2.2 Prenatal Diagnosis

With regard to prenatal diagnostic findings, it should be a general rule to provide truthful information – on the possibility of disease as well as on the possibility or impossibility of having a normal child in a subsequent pregnancy. Medical geneticists do take the possibility of decreased fertility after abortion into account, because there is a risk of permanent dilatation of the cervix from the abortion procedure, causing cervical insufficiency and miscarriage of future pregnancies. Although the risk from a single abortion procedure may be negligible, the risk increases after multiple abortions. The risk of disease should never be played down, and parents wishing abortion should be supported. If, on the other hand, parents decide to accept the child, this should be an informed decision. They must be assured that they will receive all possible medical and social support in case the child has a genetic disease.

The medical geneticist often has to decide whether deviating gonosomal findings should be disclosed at all and how. Provided pregnancy is accepted by the parents following disclosure of 45, X or 47, XXY findings, would such knowledge endanger the child's normal development by altering the behavior of one or both parents or causing stigmatization? If parents know, is it always possible to guide them in a way that causes no damage to the child? What will happen if a child learns about its chromosomal status from someone else? Disclosure of findings may entail loss of identity and a burden on the child's life.

Geneticists in the GDR agree not to do prenatal diagnosis without medical indications. A request for prenatal diagnosis for sex preselection will be rejected without hesitation, as long as it is not medically indicated. Abortion of a healthy fetus of an undesired sex cannot be ethically justified, especially as in this society both sexes enjoy equal opportunities. There is also the risk of possible infertility in the wake of repeated abortions.

In cases in which prenatal diagnosis is desperately desired by a pregnant woman, without any medical indication, efforts will be made to relieve her anxiety and to dispel false ideas about prenatal diagnosis. In exceptional cases, such psychological approaches to the problem will not work, and overriding anxiety may become a psychological indication.

Prenatal diagnosis should not be unconditionally linked with consent to abortion, not even in cases of severe defect. If, however, the woman has made explicitly clear her decision to carry the pregnancy to term, the risk associated with amniocentesis should weigh heavily against its performance. On the other hand, the information about fetal damage obtained from prenatal diagnosis may be helpful to the obstetrician.

## 2.7.2.3 Genetic Screening

Several ethical problems arise in screening. No one in the GDR, with its ethnically uniform population, would see any ethical problem in screening all newborns for phenylketonuria. Quite a different situation may result from screening for genetic causes of possible deviance or conspicuously antisocial or dangerous behavior. If, for example, a screening test for alcoholism is developed (screening for certain alleles of the $C_2H_5OH$ catabolism as ADH, ALDH etc.), applicable during infancy, what would be the most ethical approach?

Pre-employment medical examination is an integral component of the compulsory occupational health system of the GDR. Expansion of occupational health checks to include genetic aspects, if these are to the benefit of the proband, can be supported without reservation. Findings will be discussed with the person concerned. Unfitness will entail re-assignment. There is no unemployment in the GDR. Yet, all examinations of this kind must be voluntary. They must be so widely available that involvement is ruled out only by explicit refusal. Relevant findings with potentially severe consequences for population genetics or for high-risk groups should be a motivation to offer counseling to the probands concerned. Data on an individual must not be accessible to anyone else.

## 2.7.2.4 Other Contexts

The term "hereditary disease" still is falsely and negatively interpreted and perceived, not only by the general public, but also among many clinical practitioners. A genetic diagnosis is still quite often accompanied by careless attribution of guilt and superficial "advice" reflected in statements such as: "You will never have a healthy child." "This family is degenerate." "XYY represents a criminal character." Enlightenment and education are ethical challenges for the medical geneticist. Geneticists have to reemphasize, time and again, that a genetic defect cannot be culpably acquired by misbehavior.

## 2.7.3 Consensus and Variation in the GDR

Twenty-one persons answered the questionnaire, a response rate of 80%. Some portions of the questionnaires did not apply to the specific situation in the GDR, which is characterized by centralized organization of an almost entirely state-run health system. Health care is absolutely free of charge, with very few exceptions. This is why some of our colleagues had difficulties in forming opinions on certain issues.

For example, under GDR conditions, when cooperation is refused by the proband, counseling depends strongly on whether or not relatives show up voluntarily. General counseling is not practical unless relatives are cooperative. Differences in replies to the questions on patient confidentiality versus duties to relatives at risk reflected a spectrum of more active and less active approaches to family counseling rather than discrepancies on principle. Disclosure to clients seeking advice should be limited by their ability to tolerate the information and their comprehension of details. This problem is not specific to genetic counseling. Similar situations are quite frequent in medical practice in general. The approach depends upon the individual situation, and there can be no standardized answer to such questions.

With regard to a balanced translocation detected in one parent of a Down syndrome child, 13 (65%) would disclose the carrier status under all circumstances, whether requested or not. Eight (40%) would also undertake complete briefing of all relatives at risk of having a Down child. Six (30%) would try to find out from parents, prior to the blood test, whether they wished to know which of them was the carrier and would disclose no information unless requested to do so. One would not disclose carrier status unless asked to do so. All respondents rejected the idea of giving false information (both are carriers).

With regard to the XY female, only four (19%) would disclose her chromosomally male gender.

Secrecy on certain details was basically considered as justified, if the truth might place intolerable psychic burdens on the client. Secrecy was more often the option in cases where openness might entail an identity crisis, for example, in a chromosomally male woman, as compared to a situation where an alternative (prenatal diagnosis) might be offered to resolve the client's problem. The giving of false information was generally rejected.

**Conflict between patient confidentiality and responsibility to endangered relatives**
There was no consensus about questions touching on the relationship between professional secrecy and the duty of disclosure. When it came to informing rela-

tives of a Huntington patient, against the patient's explicit request, nine respondents (43%) rejected disclosure unconditionally by making reference to professional secrecy. Yet, some of them made it absolutely clear that they would try their utmost to persuade the patient to agree to disclosure to relatives. Nine (43%) would inform relatives even if they did not ask.

Seven respondents (33%) believed in unconditional professional secrecy in the context of hemophilia. Seven (33%) would inform relatives even if they did not ask, and another six would disclose such information only when asked to do so. One respondent would inform the patient's referring family doctor.

In cases of false paternity, 17 (81%) would tell the mother alone, without her husband present. Three would tell the couple that they had not been able to discover which of them was genetically responsible, and one would tell the couple that they were both genetically responsible.

With all due respect for professional secrecy, the majority of geneticists would also give due consideration to their responsibility to promote optimum prevention and prophylaxis. Efforts would be made in such situations to find a solution somewhere in the middle between professional secrecy and the duty to prevent harm, with information provided but reduced to a minimum. A sizeable minority insisted on professional secrecy without limitation, but fewer did so in situations where an alternative could be offered by counseling.

### Diseases with variable expressiveness
Tuberous sclerosis is a typical example of this group of diseases. The majority of geneticists approached in the poll would discourage an affected man or woman from having children or would be in favor of thorough discussion of risks. Contraception would be discussed for both male and female carriers and artificial insemination would be suggested if the male partner was affected. Vasectomy, tubal ligation, and surrogate motherhood were advised against or not discussed by the majority of respondents. Adoption was discussed as a possibility, but was explicitly recommended only by a minority. The trend toward comprehensive information and rejection of irreversible intervention predominated for diseases with variable expressiveness. Measures with direct impact upon the personal welfare of third persons (surrogate motherhood) were mostly rejected or not mentioned at all.

### Prenatal diagnosis

### Uncertain information from prenatal diagnosis or findings of questionable scientific value
Fifteen respondents (71%) would tell their clients that their colleagues disagreed about the interpretation of conflicting prenatal diagnostic findings. Two would suggest the possible presence of an abnormality, and four would tell parents that there was definitely an abnormality.

In the case of XO or XYY fetuses, the majority did not take clear-cut positions in counseling or preferred an optimistic interpretation. Ten recommended termination of pregnancy in response to suspicion of a small neural tube defect, while another ten would disclose the findings but refrain from making a recommendation. Only one was unambiguously in favor of carrying the pregnancy to term.

In all cases in which results recorded from prenatal diagnosis were not conclusive, most believed in providing full information to their clients in an attempt to get them involved in decision-making.

### Scope of prenatal diagnosis

The majority of respondents [20] rejected prenatal diagnosis for maternal anxiety, with almost all calling for thorough discussion with the client concerned. Regarding parents who refuse abortion, eleven geneticists were in favor of prenatal diagnosis and ten were against. However, most of the latter would discuss the problem thoroughly with the pregnant woman. Prenatal diagnosis for sex preselection, in the absence of X-linked disease, was almost totally rejected, with two exceptions.

In cases of new/controversial interpretations of diagnostic findings in low AFP, 15 would explain the situation to their clients but would not try to persuade them in favor of or against prenatal diagnosis. Five would recommend prenatal diagnosis.

The question of a commercial laboratory is not relevant to the GDR. Two respondents therefore declined to answer at all. The majority of the others favored a ban on such commercial activities. A minority considered it justifiable for such a commercial laboratory to perform prenatal diagnosis for maternal anxiety (eight) or for parents who refuse abortion (seven). There was opposition to a commercial laboratory performing prenatal diagnosis for sex preselection and to any laboratories not associated with a medical genetics unit to interpret results.

In the self-expressed views of geneticists regarding indications for prenatal diagnosis, a fairly unambiguous trend has become visible: medico-genetic reasoning should be decisive in determining indications. Other reasons (including parents' desire for a child of one sex) should not be accepted, because of the risk involved in the procedure. Providing full information was again considered a priority.

### Screening methods and presymptomatic tests

*Screening methods.* General mass screening for phenylketonuria was introduced in the GDR in 1970. The success so far recorded has contributed to a positive attitude towards legally-required screening. Sixteen respondents favored mandatory screening for susceptibility to occupationally-related disease, while four favored voluntary testing. The patient, his or her doctor, and the local health authority should have access to results of this screening. (Differentiation between these three levels of recipients of information is irrelevant to people in this country, since the public health service of the GDR is almost exclusively state-run). The majority of respondents would not require the worker's approval of access by these parties. Other institutions (employer, insurer) should not be informed. This question applied only to a limited extent to the situation in the GDR and, therefore, was not answered by all the respondents. The majority of respondents supported the introduction of mandatory screening of all newborns for cystic fibrosis, provided that the test distinguished between heterozygotes and homozygotes, and that there were practical consequences for medical care.

*Presymptomatic tests.* Most of our colleagues believed that only the proband, the spouse, and relatives at risk should have access to the results of a presymptomatic test for HD. This access should be only with the proband's consent. Other institutions (school, insurers, employer) should not be informed, though a minority considered disclosure acceptable with the proband's consent. Only two were in favor of compulsory disclosure to health insurance companies.

*Situations of greatest ethical conflict.* Two-thirds of all respondents selected two cases as giving the greatest ethical conflict. These were confidentiality of a Huntington disease patient versus duties to relatives at risk, and counseling about fetuses with XO or XYY. The question giving the least ethical conflict was sex preselection at parents' request.

*Future priorities.* There is worldwide demand for expansion of genetic services and intensification of research for treatment of genetic diseases. A number of colleagues, however, underscored the importance of other issues, such as screening for genetic susceptibility to cancer and cardiac diseases, environmental damage to the unborn child, and screening for identification of carriers of genetic disorders. Yet, genetic screening on the job, sex preselection on parents' request, experimental research on human embryos, zygotes, and fetuses, long-term eugenic concerns, and allocation of limited resources received altogether lower ratings or were rejected as not being justifiable. Assessment of national priorities was very similar.

*Positions on counseling.* Problems of the individual relating to the prevention of diseases and defects ranked at the top of the list of priorities. People coming for advice must receive help in coming to terms with their own problems and in understanding genetic issues. Greatest importance, accordingly, was attributed to prevention of disease or abnormality, helping individuals or couples adjust to or cope with their genetic problems, removal or lessening of patient guilt or anxiety, and helping individuals or couples to achieve their parenting goals. Seventy-one percent of respondents, on the other hand, thought that reduction of the percentage of carriers of genetic disorders in the population was not important.

The attitude of the counselor to the client seeking advice is of decisive importance to an adequate relationship of confidence. It is a major criterion by which to measure a person's ethical position, and it must be characterized by respect for the client's personhood and independent opinion, whatever it may be. The position of genetic counselors in the GDR is fairly coherent on this point. Acceptance of the patient's decision is an unambiguously visible trend. Indirect persuasion, by suggesting what most other people or the counselor personally would do, should be limited to extraordinary situations. Almost all respondents rejected making decisions for clients. Only two of 22 felt that such action might be justified in rare cases.

To help resolve problems of families with genetic diseases is the only purpose of genetic counseling. Voluntariness and respect for human dignity are the supreme commandments. A fundamental contradiction is implied in the postulation of mandatory screening programs as aids for individual decision-making.

## Comparison with other countries

Geneticists in the GDR held an independent view on many issues. In diseases that are not diagnosable prenatally, such as tuberous sclerosis, 60% of GDR respondents would dissuade carriers from having more children. The international figure was 19%. Between 50% and 60% would advise contraception, while 14% would do the same internationally. Adoption would be advised by 20% to 30% in the GDR, but only by 3% outside the GDR. In cases of low alpha-fetoprotein values, 23% in the GDR would recommend prenatal diagnosis, but only 9% would do so internationally. In all, 48% in the GDR would advise abortion in response to increased alpha-fetoprotein values without sonographic detection of a malformation. It may be of interest that almost identical figures for these questions were recorded in Hungary, with a major difference only on the last question (only 27% in Hungary recommended abortion). The majority of GDR geneticists were in agreement with colleagues around the world about approaches to counseling. They advocated that clients should not be influenced in making decisions. Presentation of examples of what others have done or of one's own opinion was accepted relatively often, but clear-cut recommendation was, basically, rejected (in contrast to Hungary).

Prenatal diagnosis without medico-genetic indication was rejected by most of the genetic counselors in the GDR, though a smaller number of respondents would refuse the request of parents who oppose abortion. Again, the Hungarian figures were similar to those for the GDR, in contrast to most other countries. Screening of newborns by law for cystic fibrosis, if and when this becomes possible, was supported by 67% of the GDR geneticists. This was the highest percentage of all countries, except for Hungary (67%). Answers may have been based on the excellent experience with nationwide screening for PKU in the GDR since 1970.

Vasectomy was rejected or not discussed at all by 100% of counselors, a higher percent than in any other country. Tubal ligation was rejected or not discussed by 70%, a higher figure than in any other country except Japan (81%). Surrogate motherhood was rejected or not discussed at all by 95% of GDR geneticists (but only by 54% internationally).

## 2.7.4 Cultural Context of Medical Genetics in the GDR

The historical, social, cultural, and religious background against which ethical views and answers were formed is characterized by the following peculiarities:

1. Experience with National Socialism, 1933 to 1945, and World War II;
2. Existence of a socialist system;
3. Continuity of a cultural heritage of Central European making.

1. The misuse of genetics and the crimes committed against so-called "genetically spoiled" individuals and their families during the era of National Socialism have been deeply imprinted in the minds of the general public and, particularly, in the minds of medical doctors and scholars. That is why people are sensitized and re-

spond with great vigilance to problems relating to eugenic issues or to discussions on sterilization and other variants of discrimination against special groups in the population. Even now, it happens in counseling practice that in the course of recording genealogical trees, say, of psychiatric patients, ancestors are discovered who had been killed in National Socialism for eugenic purposes or in euthanasia programs. It is for these reasons, and owing to persistent antifascist education over the past decades, that major emphasis in counseling is laid on the patient's or client's individual freedom of decision-making. It is for the same reasons that reservations are widespread against any form of irreversible sterilization.

Public opinion, in general, is not as clear-cut. There still is prejudice against "people afflicted with genetic disorders," and the term "hereditary disease" has to be avoided or replaced by a euphemism in counseling sessions, since it is burdened by a past in which it was not merely a judgement of value but sometimes also a death sentence on probands and their families.

2. Public health is state-run and state-financed in the GDR, as in other socialist countries. This does not rule out the existence of denominational or other cooperative health centers, but there is neither financing from private sources nor private payment for health services. Hence, genetic examinations, including prenatal diagnosis, are possible only on the basis of a medical indication. Patients cannot "buy" these services without such indications. Such strict rules on indication depend for implementation on medical and genetic counseling prior to and after an intervention. The availability of genetic counseling is absolutely unproblematic, because every GDR citizen is protected by compulsory social insurance. Due to full employment as well as to state-guaranteed protection against dismissal in cases of genetic susceptibility to occupationally-related illness, there is no ground for fear of financial or social consequences of occupational screening. Susceptibility will entail reassignment to a safer job, but not dismissal.

3. The Marxist-socialist system of the GDR carries on the positive cultural traditions of Central Europe. Nine million of about 17 million inhabitants are members of one of the Christian denominations. Other religions do not play a role in the GDR. Only 1.2 million of those nine million Christians are Roman Catholic. There was no Catholic among the geneticists approached for this study, which is not surprising, given the low percentage of Catholics in the GDR population. The numerical ratio of counselors with Lutheran background to atheists was approximately identical to that in the total population. There was no basic difference between both Lutherans and atheists on ethical principles, nor was a difference to be expected, since Lutherans are known to take no strongly-demarcated positions on issues like contraception or abortion.

## 2.7.4.4 Abortion Laws in the GDR

Abortion, according to GDR law, is fully within the discretion of the woman concerned up to the twelfth week of gestational age. Once that deadline is past, the woman has to make an application for approval by a medical panel. According to cultural traditions, there is no stereotyped preference for one sex in parents' aspirations. Hence, there is no cause to fear abuse of chorionic biopsy during the first twelve weeks of pregnancy.

In conclusion, there is still a historically substantiated suspicion about genetic measures among the general public and the medical profession. However, that suspicion should be interpreted as a form of permanent self-control rather than as a scientific disadvantage.


## 2.7.5 Ethical Issues and Future Trends

Continued qualitative and quantitative expansion of prenatal diagnosis by chorionic biopsy and more subtle ultrasonographic diagnosis will be accompanied by the emergence of new ethical questions. Some problems will be resolved without deliberate intervention, by new insights and new experience.

1. Among the technical advances giving rise to new ethical issues will be the following:

DNA analysis with genomic diagnosis in the context of counseling, prenatal diagnosis, and screening, with gene therapy through transfer to somatic cells and gonocytes;

Improvement of more subtle ultrasonographic diagnosis will help to detect disorders in the fetus in advanced pregnancy, beyond the 24th week;

In vitro fertilization and extended survival of small embryos will pose at least two questions: How to terminate their development? What will then be the meaning of abortion?

2. The most intricate ethical problems will emanate, no doubt, from use of DNA analysis in genomic diagnosis and, possibly, in genetic therapy on somatic cells or gonocytes. Genomic analysis can help to predict susceptibility in human beings, before symptoms become perceptible from physical appearance or behavior. The same will be true for hereditary disorders leading to mental retardation. This may lead to discrimination against the individuals concerned. There will be problems related to the individual's right to examination, right to ignorance, preservation of individual integrity, and the individual's right to make all decisions voluntarily on the basis of sufficient information.

The desire for the perfect child is being articulated with growing emphasis, along with widening possibilities in medicine, increased expectations, and deliberate family planning. Difficult situations will emerge from delayed detection of a defect at a highly-advanced gestational age (for example, an accidental diagnosis beyond the 24th week by advanced ultrasonography) or even after childbirth. Will the late detection of a defective child have a changing impact upon attitudes towards pregnancy? Will it always be considered as humane that a knowing woman has to carry pregnancy to term against her own desire, say, beyond the 26th week of gestational age, and has to give birth to a severely malformed child? Such pregnant women need special psychological surveillance.

Gene transfer to somatic cells or gonocytes for the purpose of averting severe congenital disorders is not considered an ethical problem, given its technical practicability and good success. However, gene transfer will have side-effects. What will be their nature and consequences? Are they more acceptable than a genetic disorder would be?

However, there are other questions which might be more problematic in the future: What is the definition of illness requiring therapy? What is the definition of normal? What can be tolerated as normal? Under what circumstances should treatment be given or pregnancy terminated? How should medical abortion be judged, if it became possible to bring an eleven-week fetus to full maturity outside the mother's body?

3. Medical ethics is a subject which has been treated in a general fashion over the years. Yet, history has taught us that the Hippocratic Oath has not prevented grave mistakes, inhuman action, and even crime. Ethical problems have become more strongly a focus of concern as a result of this historic experience and developments in the medical sciences. There are many books and other publications on ethics in the GDR (see Bibliography). Efforts are being made to establish humanist positions in working committees and expert panels on ethics, including philosophers, physicians, geneticists, lawyers, and psychologists.

The impossibility of allowing commercial interests to penetrate genetics in the GDR, and a national policy under which man is the measure of society are important sources of humane action in this country.

All geneticists are given the opportunity and are even called upon to deal with ethical issues and to seek professional upgrading in this area. Postgraduate courses and a monthly lesson in Marxist philosophy are provided.

The specific commitment of all geneticists to the prevention of nuclear and any other war is a predominant ethical motivation for all of us to continue and improve our beneficial work and never to be confronted with the challenge of having to give treatment and counsel to victims of war or to human beings damaged by nuclear, biological, and chemical weapons.

4. Variations in view, referred to in Section 2.7.3, will continue to exist. There is far-reaching agreement on underlying principles. The amount of controversy still existing will, hopefully, be diminished, especially as some geneticists in the GDR are newcomers to this field and have not had a long time for discussion of ethical problems.

5. There is good reason for optimism regarding the potential of our society to prepare a good ethical road for medical genetics. The replies of our colleagues to the questionnaire also revealed that certain social conditions relevant to ethics do not exist in the GDR. These include anxiety about being fired, unemployment in general, discrimination against the female sex, and commercial manipulation of medical services for those who can pay the price.

# References

1. Bach H [1983] Zur Entwicklung und gegenwärtigen Situation des Humangenetischen Beratungsdienstes in der DDR. Dt Gesundheits-Wesen 38: 51–54

# Bibliography on Ethics and Human Genetics in the GDR

Dietl HM (Hrg.): Eugenik. Entstehung und gesellschaftliche Bedingtheit. Medizin und Gesell-schaft Bd. 22. VEB Gustav Fischer Verlag, Jena 1984

Dietl HM, Gahse H, Kranhold H-G: Humangenetik in der sozialistischen Gesellschaft. VEB Gustav Fischer Verlag, Jena 1977

Dörfler W: Molekularbiologie und Medizin. Internist 27 [1986] 78–86

Esche H: Gentechnologie, Grundlagen und Anwendung. Internist 27 [1986] 87–92

Gahse H, Kranhold H-G: Ergebnisse einer empirischen Befragung verschiedener Bevölkerungs-gruppen über Kenntnisse und Einstellung zu Erbkrankheiten und ihre Behandlungsmöglich-keiten und zur humangenetischen Familienberatung. Z ärztl Fortbild 69 [1975] 267–272

Geissler E, Kosing A, Ley H, Scheler W (Hrg.): Philosophische und ethische Probleme in der Molekularbiologie. Akademie-Verlag, Berlin 1974

Geissler E, Scheler W (Hrg.): Genetik engineering und der Mensch. Akademie-Verlag, Berlin 1981.

Henning G: Kinderwunsch-Wunschkind? Weltanschaulich-ethische Aspekte der Geburtenrege-lung in der DDR. Dietz-Verlag, Berlin 1984

Henning G, Reinhardt M, Knappe M, Wolf H-J: Gedanken und Vorschläge zur weiteren Op-timierung der Familienplanung Dt. Gesundheitswesen 39 [1984] 12, 465–468

Körner H, Körner U: Zu ethischen Fragen in der humangenetischen Beratung und pränatalen Diagnostik. Dt. Gesundheitswesen 35 [1980] 235–238

Körner H, Körner U: Medizinische und ethische Probleme in der humangenetischen Beratung und pränatalen Diagnostik. In: Körner U, Seidel K, Thom A: Grenzsituationen ärztlichen Han-delns. Medizin und Gesellschaft Bd 13. VEB Gustav Fischer Verlag, Jena 1981 (1983 2. Aufl., 1984 3. Aufl.), 80–93

Körner U, Körner H: Die Frage nach dem Wert und Sinn des Lebens in der medizin-genetischen Familienberatung. Z ärztl Fortbild 78 [1984] 549–551

Körner U, Körner H: Ethische und methodische Aspekte der in vitro-Befruchtung beim Men-schen. Dt Gesundheitswesen 39 [1984] 1067–1072

Körner U: Moral und Ethik in der Medizin. Z ärztl Fortbild 80 [1986] 961–964

Körner U: Positionsbestimmung zur In-vitro-Fertilisierung und zum Embryotransfer beim Men-schen. Zent bl Gynäkol 108 [1986] 529–532

Körner U: Vom Sinn und Wert des menschlichen Lebens. Dietz-Verlag, Berlin 1986

Körner U, Seidel K, Thom A: Grenzsituationen ärztlichen Handelns. In: Baust G, et al: Medizin und Gesellschaft Bd 13. VEB Gustav Fischer Verlag, Jena, 3. Aufl 1984

Luther E (Hrg.): Beiträge zur Ethik in der Medizin. Medizin und Gesellschaft Bd. 19. VEB Gustav Fischer Verlag, Jena 1983

Luther E (Hrg.): Ethik in der Medizin. VEB Verlag Volk und Gesundheit, Berlin 1986

Metzke H, Hinderer H: Ethische und juristische Probleme der Familienerfassung zur genetischen Beratung. Ergebn experiment Med 45 [1985] 39–42

Presber W, Löther R (Hrg.): Sozialistischer Humanismus und Betreuung Geschädigter. Medizin und Gesellschaft Bd 14. VEB Gustav Fischer Verlag, Jena 1981

Reif M, Baitsch H: Psychologic issues in genetic counselling. Hum Genet 70 [1985] 139–198

Witkowski R, Prokop O: Genetik erblicher Syndrome und Mißbildungen. Wörterbuch für die Familienberatung. Akademie-Verlag Berlin, 1. Aufl. 1976

# 2.8 Ethics and Medical Genetics in Greece

L. Velogiannis-Moutsopoulos and C.S. Bartsocas

## 2.8.1 Medical Genetics in Greece

### 2.8.1.1 Scope of the Problem

Health has been highly valued in Greece from the time of antiquity: Gorgias, the famous pre-Socratic philosopher, is credited with saying, "the highest blessing possible for a man to possess is the health of the body" [52]. Since that time, the common greetings in Greece have been wishes for good health: "Health to you" or "May you go well".

Following many centuries of foreign occupation, Greece emerged as a new independent nation about 165 years ago. The new nation had a long way to go to combat poverty, illiteracy and changes of social structure in order to reach today's state of development. Financial difficulties, geography, wars and other problems always restricted allocations to the health sector. This created special problems for the development and the provision of adequate medical and social services, including genetic services.

A remarkable improvement in health care occurred in the late 1950s, with greater extension of services to the inhabitants of remote areas, such as the islands and mountainous regions. The diminishing number of children per family (1.7 according to the 1981 population census) and a bell-shaped population curve contributed to a realization of the need for organized genetic services, specially trained scientists to staff them, and investigation of the locally prevalent hereditary diseases, mainly the hemoglobinopathies.

**Number of Births per Year, 1975–1985**
With the improvement of the standard of living and the educational level of the population, the increasing professional involvement of women and the increasing demands of a technological society, the number of births has steadily decreased from year to year (Table 2.8.1).

It should be stressed here that although abortions were illegal until 1986, induced termination of pregnancy has been practiced as the most popular means of birth control. It has been estimated that there are three times as many abortions in Greece as live births [41].

**Incidence of Genetic Diseases and Congenital Malformations in Greece**
Thus far there are no registries of genetic diseases in Greece. Periodic surveys of congenital malformations showed a significantly lower prevalence of neural tube

**Table 2.8.1.** Live births – Numbers and rates: 1975–1984[1]

| Year | Live Births | |
|------|-------------|---|
|      | Numbers | Per 1,000 inhabitants |
| 1975 | 142,273 | 15.73 |
| 1976 | 146,566 | 16.00 |
| 1977 | 143,739 | 15.51 |
| 1978 | 146,588 | 15.66 |
| 1979 | 147,965 | 15.66 |
| 1980 | 148,134 | 15.36 |
| 1981 | 140,953 | 14.48 |
| 1982 | 137,275 | 14.01 |
| 1983 | 132,608 | 13.47 |
| 1984 | 125,724 | 12.70 |

[1] Vital Statistics, Athens (1985)

defects than in northern European countries, but similar ratios for facial clefting, congenital dislocation of hip, pyloric stenosis, and other disorders [7, 40].

Since thalassemia has been and still is a serious social and medical problem in Greece, epidemiological surveys carried out in the 1960s showed a prevalence of 7.7% for beta-thalassemia genes in the population [30]. Recent studies show a similar prevalence for alpha thalassemia genes (8.4%) [22]. The thalassemia genes occurring in Greece are heterogeneous and call for great care in the identification of carriers and prenatal diagnosis. The sickle cell anemia gene is less frequent, found in about 3% of the population. Nevertheless, its coexistence with a thalassemia gene in the same individual causes microdrepanocytic anemia, often as serious as homozygous beta-thalassemia.

The incidence of the glucose-6-phosphate dehydrogenase deficiency (G-6-PD) gene is estimated to be 3% in Greece [7]. Deficiency of the G-6-PD enzyme is a potential hazard for kernicterus in jaundiced newborns and favism in children and adults.

Although the mean prevalence of the beta-thalassemia genes is approximately 8%, the figures vary widely among the various regions of the country, ranging from 3.3% to 14% [12, 45]. On the basis of these figures and the fact that there are approximately 120,000 live births per year, it is estimated that 1,000 couples are at risk of giving birth to infants presenting hemoglobinopathies each year [39]. The incidence of heterozygotes for sickle cell anemia is very low, as stated above. However, the disease is endemic in previously malaria-stricken regions of the country, where up to 20% may be carriers. In the Kopais Lake region, for instance, where prevalence of the sickle cell gene is approximately 23%, 1% of the live-born children used to be affected [46].

**Childhood Mortality and Congenital Malformations**

A remarkable change in causes of childhood mortality occurred in Greece during recent decades. Infectious diseases are no longer significant causes of death, and there is an increasing incidence of genetic disorders. The leading causes of infant and childhood mortality are presented in Table 2.8.2. The growing women's libe-

**Table 2.8.2.**  Leading causes of infant mortality[1]

|  | % of deaths |
| --- | --- |
| 1. Prematurity | 37 |
| 2. Asphyxia | 12 |
| 3. Respiratory diseases | 9 |
| 4. Congenital heart diseases | 6 |
| 5. Other | 36 |

[1]  National Statistical Service of Greece (1978)

**Table 2.8.3.**  Distribution of birth ratio in Greece in relation to maternal age

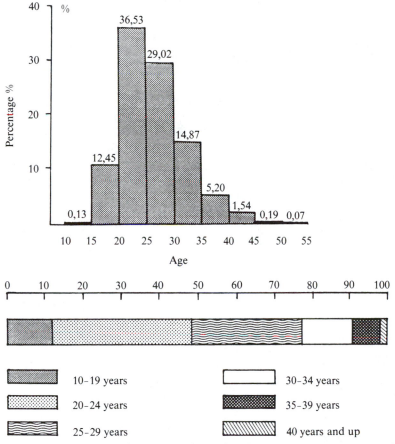

Schematic presentation of the percentage of births in Greece during 1980, in relation to maternal age.

ration movement in Greece, the low birth rate, and the large number of women who have induced abortions (an estimated 300,000–400,000 illegal abortions are performed annually) indicate that more women will have children in advanced age, because they will complete their education and develop professional skills before they marry. Many more women in Greece are deciding to have children after

211

the age of 30 or 35. On the basis of 120,000 live births per year, it is estimated that 1,000 children with Down syndrome would be born per year, in the absence of prenatal diagnosis programs [39].

An increasing number of women are career-oriented, and family planning is beginning to influence childbearing in Greece. The modern Greek woman is better educated, more informed, and seeks professional advice more often than before on matters of hereditary disease, congenital malformations and mental retardation, should a family history be positive for these.

In 1980, 20.5% of total births were to women aged 30 to 39 (Table 2.8.3). This percent is expected to increase dramatically in the future, as women devote the years between 20 and 29 to career development and defer child-bearing to later ages.

## 2.8.1.2 Organization of Clinical Genetic Services in Greece

The first genetic counseling centers began to offer their services in the early 1960s. They functioned as cytogenetic services in the Children's Hospital of Athens. A few years later neonatal screening for phenylketonuria was applied by the Institute of Child Health to cover the entire country. Screening for hypothyroidism and later on for G-6-PD deficiency were added in the 1970s. Their impact was remarkable, as in all other countries, in diminishing hospital admissions of mentally retarded children with PKU or hypothyroidism.

Unfortunately, in spite of individual efforts, Medical Genetics in Greece has not achieved the same level of recognition as it has in other countries [49]. Its level of teaching in medical school is insufficient and the Greek state does not recognize medical genetics as a separate medical specialty. Several well-trained geneticists work in Greece offering important services in cytogenetics, hematological genetics, and birth defects. It is, however, evident that the country lacks formal clinical genetics centers. Almost all genetic services are in the Athens area, and the number of physicians in full-time clinical genetics is extremely limited. Also the ratio of physicians to technical personnel is disproportionally small, antieconomic and basically dysfunctional (Table 2.8.4).

There is, however, a fairly well-organized network of 19 centers across the country that offer screening for hemoglobinopathies. Nonetheless, the largest center for

**Table 2.8.4.** Existing staff and needs for personnel in genetic centers[1]

| | Clinical Geneticists | Cytogeneticists | Biochemists | Biologists | Social workers | Genetic Nurses | Technicians | Secretaries |
|---|---|---|---|---|---|---|---|---|
| Type of personnel needed | 6–8 | 6–8 | 6–8 | 15–20 | 6–8 | 6–8 | 40–50 | 20–25 |
| Existing personnel | 24 | 14 | 4 | 9 | 2 | 3 | 39 | 4 |
| Full-Time | 2 | | 2 | 8 | 2 | 3 | 6 | |
| Part-time | 22 | | 2 | 1 | | | 33 | |

[1] Vasilopoulos D (1985)

212

**Table 2.8.5.**   Genetic Services in Greece[1]

| | Clini-cal genetics | Cytoge-netics | Bioche-mical genetics | Molecu-lar ge-netics | Immuno-genetics | Hemato-logical genetics | Prenatal diagnosis |
|---|---|---|---|---|---|---|---|
| "P. & A. Kyriakou" Children's Hospital, Athens | + | + | + | – | + | + | – |
| IKA Genetics Center, Athens | + | + | – | – | – | + | – |
| Institute of Child Health, Athens | + | + | + | + | – | – | – |
| Neurology Service, Univ. of Athens | + | – | – | – | – | – | – |
| First Pediatric Service, Univ. of Athens | + | + | + | + | – | + | + |
| First Medical Service, Univ. of Athens | + | + | – | + | – | + | +* |
| Alexandra Maternity Hospital, Athens | + | + | – | – | – | – | + |
| Stomatology Service, Univ. of Athens | + | + | – | – | – | – | – |
| Pediatric & Biology Services, Univ. of Patra | + | + | + | + | – | – | – |
| General Biology, Univ. of Ioannina | – | + | – | – | – | – | – |
| "Agia Sofia" Hospital Univ. of Thessaloniki | + | + | – | – | – | – | – |

* Hemoglobinopathies, cystic fibrosis only.
[1] Vasilopoulos D (1985)

counseling and screening for hemoglobinopathies with referral services to related centers for prenatal diagnosis is in Athens, as a division of the First Medical Service of the University of Athens. Collaborating with the First Obstetrics and Gynecology Service of the University of Athens for fetoscopy and chorionic villi sampling, the center provides screening for hemoglobinopathies, counseling and prenatal diagnosis.

A survey of the centers for genetic services in Greece showed that there are 12, most of them associated with the Universities (Athens, Patra, Ioannina, Thessaloniki), and an additional private center, which was founded in Athens in 1986 [19]. The genetic services offered are listed in Table 2.8.5.

It is evident that cytogenetic studies and clinical genetic services are offered in the majority of the centers. Some centers include biochemical facilities for investigation of amino acid metabolism disorders, organic acidurias, lysosomal disorders, or urea cycle disorders. A major contributor to diagnosis of inherited metabolic disorders is the Institute of Child Health, an independent, state-supported institution, which carries on the neonatal screening programs of Greece. Genetic counseling is formally given at most of the centers listed, but private pediatricians, obstetricians, or hematologists occasionally provide counseling services.

Counseling in Greece is provided almost exclusively by physicians. Counseling for chromosomal, metabolic disorders and congenital malformations is provided by physicians in public and private sectors. The center for prenatal diagnosis for hemoglobinopathies provides the most appropriate counseling for these conditions. Considering the workload, and the fact that the majority of geneticists work in Athens, it is very doubtful whether needs for counseling in Greece are properly met. There is no formal training for clinical geneticists or genetic counselors. Most geneticists received their training in genetic centers overseas.

Postnatal chromosome studies in Greece include blood karyotypes in children with malformations or mental retardation, individuals or couples with recurrent miscarriages or infertility, bone marrow and tumor karyotypes.

Investigation for genetic disease is carried out in most children's hospitals or pediatric departments. If specialized biochemical (lysosomal, metabolic) or other studies are required, blood or biopsy samples are forwarded to centers providing the services needed, such as the Institute of Child Health, or occasionally specialized foreign centers.

## Health Care System in Greece: Financing Genetic Services and Abortion

Greek society combines a partially socialistic political and economic structure with elements of a liberitarian society. Unlike capitalistic societies, societies with socialistic structures focus on a broader societal perspective, rather than on the interests of the individual. It follows that Greece never experienced a purely market-oriented type of health services delivery system. For many years, Greece has had a system under which every citizen was covered by health insurance. Almost 99.8% of the population has insurance coverage. Very recently Greek policy-makers recognized an explicit right to health care (Law 1278/82 – 1397/83). Subsequently, the cost of the use of genetic services, prenatal diagnosis, and abortion, if needed, is covered by health insurance. The Ministry of Health, Welfare and Social Insurance is responsible for public health, medical care, social welfare and social security. In addition to the national insurance system, physicians are free to practice privately, if they are not working full-time for the National Health System. They charge fees according to their professional status and they do not have admitting privileges to government hospitals or to university hospitals, which are all state-supported. According to the constitution, universities are public. Private hospitals exist throughout the country, with quality varying from poor to excellent. A few physicians who are in private practice had post-graduate training in genetics in countries with developed scientific programs and perhaps have better skills for counseling. The competition between the private and public sectors of health care, along with other deficiencies in the health system, creates lack of trust among health care consumers. This lack of trust drives them to foreign countries (especially the United Kingdom) for more effective medical services. Usually expenses incurred abroad are reimbursed by national insurance. From 1974 to 1981, the number of health consumers who sought foreign medical services and were covered by national insurance increased by 647% [9]. The policy in Greece is that if an important service is not offered in the country, national insurance can cover the expenses of the health consumer abroad if a committee approves it. Prenatal diagnosis of hemophilia was one example.

If the funds allocated for covering health expenses in other countries were allocated to build services and train staff in Greece, this might be a more efficient way to solve health care problems.

**Table 2.8.6.** Development of Amniocentesis in Greece 1976-1984

| Year | Number of amniocenteses | % of increase in 4 year period | % of increase annually |
|------|-------------------------|-------------------------------|------------------------|
| 1976 | 5 | | |
| 1980 | 450 | 890 | 220 |
| 1984 | 1,000 | 120 | 30 |

## 2.8.1.3 Prenatal Diagnosis

Most amniocenteses in Greece are performed on women with increased risks for chromosomal anomalies, such as chromosomal imbalance or age 35 years and older. The remaining procedures are performed for the detection of other genetic diseases, such as metabolic disorders, and neural tube defects. Amniocentesis is also performed for fetal sex determination in pregnancies at risk for X-linked hereditary disorders. Frequently the amniotic fluid is withdrawn in regional hospitals across the country or private facilities and is forwarded to the three appropriate laboratories in Athens.

**Policy in Greece for the Use of Genetic Services and Prenatal Diagnosis**
Prenatal diagnosis by amniocentesis became available in Greece in 1976. There has been a dramatic increase in the number of couples seeking prenatal diagnosis (Table 2.8.6). More than 50% of couples who have had an abortion after prenatal diagnosis have tried again to have a healthy child. Physicians counseling couples with affected fetuses reported only two instances in which parents decided to carry the fetus to term.

**Prenatal Diagnosis by CVS**
By the end of 1984, 110 chorionic villus samplings (CVS) had been performed for chromosomal disorders, and 30 healthy children had been born following CVS (Dr. A. Metaxotou: personal communication, 1987, Saint Sophia Children's Hospital).

Although CVS is a relatively new procedure, and its socio-economic impact has not yet been evaluated in Greece, it is likely that its benefits will be great, because the procedure is less complicated than amniocentesis, less risky, shortens the waiting time, and relieves the anxiety of the couple involved. It is expected that demand for it will increase progressively.

**Policy on Indications for Prenatal Diagnosis**
The policy to limit prenatal diagnosis to women over 37 changed recently, and now most women over 35 are accepted. There is no national policy on indications for prenatal diagnosis. The matter is under study, however, by a special Committee on Genetics, which was recently formed by the Ministry of Health. The existing centers try to handle all cases at risk, although the limited personnel and funds may present difficulties in scheduling women who appear in advanced stages of pregnancy.

## 2.8.1.4  Cost-benefit of Prenatal Diagnosis and Genetic Counseling

The prevailing theory that has guided the practices of the Greek medical profession is the theory of "measurable human worth." This is the belief that where human life is involved, the benefits are infinite and therefore the costs are irrelevant. This view, however, neglects the fact that the resources available for disease control programs are limited [48]. Indeed, in developing countries like Greece, with limited resources allocated to health care (Table 2.8.7), if we use an extraordinary amount of resources to save a single life, we contribute to the loss of many more lives by denying resources to other uses. Thus, the truly moral problem is to select appropriately among alternative goods, by weighing their social, ethical, and economic impact [48]. The purpose of the cost-benefit analysis is to provide a rational basis for health policy decisions and not to monetarize human suffering. For instance, cost-benefit analysis provides information about the benefits society would forgo by allocating resources to antenatal intervention instead of educational programs. Although a decision to undertake antenatal intervention is highly individualistic, it has a great societal impact that entails economic costs as well as psychological costs. It is possible to determine the direct economic cost of caring for an individual affected with a genetic disease, but the evaluation of suffering in terms of psychological constraints (indirect cost) is hard to assess in measurable terms. Avoidance of suffering is a rational approach, and we predict that it will be the future approach for a dramatically increasing number of couples. Our prediction is grounded on the increasing demand for prenatal diagnosis all over the world, as the survey reported in Part I.

**Chromosomal Abnormalities: Prenatal Diagnosis by Amniocentesis**
Although there are no current studies in Greece comparing the economic cost of prenatal diagnosis with the costs of caring for individuals affected by genetic disease (except those with thalassemias) studies from the United States provide some

**Table 2.8.7.**  Total National Investment for Health Care in Greece

| Year | | (Private investment excluded) | |
|---|---|---|---|
| | | % G.N.P. | % of Budget |
| 1975 | | 2.23 | 15.1 |
| 1976 | | 2.45 | 16.5 |
| 1977 | | 2.63 | 17.1 |
| 1978 | | 2.8 | – |
| 1980 | | 3.3 | – |
| 1981 | | 3.8 | 19.7 |

| | G.N.P. (U.S.A.$) (in millions) | Federal budget (in millions) | Federal budget for health (in millions) | Interest in health care* |
|---|---|---|---|---|
| Greece | 28,699 | 11,300 | 462 | 1.6 – 4.00 |

* The method of measuring the country's interest in health care is based on the use of Federal Health Budget/G.N.P. ratio

216

**Table 2.8.8.** Amniocenteses Needed per Year to Serve Population at Risk for Advanced Maternal Age[1]

| % of population to be served | No. of amniocenteses needed |
|---|---|
| 100 | 10,360 |
| 80 | 8,288 |
| 60 | 6,216 |
| 40 | 4,144 |
| 20 | 2,072 |
| 10 | 1,036 |

[1] Defined as women $\geq$ 35

guidelines. It has been shown, for instance, that the cost of caring for children with Down syndrome and other chromosomal abnormalities is 32 times greater than the cost of prevention of the disease through prenatal diagnosis [35, 47]. If we take into consideration: a) that the ratio of income per capita between the United States and Greece is 2.7 to 1; b) that the cost of institutional beds is approximately US $20/day and of hospital beds $110/day in Greece; c) that the average salary of a resident in Greece is approximately $8,000 per year; d) that individuals with chromosomal abnormalities usually have many health complications and as a result many hospitalizations; and e) the fact that their average life expectancy is 20 years, we can arrive at some preliminary conclusions about the socio-economic impact of genetic diseases in Greece, not to mention the immense psychological cost and the cost from the lost productivity of caregivers and family members (indirect costs).

The need for further development of services (obstetric centers and laboratories) is imperative for several reasons:

a) There are 10,360 women over 35 at risk because of advanced maternal age (Table 2.8.8). Of 148,000 total births, 10,360 (7%) were to women over 35.
b) There is a considerable proportion of couples at risk for genetic disorders diagnosable prenatally where the woman is under 35.
c) The utilization rate of amniocentesis in Greece is expected to increase further, first because a higher percentage of women will decide to bear children at later ages, second because consumers of genetic services will become better informed about the benefits of these services. The possibility of a lower fertility rate in the future is not expected to have much influence on the utilization of prenatal diagnosis, because the fertility rate in Greece is already at its lowest limits. Moreover, the survey in Part I revealed that Greek respondents indicated, as the three first priorities for Greece, carrier screening, increased demand, and the allocation of limited resources.
d) A cost-benefit analysis has shown the benefits of prevention.

**Hemoglobinopathies in Greece: Prenatal Diagnosis by Fetoscopy and Placental Aspiration**
The most common deleterious genes in the Greek population are the genes for alpha and beta thalassemia (Table 2.8.9). Couples undergoing prenatal diagnosis for

**Table 2.8.9.** Distribution of Pathogenic Genes Among 1493 Individuals at Risk for Hemoglobinopathies 1977 – 1983[1]

| Gene | Number (%) |
| --- | --- |
| $\beta^{th}/\beta^{th}$ | 1,251 (83.8) |
| $\beta^{th}/\delta\beta^{th}$ | 56 ( 3.8) |
| $\delta\beta^{th}/\delta\beta^{th}$ | 5 ( 0.3) |
| $\beta^{th}/\beta^s$ | 143 ( 9.6) |
| $\beta^s/\beta^s$ | 27 ( 1.8) |
| $\beta^{th}/\beta^d$ | 3 ( 0.2) |
| severe $\alpha$-thal | 8 ( 0.5) |

[1] Loukopoulos et al. (1984)

hemoglobinopathies have a 25% chance of having an affected offspring. The financial aspects of thalassemia major in Greece have been demonstrated in several studies.

In brief, it has been estimated under prevailing conditions that each newborn with thalassemia major would cost about US $5,000 per year over the 20 or more years of life expectancy, that is, a total minimum of U.S. $100,000. Complete prevention would avert almost 200 new cases per year. According to the same estimate, the budget for such a preventive program is on the order of U.S. $1,000,000 annually. Therefore the financial benefit appears to be at least 20 times higher than the estimated cost and leaves no doubt about the merits of prevention for the public health system [28].

It appears that preventive measures for hemoglobinopathies in Greece are efficient and effective. This reflects the efficacy of prevention programs as a whole and not prenatal diagnosis only [28]. Although the existing program of prevention is cost-effective, there is still room for improvement. For instance, more effective planning and organization will improve the effectiveness of the available resources.

Since increased demand for genetic services in general is the first future priority among the countries participating in the survey in Part I, it is in accordance with the principles of social utility and respect for human dignity that nations be prepared to handle this demand. Greek society indeed shows a strong concern for prevention. There is concern that resources allocated to the health sector (and as a result to genetics services) are limited, while the economic benefits of prevention are great.

## 2.8.1.5 Abortion

Abortion on request (for social reasons) became legal in Greece in June, 1986 (Law 1609/1986). It is estimated, however, that in previous years 300,000–400,000 illegal abortions were performed annually. Older studies reported that a few Greek women residing in rural areas had had up to 30 abortions induced, in most cases primitively [9], and that more than 29% of women had had at least one abortion [41].

As a result of the increasing demand for prenatal diagnosis since 1976, the Greek government enacted a law (821/1978) permitting abortion if the results of prenatal diagnosis were positive for a malformed or defective fetus. Considering the religious and cultural background of Greece, there is an irony in the way Greek women contemplate abortion. Many Greek women, despite their strong religious background, have been more motivated to practice abortion than contraception [13]. It is unfortunate that, due to lack of planned parenthood programs, women were not familiar with contraceptive methods. We do not intend to analyze and justify the attitudes of Greek women towards induced abortion on socioeconomic grounds. We simply associate these attitudes with the increased demand for prenatal diagnosis and the feminist movement toward equal rights with male partners.

The large number of induced abortions, despite the fact that they were illegal, the increased demand for prenatal diagnosis, the fact that abortion may follow prenatal diagnosis, and the low fertility rate all suggest that:

a) There are not effective programs for family planning in Greece.
b) There is no effective public support for working mothers.
c) The drive for independence, liberation, and education in women is stronger than in the old tradition, whose influence appears to be decreasing.

No public debate took place, nor was social conflict experienced before second trimester abortion became legal in cases where the fetus was defective. The Greek Orthodox Church took no overt position against it (as it did recently against the legalization of abortion for social reasons), but neither did it approve it.

Guilt, depression, anger, and denial, the feelings that were demonstrated to be the prevailing problems in selective abortion, have not been studied widely in Greece. Couples are not followed up after prenatal diagnosis, and if they decide to have an abortion they are advised where to have it, but they are not counseled after the abortion. Studies have indicated that appropriate counseling and perhaps psychiatric assistance before and after selective abortion provide significant support for troubled parents [14]. Therefore there is a need for follow-up studies in Greece.

## 2.8.2 Ethical Problems Faced by Medical Geneticists in Greece

Genetics has a definite ethical component. Many ethicists, such as Aristotle, Plato, and the Sophists [5], explicated the relationship between deterministic scientific theories and philosophical conceptions of individuality, moral freedom and responsibility. The development of prenatal diagnosis and the ability to screen prospective parents for genetic disease are major milestones in applied human genetics. These technologies have not yet been adequately assimilated into the ethics of Greek society, nor do most people have access to them. They are likely to create

219

conflicts of values and interests. Since the existence of moral rules and ethical principles helps to resolve conflicts, it is logical that Ethics, which is the systematic study of morality, play a central role in applied human genetics. The areas of applied human genetics (counseling, screening, prenatal diagnosis and abortion of a defective fetus) involve choices and decisions that reflect the values, traditions and commitments of individuals involved. All the above techniques of reproductive medicine have been introduced in Greece during the last decade. A full discussion of the moral problems, choices, and decisions that the delivery of genetic services creates in Greece will follow. We shall try to concentrate on and analyze the problems that present the most difficulties and complexities, and which are dominant in our culture. For that purpose, we will use the results of the questionnaires and any other existing resources.

Because the assumption is that all areas of human genetics manifest some common problems in different cultures, our aspiration is to help in the critical analysis of choices and decisions and to provide some guidance and support for individuals involved in decisions.

## 2.8.2.1  Counseling

Given the magnitude of the medical, personal and social problems associated with genetic disorders, it is clear why counseling is an important element of genetic services. Genetic counseling may be considered a special medical act, differing from the conventional doctor-patient relationship in the following respects: 1) The disorders involved are a consequence of a genetic abnormality; and 2) the focus of the decision to be made is usually prospective (future childbearing). Consequently, to achieve its goals (correct information, comprehension of the facts, adjustment to the disease) counseling should be performed by appropriately trained counselors.

It is unethical to misinform people (because of lack of knowledge) and morally self-defeating to ask people to make decisions as important as reproductive decisions based on false premises. Because of the high degree of anxiety and feelings of guilt and denial experienced during the counseling process, and because emotions differ in the context of cultural or religious background, it is important for the counselor to be aware of these differences.

**The Situation in Greece**
There are 24,000 physicians in Greece. Nevertheless, only 15-20 are practicing genetics, and clinical genetics is not a recognized medical specialty (Table 2.8.4). Studies elsewhere have shown that about 8% of the population needs genetic counseling. In Greece there is a need for 800,000 counseling sessions [49]. Obviously there is a major shortfall of geneticists, and the described need cannot be met. In addition, there are no special programs for training counselors or studies examining the psychodynamics of the counseling process or its effectiveness.

If we accept the communication of "relevant information" as a very important element in the counseling process, then two major ethical problems are involved, "truth telling" and "the confidentiality issue". Traditionally, medical professionals in Greece believed that unpleasant truth would hurt the patients physically and psychologically. Social changes, however, such as the spread of the concept of individual autonomy and the declaration of human rights in many parts of the world, presuppose autonomy and responsibility in every aspect of human behavior.

In addition, studies outside Greece have shown clearly that truth-telling and disclosure generally have positive psychological effects on the patient, and most patients have stated a psychological need for information [37]. In the Greek medical profession, there is a prevailing paternalistic approach to patients [32]. Despite the fact that physicians in Greece are under no ethical or explicit legal obligation to withhold the truth, especially an unfavorable diagnosis, traditionally physicians would withhold any truth that they believe would cause harm to their patients or to patients' family members.

Most physicians take for granted the right to decide what to disclose to their patients. The principle of beneficence would take precedence over the principle of autonomy or respect for persons. Most physicians in Greece would disclose ambiguous laboratory results, conflicting diagnostic findings, or controversial interpretations of the results. In the case of XY genotype in a female, Greek physicians, along with physicians from six other countries, had a strong consensus not to disclose. Their reasons for nondisclosure were grounded primarily on the principle of beneficence and on their concern for the family unit.

Sometimes counselors face a conflict between a duty to respect confidentiality and their broader social responsibility. Whether physicians have a right or a duty to disclose information to third parties, if they are at risk, will depend on balancing the other obligations involved. Although the rule of confidentiality is a very important obligation of the counselor, this obligation may have to yield to the counselor's role as citizen and as protector of the welfare of others. The response in Greece was indecisive. It proves that traditional adherence to the rule of confidentiality (even the law exempts physicians from testimony about any confidential information entrusted to them) has been abandoned and a consequentialistic approach to the issue has begun to replace it.

Can we derive moral imperatives from studies of attitudes? Not always, because it is obvious that the majority of persons can on occasion be morally wrong. Since morality is social in its origins and functions, however, and moral rules are destined to function within a given society under particular circumstances, we should take into account the values that operate in a society at a given time [18, 20]. Our culture's hierarchy of institutions and values places the family unit in a high position.

In cases of false paternity, physicians have a conflict between their duty to respect the confidences of patients and their broader social responsibility towards the unborn child and the husbands of their patients. There is no way to avoid this conflict, if attempts to obtain the mother's permission to disclose the information fail [8]. The deceived husband is morally wronged, but no risk of physical harm to him and his descendants is involved. Although deception involving innocent persons is hard to justify, the survey in Part I showed a 96% consensus around the world not to disclose to the husband. The widespread agreement expressed inter-

221

nationally to safeguard the patient's right to privacy and to protect the family unit, supported by the legal protection in Greece of information of a confidential nature, grants physicians a moral right not to disclose false paternity to the husband. Although the duty of non-maleficence is more stringent than the duty of beneficence, it is clear that the harm produced by nondisclosure is considered by society to be less than the harm that would be produced by disclosure [8]. Both utility and autonomy provide a warrant for keeping the rule of confidentiality in this case.

Another ethical issue associated with counseling is the issue of *autonomy* of counselees. An autonomous person determines his or her course of action without constraints from psychological or physical limitations. For the last century, in most parts of the world the principle that has guided reproductive decisions has been the principle of autonomy, interpreted as "reproductive freedom". Non-directive counseling respects the autonomy of counselees and is in accordance with the principle of reproductive freedom [38]. The survey in Part I shows that some countries (Greece included) still use directive counseling to a greater or lesser degree (Table 1.14). These findings substantiate the fact that in Greece counselors act upon the notion of paternalism. The principle of beneficence takes precedence over the principle of autonomy. It appears that Greek geneticists mistakenly believe that to benefit and care about someone necessarily entails a duty to protect him or her from decisions that, according to geneticists' views, are harmful. In our view, to care for others rather entails an effort to help them to maintain an independent existence and a physical and psychological integrity [37]. We hope that other social changes and a critical analysis of the results of the study will create a movement towards reassessing traditional practices in Greece.

## 2.8.2.2 Prenatal diagnosis

There are two issues in prenatal diagnosis in Greece that raise ethical questions: 1) the issue of access to the service, and 2) the issue of risks.

### Access – Justice
Assuming that the demand for prenatal diagnosis will increase in Greece, the ethical question is: How will the issue of fairness of access be addressed by physicians and agencies that provide diagnosis? To provide important health services on the one hand and on the other hand to deprive some individuals or groups of access to those services is a double standard of medical practice not morally acceptable. This occurred in Greece initially by not informing patients about the benefits or services available or because of centralization of services. To insist on fairness of access to an important diagnostic tool such as prenatal diagnosis is to insist that the practice of medicine be responsive to basic ethical principles of justice and respect for persons [15]. The role of the government in Greece is critical because it funds the services. Therefore, it is responsible for coordination, monitoring and making services available to families who need them. Access to prenatal diagnosis for persons who are at risk constitutes a requirement with strong moral claims. Prenatal diagnosis is included in the category of basic and necessary health ser-

vices. A "minimum of health care" is not provided if there is not fairness of access to prenatal diagnosis, including selective abortion [19]. Questions can be raised about the appropriateness of providing services in the following controversial circumstances: a) when couples declare their intention not to abort: b) when they want to select the sex of their child; and c) when there is anxiety but no medical indication.

A majority of respondents from Greece indicated that they would not provide prenatal diagnosis in the latter two situations. There was no consensus about the first situation (parents who refuse abortion). Under current conditions in Greece, with facilities with questionable capacity to handle the increasing number of requests, refusals of service for non-medically justified reasons are ethically acceptable. We do not intend to argue that such restrictions, which unfortunately interfere with parental choice and reproductive freedom, constitute an ideal social policy. They are acceptable, however, until questions of access, supply, and demand are resolved.

## The Risk Factor in Prenatal Diagnosis
The risks of prenatal diagnosis (risk of spontaneous abortion, maternal health complications, psychological risk, and risks of technical errors) produce ethical as well as legal problems. Studies assert that Greece is following the international

**Table 2.8.10.** Risk from Prenatal Diagnosis for Hemoglobinopathies, First Department of Medicine, Univ. of Athens Laikon General Hospital, Athens, Greece[1]

| Year | Failure of diagnosis % | Fetal loss % | False negative results % |
|---|---|---|---|
| 1977–1980 | 2.0 | 28.6 | 1.8 |
| 1981–1984 | 0.33 | 1.8 | 0.28 |

[1] Loukoupoulos et al. (1984)

**Table 2.8.11.** Decrease in the Fetal Loss Rate Following Fetoscopy, in Athens Thalassemia Control Progam[1,2]

| Year | Number of cases | Fetal losses | % Fetal losses |
|---|---|---|---|
| 1977 | 14 | 4 | 29.0 |
| 1978 | 87 | 10 | 11.5 |
| 1979 | 130 | 7 | 5.5 |
| 1980 | 209 | 10 | 5.0 |
| 1981 | 294 | 9 | 3.0 |
| 1982 | 354 | 3 | 1.0 |
| Total | 1,088 | 43 | 4.0 |

[1] W.H.O. "Report of Serono Meeting", Geneva, 2–4 May 1984. Perspectives on fetal diagnosis of congenital disorders
[2] W.H.O. Hereditary Diseases Programme, Division of Noncommunicable diseases

standards of risk for fetal loss and medical errors following prenatal diagnosis (Tables 2.8.10 and 2.8.11 [28]). In some cases, it exceeds them. We believe that the risk described is ethically acceptable, because it is communicated and informed consent is obtained. Permission to take the risk is grounded on the principles of utility and non-maleficence. Greater harms will be avoided, namely the harms of genetic diseases and parental anxiety. We assume, from our oral communication with Greek geneticists, psychologists, and social workers, that the risks of prenatal diagnosis are fully disclosed before the procedure. The process of communicating the risks, however, needs further study.

## 2.8.2.3 Screening

Screening raises ethical issues similar to those discussed above. A few other considerations arise: Whatever the biological reality, there is a certain public conception of genetic diseases that renders screening for them qualitatively different from other procedures [42]. Screening for genetic diseases is a uniquely sensitive and delicate area of health care, one that ought to be bound with special ethical restrictions.

Studies have confirmed that screening is a new and not yet evaluated medical procedure with unknown socio-psychological risks, including stigmatization, potential social ostracism, fear, and anxiety [17, 46]. Therefore screening can be understood as a research procedure as far as informed consent is concerned.

Greek society had two largely negative experiences with mass screening programs in the past. The first experience was with the Stamatoyannopoulos study in Orchomenos, in the early 1960s [46]. In this study, Stamatoyannopoulos and associates carefully designed and executed a screening program for sickle cell trait. Seven years later, when the results were evaluated, it was found that a) carriers of sickle cell trait had become socially stigmatized; b) new anxieties had been introduced into the community to the extent that people lied to prospective mates about their trait status; c) the number of carrier-carrier matings was the same as before the screening program. Although the educational effort was conducted by world authorities in the field, it did not lead to objective and rational decision-making, but to the creation of a new stigmatized status [23].

The second experience was with an unsuccessful law enacted in 1968, but never enforced or respected by Greek citizens (Law 300/1968). Its rescission was debated for a long time and finally occurred on March 21, 1980. This law obligated couples to obtain a premarital certificate stating that they had been screened for venereal diseases, tuberculosis, mental illness, leprosy, alcoholism, heart and blood disorders [43]. Although free screening was provided by government health insurance, it is common knowledge that couples were paying private physicians to provide premarital health certificates without appropriate screening.

The results of the Greek experience convince us that coercive laws and knowledge alone do not produce the expected results in the absence of appropriate education. The results in Greece may not apply elsewhere. They may reflect Greek mentality or the unavailability of prenatal diagnosis at the time. According to the survey, Greece supports voluntary screening in the workplace, voluntary screening for cystic fibrosis and no automatic access for insurance companies to the results of occupational screening. The latter question does not apply in Greece because all insurance is funded by the government and individuals cannot be rejected on the basis of their health.

However, Greek respondents suggested that: a) patients should be informed of the results of presymptomatic testing for Huntington's chorea even if they do not wish to know; and b) their spouses should have automatic access to results. The reasons given for informing patients were: "Preparation for the future" and "duty to know". These reported reasons are consistent with the paternalism displayed in the counseling process but not consistent with the equally paternalistic attitude of non-disclosure of a potentially harmful truth. The reasons given for telling the patient's spouse (family planning, preparation for the future) are not consistent either with paternalistic attitudes of non-disclosure or with the approach taken in the case of false paternity, grounded on the right to privacy and confidentiality. There might be three possible reasons for automatically informing patients and their spouses:

a) The fact that HD is rare in Greece and geneticists have no experience with it;
b) The lack of facilities for caring for persons with genetic diseases;
c) The intimate experience of suffering from hemoglobinopathies and the feelings of stigmatization when a seriously handicapped child is born.

## 2.8.3 Consensus and Variation Among Medical Geneticists in Greece

See 2.8.2.1–2.8.2.3 above for a discussion of the survey results.

## 2.8.4 Cultural Context of Medical Genetics in Greece

Greek geneticists rated "long-range eugenic concerns" relatively high (fifth) as a future priority for Greece. This did not surprise us, because physical well-being has been valued for millenia by Greek society and is even more valued now that the family size and the birth rate have declined to 1.1 children per family [9]. In addition, although "eugenics" has a bad connotation in most languages and cultures, in the Greek language it describes the good health of progeny. The notion of eugenics in the Greek language is not related to improvement of the race.

We believe that Greek geneticists do not differ significantly from internationally accepted standards in their practices. Nevertheless, there seems to be a degree of modified paternalism, which is evident from the relative directiveness in counseling. This form of paternalism, however, is not as intense as in the everyday medical practice of selective truth-telling.

225

Studies of population attitudes indicate that the Greek personality has some unique characteristics that result from established traditional culture. These include a lack of psychological sophistication, a high degree of dependency, a low level of interpersonal communication, a lack of introspection, mistrust, resistance to self-analysis, and narcissism. Furthermore, Greek patients very often develop denial mechanisms about their illnesses and seek medical advice when it is too late for effective treatment [9, 32, 43]. These characteristics evidently have a negative influence on the effectiveness of medical care and prevention, and they should be studied carefully, along with modes of altering the behavioral patterns and educational level of the Greek population [2, 31, 44].

## 2.8.4.1 Sources of Support

Although there are no medical documents to assist medical geneticists, other than the formal professional Medical Code of Ethics, Greek geneticists follow internationally-accepted policies, according to the countries where they receive their training. They eventually teach these policies to younger colleagues. More detailed discussion follows in section 2.8.5.

An Association of Greek Medical Geneticists was formed in 1982, with the purposes of generating legislation and advancing the practice of Medical Genetics in Greece. At present, it consists of 35 members, although several are hematologists dealing only with hemoglobinopathies.

## 2.8.4.2 Major Controversies

The sharpest controversy so far has dealt with the acceptance of prenatal diagnosis by older physicians. In fact, back in 1976 it was considered as a means to promote legalized abortions rather than to provide possibilities for the birth of normal newborns. Eventually more and more physicians accepted the safety, the accuracy, and the positive consequences of prenatal diagnosis. The Church kept a rather neutral position, although, as already stated, it never endorsed abortion following prenatal diagnosis.

## 2.8.4.3 National Expenditures for Medical Genetics

Greece allocates a low proportion of financial resources to the health sector (Table 2.8.7). Only 0.5% of the total G. N. P. was allocated to social services in general before 1968. A development plan for Greece later called for a significant increase, but after a national crisis in 1974, the greater portion of national resources was allocated to the defense of the country.

It is doubtful whether the low priority given to social services in Greece can be justified [1]. On the basis of a moral and legal right to health care, the Greek government acts unjustly if it does not provide sufficient money for at least a decent minimum [19].

Social services, including genetic services, receive a low priority partly because of the relatively low educational and cultural level of the population and insufficiently organized services across the country. Although it is impossible to measure total public and private expenditures on genetic services in Greece, we assume with certainty that they should be greater. It is encouraging, however, that the percentage of G. N. P. and the funds allocated to subsidize health insurance have increased in recent years and are expected to increase more. Moreover, there should be educational programs to inform the public about the availability of genetic services, the risks and benefits of the procedures and the consequences of prenatal diagnosis and induced abortion [24, 41].

## 2.8.4.4 Abortion Laws in Greece

Abortion on request (for social reasons) became legal in Greece in June, 1986 (Law 1609/1986). Abortion has been legal since 1978, through the second trimester, if the prenatal diagnosis showed a malformed or defective fetus (Law 821/1978). See section 2.8.1.5. above.

## 2.8.4.5 Studies of Effectiveness of Genetic Services

Most studies of the effectiveness of genetic services in Greece deal with the scientific aspects, particularly of the hemoglobinopathies [12, 26, 27, 28, 34, 43, 45]. There are a few studies, however, discussing the psycho-social aspects of prenatal diagnosis [6, 29]. All support findings of studies conducted elsewhere, that educated families at higher socioeconomic levels display support for interference with natural processes to prevent the birth of defective children, benefit more from prenatal diagnosis and counseling, and experience less anxiety and fear about medical intervention and prenatal diagnosis techniques [11, 24, 33].

## 2.8.4.6 Need for New Laws

Although the only existing laws deal with abortion of malformed fetuses (Law 821/1978), we expect more legislation regarding genetic services in the near future. An advisory committee to the Ministry of Health, Welfare and Social Services is studying guidelines for genetic services. The committee consists of physicians, biochemists, and biologists working in genetics. Its purposes are developing scientific quality control and ethical guidelines and proposing legislation for the practice of genetics in Greece.

We believe that we urgently need legislation, not only for the practice of medical genetics, but for the application of newer methods of technologically assisted reproduction, such as IVF. Our past experience with laws in the area of health care convinced us that coercive laws and knowledge alone do not produce the expected results without the appropriate education. They may even lead to ethically unacceptable eugenic measures, as was demonstrated in the Orchomenos study (Section 2.8.2.3.1.[10]).

## 2.8.5 Ethical Issues and Trends in Medical Genetics in Greece

Medical genetics in its modern setting affects an increasing number of individuals and presents new and more complex ethical dilemmas than it did in the past. These genuine dilemmas call for solution, and often there are no sources to draw upon for ethical guidance. For this purpose society modifies its ethical principles and rules and sometimes creates new ones to guide the new practices. Ethics as a social institution also undergoes evolution, along with science, technology, and law [16].

Greece is a developing nation and it will predictably incorporate scientific advances more slowly than developed nations. (For instance, prenatal diagnosis has been used in the United States since 1968, but in Greece the first four amniocenteses were performed in 1976). If scientific progress continues to be as slow in Greece as in the past, Greece will probably remain 5–10 years behind developed nations. The fact that most Greek physicians had their post-graduate training or at least some scientific experience in other countries (United States, Northern Europe) suggests that Greek health delivery practices will continue to be influenced by foreign practices.

The most important future priority in human genetics in Greece will be screening the population for carriers of hemoglobinopathies. The choice of carrier screening as the first priority may reflect:

1. The belief that rigorous population screening will serve as a preventive measure and will limit demand for other forms of genetic services. Preventive modes of genetic services are more suitable than treatment, according to Greek health care standards of practice. Greece is not fully prepared to handle the future increased demand for genetic services, and the development of new treatments will be delayed. In this situation, screening enhances reproductive options.
2. Greek geneticists' broader concern about the need for prevention in health care and lack of appropriate services. Because of inadequate knowledge, Greek patients sometimes seek medical advice too late for effective treatment [43].
3. The fact that economic development is not expected to improve significantly for the next 10–15 years, and resources will continue to be scarce. Other needs, such as organization of more effective emergency services, development of more effective cardiovascular units, and decentralization of services, are considered to be more important priorities than the development of genetic services.

One of us (L. V. M.) recently considered the ethical priorities for genetic services in Greece in a Ph. D. thesis [50]. The basic argument was that the priority of genetic services must be considered within the framework of an overriding imperative for a Greek system of health care that provides fair access to a "decent minimum" of medical care [19]. The ethical reasons for the allocation of funds for genetic services were based on ethical principles such as non-maleficence, beneficence, justice, reproductive freedom, and utility. We assigned a moderate to high priority to genetic services in Greece, and made recommendations about the decentralization of genetic services and long-term follow-up evaluation. Prevention seems to be the most efficient strategy in macro-allocation of funds for health care in developing countries like Greece. Genetic services are preventive rather than curative measures. Studies of the efficiency of the various modes of prevention should be conducted in the near future.

Genetic services, including prenatal diagnosis, will have a moderate rank among other social and health care priorities because the incidence of genetic diseases is not very high, treatment is very expensive, and the prospect of successful treatment is low [50]. There should be emphasis on the prevention of genetic disease through educational campaigns in schools, universities, media, societies formed by affected individuals, and family planning programs. Knowledge of biology and genetics may eventually lead to prevention of genetic diseases. Prevention through education seems efficient and does not require large expenditures. The future agenda in Greece will also require studies of improvement, coordination of existing facilities, decentralization, and efficiency [43]. Greek citizens will become more sophisticated consumers of prenatal diagnosis. This will increase pressure to use genetic services. Because resources are rationed, a portion of the demand will be unsatisfied and ethical issues of fairness of access and micro-allocation will become imminent.

Micro-allocation decisions usually take place when a scarce procedure gains acceptance and its availability is limited. Under such circumstances, issues of fairness of access may lead society to alter its macro-allocation policies in order to increase the supply of scarce resources and relieve medical professionals and administrators from the anguish of "tragic choices" [8]. This may be the case in Greece. There is an additional reason for health care administrators to consider seriously policy decisions concerning genetic services in Greece. Our recently reformed health care system presupposes that the basic medical needs of every citizen ought to be met and grants a legal right to health care for each citizen (Law 1397/83 article 1, part 1, 21 [21]). The recognition of a right to health care under our reformed new system will be an empty right if we do not provide the appropriate funds to make the services available. Prenatal diagnosis in Greece will be a basic health need for several reasons:

a) A significant percentage (8% of the total population) carries the thalassemia gene.
b) More couples will be at risk for having a child with chromosomal imbalance because a larger percentage of older women may have children.
c) There is a lack of appropriate institutions for hospitalization of handicapped children.

d) Greek families tend to feel extremely stigmatized after the birth of a seriously handicapped child.

e) The decreased family size (Table 2.8.1.) will make the preventive approach to congenital diseases more important [50].

f) The number of healthy carriers will increase as more couples at risk undertake pregnancies and use prenatal diagnosis.

Greek policy-makers in the future should base their decisions on the above considerations. Policy-making decisions should conform with generally-accepted social and ethical principles within society, and the decisions should reflect the community's priorities and hierarchy of ethical principles [52]. Our system is fair and in accordance with the principle of justice and respect for persons if couples with greater medical need and less economic ability to pay benefit more from genetic services. For instance, if all requests for prenatal diagnosis cannot be handled, it may be appropriate to give priority to women who cannot seek medical advice from the coexisting private health care sector. Public policy decisions in health care matters should try to narrow the range between the poor and the rich. Especially in developing countries like Greece, where educational and economic differences are more apparent and health care costs are distributed throughout society, this goal becomes imperative [3].

First trimester fetal diagnosis by CVS will receive increasing attention in Greece, because early diagnosis has more acceptable medical and psycho-social implications:

a) it reduces parental anxiety and psychological conflict by yielding rapid results;

b) it provides greater privacy because the pregnancy is not publicly known;

c) there are fewer medical risks, because the selective abortion is performed at 9 to 10 weeks; and

d) it is accepted with less difficulty by most cultures or religions.

Healthy children have been born after CVS. Since prenatal diagnosis by CVS has socially desirable effects, CVS should be promoted by Greek health policy makers through educational campaigns in order to encourage couples at risk to ask for advice as soon as possible.

**Future Approaches**

Greek geneticists' dominant approach to ethical problems in practice differs from the everyday practice of other medical professionals. The latter are guided by principles of beneficence, non-maleficence, and the paternalistic concept that physicians have the right to decide for patients in moral conflicts. Therefore physicians do not routinely practice disclosure, and at times they even make major decisions for patients without consulting them [51]. Geneticists, however, as the survey in Part I reveals, practice full disclosure of findings in screening and prenatal diagnosis. Moreover, geneticists who are physicians are the least paternalistic and directive of all physicians [37, 51]. The dominant paternalistic tradition in medicine still exerts an influence on medical geneticists, however. This influence can be seen in geneticists' lack of consensus about full disclosure in some cases, and also in their

consensus not to disclose XY genotype in a female and not to present some reproductive options to tuberous sclerosis carriers. The older dominant paternalistic tradition, however, is giving way to more respect for parental autonomy, in the context of genetic counseling.

Greek geneticists currently draw for ethical guidance upon:

a) traditional morality;
b) their moral intuitions;
c) their professional codes; and
d) their colleagues' experiences abroad.

Although Greek patients lack psychological sophistication and cohesiveness in the
physician-patient relationship [23, 44], more studies are needed to assess the understanding and sensitivities of the Greek population to issues related to human
genetics. Ideally, geneticists and other physicians ought to relate their medical
judgment to studies of patient attitudes about informed consent and other ethical
issues. Data in ethics are as important as data in science. Until such data are available, Greek geneticists will continue to draw upon traditional ethical resources for
professional autonomy. They will also draw upon newer beliefs about parental autonomy and enlarged reproductive freedom. The amalgam of old and new creates
a richer set of resources than practitioners may realize exists until more conscious
reflection takes place.

Since the agenda of medical genetics in Greece will probably not change dramatically, the most important issues for the near future will be the expansion of
existing facilities and the effort to respond to increased demands for prenatal diagnosis. If demand exceeds supply, the principle of justice will be the most crucial
principle to draw upon. There will be innovations in medical ethics regarding full
disclosure and diminishing paternalism. The technical expertise of Greek geneticists is already on the same level and in some areas even exceeds the experience of
other nations. This technical excellence in the detection of hemoglobinopathies
will invite continued international collaboration for data collecting and scientific
progress.

As we look ahead, we are optimistic about our culture's abilities to guide human genetics in ethically acceptable ways. Greek culture is clearly flexible and
democratic, because thus far it has disseminated the most beneficial aspects of
medical genetics (screening, prenatal diagnosis, counseling). Furthermore, ethical
requirements for current practices are in place, albeit in a state of evolution. Greek
culture will predictably continue the long-term trend toward enhancement of reproductive freedom. On the other hand, our culture will define and prohibit undesirable potential uses of medical genetics, such as coercive uses of genetic knowledge for eugenic population screening or stigmatization of carriers. Generally
speaking, it will avoid any restriction of reproductive autonomy and will also
avoid paternalistic practices.

How do we know that our society is capable of delineating such moral guidelines and keeping them clear? We can point to the following evidence:

a) the influence of the old paternalistic tradition is diminishing;
b) we are adopting new techniques and accepting the challenges that they pose;

c) We are aware of the acceleration in the number and types of ethical problems posed by the new genetics and are developing approaches to these problems. The survey reported in this book is expected to provide future guidance for difficult moral choices in human genetics.

On the basis of a moral premise that human beings have "relatively similar needs," general ethical guidance will be applicable to Greek society as well.

An international approach to the understanding of ethical problems may provide, after an in-depth analysis of the inevitable cultural differences, a precedent for ethical problem-solving within each nation.

# References

1. Abel-Smith B [1966] Labour's social plans. Fabian Tracts, London, p. 369
2. Anaplioti-Vazaiou I [1983] International acceptance of health and national health systems. Athens
3. Anderson OW [1978] Health policy in international perspective. In: Reich WT (ed) Encyclopedia of bioethics. Free Press, New York, p 653-654
4. Antsaklis A, Politis J, Karayannopoulos C, Kaskarelis D, Karabara PH, Panourgias J, Boussiou M, Loukopoulos D [1984] Selective survival of only the healthy fetus following prenatal diagnosis of thalassemia major in binovular twin gestation. Prenatal Diag 4: 289-296
5. Aristotle, Ewing AC, Edwards P, Baylis CA, Chisholm RM [1974] Responsibility and freedom of the will. In: Frankena WK, Granrose JT (eds). Introductory readings in ethics. Prentice Hall, Englewood Cliffs, pp 265-294
6. Bartsoca A, Giakoumaki E, Antsaklis A, Tzingounis V, Aravantinos D [1986] The impact of fetoscopy on Greek women. In: Psychosomatic medicine past and future, 16th European Conference on Psychosomatic Research, 6-11 Sept 1986. Psychico, Athens
7. Bartsocas CS [1984] Red-cell enzymopathies: Management and screening. In: Benson PF (ed) Screening and management of potentially treatable genetic metabolic disorders. M.T.P. Press Ltd, Lancaster, pp 79-114
8. Beauchamp TL, Childress JF [1979] Principles of biomedical ethics. Oxford University Press, New York, pp 209-217
9. Blum R, Blum E (eds) [1965] Health and healing in rural Greece. Stanford University Press, Stanford CA
10. Capron AM [1976] Legal rights and moral rights. In: Humber JM, Almeder EF (eds) Biomedical ethics and the law. Plenum Press, New York, pp 387-388
11. Carter CO, Frazer Roberts JA, Evans KA et al [1971] Genetic clinic: a follow up. Lancet i: 281-285
12. Choremis C, Fessas P, Kattamis C, Stamatoyannopoulos G, Zannos-Mariolea L, Karaklis A, Bellos G [1963] Three inherited red cell abnormalities in a district of Greece: thalassemia, sickling and glucose-6-phosphate dehydrogenase deficiency. Lancet i: 907-909
13. David HP, Friedman HL, Van der Tak J, Sevilla MJ (eds) [1978] Abortion in psychological perspective: trends in transnational research. Springer, New York, pp 225-241, 284-300
14. Fletcher JC [1972] Moral problems in genetic counseling. Pastoral Psych 23 [223]: 47-60
15. Fletcher JC [1979] Prenatal diagnosis of the hemoglobinopathies: ethical issues. Am J Obstet Gynecol 135 [1]: 53-56
16. Fletcher JC [1986] Moral problems and ethical guidance in prenatal diagnosis: past, present, future. In: Milunsky A (ed) Genetic disorders and the human fetus, 2nd ed pp 848-849
17. Fletcher JC, Robbins RO, Powledge TM [1974] Informed consent in genetic screening programs. In: Bergsma D (ed) Ethical, social and legal dimensions of screening for human genetic diseases. Birth defects series 6, Alan R Liss, New York, pp 137-144
18. Frankena WK [1973] Ethics. Prentice-Hall, Englewood Cliffs, pp 38-39

19. Fried C [1978] Equality and rights in medical care. In: Beauchamp TL, Walters L (eds) Contemporary issues in bioethics. Dickenson Publishing Co, Encino, CA, pp 366–370
20. Hare RM [1975] The language of morals. Oxford University Press, London
21. Iatridis SG [1987] Health care systems in Greece. Lancet i: 792–794
22. Kanavakis E, Tzotzos S, Liapaki A, Metaxotou Mavromati A, Kattamis C. [1986] Frequency of α-Thalassemia in Greece. Am J Haematol 22: 225–232
23. Kenen RH, Schmidt RM [1978] Stigmatization of carrier status: social implications of heterozygote genetic screening programs. Am J Pub Hlth 68 [11]: 1116–1119
24. Leonard CO, Chase GA, Childs B [1972] Genetic counseling: a consumer's view. New Engl J Med 287 [9]: 433–439
25. Levin AA, Schoenbaum SC, Monson RR, Stubblefield PG, Ryan KJ [1980] Association of induced abortion with subsequent pregnancy loss. JAMA 243 [24]: 2495–2499
26. Loukopoulos D [1985] Prenatal diagnosis of thalassemia and of the hemoglobinopathies; a review. Hemoglobin 9 [5]: 435–459
27. Loukopoulos D, Kaltsoya-Tassiopoulou A, Fessas PH [1983] Prevention of thalassemia in Greece. Schweiz Med Wschr 113: 1419–1427
28. Loukopoulos D, Karababa P, Antsaklis A, Panourgias J, Boussiou M, Karayannopoulos K, Politis J, Rombou D, Tassiopoulou-Kaltsoya A, Fessas P [1984] Prenatal diagnosis of Thalassemia and H S syndromes in Greece: an evaluation of 1500 cases. In: Fifth Cooley's Anemia Symposium. Ann New York Acad Sci 445: 357–375
29. Macri I, Houdoumadi A, Giakoumaki E [1982] Prospective mothers: anxiety, knowledge about health and acceptance of professionals. Iatriki 42: 378–388
30. Malamos B, Fessas P, Stamatoyannopoulos G [1962] Types of thalassemia trait carriers as revealed by a study of their incidence in Greece. Br J Haematol 8: 5–14
31. Manos N [1979] Brief communications, an outpatient psychotherapy group in Greece. Int J Group Psychother 29 [2] pp 251–255
32. Manos N, Christakis J [1981] Attitudes of cancer specialists toward their patients in Greece. Int Psych Med 10 [4]: 305–313
33. Margolin CR [1978] Attitudes toward control and elimination of genetic defects. Soc Biol 25 [1]: 33–37
34. Markova I, Forbes CD, Aledort LM, Inwood M, Mandalaki T, Miller CH, Pittadaki J [1986] A Comparison of the availability and content of genetic counseling as perceived by hemophiliac men and carriers in the USA, Canada, Scotland and Greece. Am J Med Genet 24: 7–21
35. Milunsky A (ed) [1977] Prenatal diagnosis of hereditary disorders. CC Thomas, Springfield, IL, p 167
36. Modell B [1986] Some social implications of early fetal diagnosis. In: Brambati B, Simoni G, Fabro S (eds) Chorionic villus sampling. Marcel Dekker, New York, pp 259–274
37. Moutsopoulos L [1984] Truth telling to patients. Med Law 3: 237–251
38. Murray RF [1978] Genetic counseling. In: Reich WT (ed) Encyclopedia of bioethics. Free Press, New York, pp 559–566
39. National Statistical Service of Greece, 1978
40. Pantelakis SN, Karageorga-Zagona M, Bartsocas CS [1973] Incidence of congenital malformations in Greece. Excerpta Medica ICS 297: 93
41. Pantelakis SN, Papadimitriou GC, Doxiades SA [1973] Influence of induced abortions on the outcome of subsequent pregnancies. Am J Obstet Gynecol 116 [6]: 799–805
42. Powledge TM [1978] Genetic screening. In: Reich WT (ed) Encyclopedia of bioethics. Free Press, New York, pp 567, 568, 572
43. Ritsakis-Wood A [1970] (ed) An analysis of the health and welfare services in Greece. Center for Planning and Economic Research, Athens, pp 17, 78–110, 180–182, 280
44. Samouilidis L [1978] Psychoanalytic vicissitudes in working with Greek patients. Am J Psychoanal 38: 223–233
45. Schizas N, Tegos K, Voutsadakis A, Arabatzis G, Angelopoulos P, Chrysanthopoulos K, Athanasiadou A, Rombos J, Skarlos D, Davakis M [1977] The frequency and distribution of beta-thalassemia and abnormal hemoglobins in Greece: a study of 15,500 recruits. Hellenic Armed Forces Med Rev 1 [11]: 197–209
46. Stamatoyannopoulos G [1974] Problems of screening and counseling in the hemoglobinopathies. In: Birth Defects: Proceedings of the Fourth International Conference, Vienna, Austria, 1973. American Elsevier, New York, pp 268–276

47. Swanson TE [1970] Economics of mongolism. Ann NY Acad Sci 171: 679–682
48. Swint MJ [1982] Antenatal diagnosis of genetic disease: economic considerations. In: McNeil JB, Cravalho EG (eds) Critical issues in medical technology. Auburn House, Boston, pp 327–342
49. Vasilopoulos D [1985] Genetic diseases and community. Medipress, Athens.
50. Velogiannis-Moutsopoulos L [1984] Ethics and public policy: ethical priorities for genetic services in Greece. University of Ioannina, Ioannina
51. Velogiannis-Moutsopoulos L, Fletcher JC, Koutselinis A [1985] Psychological approach of the terminal patient. Materia Medica Greca 13 [1]: 67–70
52. Woodhead WD (ed) [1978] Gorgias. In: Hamilton E, Cairns H (eds). The collected dialogues of Plato, 9th ed. Princeton University Press, Princeton, NJ, p 229

# 2.9 Ethics and Medical Genetics in Hungary

A. Czeizel and G. Adam

Ethical views and problems of medical genetics, mainly of genetic counseling in Hungary, a Central East-European country, were summarized previously in a monograph (Czeizel 1983, 1988).

## 2.9.1 Medical Genetics in Hungary

The concept of heredodegenerative diseases was established by the Hungarian Ernö Jendrassik in 1902. After a promising start, medical genetics in Hungary was crushed for a long period by political events, e.g., German Nazis, the Second World War, and Lysenkoism. During the 1960s a new generation revived medical genetics and achieved important goals in the 1970s. However, medical genetics in Hungary has not reached the level of an independent specialty in medicine.

### 2.9.1.1 Scope of the Problem

As shown in Table 2.9.1, from 1975 to 1985, Hungary maintained a steady population size of 10.5–10.7 million with a dramatic drop in live births. The rates of recognized spontaneous abortions and stillbirths were 13.1% and 0.8%, respectively, in this ten-year period (Czeizel et al. 1984; not shown in table). Induced abortion decreased considerably, but the proportion of abortions for medical indications increased significantly. Infant mortality figures show a decreasing trend, yet Hungary's infant mortality significantly exceeds that of most developed countries. As shown in Table 2.9.1, the rate of occurrence of congenital anomalies and some

Table 2.9.1. Pregnancy Outcomes in Hungary, 1975–1984

| Year | Livebirths | Congenital Anomalies | | Infant Mortality Rate/1,000 Live Births | Induced Abortions | Induced Abortions for Medical Reasons | |
|------|-----------|------|------|------|------|------|------|
| | | % | No. | | | No. | % all Abortions |
| 1975 | 194,240 | 3.53 | 5,380 | 32.8 | 96,212 | 10,234 | 10.9 |
| 1976 | 185,405 | 4.05 | 5,528 | 29.8 | 94,720 | 9,737 | 10.3 |
| 1977 | 177,574 | 4.03 | 4,660 | 26.2 | 89,096 | 10,266 | 11.5 |
| 1978 | 168,160 | 4.29 | 4,097 | 24.4 | 83,545 | 10,660 | 12.8 |
| 1979 | 160,364 | 4.27 | 3,844 | 24.0 | 80,767 | 13,111 | 16.2 |
| 1980 | 148,673 | 4.68 | 3,443 | 23.2 | 80,882 | 12,630 | 15.6 |
| 1981 | 142,890 | 4.29 | 2,970 | 20.8 | 78,421 | 12,405 | 15.8 |
| 1982 | 132,559 | 4.61 | 2,676 | 20.0 | 78,682 | 11,852 | 15.1 |
| 1983 | 127,258 | 4.75 | 2,423 | 19.0 | 78,599 | 11,660 | 14.8 |
| 1984 | 125,359 | 4.30 | 2,558 | 20.4 | 82,191 | 12,041 | 14.7 |

**Table 2.9.2.** Birth Prevalence and Estimates of Detriment for Common and Moderately Frequent Congenital Anomalies in Hungary in the 1980s

| ICD Code | Common congenital anomalies | Birth prevalence | Livebirth prevalence | Total years lost | Total years of actually impaired life |
|---|---|---|---|---|---|
| 740.0 | Anencephaly | 7.5 | 2.0 | 140 | – |
| 741.0 | Spina bifida cystica | 9.1 | 8.3 | 407 | 148 |
| 742.0 | Encephalocele | 1.9 | 1.7 | 74 | 41 |
| | Neural tube defects | 18.5 | 12.0 | 621 | 189 |
| 745.3 | Common ventricle | 13.9 | 7.4 | 92 | 0 |
| 745.4 | Ventricular septal defect | | | | |
| 749.1 | Cleft lip | 10.6 | 10.4 | 22 | 141 |
| 749.2 | Cleft lip with cleft palate | | | | |
| 750.5 | Congenital hypertrophic pyloric stenosis | 15.1 | 15.1 | 0 | 0 |
| 751.5 | Undescended testicles (after 3rd month) | 36.0 | 36.0 | 0 | 980 |
| 752.6 | Hypospadias | 22.4 | 22.0 | 0 | 308 |
| 754.3 | Congenital dislocation of hip and/or Ortolani click | 257.7 | 257.7 | 0 | 180 |
| 754.5 | Talipes equinovarus | 15.2 | 13.0 | 0 | 101 |
| 758.0 | Down syndrome | 11.7 | 11.7 | 283 | 536 |
| 550.0 | Congenital inguinal hernia | 110.4 | 110.4 | 4 | 0 |
| *Moderately frequent congenital anomalies* | | | | | |
| 742.1 | Microcephaly | 2.0 | 1.8 | 75 | 49 |
| 742.3 | Congenital hydrocephaly | 7.6 | 5.3 | 362 | 9 |
| 745.0 | Common truncus | 1.7 | 1.5 | 60 | 45 |
| 745.1 | Transposition of great vessels | 2.9 | 2.9 | 62 | 141 |
| 745.2 | Tetralogy of Fallot | 3.6 | 3.6 | 34 | 131 |
| 745.5 | Atrial septal defects, type II | 7.4 | 7.4 | 43 | 0 |
| 746.3–4 | Aortic stenosis | 5.0 | 5.0 | 143 | 82 |
| 747.0 | Patent ductus arteriosus | 7.4 | 7.4 | 48 | 0 |
| 747.1 | Coarctation of aorta | 3.2 | 3.2 | 85 | 0 |
| 747.3 | Pulmonary stenosis | 2.9 | 2.5 | 23 | 76 |
| 749.0 | Cleft palate | 4.2 | 4.1 | 12 | 83 |
| 750.3 | Oesophageal atresia/stenosis ± TE fistula | 1.8 | 1.8 | 52 | 22 |
| 751.1 | Atresia/stenosis of small intestine | 1.6 | 1.6 | 69 | 0 |
| 751.2 | Atresia/stenosis of rectum and anal canal | 1.8 | 1.8 | 49 | 0 |
| 752.0 | Renal agenesis/dysgenesis | 2.3 | 2.0 | 71 | 21 |
| 753.1 | Cystic kidney disease/type I | 1.4 | 1.4 | 56 | 13 |
| 753.2, 6 | Obstructive defects of urinary system | 1.1 | 1.1 | 28 | 34 |
| 755.0 | Polydactyly | 3.0 | 3.0 | 0 | 0 |
| 755.1 | Syndactyly | 2.6 | 2.6 | 0 | 0 |
| 755.2–4 | Reduction anomalies of limbs | 3.8 | 3.7 | 0 | 78 |
| 756.0 | Anomalies of diaphragm | 1.6 | 1.5 | 36 | 0 |
| 756.7 | Anomalies of abdominal wall: exomphalos/gastroschisis | 2.0 | 1.8 | 18 | 22 |
| *All other congenital anomalies* | | *142.9* | *145.1* | *2,484* | *1,207* |
| Grand Total | | 614.9 | 597.4 | 4,828 | 4,448 |

genetic diseases with early onset is relatively high for recent years. However, the expected occurrence rate is about 6%.

As shown in Table 2.9.2, from epidemiological studies, the true birth prevalences of common and moderately frequent congenital anomaly types in Hungary are known. The group of congenital anomalies is the eighth leading cause of death and the second in infant mortality, accounting for 23% of all infant deaths in the 1980s. Congenital anomalies cause altogether nearly 5,000 years of lost life and about 4,500 years of actually impaired life within the Hungarian population in each year (Czeizel and Sanikaranarayanan 1984).

## 2.9.1.2 *Organization of Medical Genetic Services in Hungary*

There are no independent institutions of medical genetics in Hungary, either in medical education or in medical services. Three levels of medical genetic services can be identified within Hungarian medical and educational institutions.

First, *clinical genetics* is pursued in the majority of pediatric inpatient clinics of medical universities, e.g., Budapest, Debrecen, Pécs and Szeged, by some qualified medical geneticists. Four gynecological-obstetrical inpatient clinics of medical universities have prenatal diagnostic centers.

Second, *genetic counseling* outpatient clinics have been part of the National Mother and Child Care System since 1976, under the direction of the National Institute of Gynecology and Obstetrics. This decision has caused tension because the methods and material of genetic counseling outpatient clinics differ significantly from those of gynecology and obstetrics. Also, this structure makes it difficult to achieve consensus and adopt common standards for genetic counseling. At present there are 15 genetic counseling outpatient clinics in Hungary: six in Budapest, with a population of 2 million, and nine in country towns. The directors of each genetic counseling clinic are medical doctors: seven pediatricians, five gynecologists, and three medical geneticists. Nearly all genetic counseling outpatient clinics have suitable cytogenetic and clinical facilities as well as auxiliary personnel. The genetic counseling outpatient clinics cover a defined territory; however, some have special profiles. The number of new counselees has continued to increase. At present eight new counselees per 100 live-born infants are recorded annually.

The most frequent indications for genetic counseling are: previous unsuccessful pregnancies, mainly malformed babies; totally or partially genetically determined disease of parents; suspected genetic disease in other family members; infertility; advanced maternal age; and consanguinity. In Hungary, counseling about teratogens is also given by genetic counseling outpatient clinics, and this special group represents a significant percentage of counselees.

Third, the laboratory background of medical genetics involves 13 well-established medical cytogenetic laboratories in Hungary. Nine are within or closely connected to genetic counseling outpatient clinics, three work in tumor cytogenetics and one in the Pediatric Inpatient Clinic in Debrecen. The mean annual number of chromosome examinations is about 2,800, mainly from peripheral blood cultures.

There are two well-established biochemical laboratories for medical genetic problems (pediatric clinics in Pécs and Szeged). Hopefully, the Central Biological Institute of the Hungarian Academy of Sciences in Szeged will also lead in basic research in medical genetics. Finally, newborn screening for phenylketonuria, galactosemia, congenital hypothyroidism and serum alphafetoprotein in pregnancy should be mentioned. Research in genetic disease is done mainly in the institutions named above. The WHO Collaborating Centre for the Community Control of Hereditary Diseases (Budapest) has four tasks:

1. To initiate delivery of preventive genetic services as a community program.
2. To develop approaches for the relevance, effect, and impact of the Hereditary Diseases Control Program.
3. To test the preventive effects of periconceptional use of vitamin supplementation in pregnancies with and without risk for neural tube defects.
4. To act as a resource for the European Regional Office program on genetic counseling.

## 2.9.1.3 Prenatal Diagnosis

Four prenatal diagnostic centers within obstetrical inpatient clinics use chorionic villi samples and transabdominal amniocentesis after ultrasound examination for prenatal diagnosis. A national policy on indications for prenatal diagnosis exists in Hungary. The general principle is that prenatal diagnosis is indicated in cases of ≥ 2% risk of severe fetal disorders not treatable with great efficacy. Six concrete indications are accepted: [1] X-linked recessive disorders; [2] autosomal recessive disorders; [3] unbalanced or balanced chromosomal aberrations in the parent; [4] recurrence risk of neural tube defect or high maternal serum AFP-value if ultrasound examination cannot diagnose neural tube defect; [5] maternal age over 39, or between 35 and 39 depending on the individual situation; and [6] special cases, e. g., psychological indication after a previous child affected by trisomy 21. In general, when problems arise, heads of prenatal diagnostic centers consider the maternal indications of amniocentesis or chorion biopsy. Recently DNA probes of cystic fibrosis, hemophilia A and Duchenne-type muscular dystrophy were introduced in Debrecen and Szeged.

## 2.9.1.4 Cost-Benefit of Early Diagnosis and Genetic Counseling

Economic aspects of the Hungarian medical service system have rarely been evaluated. Data on lost life-years and impaired life are available for congenital anomalies and shown in Table 2.9.2. The cost of the prevention of severe neural tube defects by maternal serum AFP screening was calculated to be only 10% of the cost of medical treatment, care and habilitation of persons affected (Czeizel and Klujber 1978).

238

## 2.9.1.5 Abortion

The 1956 Abortion Law allowed women to decide whether or not to terminate pregnancy. Consequently, the rate of legally induced abortions increased continuously to a peak of 206,800 in 1969. The Abortion Law was modified in 1974 to limit social indications and broaden medical indications. Today, a district "abortion committee" allows induced abortion for the following medical reasons: severe fetal disorders, high maternal risk, rape, incest, women over 35 years of age; and for the following social reasons: extramarital pregnancy, having three or more children, having two children and a third pregnancy that resulted in a stillbirth or in a spontaneous or induced abortion, or lack of housing. Medical geneticists in genetic counseling outpatient clinics may refer for termination before the twelfth week of gestation cases of $\geq 10\%$ risk of severe fetal disorder which is not treatable after birth with great efficacy and not diagnosable prenatally. They may refer for termination before the twentieth week of pregnancy in cases of prenatally diagnosed diseases and/or a $\geq 50\%$ risk of severe, untreatable fetal disorders, e.g., male sex in severe X-linked disease. They may refer without limitation of gestational time in prenatally diagnosed disorders incompatible with life. The occurrence of medically indicated induced abortions was low (about 3%) until 1973, then increased significantly in two steps as shown in Table 2.9.1. A significant problem is the unreasonable exaggeration of potential teratogens, which leads to the termination of approximately 5,000 desired pregnancies annually (Czeizel 1983).

## 2.9.2 Ethical Problems Faced by Medical Geneticists in Hungary

### 2.9.2.1 Genetic Counseling

The first genetic counseling outpatient clinic was established by G. Lenart in 1963 and was followed by several others. At that time, the traditional non-directive method of genetic counseling was employed, i.e., to give only information without advice. However, Hungarian consultands were dissatisfied with this approach and expressed a desire for more help from the counselors than mere information. They appealed for advice to make an appropriate choice among options. Gradually, we rejected neutral and defensive nondirective counseling and a system of "information-guidance" counseling was established (Czeizel et al. 1981). This term was coined with the help of the late C. Carter. First, the nosological, i.e., etiological diagnosis of the proband must be sought by case history, pedigree, and further genetic and other examinations as needed. Twenty percent of nosological diagnoses were made in connection with genetic counseling. Unfortunately, in about 20% of consultands, no nosological diagnosis of any kind could be made in the probands beyond a clinical classification. Second, medical and social perspectives of planning a child or further children were provided, including: [1] the burden of expected disorders; [2] the possibility of treatment; [3] the possibility of prenatal diagno-

**Table 2.9.3**  Distribution of consultands according to five categories of advice

| Category | Meaning | % |
|---|---|---|
| Advice I | No essential problem, pregnancy is recommended | 60 |
| Advice II | Pregnancy is recommended after some preparations | 25 |
| Advice III | Pregnancy is recommended with prenatal fetal examination | 5 |
| Advice IV | There is some problem, pregnancy requires consideration | 5 |
| Advice V | There is a serious problem, pregnancy is not recommended | 5 |

sis; [4] the specific genetic or teratogenic risk; [5] the maternal risk during pregnancy; [6] the effect of affected parent(s) on the postnatal development of children; and [7] the socioeconomic situation of the family, including the number of children already born. Third, after the above information, if consultands want to know our advice, we summarize it. When we asked consultands' opinion and evaluation of our counseling, their main objection (18%) was exaggerated "diplomacy." Many prospective parents expected not only information and advice, but also definite instructions from the genetic counseling service, which then would virtually make the decision for them. Their position is partly reassuring, since no one objected to excessive interference with their private lives. But it is also a call for caution, since medical geneticists should by no means assume the decision for parents. Genetic counseling is always individualized; however, five general categories of advice can be grouped (Table 2.9.3).

In practice we summarize our Advice I in the following way: "If I were you I would have a baby without any anxiety," or in the case of Advice V: "In your place I would not dare to have a baby – at least not for the time being – because of the significant danger." After Advice I and II, 95% of consultands have a baby. This figure exceeds significantly rates of non-directive genetic counseling, and it helps Hungary's pronatalist policy. The percent of affected newborns was 4.0 after Advice I and II, which is equal to the recorded figure of congenital anomalies in Hungary. After the "dissuading" advice IV and V, 40% of consultands were deterred. The latter compliance rate is similar to the figure for the non-directive counseling in some western countries (Carter et al. 1971). Thus, we dare hope that our information-guidance method does not harm human rights and better fits the wishes of our consultands. As a matter of fact, this method suits the original Galtonian idea: the task of medical geneticists is to provide information and counseling; however, the decision is the right and responsibility of consultands. We are concerned that non-directive counseling might result in lack of help rather than active medical and social help. Unfortunately, 44% of babies born after Advice V were affected with serious disorders. This figure was about 20% after Advice IV. After Advice III, 90% of our consultands were undeterred. Each nation has to find an optimal method in genetic counseling that corresponds best to both the expectation and the cultural tradition of the population and to the protection of human rights.

## 2.9.2.2 Prenatal Diagnosis

The majority of Hungarian medical geneticists feel that the "secondary" prevention of severe abnormalities detected through intrauterine fetal examination is an
important task. Of course, such an intervention can be done only voluntarily, at
the request of the parents, and the selective abortion is performed only on the basis of maternal decision. Occasionally, an unexpected difficulty arises when the
examination performed upon appropriate indication makes it possible to rule out
the expected disorder but accidentally sheds light on another abnormality. If this
is severe and untreatable, there is no problem, and the diagnosis can be considered lucky. What may cause a problem is when the newly-discovered abnormality
is not severe, but does have some medical and/or social consequences, e.g., Klinefelter syndrome, XYY condition, or the absence of left hand.

## 2.9.2.3 Genetic Screening

In my opinion, the most important ethical issue is the allocation of genetic services. The medical health system in Hungary provides only a fraction of the most
accessible forms of genetic services. For example, both maternal serum AFP and
prenatal chromosome examination of women over 40 are scarce resources. Only
23% of women of advanced age were screened in 1984–85. Also, false negative
findings in serum AFP are high.

## 2.9.2.4 Other Contexts: Artificial Insemination

According to regulation No. 12/1981 of the Minister of Health: "Heterolog artificial insemination is ... warranted in the case of a married woman under the age of
40 ... for whom the medically confirmed probability of having a healthy child with
her husband is negligible." Some single women over the age of 40 applied to use
this method in order to become pregnant, but we had to refuse their request. In the
author's opinion, the present regulation does not correspond to international medical rules, e.g., the Geneva Convention, which does not allow any discrimination
in the treatment of patients. Surprisingly, a few recipient couples wanted to select
their donors according to their religion. The request posed serious problems from
two aspects. From biological and social perspectives, all human beings belong to
the same species, Homo sapiens. No differentiation in value can be made among
people based on origin and religion. Another practical problem was that official
regulations after World War II forbade registration by religion in Hungary. Still, in
keeping with their principles, doctors should help patients. Thus, when we examine prospective donors, we now explain such requests and record the religion
of the donor if he is willing to disclose this information voluntarily. On account of

241

Hungary's pronatalist policy, surgical sterilization in males was not allowed until September 1987, despite the relatively frequent request for it. This example of a cultural difference should be noted by readers.

## 2.9.3 Consensus and Variation

In this study, 18 questionnaires were sent to medical genetic centers, including 15 genetic counseling clinics and three pediatric institutions without genetic counseling clinics. According to an agreement or a preliminary discussion concerning the study, each institution received only one questionnaire, because in the opinion of the heads of these units, all medical geneticists within a given institution should have the same approach. This decision is a question for debate, but required the author's compliance. This method means that the findings of 15 questionnaires represent, not 15 persons, but 15 groups involving about 50 qualified or non-qualified medical geneticists.

The variations in approaches to these problems have exceeded our previous expectation. Of course, it is necessary to find a good balance between freedom of medical decision-making (considering the individual circumstances of consultands) and acceptable individual differences among experts' ethical, political, and other attitudes as well as well-established scientific and ethical facts and ideas. However, in the author's opinion, variations in some replies to the questionnaire indicate some misunderstanding or lack of consensus. This supposition was confirmed by a working conference of participants held after the evaluation of the study. First of all, it appeared that the consensus is greater than we initially supposed, because some of the responses listed in the questionnaires were essentially similar in meaning. By combining responses with similar meanings according to the format in the introductory chapter, we found that there was strong ($\geq 75\%$) consensus about 5.17 (36%) of the 14 clinical cases. These were Case 1, false paternity (93% would protect mother's confidentiality); Case 5, XY female (80% would *not* disclose); Case 6, conflicting test results (93% would disclose); Case 7, new/controversial interpretations (87% would disclose); Case 10, prenatal diagnosis for maternal anxiety (80% would refuse); and Case 14, presenting reproductive options for female carriers of tuberous sclerosis (77% would present sterilization). There was a moderate consensus (67%–74%) in regard to 3.03 (22%) of the 14 cases. These were Case 3, hemophilia A (73% would disclose diagnosis to relatives at risk); Case 4, parental translocation (73% would *not* disclose); Case 12, XYY fetus (67% would be nondirective); Cases 13 and 14, presenting reproductive options to carriers of tuberous sclerosis (69% would not present contraception to male carriers, 73% would present contraception to female carriers, and 69% would *not* present surrogate motherhood). In all, there was strong or moderate consensus with regard to 58% of the clinical cases. Some problems were connected with confusion about whether the existing official rules or the personal opinion of genetic counselors should be decisive in the replies. For example, in Case 2 (Huntington disease) four participants selected disclosure, although the Hungarian Health Rule does not allow doctors to inform other relatives of the family without the permission of the client. If they do, it will have legal consequences without any doubt. In the case of diagnosis for maternal anxiety, three participating groups said that they would perform it, which is against the official Hungarian regulation. As to the evaluation of Hungarian experts' view of sex selection, which is not allowed in Hungary, five points are relevant. First, there is an obvious difference of opinions: nine in favor versus six against. Second, some of us are willing to consider this parental request only after two or more same-sex children, e.g., as in Case 10: a couple already have four girls and if the fetus is a girl, they will abort it. Third, this policy could moderate the decrease in births (i.e., we can save half of the fetuses from abortion). Fourth, this intervention will not change the sex ratio of newborns because in our experience, as many couples will desire daughters as sons. Fifth, children who grow up with siblings of the other sex are more sociable than others. The above discrepancies clearly indicated that some genetic counselors are not satisfied with the existing regulations. Of course, everyone may have their own ethical ideas, but in practice it is not possible to go against the accepted official rules. A further difficulty arose concerning questions providing choices (vasectomy, surrogate motherhood, donor egg, and in vitro fertilization) that are not available in Hungary.

The distribution of replies to questions about counseling approaches was surprising, because it indicated that some participating geneticist groups did not understand or did not follow the previously accepted consensus about the so-called information-guidance method. However, as the working conference of participants proved, the explanation was a linguistic misunderstanding. Some participants did not realize that the reply "e" to Question 25 (see questionnaire in Appendix) means "Advise patients what they *should* do." However, after the discussion of the accurate meaning of replies to this question, some participating groups changed their replies from "e" (advise patients what they ought to do) and "a" (tell patients that decisions are theirs alone and refuse to make any for them) to "d" (inform patients what you would do if in their situation). The latter response fits well our information-guidance method. The discussion of participating groups clearly indicated that we deliberately want to follow an *intermediate* method between non-directive and directive counseling.

All of these findings confirm that the absence of institutions that would provide an ongoing opportunity to discuss these problems causes serious difficulties in the activity of medical genetic services.

## 2.9.4 Cultural Context of Medical Genetics in Hungary

In Hungary, the medical health system is nationalized. All available medical services belong to the Ministry of Health. The main policy of the Hungarian health system is the prevention of disease by maintaining equality of free health care in each region. Within this centralized and hierarchical system there is a possibility to provide higher levels of medical services in specialized institutions. Genetic counseling outpatient clinics are under the direction of obstetrics and gynecology. Genetic research is regulated by the National Institute of Pediatrics. However, there is a Society of Human Geneticists.

## 2.9.4.2  Major Controversies

The sharpest ethical controversies in medical genetics concern the *balance of individual and social interests*. In Hungary, as in general, three human rights are usually mentioned in connection with family plannning.

1. "A person's right to shape his/her own life," i.e., it is each person's right to be allowed to live according to his/her wishes and decisions.
2. The "right to have children," i.e., everyone has the right to procreation.
3. The "right to health."

In the course of genetic counseling, these rights are often in conflict with each other and with the interests of society.

## 2.9.4.4  Abortion Laws

See Section 2.9.1.5 above.

## 2.9.4.6  Need for New Laws

The rights of fetuses/babies conceived and born have only recently been formulated. The right to be healthy and to receive adequate medical services is also a basic human right, which is also confirmed by our Constitution. Therefore, everybody has the right to receive effective therapeutic and preventive medical service to preserve his or her health. The right to be healthy certainly applies to the fetus and to the newborn, too. The implementation of these general principles and rights means, in our case, that everyone has the right to be born healthy, and specifically, the *"right of the offspring to be born healthy."* Of course, the fetus/newborn is unable to assert and to defend its right, so this responsibility belongs, naturally and legally, to parents. In fact, the wish to have children almost always means, tacitly or expressly, hope for healthy offspring. However, in some cases, undertaking pregnancy means considerable danger for the offspring. In such cases, a peculiar situation arises, since the prospective parents' interest and right to have children becomes opposed to the offspring's interest and right to be born healthy. Most prospective parents refrain from having children in these cases. Obviously, they might become the best possible parents, since they are capable of subordinating their own wishes to the interests of their children, i.e., to their right to be born healthy. A smaller proportion of prospective parents decide to have children in spite of the significant, or even considerable, danger for the offspring. This means that they consider their own wishes and right to have children more important than their children's interest, or their right to be born healthy. More than half of the children in such cases are born healthy, making the parents' decision acceptable. They decided on having children, in spite of considerable danger, after much reflection and agony. Thus, the essence of family planning, responsible parenting, is fulfilled.

In a few cases, however, prospective parents are incapable of understanding the responsibility of having children, and the offspring's right to be born healthy is violated out of ignorance, incomprehension, and sometimes even conscious irresponsibility. Such incompetent couples are mainly alcoholic, mentally retarded or psychiatric patients. Aware of cases involving incompetent parents, many people, especially physicians, are demanding increased social intervention in the form of birth control by administrative measures, mandatory sterilization, etc. Their reasoning is as follows: on the one hand, in the case of communicable diseases, society accepts, without hesitation, the protection of the community's interests. The red slips on the doors of homes with children suffering from a communicable disease, quarantines, and compulsory immunization are clear manifestations of this principle. Let us take a concrete example. If someone contracts a venereal disease, e.g., lues, he or she is legally bound to go for treatment to an institute for venereal diseases. Non-compliance results in a police summons. The risk of transmission of VD by sexual intercourse is "only" 25–30%; early damage cannot be called very severe, and, more importantly, it is treatable. Many types of hereditary damage, on the other hand, are clearly severe and cannot be treated at present. The risk of transmission from parent to child is often higher than 25–30%. Nevertheless, no one has the right to influence the parents in order to limit the transmission of genetic disorders. Yet, the similarity between the two biological processes cannot be overlooked. In both cases one person transmits a "pathogen," i.e., virus, bacterium, parasite or defective gene to another. Why does society act in the common interest at the cost of the individual's rights in the case of a communicable disease, and why doesn't it protect the children from their parents? The health of the offspring is at least as important for society as the health of adults! Furthermore, adults are capable of defending themselves, while the fetus or newborn or child cannot. Does society regard children as the parents' private property? Not at all, as proven beyond any doubt by social protection afforded to the child already born. Parents may not consciously damage the health of their children by beating, starving, etc. Why would they then be allowed to endanger their offspring by transmitting their defects? It could be argued that a person suffering from a communicable disease can transmit it to a great number of people, while heredity, especially in today's smaller families, affects only a few. It is true that communicable diseases spread horizontally, making more people sick, while genetic disorders are transmitted vertically, making the consequences harder to follow. However, the genetic damage caused in the offspring is manifested through countless generations, therefore, the number of victims may be enormous. For example, one of the most frequent and troublesome genetic diseases in South Africa, porphyria variegata, affecting thousands of people, is the result of a single immigrant's genes. Our opinion is that the difference in medical and social treatment given to these two groups of diseases is explained mainly by the time factor. Contagious diseases have been killing people for thousands of years; the possibilities of prevention have been known for more than a hundred years. Awareness of hereditary problems is almost as old as mankind but the methods of prevention are being outlined

only in our days. We need time and patience to work out proper and effective prevention. On the other hand, legal regulations also offer a way to protect the interest of children born to people unable to comprehend their parental responsibility.
Due to their disorders, the mentally diseased, mentally retarded and alcoholics are
incapable of understanding and complying with certain socially important and accepted principles. Therefore, they must be treated differently. Even the need for legal regulation may be considered, especially because it has already been established in matters pertaining to property rights. A short summary follows of the main
provisions of the Hungarian judicial practice in regard to such matters.

In terms of legal competence, persons can be divided into three categories: [1]
the legally competent, [2] those with limited legal competence, and [3] the legally
incompetent. Of special interest are the two latter groups.

12/1/ of the Civil Code states: "A minor who has turned fourteen and is not legally incompetent, has limited legal competence." 13/1/ states: "The individual of
legal age placed under guardianship by the court is considered of limited legal
competence. /2/ The court places under "guardianship with limited legal competence" those people of legal age, whose capacity, necessary to manage their affairs,
is impaired to a great extent either permanently or temporarily, although recur-
ringly, due to their mental state, mental retardation or some kind of addiction."

15/2/ states: "The minor of legal age who has not completed his/her fourteenth
year is considered legally incompetent." 16/1/ states: "Any person placed under
guardianship without legal competence by the court is considered legally incompetent. /2/ A person without legal competence, who permanently and completely lacks the capacity necessary to manage his/her affairs due to his/her mental state or retardation is placed under guardianship by the court." Finally,
according to 17: "Even without being under guardianship, a person is considered
legally incompetent if he/she is in a state completely lacking capacity to manage
his/her affairs." Thus, the court places under "guardianship without legal competence" those of legal age who permanently and completely lack the capacity necessary to manage their affairs due to their mental state or retardation. When the
aforementioned conditions exist simultaneously, the court must formally decide
whether the person in question has limited legal competence or is incompetent
and should be placed under guardianship.

On a higher level, the common denominator of limited competence and in-
competence is that the person lacks the "volitive power" or this power is inadequate. From the point of view of volitive power, the difference between people
with limited competence and no competence is in degree rather than in substance.
The basic identity of these two categories is expressed in general practice, according to which the validity of statements both by people with limited competence
and by those lacking legal competence requires the participation of the legal rep-
resentative/parent/guardian.

According to 12/1/: "The approval of the public guardianship authority is required to validate the statement of the legal representative, if the legal statement
refers to:

A. The support of a person with limited competence or lacking legal competence;
B. The inheritance rights or obligations of a person with limited competence or lacking legal competence;
C. Property with value exceeding the amount established by special regulation."

An earlier edition of the Civil Code defined this value as 10,000 Hungarian florints, i.e., about $200 U.S. Despite such legal requirements, the mentally ill, retarded, and alcoholics have the right to have children even it it means severe health, genetic, and familial-social harm to the offspring. Is a child worth less than F. 10,000? We know a case in which a mentally retarded couple have 16 children. Are they not worth F. 10,000? Of course, this absurdity can be acceptable to no one, but this is what the one-sidedness of legal regulations suggests. We desire not to be misunderstood. Regulation by law has only a limited role in securing the offspring's right to be born healthy. Still, in certain cases, when it becomes evident for the specialist/social worker/physician that a person is not capable of responsible family planning and child-rearing due to his/her mental disease or retardation, then this specialist should be able to initiate a procedure to verify that person's limited competence or incompetence after a certain number of children if it is justified by the child's state of health, mental retardation, or by the lack of proper family care, e.g., in the case of parents with mental disease. If limited competence or incompetence is confirmed, the guardianship authority could prescribe the application of an intrauterine contraceptive. No one can recommend such regulations lightheartedly, but the protection of the offspring's health is such an important social and biological issue, that we should use such means to secure the desired results. Because of genetic risk, many of the children born into these families will be mentally retarded or mentally ill. However, the social risk to which they are exposed represents an even greater danger. The unfavorable family situation, lack of suitable parental care and of favorable social-cultural circumstances make it likely that the latent predisposition will actually manifest itself in a disorder.

Of course, it should also be asked who has to assure the offspring's right to be born healthy? The authorities now leave the right to have children to parents. We introduce here the principle of family planning or having children with responsibility. With the widespread use of modern and effective contraceptive devices, the family, i.e., the individual, can decide whether or not to have children. Therefore, logically and legally, the parents have a duty to assure the right of the offspring to be born healthy, i.e., the health of the embryo-newborn. Thus, family planning means not only how many children are to be born and when, but also assuring the health of these children to the greatest possible degree. This can be done only if the future parents ("family planners") undertake conception, pregnancy and childbirth with a sense of responsibility, by considering the right of the offspring to be born healthy and to be able to develop their congenital capabilities. Most family planners are suitable future parents. However, some persons do not practice responsibility in bearing children. They are unfamiliar with or do not use modern contraceptive methods and do not respect the basic human right to be born healthy. In such cases, the justification of the family's right to have children is questionable in the light of society's interests.

Many governments already regulate the quantitative aspect of family planning. To assure the health of the offspring is equally important. Therefore, we could imagine – in some exceptional cases – legislation to assure the birth of healthy children. Medical prevention in this case should mean extending the protection of the future generation to the period before conception and during pregnancy. The interests of society and the right of the offspring to be born healthy can make such prevention possible within the spirit of humanism.

## 2.9.5 Ethical Issues and Future Trends

There is some delay in the introduction of new genetic techniques in Hungary. Many deserving persons are deprived of genetic services by this delay, but one advantage is time to study medical and ethical problems before their introduction. All resources for medical genetics are provided by official budgets of the government in Hungary. In Hungary, 3-4% of the Gross National Product is spent on health care. Preventive health programs including genetic services would require a higher proportion.

The most serious ethical issues in medical genetics today and in the future are lack of resources to allow the timely utilization of comprehensive medical and genetic services. Concurrently, the problems of many couples of low socioeconomic background must be addressed while helping them decrease their higher genetic risks.

Our goal is an appropriate and humane social regulation of family planning. Appealing to public opinion and to basic principles of medical ethics are necessary to reach the goal. There is no need or justification for general and radical administrative regulations. Aside from rare exceptions, the solution lies in educating and informing the public on health matters by reconciling the right to have children with the right to be born healthy. The right to have children is well known; we share Galton's view, i.e., physically handicapped, blind, deaf, or mentally retarded people may have children, even if we fear the recurrence of the disorder in their offspring. Even though in the case of the mentally retarded, it would be in the interest of society to limit childbearing, to have children is a general human right, in which the decision belongs mostly to the individual. The question is: how far should this right be respected? It is fair that the mentally retarded and mental patients be allowed to exercise their right to have children if they have the emotional need and the sense of responsibility. Some patients, however, are incapable of understanding and realizing the responsibility involved and the children become only the accidental byproducts of their sexual lives. This is why it would be appropriate to further regulate and limit the number of their children, which otherwise could reach 4 or 12. A great number of their children – the survey of the mentally retarded conducted in Budapest indicates 60% – end up in government-supported institutions, where they stay at least for some period of time. Quite a few of them have to be institutionalized for the rest of their lives. The care for such a child is close to F. 100,000, about $2,000 U.S., a year. Limitation of the number of children considerably exceeding the general average can be the only objective.

In essence, such families should be encouraged to practice up-to-date and effective birth control after the birth of two, perhaps three children, which corresponds to the general average. Sterilization, which is unusual and therefore regarded as discriminatory in our country, would by no means be the appropriate method. Intrauterine contraceptives provide safe protection. Specialists all over the world find this method, along with sterilization, most appropriate for biologically endangered people, mental patients, the mentally retarded, and alcoholics. In these cases, we should increasingly try to enforce the offspring's right to be born healthy and the interest of society by medical information and education, since the offspring's health and good "start" is one of society's basic needs. Undoubtedly, this poses some ethical problems, but in our opinion, the miserable life of 4-12 children irresponsibly conceived is a much more severe medical, and especially social, danger.

# References

Carter CO, Fraser-Roberts JA, Evans KA, Buck AR [1971] Genetic clinic: A follow-up. Lancet i: 281-285

Czeizel A [1983] Evaluation of medical indications in induced abortions [Hungarian]. Orv Hetil (Medical Weekly) 124: 1297-1302

Czeizel A [1988] The right to be born healthy: the ethical problems of human genetics in Hungary. Alan R Liss, New York [Hungarian edition, 1983, Budapest]

Czeizel A, Bodnar Z, Rockenbauer M [1984] Some epidemiological data on spontaneous abortion in Hungary, 1971-80. J Epid Comm Health 38: 143-148

Czeizel A, Klujber L [1978] A cost-benefit analysis of prevention of open neural tube defects based on maternal alpha-fetoprotein screening [Hungarian]. Transfusion 11: 41-48

Czeizel A, Metneki J, Osztovics M [1981] Evaluation of information guidance genetic counseling. J Med Genet 18: 91-98

Czeizel A, Sankaranarayanan K [1984] The load of genetic and partially genetic disorders in man. I. Congenital anomalies: estimates of detriment in terms of years of life lost and years of impaired life. Mut Res 128: 73-103

# 2.10 Ethics and Medical Genetics in India

I. C. Verma and B. Singh

## 2.10.1.1 Scope of the Problem

There is a general impression that genetic disorders are not important in developing countries. However, an analysis of data from India (Table 2.10.1) indicates that the frequency of genetic disorders is similar to that in the developed countries [31]. Factors such as the selective pressure exerted by falciparum malaria in the distant past, the practice of consanguineous marriages in many communities, and a huge population with a high birth rate have led to the presence of a large number of patients with genetic disorders, mental retardation and congenital malformations. Table 2.10.1 summarizes the data on the frequency of genetic disorders in India.

Based on the 1981 census data, it can be estimated that 0.832 million infants with genetic disorders/malformations are born every year. The number would be even higher if the projected figures for 1987 are considered [12]: population 776.3 million, birth rate 32.7/1000, annual births 25.39 million, infants affected at birth 0.93 million. The present [1985] infant mortality rate is 95 per 1000 births [15], of which only 1% is contributed by congenital malformations [8]. However, the health scenario is changing very rapidly. The government is energetically establishing primary health care facilities in all rural areas, and zealously pursuing a universal program of immunization [12]. These measures are expected to reduce drastically the mortality due to communicable diseases, and would thus lead to the emergence of congenital malformations as significant causes of infant mortality.

**Table 2.10.1.** Genetic Disorders in India[1]

| Disorder | Prevalence % | Total No. (Millions) |
|---|---|---|
| *Affected at birth* | | 0.832 |
| Congenital anomalies | 2.5 | 0.569 |
| Single gene | 0.6 | 0.136 |
| Chromosomal | 0.56 | 0.127 |
| *In general population* | | |
| Behavioral and C.N.S. disorders* | 1.5 | 10.650 |
| Late onset multifactorial disorders** | 10.1 | 27.390 |

[1] Verma 1986b; Data based on 1981 census
* Includes nonspecific mental retardation, schizophrenia, manic depressive psychosis, and epilepsy.
** Includes hypertension, diabetes mellitus, and coronary artery disease, but affecting certain age groups only

250

This trend is already visible in the urban areas where almost 13–15% of perinatal deaths are attributable to congenital malformations [32]. In an experimental rural area in the state of Haryana the introduction of simple measures such as immunization of pregnant women against tetanus, provision of a cheap delivery kit to traditional birth attendants, and distribution of oral rehydration salts increased the proportion of infant mortality due to congenital malformations from 5.4% to 11.3% [20].

## 2.10.1.2 Organization of Clinical Genetic Services

### Description of Centers and Services Offered
Due to the preponderance of communicable diseases, the Government of India has expectedly accorded a low priority to the establishment of clinical genetic services. Much of the research work in genetics was initially carried out by departments of physical anthropology in the universities and departments of anatomy in the medical schools. In the last 5–10 years, the clinical departments (notably pediatrics) have been engaged in providing genetic services. The Indian Council of Medical Research (ICMR) and the Department of Science and Technology (DST) of the Government of India have shown considerable interest in this area and have established centers of excellence to cater to the health needs of the future [16]. There are 77 genetic centers established in different parts of India. Table 2.10.2 summarizes the availability of selected services at these centers.

### Postnatal Chromosome Studies
Facilities for cytogenetic studies from peripheral blood cultures are available in about 42 laboratories. In a five-center study on "Genetic counseling" funded by the ICMR, the numbers of cytogenetic abnormalities detected are listed in Table 2.10.3.

**Table 2.10.2.** Availability of Genetic Services[1]

| Genetic service units (n = 77) | No. of units | % of all |
|---|---|---|
| Cytogenetics | 42 | 54.5 |
| Population genetics | 38 | 49.4 |
| Genetic counselling | 34 | 44.2 |
| Dermatoglyphics | 28 | 36.4 |
| Hematology & blood groups | 27 | 35.1 |
| Clinical genetics | 26 | 33.8 |
| Biochemical genetics | 25 | 32.5 |
| Birth defects | 23 | 29.9 |
| Cancer genetics | 13 | 16.9 |
| Amniocentesis | 10 | 14.3 |
| Molecular genetics | 6 | 7.8 |
| Pharmacogenetics | 6 | 7.8 |

[1] Verma 1980, modified

**Table 2.10.3.** Results of Chromosome Analysis

| | Bangalore | Bombay | Delhi | Lucknow | Pune | Total | |
|---|---|---|---|---|---|---|---|
| | | | | | | No. | % |
| Normal karyotypes | 881 | 325 | 378 | 107 | 402 | 2,093 | 75.6 |
| Abnormal karyotypes | | | | | | | |
| Autosomal | | | | | | | |
|   Numerical | 94 | 53 | 140 | 14 | 134 | 435 | 15.7 |
|   Structural | 14 | 11 | 25 | 0 | 1 | 51 | 1.8 |
| Sex chromosomal | | | | | | | |
|   Numerical | 22 | 13 | 12 | 1 | 10 | 52 | 2.1 |
|   Structural | 14 | 4 | 7 | 0 | 3 | 28 | 1.1 |
| Intersex cases | 20 | 0 | 15 | 0 | 16 | 51 | 1.8 |
| Variants | 40 | 13 | 0 | 0 | 0 | 53 | 1.9 |
| | 1,085 | 419 | 577 | 122 | 566 | 2,769 | 100 |

**Investigation of genetic disease**

Facilities for investigation of genetic disease are available in most of the teaching hospitals. Tests for biochemical disorders (consisting mostly of amino acid chromatography and routine medical biochemical tests) are available in all major hospitals. However, only 25 of 77 (32.5%) listed genetic centers [29] have these facilities (Table 2.10.2).

Hereditary anemias are a common problem in many parts of India [4]. Beta thalassemia is common in Maharashtra and Gujarat (Lohannas and Sindhis), Punjab (Khatris migrated from Pakistan), and West Bengal. Hemoglobin E is common in West Bengal and the whole of North-East India, and hemoglobin D in the Punjab. Sickle cell hemoglobin is widespread among many tribal communities living in different parts of India: in Maharashtra, Madhya Pradesh, Orissa and Andhra Pradesh [22, 28]. Fortunately, hematological laboratories exist in all major hospitals so that they can carry out investigations of cases of hereditary anemias. However, many of these do not have genetic units. Of the 77 centers listed, 27 (35.1%) are equipped to investigate hereditary anemias [29].

The Government of India has established laboratories of *molecular genetics* in 5-6 major universities in India. However, most of these are doing basic research so that the benefits of advances in molecular genetics are not yet available for patients in India.

**Genetic Counseling**

Counseling services are available in 34 of 77 (44.2%) genetic units in India [29]. In about 16 of these, the services provided are of a high order, as the units have a trained clinical geneticist, cytogeneticist and biochemist, with good back-up laboratory facilities.

The Indian Council of Medical Research funded a 3-year multicentric study on genetic counseling. Preliminary analysis of the data are summarized in Table 2.10.4. Mental retardation is the commonest cause for referral (16.1%). The second largest group comprises chromosomal disorders (12.2%). The other significant

**Table 2.10.4.** Patients Provided Genetic Counseling Classified According to Category of Disease

| Category | Bangalore | Bombay | Delhi | Lucknow | Pune | Total | |
|---|---|---|---|---|---|---|---|
| | | | | | | No. | % |
| Mental retardation (Idiopathic) | 242 | 376 | 162 | 81 | 248 | 1,109 | 16.1 |
| Chromosomal disorders | 196 | 95 | 374 | 58 | 121 | 844 | 12.2 |
| Syndromes | 229 | 220 | 127 | 50 | 52 | 678 | 9.8 |
| Repeated abortions/fetal loss/neonatal deaths | 336 | 130 | 53 | 6 | 141 | 666 | 9.7 |
| Intersex, primary & secondary amenorrhea, hypogonadism | 278 | 168 | 29 | 60 | 134 | 669 | 9.7 |
| High risk pregnancy | – | 332 | 225 | – | – | 547 | 7.9 |
| Hematological disorders | 27 | – | 13 | 121 | 320 | 481 | 7.0 |
| Neural tube defects | 65 | 86 | 170 | 42 | 33 | 396 | 5.7 |
| Multiple congenital anomalies | 18 | 77 | 116 | 32 | 24 | 267 | 3.9 |
| Metabolic disorders | 94 | 14 | 107 | 30 | 38 | 284 | 4.1 |
| Primary microcephaly | 16 | 17 | 66 | 9 | 73 | 181 | 2.6 |
| Skeletal dysplasia | 2 | 10 | 35 | 8 | – | 55 | 0.8 |
| Miscellaneous (genetic) | 223 | – | 203 | 88 | 201 | 715 | 10.5 |
| Total | 1,726 | 1,515 | 1,680 | 585 | 385 | 6,892 | 100.0 |

groups are of patients with specific syndromes (9.8%); repeated abortions, fetal loss and neonatal deaths (9.7%); primary and secondary amenorrhea, hypogonadism and sterility (9.7%); and high risk pregnancy (7.9%). Additionally, more patients of a specific group may be seen in a particular unit because of the special expertise available. For example, in Delhi high risk pregnancy constitutes a large group, in Pune hematological disorders, and in Bangalore cases of primary amenorrhea. Another factor which leads to differences is that in certain units there are other clinics for specific disorders. For example, in Delhi, at the All India Institute of Medical Sciences (AIIMS) there is a separate clinic for intersex disorders, as also for hematologic disorders. Therefore fewer patients with these disorders are seen in the genetic counseling clinic.

## 2.10.1.3 Prenatal Diagnostic Services

In the absence of a centralized registry it is difficult to estimate the number of prenatal diagnostic procedures being performed in the country. However, I would estimate that not more than 5% of the need for genetic services is being provided for.

a) Facilities for *ultrasonographic studies* are available in a majority (about 80%) of the 106 university hospitals, and a large number of private hospitals and maternity homes in all major cities. Ultrasonography is commonly used for help in the obstetric and medical management of patients. More recently, as the radiologists and obstetricians have improved their skills in interpretation, it is increasingly being utilized for carrying out prenatal diagnosis.

*Amniocentesis* was introduced for obstetric and genetic care even before ultrasonography. It is being carried out in most university and large government hospitals. A large number of obstetricians in private practice carry out amniocentesis, although there are limited private laboratories to process the samples obtained. I would estimate that about 3–4 private laboratories exist in each of the major cities like Bombay, Delhi, Madras, Calcutta and Bangalore.

*Chorionic villi aspiration* has been set up in about 12 centers, of which 8 are in government institutions and 4 in the private sector. The samples obtained in private clinics are processed in private laboratories. *Fetoscopy* is being done in only two centers in India.

b) *Indications for prenatal diagnosis.* Until 1975 the major indication for prenatal diagnosis at our center was determination of sex of the fetus (53 cases), of which the majority were for social reasons, and only a few (5, 10.6%) for X-linked disorders (Table 2.10.5). In 1983, the Government of India forbade the government/officially supported institutions from performing prenatal diagnosis of sex for social reasons. Subsequent cases at our center had the prenatal diagnosis carried out for the indications of genetic disease given in Table 2.10.5. The largest number of cases consisted of women who had previously given birth to an infant with a neural tube defect or with Down syndrome. Cases of advanced maternal age at conception were fewer than in the West, because most women are married early and complete their reproduction by the age of 35 years. Most of the genetic centers use a maternal age at conception of 35 years as a cut-off for advising amniocentesis.

**Table 2.10.5.** Indications for Amniocentesis for Diagnostic Purposes at Genetic Unit, AIIMS, New Delhi

| Indication | Before 1980 | After 1983 | |
|---|---|---|---|
| | | No. | % |
| 1. Determination of sex | | | |
| a) Social reasons | 48 | – | – |
| b) X-linked disorder | 5 | 6 | 5.7 |
| 2. Chromosomal analysis | | | |
| a) Previous child with Down syndrome | 7 | 34 | 32.7 |
| b) Advanced maternal age | 8 | 15 | 14.4 |
| c) Previous child with multiple congenital anomalies/mental retardation | | 10 | 9.6 |
| d) Repeated abortions/perinatal deaths | | 3 | 2.9 |
| 3. High risk for neural tube defect | 7 | 36 | 34.6 |
| Total | 75 | 104 | 100.0 |

c) There is no specific *national policy* on the indications for prenatal diagnosis. The indications for this in all the centers would be similar to the experience of our unit, as reflected in Table 2.10.5.


## *2.10.1.4  Cost-Benefit of Early Diagnosis and Genetic Counseling*


Newborn screening on a regular basis is not carried out in any center in India. It has been done as a research study for hypothyroidism and amino acid disorders. The frequency of neonatal hypothyroidism in India in areas non-endemic for iodine deficiency varies from 1:500 in Delhi [24, 25], to 1:2481 in Bombay [5]. The high incidence in Delhi probably reflects the presence of iodine deficiency in some parts of the city. However, the incidence of neonatal hypothyroidism in an area in Uttar Pradesh, endemic for iodine-deficiency goitre, was 1:24 births. This astonishingly high figure applies to the intense belt of endemic goitre which runs along the slopes of the Himalayas, extending over 2400 km from Kashmir in the West to the Naga Hills in the East. It has been estimated that almost 4% of the population in these areas have attendant disabilities of feeblemindedness, deafmutism and cretinism [25]. So, hardly any statistics are required to convince about the cost-effectiveness of a screening program in these areas. Pilot projects of neonatal thyroid screening have been initiated in many endemic areas. The more obvious and lasting solution to this problem – iodizing the salt – is a priority, and the Government of India proposes to iodize all edible salt by 1992 [12].

Appaji Rao and colleagues have screened 59,840 newborns in Bangalore for the presence of amino acid disorders, by chromatography of capillary blood collected from heel-pricks [personal communication]. Forty-two cases with abnormal chromatograms were detected. However, there was difficulty in followup of some of the infants, due to the parents' lack of a fixed abode.

Once communicable diseases are brought under control and the infant mortality rate falls below 60, newborn screening for genetic disorders would assume importance. The Government of India estimates that at the national level the infant mortality rate will fall below 60 by 2000 A. D. However, the infant mortality rate is nearing that figure in the urban areas in many states: Himachal Pradesh, Jammu & Kashmir, Karnataka, Kerala, Maharashtra, Punjab, Tamil Nadu, and West Bengal [15]. In Kerala it is already only 32. Populations in these states would qualify for newborn screening of genetic disorders. Communities which have a high prevalence of hereditary anemias (beta thalassemia and sickle-cell disease) would also satisfy the criteria for neonatal screening for these disorders.

As the majority of genetic counseling and diagnostic services are provided free, it is difficult to estimate cost-benefit ratios. However, Kochupillai and colleagues [18] estimated the cost of screening one newborn for functional status of thyroid by assay of thyroxine, in iodine deficient areas by radio-immunoassay to be Rs 5.31 (approximately 50 U. S. cents), based on locally developed technology. They further calculated that two babies are born every hour with serious iodine deficiency in endemic regions in India!

## 2.10.1.5 Abortion

The Ministry of Health and Family Welfare, Government of India states that "abortion is not permitted as a means for fertility regulation [11]." However, in 1971 a liberalized abortion law was introduced (Medical Termination of Pregnancy Act 1971). The primary objective was to save millions of women who used to take recourse to clandestine abortions by ill-qualified doctors or quacks.

The Government has trained almost 10,000 doctors in medical termination of pregnancy (MTP) techniques. It is proposed to make available at least one doctor trained in MTP at each of 8,500 primary health centers (each center serving a population of 30,000). Up to June, 1985, 4.1 million pregnancies had been terminated [12].

The incidence of elective abortion for 1984–85 (one-year period) and also the ratio of elective abortions to livebirths are depicted in Table 2.10.6. As a percentage of livebirths the maximum number of terminations of pregnancy occurred in Delhi state (18.67%). However, Delhi State mostly consists of the city of Delhi. It is probable that a similar situation exists in other metropolitan areas. Certainly the ratio is greater for the more progressive and prosperous states such as Kerala, Maharashtra, and Punjab. In Jammu and Kashmir, which is a predominantly Muslim state, the number of terminations of pregnancy is very low, as the Muslim religion does not permit abortion.

Most of the medical terminations of pregnancy occur at or before 12 weeks of pregnancy (84.8%), and the rest (15.2%) between 12 to 20 weeks of pregnancy [10]. In 43.2% of cases, MTP is followed by sterilization or fitting of an intrauterine de-

**Table 2.10.6.**   Medical Terminations of Pregnancy in Selected States in India[1]

|  | Population 100,000 | Birth rate /1,000 | Number of terminations | | |
|---|---|---|---|---|---|
|  |  |  | 1984–85 | Since inception (1972–73) | % of all births (1984–85 only) |
| Andhra Pradesh | 533.5 | 37.1 | 13,028 | 131,241 | 0.66 |
| Gujarat | 340.9 | 34.5 | 19,992 | 202,999 | 1.70 |
| Jammu & Kashmir | 59.9 | 31.6 | NA | 1,666 | NA |
| Karnataka | 371.4 | 28.3 | 18,300 | 151,566 | 1.74 |
| Kerala | 254.5 | 25.6 | 43,957 | 343,617 | 6.75 |
| Madhya Pradesh | 521.8 | 37.6 | 24,461 | 175,308 | 1.26 |
| Maharashtra | 627.8 | 28.5 | 95,836 | 507,102 | 5.36 |
| Punjab | 167.9 | 30.3 | 24,953 | 151,686 | 4.91 |
| Tamil Nadu | 484.1 | 28.0 | 65,754 | 443,166 | 4.85 |
| Uttar Pradesh | 1,108.6 | 39.6 | 103,285 | 783,636 | 2.35 |
| West Bengal | 545.8 | 33.2 | 34,458 | 273,401 | 1.90 |
| Delhi | 62.8 | 26.9 | 31,213 | 205,397 | 18.67 |
| All India* | 6,851.8 | 33.3 | 573,129 | 4,044,126 | 2.51 |

[1] India, Ministry of Health and Family Welfare, 1983, 1985, modified
* Includes other states and union territories. NA – Not applicable

**Table 2.10.7.** Reasons for Termination of Pregnancy (April 1981-March 1982)[1]

| Reason | % of all terminations |
| --- | --- |
| 1. Failure of contraception | 43.6 |
| 2. Grave injury to physical health | 15.6 |
| 3. Environmental reasons | 13.7 |
| 4. Grave injury to mental health | 12.5 |
| 5. Danger to mother's life | 8.3 |
| 6. Substantial risk of fetal abnormality | 4.9 |
| 7. Pregnancy caused by rape | 1.4 |
| Total | 100.0 |

[1] India, Ministry of Health and Family Welfare, 1983, p 194, modified

vice. The MTPs carried out for different maternal age groups are: less than 15 years 0.4%; 15-19 years 5.7%; 20-24 years 23%; 25-29 years 32.2%; 30-34 years 23.5%; 35-39 years 11.1%; 40 years and above 3.1% [10].

Table 2.10.7 lists the reasons for termination of pregnancy. Failure of contraception and grave injury to physical health comprise the two largest groups (43.6% and 15.6% respectively). Environmental reasons and other specific conditions leading to substantial risk of fetal abnormality were present in 18.6% of cases. These represent teratologic and genetic reasons for abortions. Therefore, the ratio of social/genetic abortions is 4.4 to 1.

## 2.10.2  Ethical Problems Faced by Medical Geneticists in India

### 2.10.2.1  Genetic Counseling

The major ethical problem in genetic counseling in India is whether it should be directive or non-directive. Most patients from the rural areas and even some from the urban areas are illiterate, have little knowledge of scientific principles, and know next to nothing about genetics. The patients themselves ask the doctor for directive advice. Under such circumstances it is difficult not to be "directive" in counseling. One has to keep in mind that: (i) most of the counselees earnestly desire to have a normal child, and (ii) they would like to maintain harmonious family relations, even if one parent is the carrier of a genetic disease. Giving directive advice under the circumstances places the counselor in a real dilemma, due to the unpredictability of reproductive outcome. Fortunately the patients accept the advice given in good faith and tend to ascribe an unwelcome "result" to the "will of God."

However, orthodox Hindus entertain many religious dogmas, and are not prepared to shake themselves wholly free from them. Many social taboos and prejudices weigh in their judgments. They are even content with adverse results, which they usually ascribe to their fate, past karmas (deeds) and even to the will of God. They do not attach much importance to the practice of scientific methods, if they

257

believe that the practice thereof involves them in "sin." That, perhaps, is the reason why many family planning methods are not readily accepted by the people in India.

## 2.10.2.2 Prenatal Diagnosis

The medical geneticist encounters two distinct classes of counselees: the orthodox and the unorthodox. The former do not like prenatal diagnosis, as they have imbibed from their past culture a sense of guilt towards this and harbour a sense of continued apathy toward the latest techniques in medicine. In rural areas, where there is a natural indifference toward modern medicine, people do not readily accept those medical therapies which they believe are not suited to their traditional practices. While it is ignorance that dominates this viewpoint, it is equally true that they regard it as unethical to break away from their past habits and accepted opinion of their community. It is because of this that often they will accept the quacks as their sole saviors, rather than seek expert medical advice. However, the unorthodox, mostly from the urban areas, easily accept prenatal diagnosis and abortion of an affected fetus, in order to prevent the burden of a child with a handicap.

The greatest ethical problem in India at present is prenatal diagnosis of sex for social reasons and abortion of female fetuses. Such tests are commonly performed by obstetricians/radiologists in private practice in metropolitan areas. The samples of chorionic villi/amniotic fluid are sent to and analyzed by private laboratories. Some of these centers advertise openly in the newspapers. The exact number of such tests performed and the number of female fetuses aborted is not known. It is estimated that many thousands of cases of post-amniocentesis female feticide have occurred in the country between 1978-82 [17]. In Bombay, a survey of 50 obstetricians in private practice showed that 42 (84%) were carrying out amniocentesis for diagnosis of sex [19].

The reasons for favoring such selection are immediately apparent. Although the Constitution of India guarantees equal rights to both sexes, and the developmental plans have been drafted to remove social discrimination, the status of women remains low in society. In the rural areas, where 78% of the population lives, women are not recognized as equal partners, due to cultural and social bias. The expense incurred by the family for the marriage of their daughter is considered as an economic burden. Therefore, girls are raised in financial and physical neglect. The birth of a baby girl is greeted in many parts of the country with silence and even sorrow. The discrimination against women is obvious if one examines the sex ratio in India (Table 2.10.8). It is apparent that the number of males per 1,000 females has been rising since 1911. The only state in which the sex ratio is less than 1,000 is Kerala [13, 33], with a figure of 967. Most authors favor the higher mortality in females as the significant reason for the sex ratio being in favor of males. Under-enumeration of females may also be a factor, as in rural areas the birth of a girl may go unreported. Ghosh [7] has high-lighted how the female child is at a disadvantage as compared to a boy with regard to : (i) biological attributes such as

258

**Table 2.10.8.** Sex Ratio in India[1]

| Year (census) | Males per 1,000 females |
| --- | --- |
| 1901 | 1,029 |
| 1911 | 1,038 |
| 1921 | 1,047 |
| 1931 | 1,053 |
| 1941 | 1,058 |
| 1951 | 1,057 |
| 1961 | 1,063 |
| 1971 | 1,075 |
| 1981 | 1,071 |

[1] India, Ministry of Welfare, 1985, modified

weight and height, (ii) food intake, (iii) morbidity, (iv) access to health services, and (v) life expectancy. Moreover, literacy is 24.8% in females as compared with 46.1% in males; the school drop-out rate is significantly higher in girls [13].

Many more such examples in all spheres of life can be cited where women are discriminated against. Moreover, the presence of at least one male child is desired by all couples to: (i) continue the family lineage, and (ii) ensure security for the couple when they are old, there being no social security system for old age in India. It is not surprising, therefore, that families resort to sex selection with preference for the male.

The Government does not favor sex selection tests. Since 1983, it has forbidden government hospitals/institutions to carry out prenatal diagnosis of sex for social reasons. Since the scale at which the tests are being done in private clinics has increased recently, the Ministry of Health and Family Welfare, Government of India, convened a conference of medical specialists, administrators, voluntary organizations and legal experts to chart out a future course of action. The experts were unanimous on the following points: (i) that amniocentesis and other tests for sex selection should be prohibited and should be performed only for diagnosis of genetic disease in approved institutions, which are regulated for this purpose; (ii) that advertisement of these tests should be banned and made a penal offence; (iii) that there is a need to generate public opinion against these tests being misused for the determination of sex and female feticide (see Section 2.10.4.6 below).

## 2.10.2.3 Genetic Screening

For the next decade or so it is unlikely that India will have the resources necessary to mount large-scale, generalized, all-purpose screening programs for genetic disease. What is likely, and also feasible, is to recognize communities or populations which have a high risk for certain diseases [30], and to initiate screening programs for specific diseases among them (Table 2.10.9). For these reasons, no ethical problems exist in this area of service.

**Table 2.10.9.** Populations in India at High Risk for Genetic Disease

| Disorder | Population | Incidence (%) |
|---|---|---|
| Beta-thalassemia trait | Punjabis, Sindhis, Oriyas, Saraswati marwaris, Lohanas, Bhanusali | 6 |
| Hemoglobinopathies (excluding S) carrier | E in Bengalis & Assamese; D in Punjabis | 1–5 |
| Sickle cell trait | Tribal communities Mahar, Bhils, Palghar, Nilgiris, Koyadora | 5–20 |
| G-6-PD deficiency in males | Punjabis, Parsees<br>Bhunusalis, Mahars, Nilgiris tribals, Santhals, Koyadora | 5<br><br>3–15 |
| Neural tube defects | North India: Punjabis, Jats in Haryana and Rajasthan | 0.4–0.5 |

## 2.10.3 Consensus and Variation in Approaches to Ethical Problems in Medical Genetics in India and Comparison with Other Countries

**Professional and Personal Data**

The response rate in India (38%) was lower than in some other countries, possibly because there are few physicians engaged solely in the practice of genetics. Most continue to see patients with general pediatric or medical problems. Therefore, they may have felt diffident in filling out the questionnaire. However, those responding are truly representative of the physicians dealing with genetic disorders in India.

The personal characteristics of the Indian participants in the study were similar to those participating from other countries. However, the majority of the counselors were Hindus (81%), three (11.6%) were Christians (two Protestants and one Catholic), one was Moslem and one Sikh.

**Approaches to Ethical Problems**

*1. Confidentiality versus Duties to Third Parties.* In case 1 (false paternity) there was a strong consensus that mother's confidentiality should override disclosure of true paternity (96%). In all, 70% would tell the mother alone, without the husband present, and 26% would lie in order to protect the mother's secret. Cases of false paternity are very few in India, because women are less emancipated here than in the West. Hence the respondents would not have had clinical experience with this problem.

In case 2 (Huntington disease) and case 3 (hemophilia A) 48% and 67% respectively favored disclosing the diagnosis to the relatives even if the client refuses to permit such disclosure. In all, 33% and 63%, respectively, would disclose to the

260

relatives even if they did not ask for the information. A smaller number opted for this course in the case of Huntington disease, because this disorder is extremely uncommon in India. A larger number favored disclosure of hemophilia A, as the treatment with antihemophilic globulin is still very expensive and unaffordable by the majority of patients, so this would appear to be a disease with a significant burden.

*2. Full Disclosure of Sensitive Information.* No consensus emerged either on disclosing information regarding which parent is a balanced translocation carrier in Down syndrome or disclosure of information regarding XY karyotype in a female. Only 44% and 52% of the respondents opted to tell everything in Down syndrome and XY genotype cases respectively. Regarding an XO fetus, the largest number (54%) favored disclosing all the facts, but providing non-directive counseling.

*3. Reproductive Options for Male and Female Carriers of Tuberous Sclerosis.* No consensus was reached on any of the options. However, it should be pointed out that the incidence of tuberous sclerosis is much lower in India than in the West. I have seen only three cases in a genetic practice of 20 years in Delhi.

*4. Full Disclosure of Laboratory Results.* There was strong consensus (89%) in favor of disclosure of conflicting test results of prenatal diagnosis for a neural tube defect in case 6. Only 17 (63%), however, would not give directive advice in this situation.

In case 7 (interpretation of low maternal serum AFP), again, there was a strong consensus (92%) in favor of disclosing a new and controversial interpretation of the results; 13 (50%) would not give directive advice.

In case 8 (colleague disagreement about ambiguous or artifactual results) 56% would tell patients about the disagreement.

The lack of consensus about whether or not to give directive advice in these three cases might have resulted from the almost complete absence of litigation by patients for giving medical misinformation or for malpractice in India. Counseling tends to be more nondirective and incline towards full disclosure in countries where the risk of litigation is high.

*5. Indications for Prenatal Diagnosis.* There was no consensus on performing prenatal diagnosis for maternal anxiety without other indications; 41% would perform it and an additional 15% would offer a referral. The commonest first reason given was removal of anxiety (7, 26%). This low percentage is probably due to the paucity of prenatal diagnostic facilities, and the need, therefore, to carry out prenatal diagnosis only for patients who need it most.

There was only a moderate consensus (17, 63%) to grant the request for prenatal diagnosis of Down syndrome requested by parents who already have a Down syndrome child but are opposed to abortion (case 9).

In case 4 (prenatal diagnosis for sex selection unrelated to X-linked disease), ten (37%) would grant the request, four (15%) would refer, while 13 (48%) would refuse. There is a lack of consensus on this issue because most counselors recognize the social benefits of having a male child. Most counselors appreciate that ethically this is incorrect, but economic and social realities override moral objections.

261

*6. Prenatal Diagnosis in a Commercial Laboratory.* There was a strong consensus for prohibiting a commercial laboratory from operating without being associated with a medical genetics unit (25, 92%), and from doing prenatal diagnosis for sex selection (81%). The responses to this issue were highly distorted by the mushrooming of laboratories carrying out fetal sexing in the cities. Such laboratories are often ill-equipped and charge heavily for their services. Rightly, therefore, most counselors have a negative attitude towards commercial laboratories.

*7. Cases Giving the Most Ethical Conflict.* There was no consensus on this question. The case which gave the greatest conflict to the most respondents (6, 24%), was disclosure of false paternity, followed by prenatal diagnosis for sex selection (4, 16%).

These responses differ from those of many nations in the West, because, as explained earlier, Huntington disease, which gave conflict in other nations, is extremely uncommon in India. Therefore the issue of information to siblings of an HD patient does not figure prominently in the responses of the Indian counselors.

*8. Cases Giving the Least Ethical Conflict.* The cases which gave the least ethical conflict were (in order of priority): prenatal diagnosis for sex selection (9, 35%), prenatal diagnosis of Down syndrome in a couple who would not abort (5, 19%), and prenatal diagnosis for maternal anxiety (3, 12%). Interestingly, this list corresponds exactly to the cases chosen as giving the least ethical conflict in the majority of countries, although no consensus was reached in India.

*9. Genetic Screening.* There was moderate consensus that mass screening for alpha-1-antitrypsin deficiency of factory workers who will be exposed to dust should be mandatory (20, 74%). This is probably based on the reality in India that it is difficult to find employment, so that to be effective such a program would have to be mandatory.

On the question of who should have access to results of genetic screening for occupational susceptibility, there was a strong consensus, as in all other countries, that the worker should have access to such results (92%).

The questions regarding allowing the employer's worker's compensation insurer or the employer's health insurer access to results are probably irrelevant in India, as such insurances are uncommon.

*10. Goals of Genetic Counseling.* The responses to these questions were similar to those from other countries. However, there were differences in comparison to other countries in the adoption of alternative approaches in genetic counseling. Telling patients that decisions are theirs alone was considered always appropriate by the majority (15, 56%). In addition, 12 (46%) thought that it was always appropriate to support any decisions the patients make. Informing patients what others have done was considered sometimes appropriate by half (13, 50%) while it was considered to be always appropriate by only 27%. Informing patients what the counselor would do was considered always appropriate by 8 (31%) respondents, and was considered sometimes appropriate by 7 (27%). Advising patients what they ought to do was considered sometimes appropriate by 10 (40%), never appropriate by 6 (24%), and always appropriate by only 4 (16%).

For many of the illiterate patients who have little knowledge of science or genetics, the counselors tended to be more directive. Also, the virtual absence of litigation encourages more directive counseling.

**Is There a Dominant Approach to Resolve Ethical Problems in Medical Genetics in India?**

Barring a few questions on which there was moderate to strong consensus (false paternity, prenatal diagnosis for those opposed to abortion, screening of factory workers and access to results of screening) no dominant approach could be discerned in the responses to most of the ethical questions in India. This lack of consensus probably results from the diversity in religions, language and ethnicity that exists in India.

First, religion has a very strong influence on ethical beliefs. However, people belonging to many different religions live in India [9], including Hindus 82.7%, Muslims 11.02%, Christians 2.6%, Sikhs 1.9% and others 1.6%. This diversity of religions is reflected among the counselors who answered the questionnaire and would contribute to a lack of consensus.

Second, Hinduism, unlike other religions, has no fixed dogmas and beliefs. Its contents have altered from age to age, and from community to community. It has steadily absorbed the customs and ideas of people of different races and cultures who have been pouring into India from the dawn of history [21, 26]. For this reason, there is a considerable diversity of perceptions regarding the contents of Hinduism. This is an important factor in the lack of consensus.

Third, Hinduism extols the realization of self, meaning that an individual can achieve personal salvation, but cannot do so for others. This encourages an individualistic approach and leads to a lack of consensus.

Last, some of the cases on which the questions are based represent disorders which are rare in the Indian population. Therefore the practical implications of the situations represented by these cases are less obvious to geneticists in India. This could be a cause of lack of consensus.

## 2.10.4 Cultural Context of Medical Genetics in India

The primary sources upon which Indian medical geneticists generally draw to resolve ethical problems are the age-old socio-cultural traditions and religious beliefs of Hinduism, since not only is it the religion of the majority of people (83%), but also many other religions like Buddhism, Jainism, and Sikhism (but not Islam and Christianity) are derived from it [27].

The earliest books on Hinduism are the four *Vedas*, or books of knowledge (*Rig*, *Yajur*, *Sama*, and *Atharva*). These were written between 2,500 BC and 600 BC by unknown Aryan scholars. The *Rigveda*, the oldest and the most important, describes a law for the maintenance of order in the universe (*rta*), and one which concerns the code of conduct for human society and ethical concepts such as kindness, charity, etc.

263

The second period of development is known as the epic or *puranic* period between 600 BC and 200 AD, during which *Upanishads* were written, as well as the two great epics of Hinduism – the *Mahabharata* and the *Ramayana*. These epics are a compendium of aphorisms and parables designed to bring ethical and philosophical precepts to the common people in a form and language they could understand. A chapter in the story of the *Mahabharata* is the *Bhagavad Gita*, considered the greatest piece of Hindu religious writing, whose central theme is that one should perform one's duty regardless of consequences and without consideration of reward. Later the dissenting schools of Jainism and Buddhism arose. After this period, Islam and Christianity were introduced into India.

These religious teachings, and the rule by numerous monarchs extending over centuries, have led to authority, divine or human, shaping the actions of the Hindus. This makes the common man expect directive counseling, which is thus more readily accepted than in other countries.

Even today an orthodox Indian seeks to resolve ethical dilemmas in terms of traditional beliefs. The doctrine of karma forms part of ethical consciousness and serves as the mainspring of ethical decision making. According to it, every deed consciously undertaken produces an appropriate good or bad result. This may ensue in the present life or in the next life. Thus, reincarnation is a logical corollary, for everyone has to be reborn in an unbroken series and experience the results of the deeds done in previous births. An orthodox Indian, therefore, feels strongly motivated by moral impulse, and does not want to have a miserable rebirth. A considerable part of the orthodox Indian populace entertains such a view, which has a powerful impact on moral consciousness. It is in terms of such a belief that an Indian would refuse to accept modern medical advances, more especially those in the field of reproduction. Thus family planning methods, amniocentesis and chorionic villi aspiration are not readily accepted. Therefore, having a large family is the rule, rather than the exception, and the birth of an abnormal child is accepted as the "will of God", or as a result of one's past deeds (*karma*). On the other hand, the urbanized Indian, with a Western-oriented education, feels the economic pressure, and displays an amazing capacity to accept technology which would either improve economic status, or reduce the economic burden. To this end, abortion of an abnormal fetus is readily accepted.

### Code of Medical Ethics

The Medical Council of India requires that every new graduate be given a copy of the code at the time of registration, and read and agree to abide by it. The code [23] declares "I pledge to consecrate my life to the service of humanity...... I will not use my medical knowledge contrary to the laws of humanity. I will maintain the utmost respect for human life from the time of conception......" This is a 12-page document which covers character and responsibility of the physician, advertising, professional services, etc; duties of physicians to their patients, to the profession at large, to each other, to the public; and lists the situations which would require disciplinary action.

In all medical schools, the medical student on graduation has to pledge the Hippocratic oath. At the All India Institute of Medical Sciences the following oath composed by Charak, a famous physician in ancient India, has to be taken : "Not for self, not for the fulfillment of any worldly material desire or gain, but solely for the good of suffering humanity, I will treat my patient and excel all".

There are currently no compulsory lectures on medical ethics in any of the schools. About ten lectures in humanities are delivered to the students at AIIMS, and some of these cover the subject of ethics. The younger colleagues learn the ethics of medical practice from the example of their seniors.

## 2.10.4.1 Sources of Challenge and Support for Medical Genetics

Medical genetics in India was started at the initiative of individual scientists and physicians within the departments of anatomy and pediatrics. The Government of India has given support through its research funding agencies, such as the Indian Council of Medical Research and Department of Science and Technology. The clinicians themselves have lent little support, due to the rarity of these disorders in comparison with communicable diseases and nutritional deficiencies, which are such common causes of morbidity and mortality. The parents' groups are not sufficiently organized to exert moral pressure on the Government to establish genetic services. Possibly the patient/parent groups should pressurize the politicians to use their influence to establish more genetic units.

## 2.10.4.2 Major Controversies

The major controversy at present is sex selection and abortion of female fetuses. See 2.10.2.2 above and 2.10.4.6 below.

## 2.10.4.3 National Expenditures for Medical Genetics

It is difficult to quantify this, but if one were to consider the amount spent purely on medical genetics it would be infinitesimally small. For reasons explained earlier, the national effort is still focussed on control of communicable diseases, immunizing all children by 1990, augmenting the nutrition of mothers and children, improving sanitation and providing clean drinking water to all the people. The Planning Commission, while formulating the VII Development Health Plan, has given consideration for the first time to non-communicable diseases such as cancer and diabetes mellitus, although the genetic disorders are not considered [14].

## 2.10.4.4 Abortion Law in India and its Application

Before 1971, abortion was a criminal offence with liability for imprisonment for three years, unless done in good faith to save the life of the mother. If carried out after 20 weeks of gestation, punishment was imprisonment for seven years (Sec-

265

tion 312). Any act done with the intention of preventing a child from being born alive, or causing it to die after birth, unless it was done to save the life of the mother, was punishable by imprisonment up to life (Section 315).

Despite such stringent legal provisions, a large number of abortions were carried out. The single state of Maharashtra was responsible for about 0.5 million abortions every year, and on the national level, there were probably around 5 million abortions every year. Considering this social reality, the Government introduced the Medical Termination of Pregnancy (MTP) Act, 1971. This act was perceived as a health care reform to save millions of women who used to take recourse to clandestine abortions by ill-qualified doctors or quacks, in unhygienic conditions. The Government did not introduce it as a means of fertility regulation.

The MTP Act lays down certain conditions under which an abortion can legally be conducted. Section 3 authorizes a registered medical practitioner to terminate a pregnancy which does not exceed 12 weeks, with the woman's consent, or, if she is below 18 years of age or a lunatic, with the written consent of her guardian. If the pregnancy exceeds 12 weeks but not 20 weeks, it requires the agreement of two registered medical practitioners. Their opinion favoring termination must be based on the following conditions:

(i) that continuance of the pregnancy would involve a risk to the life of the pregnant woman or grave injury to her physical or mental health, or, (ii) that the child when born may suffer from physical or mental abnormalities. When a pregnancy is caused by rape, the presumption that the doctor would have is that the pregnancy constitutes a grave injury to the woman's mental health. If a married woman pleads for the termination of pregnancy on the ground that it has occurred as a result of failure of any device or method used by her or her husband for the purpose of limiting the number of children, the doctor has the discretion to terminate it on the ground that unwanted pregnancy may be presumed to constitute a grave injury to the mental health of the woman. Section 4 provides that pregnancies can only be terminated at government run hospitals or at places approved by the Government. The rules also stipulate that abortions must be performed under hygienic conditions. Regulations have also been framed for the maintenance of proper records and secrecy. Under the MTP Act, all abortions require the consent of the woman, and all abortions after 20 weeks are illegal.

(iii) The law clearly permitted abortion up to 20 weeks of gestation if the fetus was considered to have a severe genetic/handicapping disorder. There is no social or religious conflict on this issue among the Hindus and all the religious groups derived from Hinduism. Among the Christians, the conflicts are similar to those in the West, and will not be discussed further.

The Muslim law, however, considers a fetus alive and growing from the moment of fusion between sperm and ovum, and interference with pregnancy at any stage of gestation would be a crime [6]. Al Imam Elmatwalli stated that "abortion is an offence which is punishable by payment of a money ransom (*diah*)," which is the ransom paid for killing an adult. The *Malakia* written by Imam Malik, a famous scholar in Islamic religion, stated clearly that "it is not permissible to interfere from the moment of fusion between sperm and ovum in the uterus [1]." According to these views, Islam recognizes the right to life of a fetus and also grants it the status of a person from the moment of fertilization. However, Islamic Law does justify abortion in extreme circumstances, such as the survival of the mother. Al Shaikh Shaltut has opined in *Al Fatawa* (judicial opinions) that the general principles of *Shariah* (religious law) opt for lesser harm if one is presented with a difficult choice between saving the mother or losing the fetus. The fetus could be sacrificed, as the mother is the source and origin (*Asl*) and is a full-fledged life, in contradistinction to a being which is still in the womb and not yet bestowed with full rights and obligations [2]. However, a few Islamic countries have liberalized their abortion laws. Tunisia legalized abortion in 1973 to reduce population growth. Kuwait amended its law in 1982, to permit abortion where either grievous bodily harm to the mother is imminent, or if the baby to be born is likely to suffer such incurable brain damage as would result in severe mental retardation. Turkey also has amended the law in 1983 to allow abortion on medical therapeutic grounds. As regards family planning and the use of contraceptives, the Koran does not appear to be dogmatic, and hence most Muslims have access to various methods of family planning.

## 2.10.4.5 Studies of Effectiveness and Acceptability of Genetic Services

There have been no published studies on evaluation of effectiveness of genetic services and their acceptability to patients. A multicentric study funded by the Indian Council of Medical Research is underway, but the results are not yet available. Generally, the parents accept genetic counseling in good faith and are very keen on prenatal diagnosis of genetic disease in order to prevent the birth of an abnormal child. This is due to the economic and social burden associated with the rearing of a child with a handicap, in a country with limited facilities and resources for rehabilitation.

## 2.10.4.6 Need for New Laws to Protect Against Possible Abuses

The Government of India is actively considering legislation against prenatal diagnosis of sex for purposes of female feticide, because this disturbing trend needs to be curbed. The Government has constituted a small committee with the following mandate: (i) to draw up the details of comprehensive legislation; (ii) to suggest inbuilt mechanisms for an infrastructure for ensuring proper implementation of the proposed legislation; (iii) to propose measures for generating public opinion against these tests, either as apart of the legislation itself or otherwise.

It is hoped that suitable central legislation will be introduced in the near future. The state of Maharashtra has already passed a bill (No. VIII of 1988) to provide for regulation of prenatal diagnostic tests for diagnosis of genetic disease, and for preventing their misuse for prenatal sex determination leading to female feticide. Most individuals in a democracy are opposed to law interfering in their lives. Yet when the conduct of the individual becomes so selfish and partisan that it violates moral and ethical principles, it needs to be curbed by introducing proper legislation. A group of leading doctors, lawyers, representatives of women's and other social organizations concurred in suggesting that the time has come to reinforce the change in attitude on the part of society with proper legislation. However, guiding the behavior of individuals in certain moral directions, contrary to the interest of the individual, has always been a difficult task. It is admitted that mere passage of legislation will not stop these unethical and morally indefensible practices. However, there is a need for the Government to make its commitment clear that discrimination against women, beginning before birth, will not be tolerated. The facilities for in vitro fertilization are available in only three to four centers; so far it has been available for very selected couples. There have been no cases of commercial surrogate motherhood or legal contracts for surrogacy. When these techniques are more freely available, then ethical problems may crop up.

## 2.10.5  Ethical Issues and Future Trends in Medical Genetics

The *prenatal diagnosis of sex* and female feticide is the most important ethical issue, not only at the present time, but it will remain so for the next decade or so. The issue is a deeper one, as it involves the social status of women in society. No amount of legislation will be able to eradicate such evil practices. Article 14 of the Constitution of India already provides for equal rights for men and women. Article 15 states that there shall not be any discrimination against any citizen on grounds of religion, race, caste, sex, or place of birth. Over the years, further legislation has been enacted to ensure equality to women. The law provides for equal rights of girls to the estates and income of their parents, which was not the case earlier. It has also been decreed that the offer and acceptance of dowry is a penal offence. Such laws have played some part in improving the status of women. I expect that more and more laws will be introduced to bring about this change. Unless the status of women improves by modification of the attitude and behavior of the people, this issue will continue to confront the public conscience. However, experience suggests that such changes are wrought very slowly in a democracy.

The *chorionic villi aspiration technique* is more readily accepted by the people than amniocentesis, because it is carried out at a much earlier stage of gestation, and the induction of abortion, if it becomes necessary, is much easier and has fewer risks. The ethical issues raised by this technique are similar to those of amniocentesis.

The *DNA analytic techniques* are not yet available as a service for the benefit of patients. However, their diagnostic precision will diminish the ethical dilemmas, because all parents fervently wish to have a normal child and to avoid adding an abnormal child to the family, for economic and social reasons. Fortunately, because of strong family ties, most parents remain deeply attached to such children. However, as the economic realities become harsher, the state may be required to look after these children to a much greater extent than is being done now. This will raise further ethical issues, and may help to usher in programs of newborn screening.

The issue of *surrogate motherhood* is beginning to be discussed in popular magazines. These issues will raise hot ethical debates in the coming decade.

A peep into the future suggests that genetic disorders will assume greater importance in terms of their contribution to morbidity and mortality. The Government is likely to invest more in facilities for diagnosis and management of genetic disorders. Will Indian society be able to cope with the ethical problems that emerge due to the new technologies of medical genetics? Or will we become giants in technology and dwarves in ethics? Although much depends upon the economic front, the strength and vitality of the Indian tradition is sufficiently strong to manage successfully the ethical issues that arise in the future and find appropriate solutions. Sri Aurobindo [3] says that the Hindu scriptures contain two types of Truths – one temporary and perishable, belonging to the period in which they were produced; the other eternal and imperishable, and applicable in all ages. These living truths have been constantly renewed and reshaped by the experiences of a developing nation. It is the latter which have sustained India in the past, to survive through the ravages of numerous invasions and maintain a vibrant society following democratic principles.

# References

1. Al Matwalli Al-Imam [1951] Elbabya fe Sharrh Altohfa (Text book on Islamic law). Vol 2, 2nd ed, Egypt. p 379
2. Al-Shaikh Shaltut [1982] cited by Ghanem I: Abortion, gestation and viability. In: Probsthain A (ed) Islamic medical jurisprudence. London, pp 60–61
3. Aurobindo S [1976] Essays on the Gita. 10th ed. Sri Aurobindo Ashram, Pondicherry
4. Chaterjee JB [1966] Hemoglobinopathies, glucose-6-phosphate dehydrogenase and allied problems in the Indian subcontinent. Bull WHO 35: 837–856
5. Desai MP, Colaco MP, Ajgaonkar AR, Mahadik CV, Vas FE, Rege C, Shirodkar VV, Bandivdekar A, and Sheth AR [1987] Neonatal screening for congenital hypothyroidism in a developing country – problems and strategies. Indian J Pediatr 54: 571–581
6. Elzouki AY [1986] Cytogenetic analysis of Down syndrome in Arab children and the problem of genetic counseling in the Islamic world. In: Neiermeyer H, Hicks E (eds) Bishop Bekkers Workshop on Genetics of Mental Retardation, Netherlands, D Reidel Publishing Co. Utrecht, Netherlands (in press)
7. Ghosh S [1986] Discrimination begins at birth. Indian Pediatr 23: 9–15
8. Holla M [1985] Vital statistics system, a major source of information on infant and child mortality. Indian J Pediatr 52: 115–126
9. India, Central Bureau of Health Intelligence, Directorate General of Health Services [1986] Health Information of India. Nirman Bhavan, New Delhi
10. India, Ministry of Health and Family Welfare [1983] Family Welfare Programme in India. Year-book 1982-83. Department of Family Welfare, New Delhi, 1983, p 194
11. India, Ministry of Health and Family Welfare [1985] Family Welfare Programme in India. Year-book 1984-85. Department of Family Welfare, New Delhi
12. India, Ministry of Health and Family Welfare [1987] Annual Report, 1986–87, p 123
13. India, Ministry of Welfare [1985] Child in India – A statistical profile. Ministry of Welfare, New Delhi
14. India, Planning Commission [1984] Report of the Steering Group on Health and Family Welfare Programmes for Seventh Five Year Plan
15. India, Registrar-General [1987] Infant mortality rates, India 1985. Indian J Pediatr 53: 459
16. Indian Council of Medical Research, Director-General [1986] Annual Report 1985–86, pp 46, 113

17. Joseph DT [1986] Amniocentesis and fetal feticide in Bombay – a report presented to Government of Maharashtra.
18. Kochupillai N, Jaysuryan N, Godbole MM, Pandav CS [1984] Benefit and cost of application of radioimmunoassay in tuberculosis and iodine deficiency disorders: two major health problems of developing countries. In: Albertini A, Ekins EP, Galen RS (eds) Cost-Benefit and predictive value of radioimmunoassays. Elsevier Science Publishers, p 203
19. Kulkarni S [1986] Prenatal sex determination tests and female feticide in Bombay. Report commissioned by Secretary, Department of Public Health and Family Welfare, Maharashtra
20. Kumar V, Datta N [1988] Community based studies on infant mortality in Haryana – methodological issues relating to reporting and causation. In: Jain AK, Visaria P (eds) Infant mortality in India – differentials and determinants. Sage Publications, New Delhi and London, pp 185–202
21. Kuppuswamy B [1977] Dharma and society. MacMillan Co. of India, New Delhi
22. Malhotra KC [1978] Medicogenetic problems among Indian tribes, an overview. In: Verma IC (ed) Medical genetics in India Vol.2. Auroma Enterprises, Pondicherry pp 81–88
23. Medical Council of India [1956] Code of medical ethics, MCI, Aiwan-e-Ghalib Marg, Kotla Road, New Delhi-110002
24. Menon PSN, Mathews AR, Verma IC [1986] Screening for neonatal hypothyroidism in AIIMS. In: Verma IC (ed) Genetic research in India. Sagar Printers & Publishers, New Delhi, p 171
25. Pandav CS, Kochupillai N [1985] Organisation and implementation of neonatal hypothyroid screening programme in India – a primary health care approach. Indian J Pediatr 52: 223–229
26. Radhakrishnan S [1960] The Hindu view of life. Unwin Books, London
27. Singh B [1984] Hindu ethics, an exposition of the concept of good. Arnold Heinemann, New Delhi
28. Sukumaran PK [1978] Hemoglobinopathies in scheduled castes and tribes of India. In: Verma IC (ed) Medical genetics in India. Vol.2. Auroma Enterprises, Pondicherry, pp 81–88
29. Verma IC (ed) [1980] Directory of Human Genetic Services in India. 1st ed, All India Institute of Medical Sciences, New Delhi
30. Verma IC (1986a) Genetic counseling and control of genetic disease in India. In: Verma IC (ed) Genetic research in India. Sagar Printers and Publishers, New Delhi, pp 21–37
31. Verma IC (1986b) Genetic disorders need more attention in developing countries. World Health Forum 7: 69–70
32. Verma IC [1987] A new perspective for congenital malformations. In: Verma IC (ed) Genetic research in India. Sagar Printers and Publishers, New Delhi, pp 174–187
33. Visaria PM [1961] The sex ratio of the population of India. Census of India.

# 2.11 Ethics and Medical Genetics in Israel

J. M. Chemke and A. Steinberg

## 2.11.1.1 The Scope of Medical Genetics in Israel

In Israel 99.7% of live births occur in hospitals. There are no available data on the incidence of genetic diseases. A monitoring system for congenital malformations exists in four hospitals, accounting for approximately 18,000 births per year. Israel is a member of the International Clearinghouse for Birth Defects Monitoring Systems. There is no reliable information on the mortality rate from genetic diseases, except for the mortality rate from congenital anomalies, as reported on death certificates to the Ministry of Health (Table 2.11.1). The reason is the lack of centralized statistical information, which is partially due to the fact that medical genetics was not recognized as a bona fide medical specialty. Table 2.11.1 demonstrates that the number of live births has remained quite stable for the past ten years (1975–1984) and the mortality rate from congenital anomalies has slightly decreased, mainly as a result of earlier and better diagnosis and improved treatment.

## 2.11.1.2 Organization of Clinical Genetic Services in Israel

Medical genetic services in Israel are organized in seven comprehensive departments, localised in teaching hospitals, affiliated with medical schools. All departments have laboratory facilities for tissue cultures and cytogenetics. Biochemical tests are usually carried out in specialized laboratories. All medical genetics de-

Table 2.11.1. Mortality Rate from Congenital Anomalies (per 1,000 Livebirths) [2]

| Year | Total No. Livebirths | Mortality Rate From Congenital Anomalies (per 1,000 Livebirths) |
|------|----------------------|----------------------------------------------------------------|
| 1975 | 95,628 | 4.3 |
| 1976 | 98,763 | |
| 1977 | 95,315 | |
| 1978 | 92,602 | 4.1 |
| 1979 | 93,710 | 4.3 |
| 1980 | 94,321 | 3.1 |
| 1981 | 93,308 | 2.5 |
| 1982 | 96,695 | 2.8 |
| 1983 | 93,724 | 3.2 |
| 1984 | 94,478 | |

partments provide genetic counseling, and most of them coordinate the multidisciplinary management of complex syndromes. Genetic counseling is also given prior to every prenatal diagnostic procedure for genetic conditions. Cytogenetic studies are also done on newborns and stillbirths with congenital anomalies, when a history of recurrent spontaneous abortions is obtained, and in most cases of idiopathic mental retardation (particularly in males, to investigate the "fragile X syndrome"). There are no private institutions or private laboratories for medical genetic services or genetic counseling.

Israeli medical geneticists are organized in two professional and scientific organizations: The Israel Society for Medical Genetics, and the Society for Human Genetics in Israel. Medical genetics has recently been recognized as a specific medical profession by the Israeli Medical Association or the Ministry of Health. Thus, it will be possible to establish training programs for M. D.'s or Ph. D.'s wishing to do a post-doctoral fellowship in medical genetics. All medical geneticists in Israel were trained abroad, mostly in the United States.

**Profile of Israeli Medical Geneticists**
There are 17 medical geneticists in Israel. Table 2.11.2 compares their characteristics to their colleagues in the world.

Israeli geneticists thus appear as an experienced, stable and responsible group as judged by age, marital status, years in the field, number of patients seen and hours spent in the field. All are Jews but most are non-observant and probably have no adequate background in the study of Jewish law (Halachah). Thus no specific Jewish philosophy and attitude came into play in their responses to the questionnaire. Their educational background is secular-Western, and the basic political attitude is liberal. It may be assumed that none of them had any formal education in philosophy, ethics, law or religion. Since no formal training programs exist in

**Table 2.11.2.** Comparison of Professional and Personal Data Between Israel Geneticists and Others

A. Professional Data

|  | Degree (%) | | | Median years in genetics | Median pts/wk | Median hrs/wk in genetics |
|---|---|---|---|---|---|---|
|  | M. D. | Ph. D. | Other |  |  |  |
| Israel | 66 | 20 | 13 | 15 (range 6–24) | 12 (range 3–18) | 40 (range 20–58) |
| World | 81 | 16 | 3 | 14 | 5 | 45 |

B. Personal Data

|  | Median age (yrs) | Sex M:F | Married (%) | Jewish religion | Politics (%) | | Both Equally |
|---|---|---|---|---|---|---|---|
|  |  |  |  |  | Liberal | Conservative |  |
| Israel | 47 | 2:3 | 86 | 100 | 66 | 6 | 28 |
| World | 45 | 3:2 | 82 | 17 | 35 | 16 | 49 |

medical genetics in Israel, there is no wide and continuous exposure to discussions regarding the ethical issues involved in medical genetics.

**Diseases, Diagnoses and Services**

During the last 15 years, medical genetics in Israel underwent constant development and progress. The National Program for the Detection and Prevention of Birth Defects has been operating since 1980. It was established by the Ministry of Health, and includes prenatal diagnosis and screening of newborns and high-risk populations [1]. Screening procedures for genetic diseases include PKU and hypothyroidism performed on every newborn (Guthrie test and T4/TSH). It is understood that newborns are also screened for congenital malformations while in the nurseries. PKU and thyroid hormones are analyzed in one central laboratory at the Sheba Medical Center, Tel Hashomer. Individuals of Jewish-Ashkenazi origin, and lately also of Moroccan origin, are offered screening for the carrier state of Tay-Sachs disease. This is also done in one central laboratory at the Genetics Institute, Sheba Medical Center.

## 2.11.1.3 *Prenatal Diagnosis*

Prenatal diagnosis of genetic disorders under this National Program is carried out according to established indications: Maternal age, previous chromosomal abnormality in an offspring or Down syndrome in the family, familial translocations, parental mosaicism, metabolic disorders, fetal sexing for X-linked recessive diseases and alpha-fetoprotein for neural tube defects and other malformations. Chromosomal analysis of fetal cells for advanced maternal age is currently recommended from age 35 years, and is subsidized by the government, starting at 37 years. Approximately 3000 prenatal tests are performed annually. As mentioned above, genetic counseling is given prior to every prenatal diagnostic procedure performed for genetic reasons.

The most common reasons for refusing amniocentesis when recommended by the geneticist are religious objections and maternal anxiety; in about 10% fetal demise is detected on ultrasound prior to the procedure, and in about 12% the test is not performed because of objections by the husband, although the husband has no legal standing in regard to an amniocentesis procedure on his wife.

In recent years chorionic villus sampling (CVS) has become increasingly popular; however, only a small proportion of eligible women prefer CVS to amniocentesis. The reason is usually fear of the higher risk of abortion following CVS.

Maternal serum alpha-fetoprotein (MSAFP) is offered in three genetic centers, but additional centers are about to join the MSAFP program: the Genetic Institute, Ichilov Hospital, Tel-Aviv; the Department of Human Genetics, Hadassah Medical Center, Jerusalem; and the Genetics Institute, Rothschild Hospital, Haifa. These institutions have the set-up and facilities to identify and follow abnormal results (low or elevated MSAFP). Glycogenoses are investigated in the Department of Pediatrics B, Soroka Medical Center, Beer-Sheva. Lysosomal diseases, mucopolysaccharidoses and mucolipidoses are studied at the Department of Human Genetics, Hadassah Medical Center, Jerusalem. The latter is also actively involved in the investigation of DNA polymorphism in cystic fibrosis (CF). This center performs prenatal diagnosis for CF in collaboration with the Clinical Genetics Unit, Kaplan Hospital, Rehovot. The latter coordinates prenatal diagnosis of CF for Israel, including second trimester analysis of amniotic fluid microvillar enzymes (performed at the Laboratory of Biochemistry, Ichilov Hospital, Tel-Aviv). All genetic centers have laboratory facilities for chromosomal analysis from various tissues, tissue culture facilities and amniotic fluid alpha-fetoprotein. Fetal blood sampling under ultrasonographic guidance is carried out in several hospitals, all subject to certification by the Ministry of Health. Fetoscopy is carried out primarily at the Hadassah Medical Center, Jerusalem.

## 2.11.1.4 Cost/Benefit of Early Diagnosis and Genetic Counseling

The national share of health expenditure as related to the gross national product (GNP) has increased in the ten years between 1975/76 and 1983/84 from 6.0% to 7.1% (Table 2.11.3). It is interesting to note, however, that the proportion of funds allocated for preventive medicine has declined in these years, from 1.0% to 0.7% (Table 2.11.3).

A cost/benefit analysis of prenatal diagnosis and the early detection of genetic disease, within the frame of the National Program, is available for the fiscal year 1985/86 [1]. It was carried out by the Ministry of Health and is based on the estimated costs of hospitalization days and/or institutionalization. The overall cost of the program was $303,000. This was divided in the following way: $225,000 was spent on prenatal diagnosis; $30,000 on Tay-Sachs carrier screening; $24,000 on congenital hypothyroidism; $24,000 on PKU. It should be noted that 10–15% of the actual cost was covered by the various institutions. Based on abnormal findings in the fetuses, 87 pregnancies were interrupted, adding a cost of $20,000. Thus, the total cost of the program for the detection and prevention of birth defects for the fiscal year 1985/86 was approximately $370,000.

The benefit of the program was calculated based on the expected cost of treatment of each case. Among the interrupted pregnancies there were 37 cases of

**Table 2.11.3.** National Expenditures on Health [2]

| Year | % of GNP | Public Clinics & Preventive Medicine (%) |
| --- | --- | --- |
| 1975/76 | 6.0 | 1.0 |
| 1976/77 | 6.5 | 1.0 |
| 1977/78 | 6.9 | 1.0 |
| 1978/79 | 7.5 | 0.9 |
| 1979/80 | 7.6 | 0.8 |
| 1980/81 | 7.1 | 1.0 |
| 1981/82 | 7.3 | 0.8 |
| 1982/83 | 7.3 | 0.7 |
| 1983/84 | 7.1 | – |

Down syndrome. The calculated cost of their management was almost $5,000,000. There were 12 cases of other chromosomal abnormalities. Thirteen pregnancies were interrupted for abnormal sex chromosomes. Since all these need medical and psychological treatment and have a normal life expectancy, their cost was estimated at approximately $400,000.

Among the 9,000 couples screened for Tay-Sachs, 15 double heterozygotes were detected. Six pregnancies were interrupted because of a fetus affected with Tay-Sachs. If they had survived for two to three years and spent approximately 50% of that time in the hospital, the cost would have been more than $300,000.

Four pregnancies were interrupted because of neural tube defects. Two of them were anencephalics, and two cases had meningomyelocele. If the latter had been born, they would have been handicapped for life and would have needed complicated treatments by several medical disciplines. The estimated amount saved was $500,000.

Five pregnancies were interrupted because of beta-thalassemia. If these fetuses had been born and had lived for an average of 20 years, they would have required ongoing medical treatment. The estimated amount saved was $1,000,000. The same applies for two pregnancies interrupted because of hemophilia.

There were five interruptions of pregnancies with fetuses affected with cystic fibrosis and five with other inborn errors of metabolism. If their average life expectancy was 15 years, requiring a daily supply of medications and special food, physiotherapy and medical treatment, the amount saved was approximately $600,000.

Screening for PKU and hypothyroidism was carried out on 96,000 newborns (95% of live births). Hypothyroidism was suspected in 44 infants, and in 32 of them the diagnosis was confirmed. The cost of lifelong treatment was close to 1/1,000 of the cost of keeping the patient institutionalized if left untreated. There were six cases of PKU, and for them, also, the cost of treatment during six years was less than 1/1,000 of the cost of institutionalization.

As mentioned above, the estimated cost of the program was $370,000. If the program had not existed and none of the pregnancies had been interrupted, the medical and other expenses for all the affected individuals would have been around $20,000,000. Therefore, it is estimated that for each $1 spent, $55 were saved.

## 2.11.1.5 Abortion

Interruptions of pregnancies are allowed according to the law passed by the Knesset (Israeli Parliament), as follows:

1. The woman is under the legal age of marriage, or over 40 years of age;
2. The pregnancy is the result of relations prohibited by the criminal law, incestuous relations, premarital or extramarital relations;
3. The fetus is likely to have a physical or mental defect;
4. Continuation of the pregnancy is likely to endanger the woman's life or health, either physical or mental.
5. Familial or social circumstances.

In 1980, the Knesset amended this law by abolishing paragraph 5. Purely familial or socioeconomic problems are no longer legally accepted causes for interruption of pregnancy. There is also a requirement for establishment of an "abortion committee" in each hospital that is certified to grant abortion requests. These committees are composed of two physicians, one of them a gynecologist, and a social worker.

Table 2.11.4 presents the number of interruptions of pregnancies as reported by hospitals.

As can be seen, the total number of pregnancies interrupted actually increased in 1984. The majority of previous "socioeconomic causes" appear to have been subsumed under indications such as "danger of mental harm to the woman" or "danger of physical or mental defect in the fetus." The ratio of abortions to live births is presented in Table 2.11.5, which demonstrates an increase in this ratio in 1984.

**Table 2.11.4.** Interruption of Pregnancies in Hospitals, by Articles of Law [2]

| Year* | Family/ Social** | Danger to Woman | Fetal Indications | Prohibited Relations | Woman's Age | Total |
|---|---|---|---|---|---|---|
| 1979 | 6,331 | 1,299 | 2,165 | 4,465 | 1,665 | 15,925 |
| 1980 | 647 | 5,157 | 2,118 | 5,005 | 1,781 | 14,708 |
| 1982 | - | 5,796 | 2,626 | 6,632 | 1,775 | 16,829 |
| 1983 | - | 5,062 | 2,377 | 6,661 | 1,493 | 15,593 |
| 1984 | - | 6,199 | 2,937 | 7,851 | 1,961 | 18,948 |

*no data for 1981.
**abolished by the Knesset in February, 1980.

**Table 2.11.5.** Ratio of Abortions/livebirths

| Year | No. of Livebirths | Total No. Abortions | Ratio |
|---|---|---|---|
| 1979 | 93,710 | 15,925 | 0.169 |
| 1980 | 94,321 | 14,708 | 0.156 |
| 1982 | 96,695 | 16,829 | 0.174 |
| 1983 | 93,724 | 15,593 | 0.166 |
| 1984 | 94,478 | 18,948 | 0.200 |

**Table 2.11.6.** Ratio of Abortions for Fetal Indications/Total Abortions

| Year | Total Abortions | Abortions for Fetal Indications | Ratio |
|---|---|---|---|
| 1979 | 15,925 | 2,165 | 0.14 |
| 1980 | 14,708 | 2,118 | 0.15 |
| 1982 | 16,829 | 2,626 | 0.16 |
| 1983 | 15,593 | 2,377 | 0.15 |
| 1984 | 18,948 | 2,937 | 0.15 |

Table 2.11.6 presents the ratio of abortions carried out for "physical or mental defects in the fetus" to the total number of abortions. It was interesting to verify whether there had been an increase in the ratio with the increasing awareness of prenatal diagnosis. As can be seen, the ratio has remained approximately the same since 1979. Thus, the increased rate of abortions is primarily due to maternal indications.

## 2.11.2 Ethical Problems

See 2.11.3 below.

## 2.11.3 Consensus and Variation in Israel

There was a strong consensus for non-directive counseling in borderline disorders such as XO or XYY. However, 20% would provide optimistically weighted information or advice about XYY as opposed to 7% for XO. These results are similar to approaches in other nations, with a somewhat larger minority in the XYY case. Perhaps the particular demographic situation of the Jews in the world at large, and in Israel specifically, has some bearing on optimism about XYY (see section 2.11.4). There were no significant differences in the counseling of male and female carriers of tuberous sclerosis (TS). There was a strong consensus for non-directive counseling about most reproductive options. There was no consensus, however, for presenting vasectomy, in the case of the male carrier, and surrogate motherhood, in the case of the female carrier. The former option is not well accepted socially in Israel and is definitely wrong according to Jewish law; the latter is not yet available or practical in Israel, and has marked legal and Halachic difficulties. A. I. D. for the male carrier and tubal ligation for the female carrier had only moderate consensus, perhaps because these are opposed to Halachah and are therefore seen as problematic in Israeli society (see section 2.11.4).

**Prenatal Diagnosis**
There was a strong consensus against prenatal diagnosis for sex selection unrelated to X-linked diseases. The moral considerations included the following: a) opposition to the abortion of a normal fetus or viewing sex selection as morally unacceptable; and b) the need for wise utilization of scarce resources, since being of the unwanted sex is not a medical condition that merits the limited time and facilities of genetic programs. Certain religious and ethnic groups have created a social environment in Israel that is against abortion. This, together with the demographic situation (see section 2.11.4), contributed to a consensus against use of abortion for sex selection.

There was a strong consensus for granting requests for prenatal diagnosis for relief of maternal anxiety in the absence of medical indications, and for women who oppose abortion. Respect for the patient's autonomy, and beneficence were the underlying moral values.

Israeli geneticists view prenatal diagnostic procedures as medical services that provide an opportunity to enhance the well-being of the client, in whatever way the client defines well-being. Individuals ought to be well-informed and able to make autonomous and noncoerced choices based on the information provided. When the procedure is aimed solely at the abortion of a healthy fetus, however, which is socially and Halachically unacceptable, it is strongly discouraged by Israeli medical geneticists.

## Genetic Screening

There was a strong consensus for voluntary mass genetic screening of workers, at least as reflected in the responses to the hypothetical case described in the questionnaire. The major ethical reason cited was the overriding value of the autonomy of the patient. There was a strong consensus against disclosure of results to the employer and to the various insurance companies and a moderate consensus against disclosure to the government health department. The potential misuse and unintended damage to the individual from disclosure of genetic screening results to third parties overrode the possible benefit to society. There was no consensus regarding access for the worker's physician. This may be because most referring physicians are employees of the public Sick Fund, and many are not involved in the care of patients.

## Confidentiality Versus Duties to Third Parties

There was a strong consensus regarding non-disclosure to the husband in cases where tests revealed false paternity. The major reason given was that protecting the mother's confidentiality and the family's unity overrode the value of truth-telling. In the socio-cultural environment in Israel such disclosures might have serious consequences not only for the unity of the family, but also for the child, who would be regarded as a "bastard" by the society [although most probably the scientific evidence would not suffice to pronounce the child a "bastard" in the Halachic sense].

There was a moderate consensus for disclosure of Huntington disease and of hemophilia A to relatives at risk, against the patient's wishes. There was greater consensus in the Huntington case, probably because of the greater severity of this disease and the unavailability of treatment. The major ethical reasons given were the duty to avoid harm and to provide health care to the family. These diseases cause serious harm and the disclosure of information can be used effectively to avert future harm.

## Full Disclosure to the Patient

There was a strong consensus to disclose scientifically unclear data (e. g., trisomy-13 mosaic; low levels of alpha-fetoprotein and association with Down syndrome) in a non-directive fashion, pointing out the fact that there is no agreement amongst scientists with regard to their significance. The major reason given was the right of the patient to know all the details in order to be able to reach informed decisions. For similar reasons there was a strong consensus to disclose fully, in a non-directive way, a small defect such as a low meningomyelocele. There was only a moderate consensus, however, to disclose fully a low-grade mosaicism of trisomy-21. It seems that immediate damage to a fetus has a stronger significance in the Israeli geneticist's mind than a potential risk.

There was a moderate consensus for non-disclosure of XY genotype in a female. The feeling was that the psychological harm inflicted upon such a person overrode the commitment to truth-telling. There was no strong consensus on this issue, because the deception might prove to be harmful; hence this dilemma was not easily resolved.

### Summary of Consensus

The response rate to the questionnaire by the Israeli group was high (88%). Since the total number, however, was only 15, the statistical validity of the opinions expressed should be regarded with caution (Table 2.11.7).

The opinions cited in this study are based on intuitive and personal approaches,

**Table 2.11.7.** Summary of the Degrees of Consensus Regarding Ethical Dilemmas

A. Strong Consensus

- non-directive counseling for borderline disorders (XO; XYY)
- reproductive options for carriers of TS to be presented in non-directive counseling (male or female carriers - equally):
  - taking their chances
  - adoption
  - contraception
  - IVF with donor eggs
- refuse prenatal diagnosis for sex selection
- perform prenatal diagnosis for maternal anxiety
- perform prenatal diagnosis for women who refuse abortion
- mass genetic screening - voluntary only
- no access to results of mass screening:
  - employer
  - all kinds of insurors
- no disclosure of true paternity
- disclose ambiguous laboratory results
- disclose conflicting results

B. Moderate Consensus

- reproductive options for carriers of TS to be presented in non-directive counseling:
  - AID (male carrier)
  - tubal ligation (female carrier)
- no access to results of mass screening:
  - government health department
- disclosure of Huntington disease or Hemophilia A to relatives at risk, even against patient's wishes
- disclosure which parent carries a balanced translocation
- do not disclose XY genotype in a female

C. No Consensus

- reproductive options for carriers of TS:
  - vasectomy (male carrier)
  - surrogate motherhood (female carrier)
- access to results of mass screening:
  - worker's physician

and are not based on in-depth discussions, either amongst the professionals themselves or with outsiders (philosophers, lawyers, religious leaders, etc.).

As can be deduced from Table 2.11.7, there was a moderate or strong consensus about many issues. On only a few issues was there no consensus.

The dominant ethical value upon which most decisions were based was the autonomy of the patient. Thus, in order for the patient to be able to reach reasonable autonomous decisions, any relevant information ought to be disclosed, even when ambiguous or controversial; counseling ought to be non-directive, presenting data and options in an objective way; "reasonable" autonomous requests for diagnostic procedures should be respected; screening should be voluntary with no access to results for most third parties.

There are, however, agreed-upon situations where autonomy is waived: disclosure of confidential information to relatives at risk; non-disclosure of XY genotype in a female; no presentation of vasectomy or surrogate motherhood as reproductive options; refusal of prenatal diagnosis for sex selection. In these situations, autonomy may be overriden by paternalism, opposition to abortion, political considerations, desire to avoid harm (nonmaleficence) or to do good (beneficence).

No official resources are available in Israel for ethical decision-making in medical genetics. Moreover, since there is no recognized program in medical genetics in Israel, there is no formal teaching or even discussion on ethical matters.

## 2.11.4 Cultural Context of Medical Genetics in Israel

Israel today is a country of over four million people, 80% of whom are Jews and 20% Arabs. The renewed state of Israel is 40 years old. In less than 15 years since its creation as an independent state, the population increased by 400%, mainly through large-scale immigration from all over the world. This population explosion is unmatched by any other country. Moreover, Israel has become a melting pot of persons of diverse cultural, moral and educational backgrounds. The renewed state of Israel was built upon the most tragic event in human history, the Holocaust, during which 6 million Jews were killed. There is an obviously strong memory of the terrible events only half a century ago, creating a strong desire for survival.

### 2.11.4.1 Sources of Challenge and Support

Israel currently is faced with many existential problems:

a) The surrounding Arab nations are in a state of war with Israel. The country has been actively engaged in wars almost every decade, and has suffered from terrorist activities almost daily;

b) Israel faces a difficult demographic problem, having a large minority of Arabs. The birth rate of Jews in Israel is 22/1,000, whereas that of the Arabs in Israel is 37/1,000. This striking demographic reality, combined with repossession or occupation (depending on the political viewpoint) of territories densely populated by Arabs, creates great concern in the Jewish state;

c) Israel suffers from a very difficult economic situation, creating a problem of allocation of scarce resources. A significant amount of the budget is allocated for military purposes, thus making provision of funds for health care even more difficult;

d) Politically, Israel is a parliamentary democracy. Israel is a secular Jewish state with certain officially accepted religious laws. Political parties in Israel are numerous. The coalitions are, thus, dependent on small parties, which are able to achieve their political and ideological aspirations, despite their relatively small size;

e) Socially, the Jewish population is currently composed of 55% Sephardic and 45% Ashkenazic in origin. Religiously, some 30% are identified with Orthodox Judaism. The impact of religion on the Israeli society, however, is much greater than this quoted percentage, because the religious groups fight strongly and loudly for their causes; politically they are usually the balancing forces between the major parties, thus having an impact on political decision-making out of proportion to their numbers. Furthermore, the role of religious authorities is generally accepted in the Sephardic community even among nonpracticing members;

f) The health care system in Israel is socialistic, accessible and almost free for all, supplying a high standard of medical care and medical research, and plagued with severe budgetary problems. Recently, the health care system has suffered a wave of strikes. Both the public and all types of health care providers are highly dissatisfied with the current situation. It seems that a radical change in the public health care system is rapidly approaching;

g) The practice of medicine in Israel is still based on two contrasting philosophies: the founders of medicine in Israel were strongly paternalistic in their approach and so educated their medical students, many of whom are currently the leading clinicians and researchers in this country. New immigrants from Western countries, particularly the USA, as well as some younger physicians who studied medicine or specialized abroad, are influenced by the Western approach to medical ethics, emphasizing strongly the autonomy and self-determination of the patients. These conflicting basic attitudes prevail also in the population at large; Western-educated and oriented people expect to participate in the decision-making process, whereas many Sephardic Jews prefer a paternalistic approach by their doctors. The religious community has a unique approach – they rely heavily on the advice of their rabbis or Chasidic leaders, so that families have turned over their decision-making responsibilities to religious authorities.

Jewish law is a normative religion that has answers and guidelines to all problems of life. The ethical dilemmas regarding medical genetic issues are basically similar to other ethical issues, and therefore can be guided and decided upon by Jewish law. A good number of the clients of geneticists in Israel are religious and obey the dictums of the rabbis in accordance with Jewish law. The geneticists themselves, however, are mostly irreligious, following the Western secular philosophy as their personal approach to the ethical dilemmas in medical genetics. This creates some tension in certain communities: on the one hand, disagreement with the counseling, particularly when it results in abortion, causes lack of confidence in physicians, and suspicion of misconduct by the medical community on the part of the rabbis and their followers. On the other hand, there is anger and occasionally hatred on the part of the medical community at large and geneticists in particular, because of their feelings that religious groups do not understand the purposes and importance of genetic services.

Medical groups, particularly pediatricians, gynecologists, and neurologists, are very much interested in the services of medical geneticists. Most of them, however, are not involved in ethical dilemmas and do not consider the related problems in advance.

## 2.11.4.2  Major Controversies

The sharpest controversy in Israel about medical genetics is related to the question of abortion: religious groups are strongly opposed to it and therefore are opposed to any counseling that may result in abortion. The original law of abortion included a controversial "paragraph 5," which approved legal abortion for socioeconomic reasons. This was particularly opposed by religious groups and the law was amended by excluding this paragraph.

## 2.11.4.3  National Expenditures for Medical Genetics

See Section 2.11.1.4 above.

## 2.11.4.4  Abortion Laws in Israel

See Section 2.11.1.5 above.

## 2.11.4.5  Studies of Effectiveness of Genetic Services

See Section 2.11.1.4 above.

## 2.11.4.6  Need for New Laws

In our opinion, most ethical dilemmas should not be solved by way of laws, since laws have a tendency to remain stationary, whereas medical problems are dynamic and change rapidly. Also, there are sharp differences between various groups, making it almost impossible to achieve agreed-upon optimal laws that will pass in the current political atmosphere in Israel. It would be morally unacceptable to formulate laws that will be based on compromises reached on political rather than ethical grounds. Ethical codes, however, and guidelines should be formulated for geneticists, after extensive discussions on a multidisciplinary basis, including the entire genetic community, representatives of interested medical societies, religious leaders, the health department, and interested lay "consumers," as well as ethicists and lawyers.

## 2.11.5 Ethical Issues and Future Trends

Most medical geneticists in Israel consider the scarce resources available for medical genetics and the increased demand for genetic services as the problems of greatest concern during the next 10-14 years. Of least concern for the future are issues such as screening at workplaces, sex selection and eugenics. Screening for genetic susceptibility to cancer and heart disease, research on the human embryo, the development of new treatments for genetic diseases, and the problem of environmental damage to the unborn are considered as major concerns for the future by only a few Israeli medical geneticists.

There was a strong consensus regarding the absolutely essential role of medical geneticists in helping individuals/couples to understand, adjust to and cope with their genetic problems in view of the current state of medical knowledge, so that they can reach well-informed, autonomous decisions. The removal or lessening of the patient's guilt or anxiety, and helping individuals/couples achieve their parenting goals are seen by most Israeli geneticists as important but not essential. The reduction in number of carriers of genetic disorders in the population and the improvement of the general health and vigor of the population are not seen as primary goals.

In the future, new technologies using recombinant DNA will pose ethical problems in the general population and within families. The discovery of affected asymptomatic individuals with genetic diseases for which no treatment is available poses severe ethical difficulties.

More effort needs to be devoted to improve techniques for prenatal diagnoses, and to make them more accurate and safer. In-vitro fertilization and surrogate motherhood are complicated ethical-legal-religious problems, which require careful and detailed guidelines.

In the near future it is expected that some of the concepts and many of the data may change, because of rapid advancements in the field, so that some issues that are considered ethical problems today may be solved, whereas other issues may arise, causing new dilemmas.

There is a need for greater awareness of the ethical dilemmas in medical genetics by professionals and by the public at large. This should enhance sincere debates and discussions, leading to better understanding of ethical dilemmas, and eventually formulating codes and guidelines. All this has a greater chance to be achieved in Israel now that medical genetics has been recognized by the health authorities as a bona fide medical specialty.

## Acknowledgements

The help and cooperation of Ms. E. Akstein, program coordinator of the National Program for the Detection and Prevention of Birth Defects, is gratefully acknowledged.
We thank our colleagues for their prompt responses to the questionnaire.

## References

1. State of Israel, Ministry of Health, Commodities and Services (Control) (Amniocentesis) Declaration, 1980: The National Program for the Detection and Prevention of Birth Defects.
2. Statistical Abstracts of Israel, Central Bureau of Statistics, Vols. 32–36, 1981–1985.

# 2.12 Ethics and Medical Genetics in Italy

F. Lalatta and G. Tognoni

## 2.12.1 Development of Medical Genetics and Medical Ethics in Italy

With the sole exception of a genetic counseling initiative established in Milan in 1947 by a woman doctor (Dr. V. Gianferrari), medical genetics long remained on the fringes of medicine and health care. Genetics is still an optional subject in the pre-graduate medical curriculum. Post-graduate courses were first set up in the mid-1970s at the University of Rome. Genetics laboratories and services have grown empirically, with no national or regional planning. The Italian National Health System gives great freedom to regional health authorities.

With very few exceptions, the Italian medical tradition has encouraged the development of empirical rather than scientific attitudes and skills. Scientific method, epidemiology, statistics, controlled trials – key words in the relations between medicine, science, and public health – are not taught in the undergraduate curriculum, and the controlled assessment of outcomes is an exception, rather than a tradition or habitual approach.

The situation is changing, but, despite solemn declarations of its priority, medical school reform is still a matter for the next two decades. As a consequence, any issue or novelty arising in medicine and requiring a local or national decision, however urgent, is faced with an empirical pragmatic attitude. In the absence of any tradition of controlled scientific evaluations, value judgments are left to individuals. Ethical committees are a rarity in hospitals or even on a regional scale. After years of proposals, no law yet regulates experimentation or requires informed consent, nor has the issue been debated by the medical profession or the public. There is no tradition of professional or independent auditing. It is not surprising that whenever the question arises of providing patients with proper information on the benefit-risk profile of a new drug or procedure, it is hard to find doctors who are ready or able to formulate the question in terms which are at the same time precise and respectful of the patient's dignity and autonomy [8, 9, 14].

### 2.12.1.1 Scope of the Problem

Tables 2.12.1 and 2.12.2 summarize the information available on natality and elective abortion for the years 1975–1984. There is no national scheme for malformation monitoring. Few registers have been set up and some of the results derived from the most extensive of them, coordinated by the Pediatric Institute of the Catholic University in Rome, are presented in Table 2.12.3.

**Table 2.12.1.** Livebirths and Stillbirths in Italy between 1975–1984

| Year | Livebirths | Stillbirths |
|------|-----------|-------------|
| 1975 | 827,852 | 9,271 |
| 1976 | 781,570 | 8,345 |
| 1977 | 742,546 | 7,219 |
| 1978 | 712,962 | 6,564 |
| 1979 | 670,221 | 5,748 |
| 1980* | 644,001 | 5,193 |
| 1981* | 621,805 | 4,870 |
| 1982* | 617,507 | 4,739 |
| 1983* | 600,218 | 4,361 |
| 1984* | 585,972 | 4,160 |

* provisional data

**Table 2.12.2.** Data on Voluntary Abortion

| Year | Legal abortions | Abortion/live birth ratio* |
|------|----------------|----------------------------|
| 1979 # | 187,631 | 13.6 |
| 1980 | 222,499 | 16.1 |
| 1981 | 224,067 | 16.2 |
| 1982 | 234,801 | 17.2 |
| 1983 | 233,976 | 16.9 |
| 1984 | 227,446 | 16.4 |
| 1985 | 210,192 | 14.8 |

* Per 1,000 live births
# First year when data became available, because of the introduction of regulatory law.

**Table 2.12.3.** Number and birth prevalence of 24 conditions selected for statistical monitoring at EUROCAT central registry. Italian Multicentre Registry 1980–1984* Total Births 591,524 ( = 19% of the whole Italian population base).

| Conditions | Number | Rate per 10,000 |
|-----------|--------|-----------------|
| Anencephaly | 160 | 2.7 |
| Spina Bifida | 236 | 4.0 |
| Hydrocephaly | 213 | 3.6 |
| Eye | 202 | 3.4 |
| Anophthalmia** | 92 | 1.6 |
| Cataract | 36 | 0.6 |
| Congenital Heart Defect | 1,876 | 31.7 |
| Cleft Palate | 304 | 5.1 |
| Cleft Lip/palate | 405 | 6.9 |
| Esophageal Stenosis | 164 | 2.8 |
| Anal Agenesis | 193 | 3.2 |
| Hypospadias | 1,103 | 18.7 |
| Undeterminated Sex | 37 | 0.6 |
| Renal Agenesis | 95 | 1.6 |
| Polydactyly & Syndactyly | 673 | 11.4 |
| Limb Reduction Defect | 384 | 6.5 |
| Diaphragmatic Hernia | 151 | 2.6 |
| Abdominal wall | 165 | 2.8 |
| Down Syndrome | 750 | 12.7 |

* Kindly provided by Dr. P. Mastroiacovo, Catholic University, Rome
** includes microphthalmia

## 2.12.1.2  Organization of Clinical Genetic Services

Medical genetic services have grown haphazardly. Half have the main or exclusive aim of supporting prenatal diagnostic activities. How genetic services are linked with obstetrics, pediatrics or other medical services depends on local arrangements. Cytogenetic services are associated in a few universities with the departments of human genetics or pathology.

Geographically, services are unevenly distributed. Only 4 of 28 are in the South. Largely because of the inefficiency of the National Health Service (NHS) set up in 1978, but also for economic reasons, at least an equal volume of work is done in a parallel private network, run by the same people who are active in the public health service.

Disease-oriented genetic services have long been functioning in various towns, and there is a strong tradition for providing services for thalassemia. Good cooperation has been achieved across the various disciplines and skills which cover the field [5, 12]. An outline of the development and effectiveness of preventive services for thalassemia appears below.

| | |
|---|---|
| *1975–1979* | Intensive sensitization campaign in some areas of the country on the need and the strategy for prevention of new thalassemia cases. An effective impact could be measured only in small and non-mobile populations, such as in the province of Ferrara. |
| *1977 to date* | Introduction and expansion of prenatal diagnosis. A mean 30% reduction of thalassemia major birth rates was estimated (from mean baseline birth-rates of 0.42/1,000 to 0.28/1,000), though the uneven quality and completeness of registration in the various areas did not allow absolutely precise estimates. |
| *1982–1986* | A mean of more than 1,000 at-risk pregnancies were evaluated every year. Only about 4 families per year with an affected fetus did not choose abortion. |
| *General comments* | A combination of prenatal diagnosis and intensive sensitization campaigns directed to the population and to obstetricians is needed to produce an effective policy. For example, Ferrara has reduced its incidence by approximately 90% in 10 years; the Region of Puglia, in the Southern part of Italy, is reaching the same target after 5 years of an intervention program; other areas with less systematic or prolonged intervention have much more uneven results. |

There is no consensus on the criteria to be adopted for prenatal diagnosis or for information programs on genetic issues. An official policy has yet to be established regarding how and to what extent the NHS should cover the cost of genetic testing. A few points are worth underlining, as they fit into the general framework proposed in the introduction. Genetic services are a growing, not yet well-established reality which occupies a small fraction of working hours. In only 50% of cases is genetic counseling associated with prenatal diagnosis.

## 2.12.2  Ethical Problems

See 2.12.4 below.

## 2.12.3  Consensus and Variation in Italy

**Results of the Survey**
Only 11/26 of those who received the questionnaire in Italy responded. We conducted telephone interviews in order to discover why more had not responded. Reasons given included the following: the questionnaire was too long; personal practice in genetics was too limited to allow the formulation of anything other than purely theoretical opinions; a questionnaire does not permit a respondent to give a reliable profile of ethical attitudes and behaviors. Nonrespondents had a reflex reaction against answering questionnaires. In Italy, questionnaires or interviews with professionals are rare. Nonrespondents also included a few who were ideologically polarized and who saw prenatal diagnosis as a powerful incentive to provide abortions without ethical criteria.

A small sample of respondents can always be judged two ways: either as those who have the strongest opinions and therefore reflect polarization in a society, or as those who are most directly engaged in ethical problems in their routine work. It was not the survey's aim to link answers to identifiable persons, but 6/11 signed their questionnaires. In any case, it would be inappropriate to impose any further interpretation by attempting to speculate about the personal or social origins of the responses.

The profile of respondents suggests a rather low intensity of activity; 7/11 worked no more than 8 hours per week, each seeing a mean of 4–9 new patients. The ratio of males to females mimicked closely the ratio in the Italian medical profession. Fairly unanimous (10/11) declaration of a Catholic background paralleled official statistics reporting the fraction of the population which is baptized. Being Catholic was more nominal than substantial; 2/10 in our sample admitted regular practice.

We cannot draw any firm conclusions from the responses of such a small sample. The addition or subtraction of just one person could modify Italy's position among the other countries with respect to specific items. It is probably more useful to dwell only on questions with a strong consensus or no consensus. The profile that emerged was in favor of the protection of the individual's right to decide on his/her own case, and against disclosure to third parties potentially interested in knowing the results of a genetic test. Whenever the geneticist was expected to take an active part in explaining the risks and in helping to formulate a decision, variability in the responses was the rule. Opinions were similarly dispersed in areas re-

288

**Table 2.12.4.** Ranked Future Priorities

| Italy | Around the world |
| --- | --- |
| 1. carrier screening | 1. increased demand |
| 2. increased demand | 2. carrier screening |
| 3. allocation of resources | 3. allocation of resources |
| 4. environmental damage to the unborn | 4. new treatments |
| 5. new treatments | 5. environmental damage to the unborn |
| 6. screen cancer, heart disease susceptibility | 6. screen cancer, heart disease susceptibility |
| 7. research on human embryos | 7. research on human embryos |
| 8. genetic screening in the workplace | 8. genetic screening in the workplace |
| 9. eugenics | 9. eugenics |
| 10. sex selection | 10. sex selection |

ferring to practices not currently available or formally allowed in Italy, such as vasectomy, which was legally approved only in 1987, or surrogate motherhood. This suggests an empirical ethical attitude rather than one formulated *a priori* (see 2.12.1 above).

This empirical attitude was confirmed in the respondents' clear-cut position against sex selection as an indication for prenatal diagnosis. It is interesting to contrast this with responses to the first, widely-publicized case of sex predetermination by semen centrifugation. It made headlines in the press, but no public position was taken by medical geneticists as individuals or as a group. The case dropped into the mass media with a cortege of dramatic and often imprecise commentaries about the manipulative potential of genetics. The facts that a) research at the boundaries of ethical/social frontiers was officially reported as taking place in Naples, which is traditionally more conservative than northern Italy, and b) that the choice was for a girl, contributed further to the creation of a wonderland atmosphere.

The ranking of Italian geneticists' future priorities for medical genetics in Italy and around the world (Table 2.12.4) offers a useful framework for summarizing the present Italian scene. Immediate medical goals appeared to have top priority: these were carrier screening and increasing demand for public resources. Medium-term medical objectives came immediately after, with the focus on selected problems (treatment) followed by broader issues (screening for cancer and heart disease) and potential risks from the environment. The relatively low priority of this last issue is worth noting, as it suggests that the medical genetics community, at least the small sample represented here, has not been deeply moved by the heated debate that flourished in Italy when a large population was exposed to the environmental accident at Seveso. As a result of the Seveso accident, the Regional Health Commission adopted a position favoring a free decision of the woman/couple with respect to voluntary abortion. The Commission based its decision on the unknown magnitude of the genetic risk associated with in-utero exposure to TCDD, the highly toxic component of defoliants sprayed in Vietnam. The decision provoked a fierce opposition from religious circles, was not clearly publicized, and was silently boycotted. The decision and the debate that followed did, however, contribute to the creation of public demand for liberalized abortion laws [2].

Geneticists' low ranking of research on human embryos, of screening in the workplace, and of eugenics may be read according to three different perspectives: issues given low rankings could be 1) "true" ethical issues, on which geneticists postpone judgment and adopt a wait-and-see attitude; or 2) approaches that geneticists oppose; or 3) areas of no immediate concern.

## 2.12.4 Cultural Context of Medical Genetics in Italy

Italy can be provisionally described as a society that moves much faster than its institutions and which, in medicine specifically, blends empiricism and immobility. The choices of individuals are more decisive in formulating attitudes through pragmatic decisions than are formal debates, legislation, and planning.

### 2.12.4.1 Sources of Challenge and Support

The ethical community in which developments occur consists almost exclusively of experts and opinion-makers from the religious and theological world, as there is no solid tradition in Italy of laypersons becoming involved in ethical issues with "strong" moral implications. Grass-roots cultural movements, with some political support within the majority Christian Democratic Party, claim to represent the traditional-orthodox Catholic position and tend to polarize debates around yes-no attitudes. Any intervention favoring life planning, including contraception, is seen as individual and public sin. These groups refer to the declarations of the Church hierarchy to support their active fight. The position of the National Conference of Bishops closely follows the official declarations of the central organs of the Church. The National Conference views with interest, however, the efforts of some moral theologians to bridge the widening gap between technological and scientific progress and the "orthodox" teaching of the Church [1, 6, 10, 11].

The uniqueness of the role of the Catholic religion in Italy is such common knowledge that it hardly needs repeating. This is not the place to document the profound dissociation between the Church's influence in shaping society's institutions and the influence of society itself on moral behavior and attitudes. The vast reach of this dissociation, with specific implications for genetics, is well illustrated by the fact that in 1974 and 1978 two laws which introduced divorce and voluntary abortion were passed, first in Parliament and then through popular referendums (1975 and 1981, respectively). These laws placed Italy among the most liberal countries in these areas. Society as a whole, in the widespread debate that accompanied the vote, appeared more respectful of personal rights and values than its religious and political representatives.

## 2.12.4.4 Abortion Laws

According to the abortion law of 1978:

1) first trimester voluntary abortion can be requested on social, economic, or psychological grounds;
2) second trimester therapeutic abortion is limited to specific circumstances, including documented serious abnormalities of the fetus or clinical risks for the mother's health. A certificate signed by the obstetrician who will perform the abortion is required. The intervention is allowed before the 24th week of gestation only in obstetrics departments affiliated with the National Health System;
3) individual doctors may refuse their services in the actual practice of abortion.

## 2.12.4.5 Studies of Effectiveness of Genetic Services

See section 2.12.1.2. for a description of studies of thalassemia services.

## 2.12.5 Ethical Issues and Future Trends

Public opinion is occasionally involved in emotional debates, when events like the one cited above on sex predetermination appear in the media. The usual relationship between public opinion, Church hierarchy, and politicians follows the scenario of the 1978–1981 debate on legislation on elective abortion (see 2.12.4.4 above). A major difference is that now women's movements are much less actively involved. In a field where decisions will depend, more than in any other previous debates in medical ethics, on the policies of "genetic experts," it is those same experts who have the foremost ethical duty to provide for informed consent and for patients' ethically autonomous behavior.

A promising recent move of the medical genetics community has been to set up a cooperative group which has started on a research project involving all those who are practicing prenatal diagnosis in the public health services. The project is part of a European effort to establish coordinated strategies for the timely evaluation of prenatal diagnostic procedures, through problem-oriented registries and randomized trials [4,7]. The initiative has had its highs and lows, but overall participation has been very positive for over one year. It appears particularly interesting that it has developed with no public support, and on a voluntary basis. This reflects growing interest in a policy of controlled evaluation of the benefit-risk profile and in the relevance of procedures to public health.

The group is at present considering playing an even more active role, formulating public statements whenever controversial topics arise [13].

The group expects to consider the following points:

1. It is important to recognize that we are actually moving, probably in an inexorable way, toward a situation in which the genetic control of populations and individuals may be a reality. This may become possible within a very short interval of time. In the meantime, a scientific and public culture is evolving that is aware of the implications of this evolution.
2. In the group's perspective, the following are equally inappropriate:
   - attitudes that minimize possible risks;
   - research restrictions based on ideologies and indefinite fears;
   - empirical wait-and-see attitudes, which let things happen with a casualness that slowly turns into regularity.
3. It is a scientifically and ethically unwise choice to put one's trust into legal regulations that do not reflect or encourage a real growth in the culture and organization of those who work in the field. Scientifically and ethically, the development of a cultural ethos that views the workers in the field as active protagonists in decisions should be preferred and stimulated.
4. An essential part of freedom and professional ethics is the formulation of criteria for *not* proceeding with lines of research that seem too risky in their social implications, when compared with the benefits expected.
5. The translation of very general and inviolable principles of respect for life into individual and social ethics is only possible in a context of the cognitive and decisional autonomy of the individual. This is only possible if individuals have free and well-informed access to all different options.
6. Defense of the freedom and right to conduct research cannot be an excuse for allowing competitive and market interests to predominate over scientific or humanitarian interests.
7. One of the professional duties of the scientific community is to refrain from expressing *a priori* moral judgments. Instead, scientists should clearly show the direction and ultimate implications of research [3].

# References

1. Baget Bozzo G [1987] Prima del bene e del male. Rizzoli Ed., Milano
2. Bonaccorsi A, Fanelli R, Tognoni G [1978] In the wake of Seveso. AMBIO 7: 234–239
3. C.E.S.C.A. [1987] A proposal for the establishment of a permanent observatory on the technical and ethical problems of medical genetics. Milan
4. Collaborative European Study on CVS and Amniocentesis. Collaborative European Study – 1st Trimester Fetal Diagnoses of Genetic Disease by DNA analysis
5. Community control of Thalassaemia as a model of genetic disease: Experience in the Lombardy region of Italy. Annual Report, Thalassemia Information Centre, Clinica Pediatrica – Università di Milano c/o Ospedale San Gerardo dei Tintori, Monza, Italy
6. Dionigi Tettamanzi PM [1985] Bambini fabbricati. Edizioni P.M., Milano
7. Durand P [1986] Chorion villus sampling in Europe. Human Reproduction, 1: 341–344
8. Franzosi MG, Sartorio PL, Tognoni G [1981] Che cosa attendersi dalla sperimentazione clinica. L'esperienza della Commissione Tecnica Consultiva della Regione Lombardia. In: Colombo F, Franzosi MG, Tognoni G (a cura): Prontuari Terapeutici Ospedalieri. Risultati e prospettive. Il Pensiero Scientifico Editore, pp 45–60

9. Franzosi MG, Tognoni G [1986] Italy. In: Inman WHW (ed) Monitoring for drug safety. MTP Press Limited, Lancaster, pp 93-99
10. Goffi T, Piana G (eds) [1983] Corso di morale. II-Diakonia (etica della persona). Queriniana, Brescia
11. Privitera S, Cirotto C [1985] La sfida dell'ingegneria genetica. In: Tra scienza e morale. Le Edizioni Cittadella, Assisi
12. Sirchia G, Zanella A, Parravicini A, Morelati F, Rebulla P, Masera G [1985] Red cell alloantibodies in thalassemia major. Transfusion 25: 110-112
13. Terzian E, Tognoni G [1987] Il ritorno della creazione. The Practitioner 100: 30-47
14. Tognoni G [1985] Sperimentare nell'uomo. A proposito di un disegno di legge. Ricerca & Pratica 2: 59-64

# 2.13 Ethics and Medical Genetics in Japan

K. Ohkura and R. Kimura

## 2.13.1 Medical Genetics in Japan

### 2.13.1.1 Scope of the Problem

Data in Table 2.13.1 about the number of births per year (1975-1985) were obtained from Vital Statistics published by the Ministry of Health and Welfare (Health and Welfare Statistics Association 1986).

The incidence of genetic diseases (Table 2.13.2) was compiled from a variety of literature resources (Ohkura 1984; Ohkura 1986). The method of ascertainment is different in each survey. No genetic disease with a particularly high incidence has been reported in the Japanese population.

The incidence of congenital malformations is shown in Table 2.13.3. The data were obtained from five different models of monitoring systems (Kurachi et al. 1986; Konishi et al. 1986; Kamiya et al. 1986; Kondo 1982; Sumiyoshi et al. 1985). These systems are comparable to those used by the International Clearing House for Birth Defects Monitoring Systems (ICBDMS).

The incidence of chromosome aberrations (Table 2.13.4) is based on several studies (Kuroki et al. 1978; Maeda 1978). The total number of cases observed includes approximately 30,000 newborn infants.

Table 2.13.5 shows the rate of childhood mortality in Japan. These statistics were compiled from vital statistics published by the Ministry of Health and Welfare (Health and Welfare Statistics Association 1986).

**Table 2.13.1.** Number of Births, Spontaneous Abortions, and Therapeutic Abortions in Japan 1975-1985

| Year | Live-Births | Spontaneous Abortions and Still Births | Therapeutic Abortions | Total |
|------|-------------|-----------------------------------------|-----------------------|-------|
| 1975 | 1,901,440 | 67,643 | 34,219 | 2,005,302 |
| 1976 | 1,832,617 | 64,046 | 37,884 | 1,934,547 |
| 1977 | 1,755,100 | 60,330 | 34,917 | 1,850,347 |
| 1978 | 1,708,643 | 55,818 | 31,645 | 1,796,106 |
| 1979 | 1,642,580 | 51,083 | 31,228 | 1,724,891 |
| 1980 | 1,576,889 | 47,651 | 29,795 | 1,654,335 |
| 1981 | 1,529,455 | 46,296 | 32,926 | 1,608,677 |
| 1982 | 1,515,392 | 41,135 | 33,972 | 1,590,499 |
| 1983 | 1,508,687 | 40,108 | 31,833 | 1,580,628 |
| 1984 | 1,489,786 | 37,976 | 34,385 | 1,562,147 |
| 1985 | 1,431,577 | 33,086 | 35,992 | 1,500,655 |

**Table 2.13.2.** Incidence of genetic disease

| Disease | per 10,000 births | per million population |
|---|---|---|
| **Autosomal dominant** | | |
| Huntington chorea | 0.3 | |
| Achondroplasia | 1 | |
| Retinoblastoma (bilat.) | 0.14 | |
| Polyposis of colon | 0.5 – 1.0 | |
| Sensorineural deafness | 0.27 | |
| Myotonic dystrophy | 0.15 | |
| Hypercholesterolemia | 10 – 20 | |
| von Recklinghausen disease | 3 | |
| Tuberous sclerosis | 0.5 | |
| Epidermolysis bullosa | | |
|     Dominant type | | 0.9 – 1.1 |
|     Simplex | | 3.4 – 2.8 |
| **Autosomal recessive** | | |
| PKU, classical type | 1/116,000 (over all 1/75,000) | |
| Maple syrup urine disease | 1/448,000 | |
| Histidinemia | 1/8,300 | |
| Homocystinuria | 1/742,200 | |
| Galactosemia | 1/1,035,700 | |
| Oculo-cutaneous albinism | 0.5 – 1.0 | |
| Sensorineural hearing loss | 1.4 | |
| Congenital muscular dystrophy | $6.9 – 11.9/10^{-5}$ | |
| Cretinism (Hypothyroidism) | 1/8,000 | |
| Wilson disease | 0.19 – 0.68 | |
| Polycystic kidney Potter I | 0.2 | |
| Retinitis pigmentosa | 0.27 – 0.85 | |
| Xeroderma pigmentosum | 0.10 – 0.25 | |
| Ichthyosis congenita | 0.001 – 0.05 | |
| Tay–Sachs disease | 0.005 – 0.12 | |
| Werner syndrome | 0.06 | |
| Holoprosencephaly | 1 | |
| Epidermolysis bullosa | | |
|     Recessive type | | 1.2 – 1.4 |
|     Junction type | | 0.12–0.14 |
| **X-linked** | | |
| Hemophilia A and B | 1/8,000 | |
|     (A:B = 5:1) | | |
| Progressive muscular dystrophy | 2.1 | |
|     (Duchenne) | | |
| Ichthyosis | 1/6,000 | |

## 2.13.1.2 Organization of Clinical Genetic Services in Japan

There are only a few well-organized or clearly independent departments or divisions in Japanese hospitals that provide comprehensive medical genetic services.

There are 47 administrative districts in Japan. In each district there is at least one medical school with hospitals (national, prefectural, municipal, and private),

**Table 2.13.3.** Incidence of congenital malformations per 10,000 births (from the data of several monitoring systems)

| Abnormality | Kanagawa (Oct.1981 -Dec.1983) | Osaka (Dec.1981 -June 1984) | Tottori (Jan.1974 -July 1983) | Japan Assoc. Mat. Welfare (1978-1980) | 16 Hospitals in Tokyo (1978-1980) |
|---|---|---|---|---|---|
| Anencephaly | 6.7 | 7.3 | 5.2 | 8.2 | 4.2 |
| Hydrocephaly | 3.6 | 3.6 | 3.7 | 4.7 | 2.4 |
| Cleft lip | 13.9 | 13.3 | 15.6 | 13.5 | 12.0 |
| Cleft palate | 4.4 | 5.1 | 7.6 | 6.2 | 6.1 |
| Spina bifida | 3.2 | 3.7 | 4.6 | 3.0 | 2.7 |
| Tracheo esophagal fistula, atresia of esophagus | 0.9 | 1.2 | 0.9 | 1.3 | 1.0 |
| Malformation of rectum and anus | 4.9 | 3.7 | 5.8 | 1.0 | 5.4 |
| Hypospadias | 3.9 | 4.4 | 3.1 | 1.7 | 1.7 |
| Reductive abnormal- ities of upper limb | | 2.1 | 1.7 | 3.8 | |
| Reductive abnormal- ities of lower limb | 4.4 | 1.4 | 1.7 | 3.8 | |
| Down syndrome | 6.3 | 5.9 | 8.9 | 3.8 | 9.2 |
| Total observed | 106,043 | 156,253 | 33,022 | 122,474 | 40,986 |

**Table 2.13.4.** Incidence of chromosomal aberrations per 10,000 births

| Type of aberration | % |
|---|---|
| 21 trisomy | 0.11% |
| 13 trisomy | 0.01% |
| 18 trisomy | 0.02% |
| other unbalanced | 0.03% |
| XXY | 0.05% |
| XXX | 0.05% |
| XYY | 0.06% |
| X | 0.08% |
| | (all include Mosaic) |

and general hospitals and centers or institutes for specific diseases. These facilities share local medical and health care services. They cooperate in academic and technical matters. For example, if two relatively large pediatric clinics exist in an area, and one has expertise in metabolic diseases, the other in cytogenetics, a patient and/or supporting case material will be transferred to the appropriate clinic for diagnosis, treatment and other care.

Any department, division, or individual physician or scientist who has a special diagnostic technique helps other physicians upon request. Karyotype analysis with banding and many other laboratory tests are provided by commercial laboratories. Therefore, it is difficult to quantify and define the organizational structure of clinical genetic services in Japan.

**Table 2.13.5.** Child Mortality (per 100,000) (1984)

| Age group | 0–4 | 5–9 | 10–14 | Total | Cause of death % |
|---|---|---|---|---|---|
| Population | 7,573,000 | 8,786,000 | 9,965,000 | 26,324,000 | |
| No. of deaths | 12,078 | 1,880 | 1,655 | 15,613 | |
| Mortality rate | 159.5 | 21.4 | 16.6 | 59.3 | |
| Congenital anomaly | 42.5 | 1.5 | 0.9 | 14.2 | 23.9% |
| Perinatal death | 50.9 | | | | |
| Accident, Intoxication, Violence | 20.9 | 8.0 | 4.1 | 10.2 | 17.2% |
| Malignancies | 4.5 | 3.9 | 3.7 | 4.0 | 6.7% |
| Disorders of central nervous system | 3.2 | 0.8 | 0.7 | 1.5 | 2.5% |
| Infectious disease | 11.6 | 1.4 | 1.1 | 4.2 | 7.1% |

Most technical services classified as genetic services are part of routine medical services with financial support provided by the health insurance systems under the supervision of the government. Very rare and/or difficult techniques are provided on request by specialists or specified laboratories.

**Postnatal Chromosome Studies**
When obstetricians or pediatricians find postnatal chromosome examination necessary, they order the examination in their own or some other laboratory, including commercial laboratories. Thus, it is very difficult to count the exact number of studies performed. However, it is estimated that about 0.5% of live births are subjected to this examination.

**Investigation of Genetic Diseases**
The clinical importance of determining diseases is increasing because of the increase in the incidence of genetic disease in the population. Many research groups have been organized by the government with financial support. One of the most comprehensive programs is the neonatal screening program for inherited metabolic diseases (PKU, galactosemia, maple syrup urine disease, homocystinuria, histidinemia, and hypothyroidism). The incidence of these diseases is shown in Table 2.13.2. The number of annual births in Japan is about 1.5 million. The number of infants born with one of these six diseases was about 400 in 1984. As a result of this screening program, 2,732 infants had been identified by March 1985.

There is no national registry system for genetic diseases in Japan, making it impossible to determine the overall incidence of genetic disease.

**Genetic Counseling**
Although activities and progress in the field of animal and plant genetics have continued since the early 1900s, human and clinical genetics have not been devel-

oped systematically. Currently, only two departments of genetics and one department of human genetics have been established among the 80 medical schools for teaching purposes. Eight schools have established a department for research or designated a separate institution for the purpose of research but not education. Therefore, medical students and post-graduate students have less opportunity to learn systematic human or clinical genetics.

Genetic counseling was typically provided for clients by a few physicians or human geneticists who are interested in this area. However, in 1977 the Ministry of Health and Welfare established a new project, "Family Planning Special Counseling Project," to provide genetic counseling services.

In this project, so far, approximately 500 physicians have been trained as genetic counselors and many of them now actively work in genetic counseling services. This project will be continued. Over 80 genetic counseling clinics are now spread throughout Japan.

The Ministry of Health and Welfare recognized that genetic counseling should be located within the mother-child health care program. Many local governments followed this policy and set up regional genetic counseling services systems. In general, persons at higher genetic risk do not openly present themselves to medical or health care services. They hide their problems out of a sense of shame. As we will explain later, this sense of shame plays an important role in many ethical decisions relating to genetic disorders. Public health nurses are the most adequate professionals to contact and work with such families because of the nature of their activities in the field. A short term (4–5 days for a basic or advanced course) training program was offered for such nurses by the Genetic Counseling Center and local governments. Nearly 5,000 public health nurses have now received training.

Each client has a unique problem and the range of problems is broad. They are not only concerned with recurrence risk, but also with the moral or ethical aspects of their decisions and their actions.

Genetic counseling clients are predominantly female. Their age range is from 25–35 to around 55. According to estimates (Ohkura K et al. 1981), the need for genetic counseling in Japan is between 20,000 and 30,000 individual client contacts per year. In some cities it is estimated that one or two in 10,000 inhabitants require counseling per year.

An important aspect of genetic counseling in Japan is counseling for consanguineous marriages, because the incidence of consanguineous marriages is still high, 3.9% for all types and 1.6% for first cousin marriages (Imaizumi et al. 1986).

## 2.13.1.3  Prenatal Diagnosis

Prenatal diagnosis in genetic services is offered in three forms: 1) amniocentesis; 2) ultrasonics; and 3) chorionic villus sampling (CVS). CVS is still in the experimental stage. Few gynecologists now attempt this technique. Ultrasonic examination is very popular and its usefulness in detection of congenital malformations is increasing. Amniocentesis in Japan is used largely to detect fetuses with chromosomal aberrations and also metabolic disorders. This procedure and diagnosis are performed by OB/GYN specialists and cytogeneticists or specialists in metabolic disorders.

According to a survey (Gomibuchi 1986), 30.9% of private hospitals and 62.4% of public hospitals are using amniocentesis for the detection of congenital anomalies. Also, 70.1% of private clinics, 83.4% of private hospitals, and 76% of public hospitals are using ultrasonic scanning for screening congenital malformations. As a result, the discovery rates of malformations in pregnancy have rapidly increased. In 1975, 11% of malformations were seen in utero; 76.8% at birth; and 11.9% after birth. In 1985, the rates were 24.5%, 53.5% and 22.0% respectively. The discovery rate in utero has more than doubled.

### Breakdown of Cases by Indication

A research group sponsored by the Ministry of Health and Welfare completed a long-term study of indications for prenatal diagnosis in 1983 (Sugawa et al. 1983). Data were obtained from six university hospitals and two other institutions. From 1970 to 1981, a total of 1,641 pregnancies in 1,465 women were subjected to prenatal diagnosis. The indications and results of these diagnoses are shown in Tables 2.13.6–2.13.10. Out of 1,641 prenatal diagnoses for 1,459 mothers (a mother may bear more than one baby during the period), 64 (3.9%) resulted in failure of the procedure. There were 43 cases for diagnosis of X-linked disorders, to save the female fetuses through sex selection. In addition, 102 abnormal fetuses were identified in the 1,535 pregnancies studied. The overall rate for detecting genetic abnormalities is estimated as 0.66%. As a consequence of prenatal diagnosis, 1,173 pregnancies resulted in normal infants at birth (71.5%), and 23 (1.4%) ended in miscarriage or fetal death. Some 93 pregnancies (5.7%) were terminated after a positive finding. The remaining 352 (21.4%), however, could not be traced, including 9 with positive findings.

**Table 2.13.6.** Indications and results of prenatal diagnosis

| Indication | No. Mothers | No. Pregnancies | No. abnormalities | % abnormal |
|---|---|---|---|---|
| Chromosome aberration Carrier of structural abnormality | 43 | 70 (4.3%) | 12 + [26]* | 54.3% |
| Chromosomal aberration in previous pregnancy | | | | |
| Down syndrome | 834 | 937 (57.1%) | 21+[2]+((2))** | 2.7% |
| others | 76 | 87 ( 5.3%) | 2 | 2.3% |
| Chromosome aberration in relative | 35 | 41 ( 2.5%) | 0 | 0.0% |
| High maternal age | | | | |
| 35 – 39 | } 239 | 135 ( 8.2%) | 0+ 1 | 0.7% |
| over 40 | | 107 ( 8.5%) | 6 | 5.6% |
| Others | 96 | 97 ( 5.9%) | 0 | 0.0% |
| X-linked disorder | 36 | 43 ( 2.6%) | 24 male | 55.8% |
| Metabolic disorder | 95 | 119 ( 7.3%) | 30 | 25.2% |
| Neural tube defect | 5 | 5 ( 0.3%) | 0 | 0.0% |

* [ ] balanced abnormality
** (( )) uncertain

299

**Table 2.13.7.** Prenatal diagnosis for chromosomal aberration

| Indication | No.exam. | Failure | Normal | Abnormal | |
|---|---|---|---|---|---|
| Previous child with Down syndrome | 937 | 36 (3.8%) | 876 (93.5%) | 25 (2.7%) | |
| | | | | +G | :12+1[a]) |
| | | | | +G,p+ | :1 |
| | | | | +G,q– | :1 |
| | | | | mosaic +21 | :1 |
| | | | | mosaic +mar | :1 |
| | | | | mosaic XO/XY | :1 |
| | | | | mosaic XO/XXY | :1 |
| | | | | mosaic XX/XY? | :1[b]) |
| | | | | mosaic XX/XXX? | :1[c]) |
| | | | | +mar | :1 |
| | | | | XXY | :1 |
| | | | | balanced translocation D/G | :2 |
| Others | 87 | 2 (2.3%) | 83 (95.4%) | 2 (2.3%) | |
| E trisomy | (31) | | | 14P+ | :1[d]) |
| D trisomy | ( 7) | | | 18P+ | :1[e]) |
| Sex–chromosome | (14) | | | | |
| Others | (35) | | | | |
| Abnormality in relative | 41 | 3 (7.3%) | 38 (92.7%) | 0 (0.0%) | |
| High maternal age 35–39 | 135 | 4 (3.0%) | 130 (96.3%) | 1 (0.7%) | |
| | | | | XX/XXY? | :1[f]) |
| Over 40 | 107 | 2 (1.9%) | 99 (92.5%) | 6 (5.6%) | |
| | | | | +G | :4 |
| | | | | +18 | :1 |
| | | | | XXY | :1 |
| Others Congenital malformation in previous child | 97 | 8 (8.2%) | 89 (91.8%) | (0.0%) | |
| Total | 1,404 | 55 (3.9%) | 1,315 (93.7%) | 34 (2.4%) | |

a) Misdiagnosis, fetus aborted XXY
b) Neonate was 46, XY, Maternal blood was mixed
c) Neonate was 46, XY, Pseudomosaicism
d) Recurrence of 14P+
e) Recurrence of 18P+, both parents normal
f) Neonate was 46, XY, Pseudomosaicism

## Policy on Indications for Prenatal Diagnosis

The common agreement among medical geneticists on indications for prenatal diagnosis is 1) the mother is over 35 or 40 years old; or 2) the couple has had a child with a chromosomal aberration; or 3) one parent is a carrier of a balanced translocation; or 4) the couple has had a child with a detectable metabolic disorder. Identification of fetal sex for sex selection purposes only is not a valid indication for prenatal diagnosis in Japan.

**Table 2.13.8.** Prenatal diagnosis for carriers of structured abnormality of chromosome

| Carrier | Karyotype | No. exam | Failure | Normal | Abnormality balanced | unbalanced |
|---------|-----------|----------|---------|--------|---------------------|------------|
| Mother | Robertsonian translocation | | | | | |
| | D/G | 33 | 0 (0.0%) | 10+1[a] (33.3%) | 13 (39.4%) | 9 (27.3%) |
| | D/D | 3 | 0 (0.0%) | 2 (66.1%) | 1 (33.3%) | 0 (0.0%) |
| | G/G | 4 | 1 (25.0%) | 2 (50.0%) | 0 (0.0%) | 1 (25.0%) |
| | Sum | 40 | 1 (2.5%) | 14+1[a] (37.5%) | 14 (35.0%) | 10 (25.0%) |
| | Reciprocal translocation | | | | | |
| | A/C | 3 | 0 (0.0%) | 2 (66.7%) | 0 (0.0%) | 1 (33.3%) |
| | B/D | 2 | 0 (0.0%) | 1 (50.0%) | 1 (50.0%) | 0 (0.0%) |
| | B/E | 5 | 0 (0.0%) | 3 (60.0%) | 1 (20.0%) | 1 (20.0%) |
| | C/C | 2 | 0 (0.0%) | 0 (0.0%) | 2 (100.0%) | 0 (0.0%) |
| | C/D | 1 | 0 (0.0%) | 0 (0.0%) | 1 (100.0%) | 0 (0.0%) |
| | C/G | 1 | 0 (0.0%) | 0 (0.0%) | 1 (100.0%) | 0 (0.0%) |
| | C/X | 1 | 0 (0.0%) | 0 (0.0%) | 1 (100.0%) | 0 (0.0%) |
| | Sum | 15 | 0 (0.0%) | 6 (40.0%) | 7 (46.7%) | 2 (13.3%) |
| Father | Robertsonian translocation | | | | | |
| | D/G | 7 | 0 (0.0%) | 5 (71.4%) | 2 (28.6%) | 0 (0.0%) |
| | Reciprocal translocation | | | | | |
| | A/B | 1 | 0 (0.0%) | 1 (100.0%) | 0 (0.0%) | 0 (0.0%) |
| | A/D | 1 | 0 (0.0%) | 1 (100.0%) | 0 (0.0%) | 0 (0.0%) |
| | C/C | 2 | 0 (0.0%) | 1 (50.0%) | 1 (50.0%) | 0 (0.0%) |
| | D/E | 2 | 0 (0.0%) | 2 (100.0%) | 0 (0.0%) | 0 (0.0%) |
| | Sum | 6 | 0 (0.0%) | 5 (83.3%) | 1 (16.7%) | 0 (0.0%) |
| | Inversion | | | | | |
| | inv (9)[b] | 1 | 0 (0.0%) | 0 (0.0%) | 1[c] (100.0%) | 0 (0.0%) |
| | inv (10)[d] | 1 | 0 (0.0%) | 0 (0.0%) | 1 (100.0%) | 0 (0.0%) |
| | Sum | 2 | 0 (0.0%) | 0 (0.0%) | 2 (100.0%) | 0 (0.0%) |
| | Total | 70 | 1 (1.4%) | 30+1[a] (44.3%) | 26 (37.1%) | 12 (17.1%) |

a) Misdiagnosis, Neonate Down with D/G translocation
b) Previous child was inv (9)
c) Neonatal death with malformations
d) Previous child was 10P trisomy

There is no national policy on indications for prenatal diagnosis in Japan. The indications mentioned above, however, were agreed on and recommended by the research group sponsored by the Ministry of Health and Welfare and also the Committee of the Japan Society of Obstetrics and Gynecology. Small variations are found in applying indication 1. Some apply the procedure to pregnant women over 35 years old, and others to those over 40 years. In relation to counseling before prenatal diagnosis, an ethical approach would require it of medical geneticists. This requirement, however, is not always met.

**Table 2.13.9.** Prenatal diagnosis for X-linked disorders

| Disease | No. exam. | Failure | Male | Female |
|---|---|---|---|---|
| Hemophilia A and B | | | | |
| Carrier mother | 16 | 0 | 9 | 7 |
| Affected father | 2 | 0 | 0 | 3 |
| Progressive muscular dystrophy, Duchenne | 16 | 1[a] | 10 | 5 |
| Other 5 diseases | 9 | 0 | 5 | 4 |
| Total | 43 | 1[a] | 24 | 19 |

a) liveborn male

**Table 2.13.10.** Prenatal diagnosis for metabolic disorders

| Disease | No. exam. | Failure | Normal | Abnormal |
|---|---|---|---|---|
| Autosomal recessive | | | | |
| Tay–Sachs disease | 24 | 0 | 18+1[a] | 5 |
| Gaucher disease | 23 | 3 | 12 | 8 |
| I-cell disease | 8 | 0 | 3+1[a] | 4 |
| GM gangliosidosis | 8 | 0 | 7 | 1 |
| Adreno-genital syndrome | 7 | 0 | 6+1[a] | 0 |
| Krabbe disease | 5 | 0 | 3 | 2 |
| Metachromatic leucodystrophy | 5 | 1 | 3 | 1 |
| Hurler syndrome | 5 | 0 | 3+1[a] | 1 |
| Galactosemia | 3 | 1 | 2 | 0 |
| Pompe disease | 2 | 2 | 0 | 0 |
| Methylmalonicacidemia | 2 | 0 | 1 | 1 |
| Niemann-Pick disease | 2 | 0 | 1 | 1 |
| Sandhoff disease | 2 | 0 | 2 | 0 |
| Xeroderma pigmentosum | 2 | 0 | 1 | 0+1[b] |
| Lactic acidosis | 1 | 0 | 1 | 0 |
| Propionic acidemia | 1 | 0 | 1 | 0 |
| Wolman disease | 1 | 0 | 1 | 0 |
| Sanfilippo disease | 1 | 0 | 1 | 0 |
| Cystinuria | 1 | 0 | 1 | 0 |
| Lysinuria | 1 | 0 | 1 | 0 |
| Methylene tetrahydrofolate formiminotransferase deficiency | 1 | 0 | 1 | 0 |
| Adenosinedeaminase deficiency | 1 | 0 | 1 | 0 |
| Sum | 106 (100.0%) | 7 (7.6%) | 70+4[a] (69.8%) | 24+1[b] (23.6%) |
| X–linked | | | | |
| Hunter syndrome | 5 | 0 | 2+1[a] | 2 |
| Menkes disease | 5 | 0 | 3+1[a] | 1 |
| Lesch–Nyhan disease | 2 | 0 | 0+1[a] | 1 |
| Fabry disease | 1 | 0 | | 1 |
| Sum | 13 (100.0%) | 0 (0.0%) | 5+3[a] (61.5%) | 5 (38.5%) |
| Total | 119 (100.0%) | 7 (5.9%) | 75+7[a] (68.9%) | 29+1[b] (25.2%) |

a) false negative
b) false positive

## 2.13.1.4  Cost-Benefit of Screening and Prenatal Diagnosis

Traditionally, Japanese culture has not been concerned with cost-benefit questions. The medical care budget was recently reduced for economic reasons. Therefore, cost-benefit, or cost-efficiency, problems will soon be open for discussion. Japanese health authorities do not justify planning genetic services by cost-benefit calculations; however, this may become an important factor.

## 2.13.1.5  Incidence of Abortion

In Table 2.13.11, the incidence of elective abortion (1975–1985) and the ratio to live births are shown. These are the figures officially reported by the government. The number of elective abortions reported, however, is thought to be much smaller than the number actually performed.

Contrary to popular views that there is unlimited access to abortion in Japan, actually, according to Japanese law, it is officially illegal to abort a fetus with a genetic disorder (see Section 2.13.4.4) as there is no provision for such abortions in Article 14 of the Eugenic Protection Law [1948]. Officially, abortion is illegal, except according to the guidelines of Article 14 (Chapter 29, Article 212–216 of the Criminal Code of Japan 1907). Therefore, no official reports or statistics exist as to the number of abortions performed due to genetic disorders.

Following prenatal diagnosis, a number of therapeutic abortions are actually performed. In such cases, the reason for abortion is reported as some other officially acceptable reason. Usually, the reason is either to protect the mother's health (permitted under legislation passed in 1948) or to avoid economic hardship if the pregnancy is continued (permitted under legislation passed in 1949). These two reasons are acceptable for social abortions performed under the Eugenic Protection Law. When a parent or his or her relative (within the fourth degree) has some disorder which is identified by the Eugenic Protection Law, a therapeutic

**Table 2.13.11.**  Ratio of Elective Abortions to Live Births

| Year | Elective Abortions (A) | Live Births (B) | A/B |
|------|------------------------|-----------------|------|
| 1975 | 671,597 | 1,901,440 | 0.3532 |
| 1976 | 664,106 | 1,832,617 | 0.3624 |
| 1977 | 641,242 | 1,755,100 | 0.3654 |
| 1978 | 618,044 | 1,708,643 | 0.3717 |
| 1979 | 613,676 | 1,642,580 | 0.3736 |
| 1980 | 598,084 | 1,576,889 | 0.3793 |
| 1981 | 596,569 | 1,529,455 | 0.3895 |
| 1982 | 590,299 | 1,515,392 | 0.3767 |
| 1983 | 568,363 | 1,508,687 | 0.3767 |
| 1984 | 568,916 | 1,489,786 | 0.3819 |
| 1985 | 550,127 | 1,431,577 | 0.3843 |
| Average | 668,102 | 1,789,217 | 0.3734 |

abortion is available. However, the number of these cases is very rare. No ratio of social abortion to genetic abortion is available because there are no statistics reported which are based on genetically defective fetuses. If it were possible to compare genetic abortion with social abortion, however, the incidence of genetic abortion would undoubtedly be quite low.

## 2.13.2 Ethical Problems Faced by Medical Geneticists in Japan

### 2.13.2.1 Genetic Counseling

Counselors face many ethical problems in coping with individual cases. There are many differences between the ethics which evolved from the long history of coping with infections and contagious diseases and the task of addressing genetically determined disorders.

In some cases, genetic information given to two parents is mutually helpful, acceptable, and beneficial. What is often acceptable information to one parent, however, is not always mutually acceptable. Parents may have divergent views.

In Japan, there is still the belief that the marriage of a man and a woman is also the union of their entire family lineage. Accordingly, counselors are aware that disclosure of painful information will be a source of discomfort and embarrassment to two large family units. This sometimes collides with the counselor's obligation to "tell the truth." For these reasons, the majority of Japanese people are afraid to have their genetic problems made known and wish to keep them secret. This attitude is based entirely on the traditional and emotional upbringing among the Japanese. The existence of such a disease in a family is thought to be shameful, not only for the person affected, but for all members of the family, like "losing face," "losing family name," or "bad blood." Therefore, a mother of an affected child often feels very guilty, as if she is to blame for the disorder. Sometimes her husband shares the guilt. These persons do not open their minds to counselors. In the early stages of a genetic counseling session, a counselor is required to work through such psychological problems, which are derived from traditional ethical thought and must be resolved.

By tradition, most people strongly desire to pass the family estate from first son to first son. Many traditional families wish to have healthy children, especially a boy. If a genetic risk is so high as to pose the alternative of not having a child, communication in the counseling session becomes very delicate and difficult.

Often clients ask and seek the decision of the counselor. This attitude is still common in the relationship between a physician and a patient. Most Japanese patients usually tend to follow their physician's guidance or decision. In the case of female clients, this attitude is often exaggerated, because they wish to escape the responsibility for making a decision about reproduction and blame for its result. Also, if a client has little capacity to understand his or her present situation and to make a decision, the counselor falls into a dilemma, since the ideal of genetic counseling is for the client to decide.

In Japan, extended families are often involved in counseling, whereas in many Western countries, counseling primarily involves couples only. Ethically, a counselor must frequently deal with the rights of an individual in relation to the welfare of the many relatives.

## 2.13.2.2 Prenatal Diagnosis

The purpose of prenatal diagnosis is the detection of fetal abnormality. Rarely, treatment of the fetus results. At present, however, abnormal findings most often result in abortion. There are two important ethical problems in prenatal diagnosis. First is the dignity of and respect for the affected fetus. The second problem is a quality of life question (i.e., what is an "unacceptable" abnormality?).

In Japan a social elective abortion is easy to obtain. The number performed is more than one-third of live births, due to the application of Article 14 of the Eugenic Protection Law [1948] as mentioned above. Medical geneticists are seriously concerned about the high incidence of social abortion according to the Eugenic Protection Law and the lack of any legal basis for abortion for genetic indications. And also, there is no agreement about the sort of disorders that will be subjected to selection for abortion.

Most obstetricians emphasize the efficiency of prenatal diagnosis. Also, more accurate technology for diagnosis will be developed, such as DNA probes. Evaluation by this procedure will inevitably create new ethical problems. For example, fetuses with very minor abnormalities or deviations or carriers of genetic disease could become targets of obliteration. This concern creates a very large ethical issue.

## 2.13.2.3 Genetic Screening

In Japan there are several screening systems, not only for genetics but also for general heath care. These systems were established by law or regulation. Such screening always creates the potential problem of invidious distinctions and discrimination against individuals. In spite of the original intention, screening sets norms or standards that lead to stigmatization or discrimination against individuals. For example, under the School Health Act, all school children have long received a screening test for color vision. In Japan, this anomaly excludes the color-blind from several courses of study at many universities and colleges. It also excludes them from several occupations, including driving busses or teaching school. Strong criticism of such screening and discrimination is now coming from ophthalmologists, medical geneticists, and others, and discriminatory regulations are gradually being overcome.

Another severe problem regards reproduction of females treated for PKU. The first cases identified are now at marital age and many others will be soon. If a treated female free from the manifestation of PKU is going to marry, any children would be subject to risk. Her potential for producing a retarded child (maternal PKU) raises many questions. Although there is a possibility of preventing retardation in the child by controlling the mother's blood phenylalanine levels through a low phenylalanine diet begun before conception and continuing throughout pregnancy, it is very difficult to put prospective mothers with PKU on the diet early enough to prevent fetal damage.

The purpose of genetic screening should be assessed while considering the rights of the individual. Such screening proceeds under the beautiful phrase "for social benefit," but may involve careless management of individual cases. It is a significant ethical problem faced by geneticists.

## 2.13.2.4 Other Contexts

In the traditional family structure of Japanese society, each person is expected to behave in a modest, nonassertive way, striving for harmony in relationships with others, particularly with professionals such as physicians, government officers, and superiors in the workplace. Confrontation in human relationships is discouraged; instead, Japanese people work together, focusing on "common elements." The tendency to identify with others as a part of a family or organization, or as a member of the society, contrasts dramatically with the American notion of being a different or unique individual. "Different" means strange in Japan and this strangeness is a negative value in Japanese culture. This is the reason why the Japanese do not usually voice too many differences of opinion with one another. That is, one reads another's mind or thought without detailed debate or discussion. Accordingly, ethical issues are not subjected to thorough discussion to achieve a common agreement or to clarify the differences between ethical principles.

The Japanese mentality, nurtured in the Confucian ethos to respect law, order, authority, and social status, did not change even after the rapid modernization of Japanese society, with its emphasis on science and technology. Reflecting ancient social values and human relationships, until very recently physicians in Japan have typically behaved in a paternalistic and authoritative way toward patients and family members. Patients also feel inclined to obey prestigious physicians.

In the field of clinical medicine, the clinical geneticist has a fundamental knowledge, but there is a wide gap between clinicians and medical geneticists concerning the ethical issues faced by medical genetics. Most clinicians center their professional interest on the individual patient, to the exclusion of the patient's relatives. Medical geneticists, however, must always consider not only the patient but also the relatives at risk for genetic disorders. Medical geneticists also hold different views from clinicians about the "quality of life" of persons with genetically determined disorders.

## 2.13.3 Consensus and Variation in Japan

The completeness of Japanese responses to specific parts of the questionnaires is compared with completeness of responses outside Japan in Table 2.13.12. The left-hand column describes the percent who responded to the 25 questions on the ethical section of the questionnaire, including clinical cases, most and least difficult cases, screening, counseling, and future priorities. The average Japanese geneticist answered 91% of the questions, with a range of 80% to 100%. The average geneticist outside Japan answered 95% of the questions, with a range of 87% to 99%. Responses to the questions about professional and personal background in the first part of the questionnaires have been excluded. Some of the 25 questions had multiple parts; therefore a total of 77 answers was requested. The completeness of responses in Japan was lower than outside Japan, but the difference was not statistically significant. The questionnaires also had a total of 37 places where respondents could give ethical *reasons* for their choices of action. Response rates to these are described in the right-hand column. The average response rate for the Japanese (61%) was significantly lower than the rate for those outside Japan (80%). It is apparent that responding in one's own words, in written English, could take considerably more time than responding to a checklist of answers. Also, some Japanese geneticists may not be accustomed to considering these delicate issues in an ethical framework.

We analyzed the degree of strong consensus ($\geq 75\%$) on 53 questions. These included 1) all 14 clinical cases, three of which had multiple parts (2, 5, and 6 parts respectively), making a total of 24 answers requested; 2) the 4 questions on screening, 2 of which had 7 and 8 parts respectively, making a total of 17 answers requested; and 3) all 12 questions on goals and approaches for counseling. The question on regulating commercial laboratories was omitted from the analysis because it is not applicable to the situation in most countries. In questions with multiple parts, each part has been counted as a percentage of the question rather than as an entire question. For example, each part of a 5-part question is counted as 0.20 of that question. As seen in Table 2.13.13, there was less internal consensus in Japan about genetic screening and clinical cases than in the U.S., Canada, or the Federal Republic of Germany (see also Part 1 of this book, Table 1.23).

Geneticists' reasons given for their choices of action were classified according to

**Table 2.13.12.** Comparison of Response Rates

|  | Ethical Questions (77 potential responses) | Ethical Reasons (37 potential responses) |
|---|---|---|
| Japan (n=51) | 90.8% (100%–80.39%) | 60.84% (88.24%–43.14%) |
| All other countries (n=631) | 94.82% (99.20%–86.84%) | 79.91% (92.30%–68.86%) |
|  | chi–square=2.49 0.20>p>0.10 | chi–square=8.394 0.01>p>0.001 |

**Table 2.13.13.** Percent of Questions with Internal Consensus in Japan and Selected Nations

| Country | % with No Consensus (<66.6%) | | |
| --- | --- | --- | --- |
| | 14 Clinical Cases | 4 Screening Questions | 12 Questions on Counseling Goals/Approaches |
| Japan | 41 | 67 | 17 |
| U.S.A. | 35 | 35 | 9 |
| Canada | 38 | 35 | 17 |
| FRG | 23 | 25 | 17 |

| Country | % with Strong Consensus (≥ 75%) | | |
| --- | --- | --- | --- |
| | 14 Clinical Cases | 4 Screening Questions | 12 Questions on Counseling Goals/Approaches |
| Japan | 58 | 33 | 67 |
| U.S.A. | 64 | 61 | 83 |
| Canada | 48 | 36 | 75 |
| FRG | 50 | 65 | 67 |

Note: Questions with a moderate consensus (66.6–74%) have been omitted from this table.

**Table 2.13.14.** Ethical Principles in Reasons for Choices of Action

| | Autonomy | Non-Maleficence | Beneficence | Justice | Nonethical |
| --- | --- | --- | --- | --- | --- |
| **Japanese** | | | | | |
| No. of responses | 581 | 317 | 191 | 56 | 90 |
| % | 0.4660 | 0.2542 | 0.1532 | 0.0465 | 0.0722 |
| **Non–Japanese** | | | | | |
| No. of responses | 11,579 | 4,652 | 3,806 | 855 | 1,055 |
| % | 0.5146 | 0.2068 | 0.1692 | 0.0380 | 0.0469 |

Note: We entered up to two ethical reasons per question for each respondent. Therefore, on each question, a respondent could have 0, 1, or 2 reasons entered. The numbers of responses above therefore reflect unequal input by different individuals. One respondent could have given 75 ethical reasons, while another gave only 1. In computations involving "multiple measurements" per respondent, chi-square and other standard measures of association do not apply.

**Table 2.13.15.** Primacy of Welfare

| | Parents | Patients | Child or Fetus | Future Generations | Geneticists |
| --- | --- | --- | --- | --- | --- |
| **Japanese** | | | | | |
| No. of responses | 202 | 178 | 74 | 13 | 30 |
| % | 0.3389 | 0.2987 | 0.1242 | 0.0218 | 0.0503 |
| **Non-Japanese** | | | | | |
| No. of responses | 3,643 | 2,744 | 513 | 81 | 271 |
| % | 0.4125 | 0.3107 | 0.0581 | 0.0092 | 0.0307 |

* See explanatory note for Table 2.13.14

308

**Table 2.13.16.** Perceptions of Conflict

| | No Conflict | Parent-Child, Fetus | Client-Family | Client-Geneticist |
|---|---|---|---|---|
| **Japanese** | | | | |
| No. of responses | 416 | 41 | 57 | 58 |
| % | 0.6922 | 0.0682 | 0.0948 | 0.0965 |
| **Non-Japanese** | | | | |
| No. of responses | 6,551 | 300 | 893 | 556 |
| % | 0.7417 | 0.0340 | 0.1011 | 0.0630 |

* See explanatory note for Table 2.13.14

the ethical principles of Autonomy, Non-maleficence, Beneficence, Justice and Strict Utilitarianism. For an explanation of the coding, see Part 1, Sections 1.7.1 and 1.7.2, and also Tables 1.31 to 1.36. Using a "multiple responses" program in SPSS-X, we added the total numbers of reasons falling under each value heading, for both Japanese and non-Japanese (Table 2.13.14). Standard measures of statistical significance, such as chi-square, cannot be applied to these summaries of values, because they reflect unequal input by individual respondents. We coded up to two ethical reasons per question for the 14 clinical cases and 2 of the screening questions, and one reason per question for each of the 15 question sections on access to results. A respondent could therefore give 0, 1, or 2 reasons per question. Therefore, some individuals may have contributed 47 responses to the summary while others contributed none. Nevertheless, we would like to make some general statements about Japanese geneticists' ethical reasoning. Their behavior has tended to minimize or prevent the infliction of harm on individuals and families (non-maleficence). We also believe that they have less respect for patient autonomy than geneticists in Western nations.

Table 2.13.15 shows whose welfare had primacy in the reasons given by Japanese and non-Japanese respondents (see also Part 1 of this book, Table 1.35). As with the previous table, statistical measures of association are not valid because of the unequal number of responses contributed by individual respondents. We believe, however, that Japanese geneticists give more emphasis to the welfare of the fetus or child and less emphasis to the welfare of the parents than non-Japanese geneticists. Japanese parents very strongly desire the welfare, health, and happiness of their children, and put the child's welfare before their own. Parents do not hesitate to sacrifice themselves for their children. Therefore, it is not surprising that Japanese geneticists perceived a conflict between parent and child or fetus (Table 2.13.16. See also Part 1, Table 1.36).

## 2.13.4  Cultural Context of Medical Genetics in Japan

### 2.13.4.1  Sources of Challenge and Support

Challenges to and support for medical genetics in Japan are found in psychological and social sources. A genetic problem in a family depresses almost every member of the family psychologically and emotionally. (In Japan the extended family is far more important, and also larger, than in the United States). The Japanese typically are not open to their need for genetic services, as described above. Latent demands for help and service are great. These "silent people" have been received quite often by public health nurses who operate most of the 850 health centers set up all over Japan [1987].

Some medical interest groups, e. g., human or clinical geneticists, pediatricians, obstetricians, and physicians who work in public health, actively encourage the national and local governments, academic, professional, and social groups to support and expand the activity of medical genetics. Political parties, religious leaders, and legal authorities (with few exceptions), however, will not address human genetics. The reason is simple. Genetic problems are difficult to understand. Also, those in positions of leadership are uncomfortable with reproductive issues and they still confuse medical genetics, particularly genetic counseling, with the Nazis' eugenic movement. Also, they are reluctant to touch upon the secrets of particular persons.

Parents and handicapped people have also been successful in forming support groups. The national government and local governments have sponsored and supported many research groups financially, and have established several groups. Research projects that they fund are directly related to hereditary diseases. The purpose of research is much more closely related to clinical interests, namely diagnostic techniques, treatment, and pathology. Such research focuses on medical aspects of hereditary diseases but not on genetic research to study genetic aspects of the disease. Recently, some groups have developed medical genetic approaches to some diseases.

The Japanese demonstrate bias and prejudice about hereditary diseases and sometimes toward affected individuals. This prejudice has influenced, not only the thought of the common person, but also professionals and the well-educated person. Therefore, government, agencies, and foundations still hesitate to support a research project on medical genetics as an independent project when there is such social stigma attached.

### 2.13.4.2  Controversies Concerning Medical Genetics

Active opposition to medical genetics has not yet occurred. Soon after prenatal diagnosis was introduced, however, a local government described it as a movement of "Don't have an unhappy child." A few handicapped groups objected very strongly to this slogan, because it characterized an affected child as an "unhappy one." Their complaint was "What is an unhappy child?" This program was terminated immediately. Afterwards, three similar programs were discontinued, on account of the same complaints. These three programs were also strongly criticized because of their emphasis on prenatal diagnosis. Other than these four controversies, no others have appeared.

In 1977, the Ministry of Health and Welfare decided to establish a new project, the "Family Planning Special Counseling Project." Under this program the Genetic Counseling Center was set up as an attached facility of the Japan Family Planning Association, Inc. in Tokyo. A large group representing the handicapped sent statements that financial support from the government should be stopped. However, the group did not ask that the activities of the Center be halted. The strongest emphasis by these groups is that the extension of prenatal diagnosis and genetic counseling may lead to killing or eliminating handicapped children and encourages abortion. They requested that government support for these services be stopped. They did not interfere with parents who used this facility and the services, however.

Currently, there are no active controversies.

## 2.13.4.3 Resources Expended by Japan in Support of Medical Genetics

All Japanese participate in one of three health insurance systems controlled by the government. Employees pay half of the insurance cost and employers pay the other half. In the case of the unemployed and owners of small self-owned businesses, the family and employees contract with the National Health Insurance, which is managed by the government. In these systems, many services related to medical genetics, e. g., prenatal diagnosis, are financially covered.

The screening expenses for inborn errors of metabolism, e.g., PKU, galactosemia, maple syrup urine disease, homocystinuria, histidinemia, and hypothyroidism, have separate budgets. As an example of government support, milk for affected children is supplied without charge through the agency with government support.

Health insurance covers 90% of medical expenses for the employee and 70% for family dependents. Also, 70% of the medical expenses for members of the National Health Insurance System are covered. In cases of some intractable diseases and specified pediatric diseases (including hereditary diseases), however, the remaining 30%, which is charged to patients or parents, is covered by national and/or local government budgets.

Research funds for medical genetics and related projects are mostly from government budgets and private foundations. It is very difficult, however, to classify the funds for medical genetics properly. Most of these projects are interdisciplinary, but some are independent projects.

The total amount of health care expense in Japan was ¥16,015.9 billion in 1985, with a GNP of ¥320,774.8 billion. The proportion of the health care outlay to the GNP is 4.99%. Several government budgets included medical genetics in 1986, but not all. Activities funded included:

| | |
|---|---|
| Screening of inborn errors of metabolism (5 disorders), hypothyroidism and neuroblastoma | ¥76.9 billion |
| Research funds for prevention of handicapped children | ¥0.6 billion |
| Research funds for several intractable diseases and specified pediatric diseases (including hereditary diseases) | ¥12.26 billion |
| Research funds for neurological diseases | ¥0.45 billion |
| Subsidy to the Genetic Counseling Center (a part) | ¥15,600,000 |

Local governments also have a budget for conducting programs related to medical genetics. It is very difficult, however, to obtain detailed information.

## 2.13.4.4 The Abortion Law in Japan

The Eugenic Protection Law, promulgated in 1948, approved abortion to protect maternal health and to prevent financial harm due to continuation of a pregnancy.

This law cites about 30 diseases or malformations that qualify one for eugenic sterilization or abortion. Only a woman who has one of the above-mentioned diseases or malformations or has an affected relative within the third or fourth degree (including her husband's relatives) is authorized to receive sterilization or abortion. And under the same condition a man is authorized to receive eugenic sterilization. This law, however, does not specifically allow abortion of an affected fetus or embryo. Usually, the OB/GYN practitioner will apply one of the two legally-allowed reasons to perform an abortion in these cases. It has been understood as a sort of emergency procedure.

This law played an important role in controlling the rapid increase in the population after World War II. The dissemination and popularization of family planning helped stabilize population growth. On the other hand, sexual freedom has become a severe social problem. A few religious groups and politicians fear moral degeneracy. They argue that this degeneracy of sexual morality is an outcome of legal and free abortion. These groups are strongly against this law with its provision of economic reasons for abortion.

On the contrary, groups that protect and emphasize the rights of women wish to continue the law. They advocate that the decision to bear a child should be made by the woman. They insist on this assurance. On the other hand, they do not agree with the addition of genetic indications to the abortion law. Their claim is based on the protection of the right to life and abuses due to sex selection. These claims are also supported by groups representing the handicapped and other interest groups. A few groups of providers of prenatal diagnosis answer their objections by showing the facts about the procedure and its use. However, they do not insist on updating the 1948 law. It is a tacit understanding that in cases of fetal defect this procedure will be performed for the reasons mentioned above. At present, there are few active discussions.

## 2.13.4.5  Studies or Evaluations of the Effectiveness of Genetic Services

In English-speaking countries, especially the United States, the term "genetic services" is used. In Japan, however, there are no adequate terms corresponding to this. What non-Japanese consider "genetic services" are integrated into OB/GYN medical services.

One large genetics program is screening for inborn errors of metabolism: 99.6% of the neonates born in 1984 and 98.6% in 1983 were screened. Screening statistics for hypothyroidism were 98.5% in 1983 and 99.9% in 1984 (Report of the Ministry of Health and Welfare 1985). The figures reflect a parental acceptance of screening programs.

Prenatal diagnosis (by amniocentesis) was accepted only as a way to diagnose and intervene directly in the birth of an affected child. Ever since the development of this procedure, however, resistance has existed for emotional and ethical reasons. It was sometimes very strong. Therefore, this technique is not yet prevalent throughout Japan. A shortage of qualified personnel to perform the procedure is not a limiting factor.

In a number of genetic counseling services, follow-up studies were carried out (Ohkura and Jikuhara 1979). The rate of response to the questionnaires was always very low in every study. Most Japanese clients do not want contact with the genetic counselor after the counseling. In some cases, clients do not declare their names and addresses, or they give a false name. Under these conditions, we were not able to obtain necessary information for evaluation of clients' decisions or attitudes following the counseling.

Although there is no direct evaluation of the service by clients, the mass media evaluates the program of genetic counseling. We conclude that most Japanese have a good understanding of and readily accept genetic services, but they do not discuss it in an overt, open way.

## 2.13.4.6  Need for New Laws

Many believe that serious and probably inevitable harm will come to society through the improper use of life science technology, although well-intended. It is often "after the fact" that the public recognizes social harm. Abuses in human genetics may occur at the hands of scientists or physicians interested in human or medical genetics but who do not have adequate preparation in this field. However, to protect against possible abuses in human genetics, we believe that legislation may not be necessary. Feedback mechanisms operating in academic societies, professional associations, and interest groups may be sufficient to prevent abuses and create ethical self-regulation of medical genetics in Japan.

## 2.13.5  Ethical Issues and Future Trends

One expected trend is the development of techniques for early diagnosis, including carrier detection. Pre-symptomatic diagnosis and carrier detection result from genotype diagnosis. An individual carrying a specified genotype may be recognized as genetically "defective." This recognition will also be by the individuals themselves. Such individuals may experience identity problems if they know their genotype. In other words, the effect of this is to distinguish and identify individuals as "different." This runs strongly counter to the Japanese concept of "sameness." Techniques will be developed very rapidly and statistics for diseases or disorders that are identified by early diagnosis will increase. The expansion and development of new techniques, however, may not be controlled. Many minor disorders will also be involved as a result of early diagnosis. Genetically determined diseases and abnormalities should be recognized as part of the genetic characteristics or attributes of the human species. It is not possible or desirable to exterminate all of them. Human beings, therefore, must accept and live with some "undesirable" genetic characteristics.

The central dilemma created by human genetics is that development of new techniques in early diagnosis, treatment, and education of the handicapped will increase the gene frequencies in future generations. There will be no escape from this problem.

Hereditary diseases are always a serious family problem. If prenatal diagnosis becomes a routine screening procedure, the rights of women and their equality could be diminished (Arditti et al. 1984).

The most serious ethical issue in Japan is the conflict of interests between a couple, sibling(s), parent(s), child(ren), other relatives, and society. There are increasing concerns among young people about first-cousin marriages. Also the secrecy and privacy relating to the genetic deficit of the particular family member is very important as it might have some grave negative effect on the marital chances of the family members. There is still subtle discrimination against those who have genetic diseases. Traditionally a genetic disorder was regarded as a shameful happening to be hidden from other people's sight. Traditional religious teaching in Japan has contributed to an idea that genetic diseases are the result of misconduct in a previous incarnation or of misbehavior by earlier generations of the family.

An anticipated issue of significance is the allocation of limited resources. In this study, Japanese geneticists evaluated this issue as not very important. However, Japan is beginning to reduce its budget for medical and health care. Priority in budgeting may soon become a serious issue.

Religious groups are not resources upon which medical geneticists can draw in resolving ethical dilemmas. Medical geneticists have not faced religious problems in their practice. Almost all Japanese clients would prefer to seek answers to their problems from the scientific, medical point of view rather than the religious point of view. The ethical concepts of Japanese medical geneticists challenge the philosophy of Confucianism, Shintoism, Buddhism, and traditional Japanese thought as described briefly above. These traditional and cultural fundamentals will not change in the near future.

The cultural background of ethics differs among nations. In Japan, Korea, and some other countries, the name of the nation or the people, e.g., Japanese, almost always means the name of a homogeneous ethnic group. Of course, there are small minority groups, such as the Ainu.

Ethical guidelines might be very important in a multi-ethnic, multi-religious and multi-linguistic nation. Ethics are essential norms to keep harmony in a pluralistic society constituted by different peoples. In contrast, in the society of the Japanese, a so-called unitary homologous nation, a strong emphasis on a particular ethical guideline would create the opposite effect, controversy and disharmony.

Disharmony would occur because a person or family with a genetic problem is almost always faced with a psychological problem. Some may also have ethical problems, such as disclosure to relatives or abortion of an affected fetus. A traditional Japanese does not point out or openly criticize the psychological or moral problems of others. Usually communication is tacit. If geneticists made some ethical guidelines clear through verbal expression, patients would become recalcitrant or defiant, and disharmony would occur. Especially for patients who already feel or know that they face ethical problems, a doctor's direct mention of or emphasis upon this ethical problem would be scratching a psychological wound, or a "wound of heart." Therefore, it is necessary for geneticists to use gentle and intelligent means of communication.

Recently, much criticism and attention have been given to several new reproductive technologies in Japan that have focussed society's attention on problems of medical ethics. In general, medical geneticists have had little experience in ethical deliberations. In the future, ethical aspects of medical and genetic problems will be emphasized more frequently. This will compel physicians to make decisions with more adequate attention to their ethical dimensions. This will change the doctor-patient or counselor-client relationship. The superiority of the professional, especially the medical doctor, will give way to an equal relationship with the patient or client. This new equality will bring with it major changes in ethics, especially increased respect for the client's autonomy.

This will not happen overnight, however. Before the attitudes of medical geneticists change significantly, there must be a change in the Japanese people's traditional way of thinking towards a more rational scientific view.

# References

Arditti R et al. (eds) [1984] Test-tube women. What future for motherhood. [Japanese ed.: Jansson Y [1986] Kyodo Tsushin-sha, Tokyo]

Gomibuchi M [1986] A consideration of the Eugenic Protection Law and fetal indication. Medical Way 3 [12]: 159-164

Health and Welfare Statistics Association [1986] Annual statistical report of national health conditions 1986. Health and Welfare Statistics Association, Tokyo

Imaizumi Y [1986] A recent survey of consanguineous marriages in Japan. Clin Genet 30: 230-233

Kamiya S et al. [1985] A field study on the occurrence of congenital malformations (Tottori area). Report of research group on the monitoring of congenital malformations. The Ministry of Health and Welfare

Kessler S (ed) [1979] Genetic counseling. Psychological Dimensions. Academic Press, New York

Kimura R [1984] The meaning of gene therapy. Japanese Journal of Nursing. 48 [9]: 1061–1064

Kondo K et al. [1982] Monitoring of birth defects at the Tokyo Metropolitan hospitals and lying-ins. Tokyo General Institute for Neurosciences.

Konishi H et al. [1986] A field study of monitoring of congenital malformations (Osaka area). Report of research group on monitoring of congenital malformations. The Ministry of Health and Welfare

Kurachi K et al. [1986] A field study on the monitoring of congenital malformations (Kanagawa area). Report of research group on monitoring of congenital malformations. The Ministry of Health and Welfare

Kuroki Y et al. [1978] Pilot study for estimation of chromosome aberration and monitoring by postnatal chromosome analysis for all newborn babies in one hospital. Report of research group on prevention of disordered and handicapped children. The Ministry of Health and Welfare

Maeda T et al. [1978] A cytogenetic survey of consecutive liveborn infants – incidence and type of chromosome abnormalities. Jap J Human Genet 23: 217–224

Matsuda T, Yoshioka A and Ohkura K (eds) [1985] Proceedings of Symposium on Application of the Knowledge of Human Genetics including Genetic Counseling for Clinical Medicine – Ethical and Psychological Dimensions. Rinsho iden kenkyu (Med Genet Res). 7: 55–155

Ohkura K [1981] Diseases of the Japanese. In: Rothschild HR (ed) Biocultural aspects of disease. Academic Press, Orlando, FL, USA, pp 295–325

Ohkura K, Handa Y, Handa T [1981] Present and future of genetic counseling. Rinsho iden kenkyu (Med Genet Res). 2: 60–138

Ohkura K, Jikuhara T [1979] Evaluation of genetic counseling. Rinsho iden kenkyu (Med Genet Res) 1: 41–47

Ohkura K, Kimura R [1987] Genetic diagnosis and therapy in bioethics – comparison between U.S. and Japan. Medical Way 4 [1]: 51–60

Sugawa T et al. Study on quality control of prenatal diagnosis. From the follow-up study of 1,641 cases. Report of research group on monitoring of congenital malformations. The Ministry of Health and Welfare

Sumiyoshi Y et al. [1985] Statistical report on the survey of external malformations by Japan Association for Maternal Welfare. Japan Association for Maternal Welfare.

Yezzi R [1980] Medical ethics: Thinking about unavoidable questions. Holt, Rinehart & Winston, New York

# Additional Bibliography on Ethics and Genetics

Arai K [1985] Examination of ethical and psychological issues in cases of genetic counseling. Rinsho iden kenkyu (Med Genet Res) 7: 68–72

Higashi K [1985] Ethical views in genetic counseling – from a survey of parents with handicapped children, through a questionnaire. Rinsho iden kenkyu (Med Genet Res) 7: 75–79

Ohkura K [1985] Application of human genetics including genetic counseling in clinical medicine – psychological and ethical view. Rinsho iden kenkyu (Med Genet Res) 6: 71–90

Ohkura K [1985] Ethical and psychological issues in application of human genetics in clinical medicine. Rinsho iden kenkyu (Med Genet Res) 7: 57–66

Ohkura K, Kimura R [1987] DNA diagnosis, gene therapy and bioethics. Medical Way 4: 51–60

Tanaka A [1985] Medical ethics in case of chromosome aberration. Rinsho iden kenkyu (Med Genet Res) 7: 81–83

# 2.14 Ethics and Medical Genetics in Norway

K. Berg and K. E. Tranøy

## 2.14.1.1 Scope of the Problem

Despite its geographical size, Norway has a population of just over 4 million, which is about half the population of the neighboring country of Sweden. The number of births per year has been declining for several years, reaching a present level of about 50,000 (Table 2.14.1). The great majority of people living in Norway today were born in Norway to Norwegian parents, but in recent years a number of foreigners have settled, mostly around the larger cities, particularly Oslo. These immigrants have on the whole adapted very well to their new home country.

The exact frequency of genetic disease or congenital malformations in Norway is not known. However, since 1967 every birth has been reported to the medical birth registry, and birth defects that can readily be observed at birth or within a few days after birth are reported. Clearly, recording at or shortly after birth will leave some conditions undetected. On the other hand, the population-based registry system in Norway should provide true figures for malformations such as anencephaly, open spina bifida, cleft palate, total cleft lip or limb reduction defects. Down syndrome will be under-reported at birth because of both clinical uncertainty and a reluctance to apply the diagnosis of Down syndrome until the results of chromosome analysis are available. The rates of selected malformations per 10,000 births in 50,594 children born in 1984 are summarized in Table 2.14.2 (extracted from International Clearinghouse for Birth Defects Monitoring Systems, Annual Report 1984). These rates are similar to the rates among 336,552 children born during the base-line years of 1967 through 1971.

The impact of congenital malformations on childhood mortality is described in Table 2.14.3. It resembles that in other countries in the region.

**Table 2.14.1.** Livebirths, Stillbirths and Infant Deaths in Norway

| Year | No. of Livebirths | No. of Stillbirths | No. of deaths in first week of life | Total deaths <1 year |
|------|-------------------|--------------------|--------------------------------------|----------------------|
| 1975 | 56,345 | 458 |     | 625 |
| 1976 | 53,474 | 400 | 318 | 561 |
| 1977 | 50,877 | 394 | 281 | 468 |
| 1978 | 51,749 | 346 | 234 | 446 |
| 1979 | 51,580 | 382 | 230 | 453 |
| 1980 | 51,039 | 363 | 205 | 411 |
| 1981 | 50,708 | 299 | 189 | 382 |
| 1982 | 51,245 | 324 | 193 | 413 |
| 1983 | 49,937 | 303 | 195 | 395 |
| 1984 | 50,274 | 261 | 190 | 419 |

**Table 2.14.2.** Selected Disorders Reported in 1984 on the Medical Birth Report Forms in Norway (n = 50,594 births)

| Disorder/Malformation | Number | Rate per 10,000 |
|---|---|---|
| Anencephalus | 10 | 2.0 |
| Spina bifida | 27 | 5.3 |
| Encephalocele | 3 | 0.6 |
| Hydrocephalus | 24 | 4.7 |
| Microtia | 2 | 0.4 |
| Cleft palate | 31 | 6.1 |
| Total cleft lip | 59 | 11.7 |
| Esophageal atresia or stenosis | 8 | 1.6 |
| Anorectal atresia or stenosis | 12 | 2.4 |
| Hypospadias | 81 | 16.0 |
| Renal agenesis/dysgenesis | 4 | 0.8 |
| Limb reduction defects | 26 | 5.1 |
| Abdominal wall defects | 55 | 10.9 |
| Diaphragmatic hernia | 13 | 2.6 |
| Down syndrome | 46 | 8.5 |

From International Clearinghouse for Birth Defects Monitoring Systems, Annual Report 1984

**Table 2.14.3.** Impact of Congenital Malformations on Childhood Mortality in Norway in 1984

| Age at death | Total Number | Number with Congenital Malformations | % with Congenital Malformations |
|---|---|---|---|
| Less than 1 year | 419 | 141 | 33.7 |
| 0–4 years[1] | 527 | 167 | 31.7 |
| 5–9 years | 49 | 6 | 12 |
| 10–14 years | 61 | 4 | 7 |

[1] Includes less than 1 year

## 2.14.1.2 Organization of Clinical Genetic Services in Norway

In Norway, health care organization and delivery have been the responsibility of the state for several decennia. Thus, hospital care as well as extensive out-patient treatment, permanent medications and expensive diagnostic procedures have been paid for by the government for many years. The general public essentially pays only for visits to doctors for acute or trivial matters and for drugs for acute disease. There has been a trend over the last several years to increase the fraction of the cost of medical care for which the public pays. However, treatment for any significant disease or extensive diagnostic procedures, including prenatal and other genetic diagnostic work-ups, is free for the individual. There is mandatory membership in the National Norwegian Health Service (NNHS).

Medical genetics became a specialty equivalent to traditional specialties such as surgery or internal medicine in 1971. This led to the establishment of a specialist's fee, based on the number of working hours actually spent on the case, which authorized specialists could charge for genetic counseling. In principle, specialists in medical genetics could start private practices and have their fee for genetic counseling paid by NNHS funds, but none of the small number of authorized specialists has thus far chosen to do so. The established honorarium has been used only sporadically by individual specialists. Counties establishing genetic counseling services will, however, predictably utilize this opportunity to have part of their expenses reimbursed by charging the NNHS for individual cases handled by specialists. Counselees are never charged for genetic counseling. In the great majority of cases, the NNHS will pay for counselees' travel from their place of residence to the specialist.

Until recently, the Institute of Medical Genetics, University of Oslo, was the only university department of human or medical genetics, but the University of Bergen now has such a department. The first department of medical genetics within the health care system was established by the City of Oslo in 1976. The department, which was integrated into the Institute of Medical Genetics, University of Oslo, was charged with the task of providing genetic counseling for the population of Oslo. Since 1981, the Department of Medical Genetics, City of Oslo, has also been charged with the task of conducting all the laboratory work necessary for prenatal diagnoses in the whole of Norway. Prenatal diagnosis is considered a government responsibility, and the state reimburses the City of Oslo for all its expenses connected with prenatal diagnosis. The medical genetics center formed by the combination of the Institute of Medical Genetics, University of Oslo, and the Department of Medical Genetics, City of Oslo, has the rank of World Health Organization Collaborating Center.

In 1986, government funds were allocated to the University of Bergen to make it possible for its Department of Medical Genetics to conduct prenatal diagnosis, and to the health authorities in the county of Troms to establish a Department of Medical Genetics at the University Hospital in the city of Tromsø.

Postnatal chromosome studies have been utilized for diagnostic purposes in Norway since 1960. Since the early 1960s the government health insurance system has paid a fixed sum per analysis to two laboratories (Institute of Medical Genetics, University of Oslo, and the chromosome laboratory at the Department of Pediatrics, University Hospital, Bergen) authorized to conduct diagnostic chromosome analysis. The greater part of the sum paid by the government for chromosome analysis is used to cover the salaries of laboratory technicians.

Some 1,200–1,300 postnatal chromosome studies are conducted annually, the majority of them at the Institute of Medical Genetics, University of Oslo. When the centers at Bergen and Tromsø become fully operative, the capacity for prenatal diagnosis should increase to 1,800 per year and the staff and other resources should be adequate for this amount of diagnostic work. Staffing of the three centers is done on the basis of the plan which the Director of Health has developed, and the estimated number of necessary staff members is based on experiences from many centers around the world.

The clinical work-up of patients with genetic disease is mainly considered as the responsibility of clinicians in the respective disciplines, but at the center in Oslo medical geneticists participate extensively in diagnostic clinical work. The work-up of the family and the extended kindred is considered the responsibility of the

319

medical geneticist in the areas where such expertise in available (Oslo, Bergen, Tromsø). Specialists from the center in Oslo visit hospital departments and institutions for the blind, deaf, or persons with other handicaps on a regular basis to provide genetic counseling.

The centers that are involved in prenatal diagnosis will be expected to provide genetic counseling for everybody who comes for prenatal diagnosis. Other than that, the need for genetic counseling is poorly covered. The City of Oslo is the only community that has an adequately staffed unit for genetic counseling to cover the needs of the population. Genetic counseling is provided also in Tromsø and Bergen, but both centers are inadequately staffed to meet the needs. For the rest of Norway, there is no established system to provide genetic counseling, but the staffs at the university units in Oslo and Bergen counsel on a voluntary basis. Since these people have other primary duties to attend to, coverage of the need for genetic counseling outside Oslo, Bergen, and Tromsø can only be characterized as inadequate.

Cases requiring more extensive counseling (not including counseling in connection with prenatal diagnosis or routine postnatal chromosome studies), with indepth family studies, number 300 or more per year at the Department of Medical

**Table 2.14.4.** Families that Received Genetic Counseling in 1984 at the Department of Medical Genetics, City of Oslo, According to Disorder

| Disorder | Number | Percent |
|---|---|---|
| Dwarfism | 5 | 1.1 |
| Skeletal disorders | 20 | 4.3 |
| Osteogenesis imperfecta | 12 | 2.5 |
| Eye disorders | 38 | 8.1 |
| Deafness | 5 | 1.1 |
| Kidney disease | 10 | 2.1 |
| Liver disease | 1 | 0.2 |
| Disorders of skin or hair | 3 | 0.6 |
| Diabetes | 17 | 3.6 |
| Huntington disease | 14 | 3.0 |
| Other neurological disorders | 44 | 9.4 |
| Cardiovascular disorders | 9 | 1.9 |
| Down syndrome | 19 | 4.1 |
| Other chromosomal disorders | 21 | 4.5 |
| Infertility, habitual abortion | 6 | 1.3 |
| Neural tube disorders | 13 | 2.8 |
| Hemophilia | 3 | 0.6 |
| Exposure to teratogens | 4 | 0.8 |
| Advanced age in pregnant women | 151 | 32.3 |
| Multiple malformations, mental retardation | 27 | 5.8 |
| Metabolic disorders | 13 | 2.8 |
| Psychiatric disorders | 4 | 0.9 |
| Immunodeficiency | 9 | 1.9 |
| Retinitis pigmentosa | 10 | 2.1 |
| Anxiety | 6 | 1.3 |
| Other conditions | 4 | 0.9 |
| Total | 468 | 100 |

Genetics, City of Oslo. This is well above an early estimate by a World Health Organization expert group that genetic counseling would be needed annually for approximately 5% of the births in the population. A breakdown of families that received genetic counseling following family studies in 1984 at the Department of Medical Genetics, City of Oslo, is given in Table 2.14.4.

The staff at the Department of Medical Genetics, City of Oslo, collaborates extensively with several societies for various diseases, such as the national societies for Huntington disease, dwarfism, muscle disorders, and hemophilia, and benefits greatly from this collaboration.

## 2.14.1.3 *Prenatal Diagnosis*

The first prenatal diagnosis was carried out in Norway in 1971. For the next ten years such examinations were carried out exclusively at the Institute of Medical Genetics, University of Oslo. This was done in an improvised way, on a voluntary basis, by devoted staff with other primary duties. The strain caused by the prenatal diagnosis work in a setting where no resources had been allocated to it grew gradually and the situation became critical in 1978-1980. The Ministry of Health had a commission examine the situation, and on the basis of its report proposed to Parliament (Stortinget) that prenatal diagnosis should be the responsibility of the government and that state resources should be allocated to the Department of Medical Genetics, City of Oslo, to make it possible for that department to conduct prenatal diagnosis on a nation-wide basis and later on a regional basis. In 1981, the proposal was carried by a majority of 91 votes to 19, the opposition consisting of the representatives of the Christian People's Party (CPP), whose leader requested that a more thorough debate about prenatal diagnosis be held later. This first allocation of funds from the government health care system to establish medical genetics services was sufficient to conduct 500 prenatal examinations per year. This figure was only about one-tenth of comparable figures for the other Nordic countries, but still represented a significant step forward. The low capacity to conduct prenatal diagnosis made it necessary to give priority to women with the highest risk of having a child with a serious genetic disorder.

In the debate that took place early in 1983 as a result of the request from the leader of the CPP, a great deal of concern surfaced. It became clear that, although prenatal diagnosis was to continue to be the responsibility of the government, Parliament wanted severe restrictions on it. It was explicitly stated that the annual number of prenatal diagnosis cases should remain at the established level of 500. Thus, the Norwegian Parliament effectively put a quota of 500 on prenatal diagnosis in a population of more than 4 million. The statements from the Parliament's Committee on Social Affairs and the debate reflected a curious alliance between people with very different political, social, and religious views. Although the Committee advocated very restrictive practices, it also stated that the overall social situation of the women should be considered and that it should be possible to have the procedure done even in the absence of the accepted medical indications. The parliamentary debate demonstrated the importance of adequate information, and

321

suffered precisely from the lack of such information. One of the leading members of Parliament effectively summed up the situation when he stated that prenatal diagnosis was an area that was not very suitable for a debate in Parliament.

In 1983, the Parliament requested that a commission be appointed to follow medical genetic services in Norway, particularly to make sure that services were offered on as just a basis as possible. This seems to be a situation unique to Norway.

It has been clear for a long time that there are extreme variations between regions in Norway in the use of prenatal diagnosis. It is hard to escape the conclusion that the extremely limited resources make it impossible to present an offer of prenatal diagnosis that reaches everybody on an equal basis everywhere in the country. The principle of equal access to health services is one of the basic principles of the NNHS. The Department of Medical Genetics, City of Oslo, reported this inequality of access to the authorities, and requested both an increase in the annual number of prenatal diagnoses, and more extensive medical genetic services. The commission established by Parliament supported the proposal. The National Director of Health developed a plan for expanding medical genetics services in Norway and submitted the plan to the Minister of Social Affairs in the Spring of 1985. Essential elements of the plans are the establishment of three to four medical genetics units attached to medical faculties of universities over a ten-year period. Implementation of the plan has started, but for financial reasons, developments have progressed more slowly than proposed by the Director of Health.

Demands for prenatal diagnosis increased drastically over the years. In 1985, Parliament resolved to expand the quota from 500 to 750–800 annual analyses and allocated the funds necessary for this to the Department of Medical Genetics, City of Oslo. In 1986, funds to establish prenatal diagnosis services in Bergen and Tromsø followed. There was hardly any debate at all in Parliament when additional funds for prenatal diagnosis were allocated in 1985 and 1986, respectively. The contrast to previous, heated debates was striking.

It is still unknown when the new units in Bergen and Tromsø will actually be able to conduct prenatal diagnosis work. In late 1987, the national quota was still 750–800 annual analyses, and all analyses were still conducted at the Department of Medical Genetics, City of Oslo.

Table 2.14.5 shows a breakdown of prenatal diagnosis cases by indication in 1985. Risk of a chromosomal disorder in the fetus remains the overwhelmingly

**Table 2.14.5.** Breakdown of Prenatal Diagnosis Cases in Norway by Indication, 1985

| Indication | Number | % |
|---|---|---|
| Maternal age 38 years or above | 560 | 79.9 |
| Previous child with trisomy 21 or other trisomies | 46 | 6.6 |
| Balanced translocation in one parent | 4 | 0.6 |
| Previous child with neural tube defect | 47 | 6.7 |
| Previous child with metabolic disorder | 10 | 1.4 |
| Others | 34 | 4.8 |
| Total | 701 | 100 |

important indication. The frequency of induced abortions caused by findings at prenatal diagnosis continues to be very small: 4–5% of the total having prenatal diagnosis.

As stated above, the Norwegian Parliament wanted both a restrictive attitude towards prenatal diagnosis and that the test should be available even in the absence of strict medical indications. In a situation where it was necessary to refuse many requests for prenatal diagnosis every week, the only acceptable practice was to favor the women with the highest risk. This led to the following indications, which have been explicitly stated in a letter from the National Director of Health to all physicians in Norway. According to this letter, the following situations warrant prenatal diagnosis in Norway:

1. A previous child with a chromosomal disorder
2. A previous child with a neural tube defect
3. A previous child with an inborn error of metabolism that can be diagnosed by prenatal diagnosis
4. A previous child with a serious X-linked recessive disease or a woman known to carry genes for such a disease
5. Known carrier state in one of the parents for a chromosomal anomaly and increased risk of unbalanced chromosomes in an offspring
6. Maternal age at delivery greater than 38 years, and therefore increased risk of chromosomal anomaly in offspring.

Since only one center actually conducts prenatal diagnosis in Norway, the above are the indications as practiced on a nation-wide basis. The "age-limit" of 38 years for prenatal diagnosis because of risk for Down syndrome in offspring is felt as extremely strict. It is well known that a significant number of women are having prenatal diagnosis conducted in the neighboring countries of Sweden and Denmark. This is considered ethically questionable, since it adds to the inequality between regions and individuals with respect to the possibility of having prenatal diagnosis performed. It is very much hoped that the new centers in Bergen and Tromsø will soon be operative, so that the nation-wide capacity will increase, making it possible to modify the present strict indications for prenatal diagnosis.

## 2.14.1.4 Concerning the Cost-Benefit Problem

No cost-benefit analysis has been conducted for prenatal diagnosis or genetic counseling in Norway. It is clear from analyses in other countries, however, that prenatal diagnosis is cost-effective when a relatively high age limit is used for the maternal age indication. With the present age limit of 38 years there can be no question about the cost-effectiveness, and this will be true even if the limit is lowered to 37 or 36 1/2 years.

Among politicians, there has been considerable resistance to taking the financial aspects into consideration, presumably because it could put a price tag on the lives of handicapped persons or lead to altered attitudes towards the handicapped. It is beautifully consistent to refuse to allocate resources on moral grounds, and then to launch moral objections against cost-benefit analyses of genetic services and "price tags" on human lives.

Genetic counseling is done on a non-directive basis, and it is not a task for the counselor to try to make the couples at risk abstain from having children. Accordingly, one cannot measure the effectiveness of counseling by evaluating restrictive reproductive practices following genetic counseling. The aim of genetic counseling in Norway is to make it possible for the couples in question to make their choices, for example concerning further reproduction, on as well-informed a basis as possible. Accordingly, it would be totally meaningless to try to evaluate the economic consequences of genetic counseling.

### 2.14.1.5 Abortion

Table 2.14.6 shows the incidence of elective abortion in Norway in 1975 through 1985. It is particularly interesting that the introduction of a liberal abortion law did not significantly change the total number of abortions in Norway. The annual number of abortions fluctuates between approximately 13,500 and 15,500, and the number of livebirths is at present around 50,000. Accordingly, the elective abortion/livebirth ratio is slightly more than 1/4.

The incidence of abortion following genetic diagnosis is negligible. Thus, with the present number of prenatal diagnoses, findings leading to pregnancy termination will be made in only 20–30 cases per year, and it is doubtful that the number will ever reach 100 per year, even with greatly expanded medical genetics services. Accordingly, there are more than 500 cases of social abortion for every abortion following explicit genetic diagnosis. In the public health statistics, "genetic abortion" appears to be more frequent. This is so because the commissions that decide whether mid-trimester abortion is acceptable (see section 2.14.4.4 below) may give *risk* of genetic disease in the fetus as the reason for pregnancy termination, without an exact diagnosis.

**Table 2.14.6.**    Elective  Abortion  in  Norway
1975–1985

| Year | Number of abortions |
| --- | --- |
| 1975 | 15,132 |
| 1976 | 14,754 |
| 1977 | 15,528 |
| 1978 | 14,783 |
| 1979 | 14,456 |
| 1980 | 13,531 |
| 1981 | 13,845 |
| 1982 | 13,496 |
| 1983 | 13,646 |
| 1984 | 14,070 |
| 1985 | 14,599 |

## 2.14.2 Ethical Problems Faced by Medical Geneticists in Norway

Some of the ethical problems that medical geneticists in Norway have to face are conditioned, wholly or in part, by what seem to be typically if not exclusively Norwegian circumstances (see 2.14.4 below).

There is an air of paradox between contemporary medical genetics and traditional Norwegian morality. Genetic counseling, prenatal diagnosis, and genetic screening have all been at the center of heated debates in Norway, but there is comparatively little written material on these issues stemming from scientific studies or surveys (Berg 1985a, 1985b, 1985c, 1985d). Public debates about ethical aspects of medical genetics have taken place mostly in newspapers, non-scientific journals, and more-or-less popular books.

### 2.14.2.1 Genetic Counseling

The predominant attitude of Norwegian medical geneticists is one of *pronounced respect for patient autonomy and self-determination, coupled with full disclosure to the patient (NOT to third parties!) if, AND ONLY IF, desired by the patient, and with a strong respect for honesty and truthfulness.* Taken together, these factors produce a typically non-directive ideal of counseling. Norwegian geneticists clearly respect the distinction between *giving advice* and *providing a basis for independent choice.*

There is little disagreement in Norwegian public opinion about the desirability of genetic counseling. The focus of public concern is the nature of the counseling. There is considerable concern and fear that such counseling is going to be DIRECTIVE, in the sense that the counselor's personal value system may appear as "scientific" advice and/or as covert pressure on counselees: "No prenatal diagnosis for you unless you are willing to choose abortion in the case of an affected fetus." Fear of pressure to choose abortion is clearly linked to the very limited Norwegian capacity for prenatal diagnosis by amniocentesis.

### 2.14.2.2 Prenatal Diagnosis

In Norway there is no prenatal diagnosis on a private fee-for-service basis. Strict *rationing* of access to prenatal diagnosis is unavoidable in Norway as long as the capacity is, by decision of the Norwegian Parliament, so severely restricted. These two facts can, of course, be traced to the Norwegian moral heritage (see 2.14.4 below). It follows that there can be no prenatal diagnosis without thorough previous counseling. So arguments based on wasteful use of scarce resources carry heavy weight in Norway, regardless of the moral affiliations of the geneticist. It IS a very scarce resource, and so the use to which it is put had better be worthwhile. This

325

does not preclude disagreement over what constitutes appropriate use. The limitations on capacity reinforce the necessity of satisfying strict requirements of fairness in selecting candidates for diagnosis in the first place. This is part of the Norwegian practice of saying NO to the use of prenatal diagnosis for purposes of sex selection only, although it is easy in Norway to find other and weightier moral arguments against sex preselection. There is nothing "pathological" or "defective" about being of one sex rather than the other. No matter how highly Norwegian geneticists value patients' self-determination, other criteria for selecting candidates for prenatal diagnosis – such as the risk of bearing an affected child – are obviously more important than self-determination when the resource is so scarce.

There is a frequently-voiced fear (perhaps "worst case scenario" is a better term) that prenatal diagnosis will be misused in the service of some large-scale eugenics scheme. The factual argument that this would not be possible, even granted a scale of resources which could make prenatal diagnosis mandatory, does not always succeed. The ethically serious consideration is fear that aborting affected fetuses on the basis of a medical diagnosis will introduce an unacceptable "moral class distinction" between "defective" versus "non-defective" humans into the Norwegian public health service.

## 2.14.2.3  Genetic Screening

In Norway, as in most other countries, there is fairly full agreement that, in those cases where screening is instituted, there should be full disclosure of all the findings to the person screened and very strict restrictions on the access of third parties to the data. The only exception to full disclosure to the person screened might be the phenotypical female with an XY karyotype, and the argument then is that such information would do more harm than good, a classic (but strong) utilitarian argument. On the whole, there is a remarkable agreement about the institution and applications of genetic screening and its findings among Norwegian geneticists.

## 2.14.3  Consensus and Variation in Norway

From a total of ten Norwegian medical geneticists there were six respondents. The reflections and conclusions reported here cannot and do not build so much on statistical data as on close reading of the six questionnaires available and, especially, on the reasons given for choices.

Two overall impressions can be summarized as follows: First, there was considerable agreement among Norwegian geneticists. Second, with fairly few exceptions, there was a corresponding consensus between Norwegian geneticists and their colleagues in other countries, although we also found areas of variation. An example of consensus was sex preselection by amniocentesis, which was unanimously and expressly rejected as unethical by all six Norwegians. The outcome would surely have been the same if all ten had given their views. On this issue, geneticists in the majority of nations were opposed, so those in favor appeared as deviants in the international perspective.

It would have been surprising if Norwegian geneticists had been out of step with their international scientific community, especially when we note that all six identified themselves as non-churchgoers and five of them said that they had no religious background at all. What was surprising, however, was that there should be such extensive consensus on highly "loaded" ethical issues among Norwegian doctors who, on the whole, still tend to regard morality and ethics as fields characterized by subjectivity, cultural relativism, and disagreement.

### Significance of Norwegian Responses

Although statistics on the basis of six responses are neither reliable nor interesting, a close non-statistical scrutiny of the material was both rewarding and suggestive. We have attempted to produce an ordered list of the medico-moral values (or norms, or principles: we do not try to distinguish among these here) held by Norwegian medical geneticists, as shown by their responses and comments on the questionnaire.

I. The primary goal of the six participating geneticists was *to help individuals and couples* adjust to and cope with their genetic problems and to understand their options as well as the present state of medical knowledge so they can make informed decisions. The unanimous votes on these two counseling goals made this quite clear (see Part 1, Table 1.17).

II. Although these goals, which are very consistent with traditional medical ethics, might be called utilitarian, they are to be achieved through *non-directive counseling and voluntary participation* of patients.

III. Problems connected with the *handling of genetically relevant information* turned out to be of central importance. The patient's right to know was frequently invoked as important to his or her welfare. It is worth noting that the client's right *not* to know was emphasized along with the right to know. This was to stress that it was not the doctor but the patient who was to decide what sort of information the doctor was to communicate to his/her clients. However, answers from some of the respondents showed that not all doctors agreed about this, and also that a radical "patients' rights" position on this issue was likely to cause practical complications. It is difficult meaningfully to claim a right not to know without knowing what it is that you want to be ignorant about, a paradox that is often, but not always, insoluble.

IV. *Autonomy* (meaning *patient autonomy*) was a very important value for Norwegian geneticists. This was hardly surprising, given a firmly non-directive ideal of counseling, in spite of the fact that the primary goal of helping individuals and couples might seem to invite a certain amount of paternalism. Although we only rarely found expressions bearing witness to more paternalistic attitudes, they were not altogether absent (see below). Some of our geneticists did seem, however, to stress patient autonomy to a point where the geneticist would seem to be entirely at the patient's service and command, though always, of course, within the limits of the law. In one case, it was hard to avoid suspicion that geneticists invoked the value of patient autonomy as a pretext for a deeper wish to escape from their not always pleasant responsibilities.

V. In this context, *the value of truth-telling (or honesty)* became important, as expected. Surprising, however, was the sophistication of those respondents who noted a morally important (and very real) asymmetry between truthtelling and lying. In some cases (but not in all!) it was indeed possible to withhold the truth without thereby lying to (i. e., inducing a false belief in) the patient. The interesting point is that among our respondents, the principle that one should *avoid telling lies* was clearly ranked as being morally prior to the principle that one should *tell the truth.* This is a possible and even reasonable position to take: the geneticist should tell patients the truth about their genetic status when they desire to have such information. But the geneticist should *never lie* to patients, no matter what sort of information or ignorance they might desire.

VI. The values of *truth-telling* and *confidentiality* must obviously be closely connected. Our respondents were in agreement with each other that disclosure (truthtelling) to third parties was not acceptable except where non-disclosure (confidentiality) would quite clearly be in conflict with the best interests of the patient or an "innocent" third person (such as the spouse in the Huntington disease case). In this case, it was clearly possible to *avoid telling lies* if information were withheld.

We must add the reminder that, given the primary goal of helping clients/patients to cope with their problems, the principles underlying this ethical system are the principles of ethical *consequentialism*, not those of *ethical deontology* (where moral norms and principles are accepted as being morally binding *per se*, and not because of their consequences). The welfare of those to whom they were committed as physicians was the guiding moral concern of these geneticists. Clearly, a deontological ethics – an ethics of strict duties – would have been far less inclined to accommodate a strongly non-directive ideology of genetic counseling.

We have already noted that some of our respondents implicitly called attention to an asymmetry between truth-telling and refusal to lie. There is a similar asymmetry between *doing good* and *avoiding harm* on which respondents explicitly relied. The consequentialism to which they adhered was anchored in the importance of avoiding harm rather than in a duty to do good. Many examples illustrating this tendency can be found in the reasons that respondents gave for their choice of answers. Thus, and we quote, "Vasectomy may be harmful" (and therefore should be rejected as an option), "The truth in this case will probably cause harm to the patient" (and therefore it should be withheld by the geneticist – in the XY female case); "Will cause the least harm to the family" (in the balanced translocation case).

**The Dominant Approach to the Morality of Counseling**
We have already indicated the dominant approach among Norwegian geneticists to the problems of genetic counseling (2.14.2.1 above). In brief, theirs was *a consequentialist approach to an ideal of non-directive genetic counseling.* There were few traces of or appeals to *a priori* moral principles. One of the rare examples concerned sex preselection, which one respondent said was simply "unethical in itself" or "highly unethical" without further argument or appeal to consequences. Perhaps the inclination of some to wish for legislation in controversial areas is the manifestation of a suppressed desire for strict and unconditional moral norms – a feature of the moral system that is incompatible, or difficult to reconcile, with an

ideal of non-directive counseling on consequentialist foundations. Even those respondents who betrayed authoritarian or paternalistic inclinations appeared to find it difficult to go against the strong present trend in favor of autonomy, which today is an outstanding trait in bioethics in particular and in Western society in general. According to one respondent who thought that there should be restrictive legislation/regulation for commercial laboratories, "Society has ... an obligation to establish general rules/norms" regarding prenatal diagnosis for maternal anxiety and sex preselection. Respect for the law is a deeply ingrained trait in traditional Norwegian culture.

However, some of our respondents had problems maintaining a fully consistent attitude about the morality they claimed to accept. Four of our respondents said that it was "never appropriate" to advise patients what they ought to do. Yet in four of the clinical cases (counseling about fetuses with borderline disorders XO and XYY, presenting options to male and female carriers of tuberous sclerosis, and counseling about a possible small neural tube defect) they answered that they would "advise" or "urge" patients to take one option rather than another. This finding is not easy to interpret. It could mean either that they had not really thought the issue through or that they did not see this as a lack of consistency. The consistency requirement is itself a norm, in ethics as well as in science, but in ethics in particular it is unclear precisely what is required of us. In any case, this raises an issue that might be worth pursuing.

The acceptance of patient autonomy as a key value in genetic counseling may itself be a source of conflict, but the contemporary trend in favor of autonomy is difficult to resist.


## 2.14.4 Cultural Context of Medical Genetics in Norway


### 2.14.4.1 Sources of Challenge and Support


**Religion and Society**

Undoubtedly, the main source of challenge and support for medical genetics in Norway is the country's religious and moral heritage.

According to a 400-year-old tradition, Norway is a Lutheran country, in much the same way as two other countries in the study: Denmark and Sweden. Norway has an established Lutheran Church, and the clergy and other church staff are state employees. Also, the responsibility to build and maintain churches resides with the government. However, the fraction of the population that may be considered as active, observant members of congregations is much smaller than the number of inhabitants who have remained members of the Lutheran state church.

The general cultural and specifically moral heritage that flows from Lutheran tradition is more influential and perceptible in Norway, however, than in other Scandinavian countries. This divergence is due to the fact that, in moral matters, a clearly puritan view is prevalent in Norway. This may create an impression of paradox in the mind of an innocent observer. For in many ways, Norway is notoriously anything but puritan. Sexual morals have been liberal if not downright lax (at least until the age of AIDS) and current legislation grants any pregnant woman the right to abortion on demand during the first trimester, at the expense of the NNHS.

Nevertheless, and for reasons that are not at all easy to understand, there exists in Norway a "moral minority" whose influence in matters of medical ethics is much more powerful than their limited numbers would suggest. (In using the term "the moral minority," we are making implicit reference, as American readers will undoubtedly realize, to the American movement that calls itself "The Moral Majority.") To most Norwegians, the views of this minority appear as a rather stern blend of puritanism and pietism. For reasons that are far from clear, this "moral minority" has some of its most important strongholds in the health professions, in particular in the nursing profession, but also among physicians, some 7–8% of whom are members of the Norwegian Association of Christian Physicians (NACP). Representatives of the same stern moral outlook are also found among members of the Norwegian Parliament, among politicians in general, and, of course, among the clergy, who are traditional providers of moral leadership in Norway. The moral minority has a stronghold in the Christian People's Party, which attracts around 10% of the votes. It is particularly strong on the western coast of Norway, where there is a fundamentalist lay movement whose influence exceeds its size.

There is little doubt that the Norwegian fundamentalist minority has a significant influence on public opinion and policy making, but it is also clear that ethical problems related to progress in medicine, genetics, and biology have received attention from a much larger fraction of the population. The fundamentalists, as well as other groups deeply involved in ethical problems, participated most actively in the debate that eventually led to a liberal abortion law in the 1970s. Some of them later focused on prenatal diagnosis and the small number of pregnancy terminations following it.

At the other end of the spectrum, the trend toward patient autonomy receives forceful support from the Norwegian penchant for *individualism*, which is a characteristic feature of the pattern of Norwegian culture. A certain moral individualism is a conspicuous and central feature of Lutheranism, at least within the frame of valid law.

## Public Debate
Legal authorities, e.g., professors in the law schools who are often consulted by the media on controversial issues of public interest, have not so far taken a very active part in the public discussion of ethical issues in medical genetics. Some philosophers have been active, especially those working in ethics. However, in contrast to neighboring Sweden, where *philosophers* have been very active in bioethics, in Norway it is to the *social sciences* that people have turned for comment and guidance on controversial issues.

## Resources Used by Medical Geneticists in Norway to Resolve Ethical Problems
The following comments are organized under two perspectives or points of view: A strictly ethical one and a health policy perspective. The two are not independent

330

of each other. The ethical perspective is less formal and explicit, but not less important than the policy perspective. Norway has very little in the way of written ethical rules to which geneticists can turn for guidance. The *Ethical Rules* of the Norwegian Medical Association, which are important, are mostly too general to answer the questions that arise in the practice of medical genetics. The Medical Research Council (MRC), through its *ad hoc* Committee on Research Ethics, has published a 17-page leaflet or manifesto on the research ethics of medical genetics, which does give some guidance (Medical Research Council 1981). However, its dividing line between genetic research on the one hand and diagnosis and therapy (counseling) on the other is not always easy to see. Various popular books on contemporary medicine and/or medical ethics contain chapters on some of the ethical problems of medical genetics, but none of these are authoritative statements. They are not even balanced or representative expressions of a consensus among professionals. It is not surprising, then, that in the comments from our six respondents there was only one reference to professional bioethics – an unspecific reference to views held by John Fletcher [1985].

The introduction in Norway of medical genetics, and of prenatal diagnosis by amniocentesis in particular, could not have come about without government funding and the approval of the Norwegian Parliament. Parliamentary debates about these issues have claimed a great deal of public attention. It takes very little to arouse a suspicion of "genetic manipulation" or "tinkering with human nature, life itself or what God has created," in Norway. The official reports of parliamentary debates and other parliamentary documents (Stortingsmelding 1981–82) contain statements on some of the principles underlying Norwegian policy in the field of medical genetics. Thus it was by explicit votes in Parliament that the total capacity for prenatal diagnosis in Norway was first set at 500 per year and later raised to some 800.

The parliamentary review committee (see 2.14.1.3 above) attracted considerable attention and interest when it was first established, but seems to have lived a quiet life since then. But it *exists* and it would surely make the headlines again if it were to find something to criticize. Given the fact that there is no private practice of medical genetics in Norway, plus the fact that Norwegians tend to be law-abiding, it is not likely that it will find attempts to circumvent the rules.

Prior to 1986, there was no systematic teaching of medical ethics in Norwegian medical schools. The answer to the question: "How do you teach younger colleagues about these ethical issues?" is that there is no distinctive formal instruction in these matters at all. That is not to say that ethical issues are not explicitly brought to the attention of both older and younger colleagues. Such activities are organized in the context of regular instruction and supervision in medical genetics, and in addition, in special seminars, informal discussions, and in connection with visits from guest lecturers, mostly from the USA.

To summarize, there is nothing in Norway like the ethics committees and Institutional Review Boards of hospitals and clinics in the USA. There is no formal bioethical authority anywhere in the Norwegian system. Formal health policy decision-making in the field of medical genetics occurs at several levels in the NNHS. The Norwegian parliament calls the tune by providing, or refusing to provide, the necessary funds. On the government administrative level there are two important organs: The National Directorate of Health (Helsedirektoratet) and the Ministry of Health and Social Services (Sosialdepartementet). Both may issue medical genetics policy directives of a national scope.

The city of Oslo is a special case. The original "home" of medical genetics in Norway is the Institute of Medical Genetics at the University of Oslo. For almost a quarter of a century, this was the only one of its kind in Norway, and the policy that was formulated and followed here was, for all practical purposes, national policy. Of particular interest is a joint statement of principles and policies for the practice of medical genetics, including prenatal diagnosis, which was developed in 1978 and which has, in fact, functioned as a general set of guidelines for the practice of medical genetics in Norway (Stortingsmelding 1981–82, pp 36–40).

## 2.14.4.2 Major Controversies

The sharpest and most heated controversies that have arisen about medical genetics in Norway have turned on two issues. One concerns the ideology of genetic counseling. Representatives of the "moral minority" and others have voiced anxiety over the insufficient non-directiveness of present counseling practices. They fear that counselors are advocating prenatal diagnosis and are not presenting other options. Some members of the Association of Christian Physicians have argued that the counselor should advise sexual abstinence for people who are at risk of having children with genetic diseases, rather than offering prenatal diagnosis during pregnancy. We believe, however, that this view is shared by only a small number of people.

The other controversy is over recourse to selective abortion after prenatal diagnosis when the diagnosis reveals an affected fetus. This is somewhat surprising in view of the fact that there is free abortion in Norway. Some suggest that the explanation is to be found in a general desire to limit the number of abortions. But the number of abortions "caused" by prenatal diagnosis is so small that this explanation is hardly a rational one. It is more likely that there is fear of having abortions done on the indication of a medical diagnosis that "pronounces" the affected fetus unworthy of life.

The skepticism among the moral minority about the use of genetic screening for public health purposes is not shared by Norwegian geneticists. This controversy is probably explained by the fact that the general public has a less than adequate knowledge of what can and cannot be done by means of contemporary genetics.

In conclusion, it is worth repeating that the "moral minority" *is* a minority. There is a very visible conflict today between the traditional cultural and moral heritage and an ongoing process of secularization. The coexistence between these two trends is often uneasy. It will probably continue to be uneasy, and, as often in the past, unpredictable with regard to outcome. No wonder that Norway is a country of surprising compromises.

## 2.14.4.3  National Expenditures for Medical Genetics

An estimated 6–7% of the gross national product is spent on health care in Norway. Resources spent on medical genetics represent a minuscule fraction of this (see 2.14.1.2 above).

## 2.14.4.4  Abortion Laws in Norway

The present abortion law of June 13, 1975 with modifications introduced on June 16, 1978 was implemented on January 1, 1979. The law gives the pregnant woman the right to choose to have a pregnancy interrupted until the end of the 12th week of pregnancy, counted from the first day of the last menstrual cycle. After that time a pregnancy may be interrupted if:

a) the pregnancy, delivery, or care for the child can damage the woman's physical or mental health;
b) the pregnancy, delivery, or care for the child can cause a difficult social situation for the woman;
c) there is a great risk that the child will have a serious disease due to inherited factors, or a disease caused by exposure to damaging elements during pregnancy;
d) the woman became pregnant under conditions that seriously violated her freedom to choose or as a result of an incestuous relationship;
e) the woman has a serious psychiatric illness or is seriously mentally handicapped.

In connection with items a, b, and c the total living situation of the woman shall be taken into consideration, including her possibilities of caring for the child. The woman's own judgement counts heavily in the decision-making. The longer the duration of pregnancy, the stronger must the reasons be for termination to be permitted. After the 18th week of pregnancy, the reasons must be very strong to permit termination. If there is reason to believe that the fetus could survive outside the uterus, permission to terminate can only be given if the continuation of pregnancy would be life-threatening to the woman.

In the guidelines for the law, a serious genetic disorder in the fetus is specifically mentioned as an acceptable reason for pregnancy interruption after the 18th week. The magnitude of the risk of a serious genetic disorder in the fetus required for second trimester termination is not stated, but the law's term "great danger" means that at the very least the risk must be significantly greater than in the population at large.

The debate concerning the abortion law of 1975 with its amendments of 1978 was very heated in Norway and probably affected politicians' views on prenatal diagnosis significantly. One is left with the impression that after the fight against a liberal abortion law had been lost, its antagonists continued their fight through resistance to prenatal diagnosis.

## 2.14.4.5 Studies of the Effectiveness of Genetic Services in Norway

There has been no systematic study of the effectiveness of genetic services in Norway. For genetic counseling, no parameter to measure effectiveness can be based on reproductive outcomes, since counseling is non-directive.

A woman must be at high risk to have prenatal diagnosis in Norway; therefore the potential cost-effectiveness of prenatal diagnosis is obvious. The high cost of keeping the handicapped in hospitals or institutions means that the annual expenses for prenatal diagnosis would probably be covered if two to three pregnancies where the fetus has Down syndrome were terminated every year. As stated in 2.14.1.4 above, cost-effectiveness is generally not considered as a relevant factor in a discussion concerning prenatal diagnosis. It may be observed, however, that the ethical committee of the MRC, in its manifesto on the ethical problems of genetic counseling, says expressly that "social and economic considerations ... are not acceptable as an ethical basis for genetic counseling."

Geneticists have the impression that the great majority of people receiving genetic counseling or prenatal diagnosis feel that the services are very helpful. The level of acceptance of prenatal diagnosis is very high in women who are offered it. This holds true even after a previous pregnancy has been interrupted due to findings from prenatal diagnosis. Thus, women who have a pregnancy interrupted because of a neural tube disorder in the fetus practically always return for prenatal diagnosis in their next pregnancies.

## 2.14.4.6 Need for New Laws

It is hard to imagine any danger of abuse in medical genetics in Norway, such as obligatory prenatal diagnosis if an affected child has been born, or a demand from society that pregnancies should be terminated if the fetus has a serious genetic disorder. Norway already has a law forbidding embryo manipulation and embryo research.

There is definitely a need for better protection of genetic information about individuals, and this protection should probably be incorporated in a new law. Traditionally, life insurance companies, pension funds, employers and certain educational institutions may request health information at intake as well as later. The life insurance companies have applicants sign an agreement that the company is free to obtain clinical and health information from any doctor or hospital. Insurance is refused, delayed, or very costly if a person is considered at significant risk.

Developments in medical genetics have produced new possibilities for discovering disease risks. Thus, the detection of genetic markers closely linked to disorders that become manifest only in middle age (such as Huntington disease) will almost certainly lead to definite disease prediction in young healthy people in families with serious dominant disorders. At present, life insurance companies and others have the right to ask for the result of any predictive test, and this of course would not benefit the person in question. Furthermore, genetic factors suggesting a predisposition toward frequently occurring disorders, such as atherosclerosis or obstructive pulmonary disease, are already known. There is every reason to expect that the new DNA technology will result in numerous possibilities for testing for predisposition to disease. There is little doubt that insurance companies and others would be most interested in information of this type. The danger is that disclosure of results of predictive tests, which can be used to one's disadvantage, may make people very reluctant to use predictive tests. Beneficial use of predictive tests, such as taking preventive measures against early coronary heart disease where there is a predisposition, could do much to reduce or postpone illness. Every effort should be taken to promote such beneficial use. This consideration argues strongly in favor of a new law that would make it unlawful for insurance companies, pension funds, employers, educational institutions and others to ask an individual who at present is healthy for the results of predictive tests or to have such tests done.

Present practices concerning the use by life insurance companies and others of clinical and health information started long before society became conscious of the right that citizens should have to protection of data concerning their health and private lives. Present practices would be impossible to introduce today. There is a need for a thorough review of these practices to see whether or not they are justified. It is of the utmost importance that the new possibilities for predictive testing resulting from research progress in medical genetics are kept outside the reach of insurance companies and other institutions. A law is urgently needed.

## 2.14.5  Ethical Issues and Future Trends

**Impact on Ethical Issues**
Important ethical and legal issues already exist in the area of predictive genetic testing (2.14.4.6). Problems caused by inadequate rules for handling of information resulting from predictive tests will doubtless increase, unless adequate legal steps are taken in the near future.

In the neighboring country of Sweden a decision has been made to screen all ten-year-old schoolboys for alpha-1-antitrypsin deficiency, a genetic anomaly known to predispose to obstructive lung disease. If the legal situation is similar to the Norwegian situation today, it is easy to predict that life insurance companies and others will in the future ask for the results of these tests. It is particularly worrisome that these tests will be conducted long before the person has an adult's right to agree to or refuse participation in a screening program.

Ethical issues related to predictive testing will persist, even if new laws are introduced. Thus, one may question the right of a person belonging to a family with a disorder such as Huntington disease to withhold the result of predictive testing from the spouse, since if the person carries the Huntington disease gene it has very serious consequences also for the spouse. More than once, people who unknowingly have married a person belonging to a family with Huntington disease have stated that they would not have had any children had they known about the disease risk.

If a person can cause great harm to many others, society may want to limit the person's right to full protection of health-related information. A bus driver or pilot with early Huntington disease could be a hazard to others, and at first glance it may seem reasonable that a physician in charge of pilots' health should have access to results of predictive tests. A system permitting this could still exclude life insurance companies and pension funds from such access. On the other hand, it could be argued that the frequent health examinations and function tests of pilots are more than adequate to detect early signs of a serious disease, such as Huntington. The best guideline seems to be a system that secures as normal a life as possible for as long as possible for at-risk individuals.

Developments in prenatal diagnosis will doubtless make first trimester chromosome and other analyses easily available. The legal situation in Norway in effect makes it possible for a couple to have an abortion if the fetus is not of the preferred sex, even if healthy. This is so because until the end of the 12th week of pregnancy, a woman can have an abortion if she asks for it. It is difficult to see how this dilemma can be handled. Withholding information about the fetus' sex until after the 12th week of pregnancy, as has been practiced in Denmark, would not be legal in Norway if the woman requested that information. It would be ethically questionable to establish such a rule in a law, since refusing to give the information would be in conflict with the principle of respect for the counselee's autonomy.

Genetic therapy is likely to become a reality in the next several years. As long as such therapy is done only on somatic cells and only for serious disorders, it is difficult to see any major ethical problems, apart from those of determining priorities between extremely expensive treatment for a very small number of patients and actions that could help many more people. Genetic therapy on embryos would be questionable, because genes introduced into the embryo could be passed on to hundreds of new generations and appear in an almost infinite number of combinations with other genes. There is a definite possibility that some of these combinations could have unfortunate consequences for the individual.

It seems likely that the introduction of genes into embryos and insertion of the genetically altered embryo into the uterus will be outlawed in many countries within the next few years. There would not be a need for genetic therapy for embryos, unless one wanted to avoid pregnancy termination at almost any cost. If knowledge about a disease is sufficiently advanced that genetic therapy of the embryo can be contemplated, it would almost certainly be possible to detect the disease by prenatal diagnosis. Such diagnosis, followed by selective abortion when the fetus is affected, would be a much more cautious approach than introducing a new gene that could be transmitted to thousands of people in the future.

When genes affecting intelligence or temperament are identified, some people might want to use prenatal diagnosis and selective abortion to make sure that they only have children with a high IQ. Such a practice would be questionable, because one cannot exclude the possible other effects of a gene that is of importance for intelligence or temperament. Furthermore, having an IQ in the middle part of the normal range rather than towards its upper end is by no means a disease. Accepting a wish for high IQ as a reason for prenatal diagnosis could lead to its use to select for other characteristics that are not related to disease.

336

## Serious Ethical Issues in Norway

The "most serious ethical issues in the near future" in Norway seem to be the following: increased demand for genetic services; carrier screening for common genetic disorders; and allocation of limited resources. This statement is a summary of the answers given on the survey questionnaire. None of the Norwegian respondents felt that sex preselection, long-range eugenic concerns, or research on the human embryo would be issues of any importance at all in Norway in the next 10-15 years. Development of new treatments for genetic disorders was, however, mentioned by three as being of the greatest importance.

## What Ethical Resources Will Medical Geneticists in Norway Draw Upon to Face These Issues?

We believe that there are four points to stress in answering this question. In the first place, we expect that the emergence of a serious and *professional discipline of biomedical ethics*, the beginnings of which are already visible, will provide entirely new possibilities for consultation and enlightened discussion of bioethical issues in the future. There is no reason to think that Norway will turn out to be different from the rest of the world in this respect. Second, the realization that modern biomedical ethics is in essence an *interdisciplinary undertaking* will recruit to the field not only philosophers, theologians, and lawyers, but also people from the health professions who will feel the need to participate actively in the growth and development of this field. Health professionals will find it ethically unacceptable to leave this field to people from non-medical professions. Third, ties with bioethics activities in countries outside Norway will be strengthened. Again, the trend is already in this direction. Finally, we expect developments within what we have called "the moral minority." As serious work in bioethics proceeds in Norway, theologians, perhaps along with members of the Norwegian Association of Christian Physicians, may be expected to join in the efforts to raise the general level of medical ethics debate in Norway to a more professional and clinically useful level. Poor arguments in ethical debates are in themselves unethical, because in the longer run they are likely to be counter-productive.

## Towards Consensus

Although it may be impossible to give a reasonable estimate of *how much* we expect the variation described in 2.14.3 to diminish, there is every reason to think that it will diminish rather than increase. So far it is a common experience, both in Norway and in other countries, that when reasonable and educated people get together to discuss bioethical problems calmly and in their proper setting, the trend towards *consensus* is much stronger than the forces that might otherwise pull us apart. In essence, Norway is a very homogeneous country, culturally AND morally. Variations within our moral scene are modest in comparison with many other countries. So we believe that future developments toward more systematic and serious cultivation of bioethics as an open and interdisciplinary field will also cement and strengthen some of the moral ties already in place. The new consensus will be on a more adequate level of conscious awareness and argumentation.

**Society's Ability to Guide Medical Genetics in Ethically Acceptable Paths**
The society at large has until now had little to offer in the way of ethical guidance for Norwegian workers in medical genetics. One of us (KB) tried to initiate a discussion of ethical issues related to prenatal diagnosis in the early 1970s (Berg 1973, 1979a, 1979b), but there was very little response. Public interest in the matter began only after the heated debate concerning the new abortion law. It seems that medical geneticists themselves have always been well ahead of the community at large in discussing ethical issues. Ethical awareness among medical geneticists in Norway as well as in many other countries seems to be the best guarantee that work will continue along ethically acceptable paths. Anxiety and inadequate knowledge among the public, however, could lead to demands for restrictive rules and prohibitions that would hurt those needing medical genetics services. It is hardly possible to imagine a development where the medical geneticists of Norway would embark upon irresponsible practices. Any failure of Norwegian society's ability to provide ethical guidance will not be on the permissive but on the restrictive side.

# Acknowledgements

Part of this paper was written while one of us (KB) was a Scholar-in-Residence, Fogarty Center for Advanced Study in the Health Sciences, National Institutes of Health, Bethesda, MD, USA.

# References

Berg K [1973] Lecture. Yearbook of the Norwegian Academy of Science and Letters, Oslo
Berg K (1979a) Den prenatale diagnostikk. Medisinsk egenlovmessighet eller etisk styring? Kirke og Kultur, 58–62
Berg K (1979b) Prenatal diagnostikk: praktiske og etiske aspekter. Kirke og Kultur, 476–488
Berg K (1985a) Etiske problemer i forbindelse med genetisk veiledning. Medicinsk Årbog, Munksgaard, København, pp 19–28
Berg K (1985b) Etiske sider ved gendiagnostikk. Forskningsnytt 29: 51–55
Berg K (1985c) Etikk og medisinsk genetikk. In: Neegaard G (ed) Moderne Medisin og Etikk, NKS Forlaget, Oslo, pp 87–104
Berg K (1985d) Hva blir engstelsens pris? Nord. Med. 100: 134–135
Fletcher JC, Berg K, Tranøy KE [1985] Ethical aspects of medical genetics: A proposal for guidelines in genetic counseling, prenatal diagnosis and screening. Clin Genet 27: 199–205
Medical Research Council, Committee on Research Ethics [1981] Etiske problemer vedrørende genetisk veiledning (Ethical problems in genetic counseling). [English summary] Oslo
Stortingsmelding 73 (1981–82) Report to parliament from the Ministry of Social Affairs on the organization of medical genetics services in Norway. Oslo

# 2.15 Ethics and Medical Genetics in Sweden

E. Bischofberger, J. Lindsten, and U. Rosenqvist

## 2.15.1 Medical Genetics in Sweden

### 2.15.1.1 Scope of the Problem

At the end of 1985, Sweden had 8.4 million inhabitants. During 1975-1984, the annual number of births varied between 92,120-104,235, of which 246-603 (3.7-5.8 per 1,000 births) were stillbirths. The perinatal and infant mortality rates varied between 7.3-11.3 and 6.4-8.6 per 1,000 births, respectively.

There is no general register of genetic diseases in Sweden, but the incidence of many disorders can be obtained from several national registers, mainly the Medical Birth Registration (since 1973), the Cytogenetic Register (since 1978), the Register of Congenital Malformation (since 1964), and the Register of Mentally Retarded Children (since 1978). Furthermore, some individual clinical scientists keep their own registers of certain genetic diseases, e.g., coagulation disorders, cystic fi-

**Table 2.15.1.** Causes of Childhood Mortality (0-14 years) in Sweden in 1984[1]

| Childhood mortality and its causes | | Age group | | | |
|---|---|---|---|---|---|
| | | <1 week | 1 week - 1 year | 1-14 years | all[2] |
| Overall mortality | No | 309[3] | 292[3] | 266 | 867 |
| | % | 3.3 | 3.1 | 0.18 | 0.57 |
| Congenital malformations | No | 117 | 105 | 30 | 252 |
| | % | 38 | 36 | 11 | 29 |
| Other causes of perinatal, neonatal, and infant death | No | 166 | 46 | 1 | 213 |
| | % | 54 | 16 | 0.4 | 25 |
| Accidents, intoxi- cation, violence | No | 0 | 7 | 99 | 106 |
| | % | 0 | 2 | 37 | 12 |
| Malignancies | No | 3 | 4 | 66 | 73 |
| | % | 1 | 1 | 25 | 8 |
| Disorders of the nervous system | No | 1 | 20 | 16 | 37 |
| | % | 0.3 | 7 | 6 | 4 |
| Infectious diseases | No | 16 | 12 | 7 | 35 |
| | % | 5 | 4 | 3 | 4 |

[1] Data provided by Anders Ericsson, the Swedish Board of Health and Welfare
[2] The mean population for 1-14 years of age was 1,434,904 and for 0-14 years of age 1,527,528
[3] The total number of births was 93,889

**Table 2.15.2.** Incidence (number per 10,000 births) of certain malformations in Sweden 1973-1984[1] (s = single, m = multiple births)

| Diagnosis[2] | 1973-81 | | 1982 | | 1983 | | 1984 | |
|---|---|---|---|---|---|---|---|---|
| | s | m | s | m | s | m | s | m |
| Anencephaly | 1.76 | 0.55 | 1.07 | 0.11 | 0.87 | 0.43 | 0.64 | 0.11 |
| Spina bifida | 3.52 | 0.49 | 3.55 | 0.21 | 2.83 | 0.54 | 2.67 | 0.32 |
| Encephalocele | 0.46 | 0.37 | 0.43 | 0.43 | 0.54 | 0.33 | 0.11 | 0.11 |
| Hydrocephaly | 1.17 | 0.97 | 1.83 | 1.07 | 1.41 | 0.54 | 1.07 | 0.64 |
| Cleft lip | 14.73 | 2.38 | 14.61 | 2.15 | 17.50 | 2.72 | 15.07 | 2.35 |
| Esophageal atresia | 1.30 | 0.94 | 1.50 | 0.75 | 1.41 | 0.65 | 0.75 | 1.07 |
| Anorectal atresia | 1.58 | 1.47 | 0.75 | 0.75 | 1.09 | 1.09 | 0.85 | 0.85 |
| Congenital heart defects | 10.55 | 4.84 | 11.82 | 4.41 | 11.74 | 3.37 | 13.56 | 3.42 |
| Diaphragmatic hernia | 1.46 | 0.90 | 0.86 | 0.86 | 1.20 | 0.54 | 0.85 | 0.11 |
| Omphalocele | 1.57 | 1.05 | 0.54 | 0.64 | 1.20 | 0.98 | 1.92 | 0.53 |
| Hypospadias | 12.09 | 0.81 | 10.53 | 0.43 | 13.26 | 0.87 | 3.07 | 0.53 |
| Limb reduction defects | 4.26 | 1.81 | 2.79 | 1.83 | 3.15 | 1.52 | 3.74 | 1.18 |
| Down syndrome | 8.53 | – | 10.42 | – | 13.80 | – | 9.14 | – |

[1] Data provided by Anders Ericsson, the Swedish National Board of Health and Welfare
[2] For details see Ericsson et al. 1977, Iselius et al. 1986, and Källén 1987

**Table 2.15.3.** Diagnosis of 425 children who were born in 1978 and who had been reported to the Register of Mentally Retarded Children at the end of 1985. A total of 93,248 children were born in 1978[1]

| Diagnosis | Number |
|---|---|
| Down syndrome | 79 |
| Other chromosome aberrations | 9 |
| Inborn errors of metabolism | 17 |
| Different syndromes, all | 11 |
| tuberous sclerosis | 4 |
| Cornelia de Lange | 2 |
| others | 5 |
| Brain malformations, all | 16 |
| hydrocephaly | 2 |
| hydrocephaly plus spina bifida | 2 |
| microcephaly | 5 |
| porencephaly | 3 |
| others | 4 |
| Prenatal causes, all | 67 |
| infections | 14 |
| multiple malformations | 14 |
| others | 39 |
| Perinatal causes | 32 |
| Postnatal causes | 19 |
| Unknown | 175 |
| Total | 425 |

[1] Data provided by Anders Ericsson and Mats Börjesson, the Swedish National Board of Health and Welfare

brosis and Duchenne muscular dystrophy. The same is true for some associations for handicapped individuals. The degree of ascertainment is bound to vary considerably under such circumstances, but for some disorders it is considered to be very high, e.g., for certain malformations (Ericsson et al. 1977, Källén 1987) and Down syndrome (Iselius et al. 1986).

Childhood mortality and its causes, as well as the incidence of different malformations and causes of mental handicap as obtained from the registers mentioned above, is presented in Tables 2.15.1–2.15.3.

## 2.15.1.2  Organization of Clinical Genetic Services in Sweden

The first Department of Medical Genetics in Sweden was founded in 1922 at the University of Uppsala. Next followed the Departments of Cell Research and Genetics at the Karolinska Institute (1949) and Clinical Genetics at the Karolinska Hospital (1970) in Stockholm. The current resources for clinical genetics services are summarized in Table 2.15.4.

The figures given in Table 2.15.4, however, reflect only part of the genetic counseling and prenatal and postnatal chromosome analyses. Genetic counseling is also provided by clinicians at different departments and hospitals around the country. Furthermore, AFP analyses of serum and amniotic fluid samples are carried out at several departments of clinical chemistry, as are analyses of different inborn errors of metabolism. Screening of newborns for certain inborn errors of metabolism is centralized in one national laboratory, while the diagnosis of neurolipidoses, coagulation and hereditary muscular disorders is centralized in specialized laboratories. Furthermore, ultrasound examinations of fetuses at risk for malformations are done by obstetricians and radiologists at many hospitals. Thus, it is not possible to give an accurate estimate of the total resources available in the country for diagnosis and counseling of all patients with all types of genetic disorders.

**Table 2.15.4.**  Resources for Clinical Genetics Services in Sweden during 1985[1]

| Resource | Number of permanent positions | Budget in millions | |
|---|---|---|---|
| | | SEK [2] | (US $)[4] |
| Physicians | | | |
| specialists | 9.6[3] | 3.3 | (0.5) |
| non-specialists | 3.65 | | |
| Other academic positions | 3.3 | 7.7 | (1.2) |
| Technical/administrative staff | 59.9 | | |
| Other expenditures | – | 3.3 | (0.5) |

[1] Data provided by the five Departments of Clinical Genetics and two additional, minor laboratories
[2] The cost for medical care in Sweden was 96 billion Swedish crowns (SEK) in 1985 (9.4% of the gross national product)
[3] Two of the specialists are professors of clinical genetics
[4] Exchange rate in 1987

On the basis of a committee report issued by the National Board of Health and Welfare (Socialstyrelsen 1976), clinical genetics was established as a separate specialty in the Swedish medical care system in 1977. The report recommended that there should be one department of clinical genetics in each of the six regions of the country, each region having 1–1.5 million inhabitants. At present there are five such departments, and each department is responsible for the organization of clinical genetic services within its region.

## 2.15.1.3 Prenatal Diagnosis

Routine analysis of amniotic fluid cells and chorionic villi are centralized in the five departments mentioned above and two additional, minor laboratories. Officially, there is no national policy on indications for prenatal diagnosis, but such a policy has developed through contacts between the laboratories within the frame of activities of the Swedish Society for Medical Genetics (a section within the Swedish Medical Society). This policy is summarized under 2.15.3.2.

The numbers of cases referred for genetic counseling and prenatal as well as postnatal cytogenetic analyses during 1985 are given in Table 2.15.5. The policy on indications for prenatal diagnosis is discussed below in section 2.15.3.2.

**Table 2.15.5.** Number of Cases Referred for Genetic Counseling and Number of Cytogenetic Analyses in Sweden during 1985[1]

| Type of service | Number of cases |
| --- | --- |
| Genetic counseling (excluding prenatal diagnosis) | 989 |
| Chromosome analysis | |
|     peripheral blood | 3,744 |
|     skin biopsy | 380 |
|     bone marrow | 608 |
|     other tissues | 178 |
| Prenatal cytogenetic analyses | |
|     amniotic fluid cells | 4,156[2] |
|     chorionic villi | 181[2] |
| Indication for prenatal cytogenetic diagnosis | |
|     maternal age over 35 years | 2,535 |
|     anxiety | 430 |
|     other | 385 |
|     not specified | 987 |

[1] Data provided by the five Departments of Clinical Genetics and two additional, minor laboratories

[2] Of the 4,337 cases studied 85 were found to have an abnormal karyotype

## 2.15.1.4 Cost-Benefit

A health economic analysis of the Swedish neonatal metabolic screening program was published in 1982 (Alm et al.). Only costs and benefits which could be expressed in terms of money were included in the calculations (e.g., hospital care, outpatient visits, and institutional care). It was found that the most effective means by which the efficiency of the screening program could be optimized was to improve the screening coverage from 98 to 100% and to reduce the number of false positive screening tests.

## 2.15.1.5 Abortion

The numbers of abortions for genetic indications after the 18th week of gestation carried out during 1976–1985 are presented in Table 2.15.6. Since abortion is free, and socially tolerated, the figures given in the table are considered to be reliable. Indications are registered only for abortions performed for special reasons. Thus, the proportion of early abortions carried out because of neural tube defects diagnosed at ultrasound screening and chromosome aberrations detected by analysis of chorionic villi is not known.

## 2.15.2 Ethical Problems Faced by Medical Geneticists in Sweden

The following major ethical problems were identified in the Swedish responses to the questionnaire used in the present survey:

**Table 2.15.6.** Number of Liveborn Children and Legal Abortions in Sweden during 1975–1985[1]

| Year | Liveborn children | Legal abortions | |
|------|-------------------|-----------------|---|
| | | total | after 18th week of gestation (with fetal abnormality) |
| 1975 | 103,632 | 32,526 | 323 (–) |
| 1976 | 98,345 | 32,351 | 331 (–) |
| 1977 | 96,057 | 31,462 | 330 (34) |
| 1978 | 93,248 | 31,918 | 333 (37) |
| 1979 | 96,255 | 34,709 | 344 (63) |
| 1980 | 97,064 | 34,887 | 338 (83) |
| 1981 | 94,065 | 33,294 | 264 (67) |
| 1982 | 92,748 | 32,602 | 256 (81) |
| 1983 | 91,780 | 31,014 | 266 (83) |
| 1984 | 93,889 | 30,755 | 269 (93) |
| 1985 | 98,463 | 30,838 | 237 (90) |

[1] Data provided by Anders Ericsson, the Swedish National Board of Health and Welfare

343

## 2.15.2.1 Genetic Counseling

- how to balance the respect for the patient's right to information about her/himself with the duty to protect relatives from harm by providing genetic information which may be useful to them;
- whether of not to disclose non-paternity;

## 2.15.2.2 Prenatal Diagnosis

- whether or not to use prenatal diagnosis for determination of sex;
- lack of resources for prenatal diagnosis (most likely due to an ongoing debate on whether more resources would result in a change in attitudes towards severely handicapped persons);

## 2.15.2.3 Genetic Screening

- the ethical problems associated with presymptomatic diagnosis of genetic disorders with late onset.

## 2.15.2.4 Other Contexts

In addition, the following situations present ethical problems to many medical geneticists in Sweden today:
- that semen, but not ova, can be used for donation, which has caused discussion about the equal value and rights of the two sexes;
- that donor semen may be used for insemination, but not for in vitro fertilization (this position might change as a result of a law in preparation).
- that research on embryos fertilized in vitro will only be allowed until the 14th day after fertilization according to preliminary norms published by the Department of Health and Welfare. It is felt that this may hamper future research on in-vitro fertilization and embryonic therapy.

## 2.15.3 Consensus and Variation in the Approach to Ethical Problems

The Swedish responses to the questionnaire were very similar to those from the other participating countries. The differences were generally small and can probably be explained by differences in available resources for clinical genetics services. The only major differences were found in the cases on prenatal diagnosis for maternal anxiety and physicians' access to the results of screening in the workplace. The answers indicated that prenatal diagnosis is performed on wider indications, and that the physician's right to obtain information about the results of occupational screening might be somewhat stronger in Sweden. The fact that the autonomy of the individual was the value that ranked highest in most answers is in accordance with this observation. The questions regarding surrogate mothers and prenatal selection of sex were found to be the most controversial issues.

## 2.15.4 Cultural Context of Medical Genetics in Sweden

**Three Contexts for Discussion of Ethical Problems**

Three contexts for discussion have been used for ethical problems in Sweden. First, several major ethical issues have been openly and widely debated in the mass media. Members of different professions, including medical geneticists as well as laypersons, have participated in this debate. Second, some issues related to certain methodologies, e.g., in vitro fertilization, prenatal diagnosis, and artificial insemination, have been subject to official reports by committees appointed by the government. Third, there are a number of institutions for ethical discussions in the country, which ensure a thorough ethical analysis and stimulate moral awareness. These activities should promote a readiness to address new problems in the hope of reaching consensus.

Resources to analyze ethical problems used by medical genetics include the following public institutions and government committees:

The National Department of Health and Social Services, the National Board of Health and Welfare (exercising the function of supervision) and the County Councils (with financial and operational responsibility for all the public health services within a region) are the main public institutions available as resources for the analysis of ethical problems in Sweden.

The *Recombinant DNA Technique Committee* (government appointed) published an official report, "Recombinant DNA Technique under Control," in 1978, which prompted the appointment of a National Recombinant DNA Advisory Committee in 1979.

In 1984, the *Gene-Ethics Committee* (government appointed) presented a report entitled "Genetic Integrity." The Committee suggested that research on embryos is acceptable, provided that it is medically well-founded and performed within 14 days after fertilization. Moreover, the committee stated that the use of DNA-based prenatal diagnosis should be restricted to severe genetic diseases, i.e., diseases that threaten the development of the fetus or the child. It also proposed that DNA-based diagnosis may be used in public health investigations of genetic diseases, provided that the investigation has a clear medical aim and that genetic information concerning the individual is reliably protected. These proposals are at present under evaluation.

*The Insemination Committee's* first official report, "Children by Insemination" [1983], led to a law on artificial insemination, which came into force on March 1,

345

1985. According to this law, the sperm donor must be identifiable and registered. Furthermore, the woman must live in a stable (heterosexual) relationship, and the insemination must be performed in a public hospital.

The Committee's second report, "Fertilization Outside the Body," proposed that in vitro fertilization (IVF) is acceptable for couples with a stable (heterosexual) relationship. Both donation of ova and sperm donation in combination with IVF, as well as surrogate motherhood, should be prohibited.

### Prenatal Diagnosis

A group of experts, including medical geneticists, appointed by the National Board of Health and Welfare, presented a report in 1982 regarding the application of prenatal diagnosis (Socialstyrelsen 1982). This report has become well-known in the medical community at large and also among a number of official organizations. The groups proposed that financial and other resources to perform amniocentesis and laboratory analysis should be offered in the following instances:

- all women 37 years or older;
- selectively between 35 and 37 years of age;
- if a woman has previously given birth to a child with a chromosome anomaly or metabolic disorder, or if such defects can be anticipated;
- if the woman has previously given birth to a child with a neural tube defect or if the AFP levels are abnormal;
- the sex of the fetus should only be determined for medical rather than for social reasons.

This program has been nationally adopted without having been enforced by the legal authorities.

The report was submitted to many legal, political, religious, and scientific institutions as well as to single individuals for consideration. About 100 responses were received. An overwhelming majority approved the following points of the proposed program:

- the pregnant woman must be absolutely free to accept or to reject prenatal diagnosis, but has no absolute right to demand it;
- prenatal diagnosis should be provided for medical indications;
- the current view is that the legal right of the woman to abortion should be maintained, no matter what reason she has for her decision. The Christian Democratic Party and the Archbishop of the Swedish Church, however, argued in favor of limiting the right of the woman in this respect;
- the right to give birth to a defective child must be respected;
- the woman should get full information concerning the results of prenatal diagnosis. Some respondents, however, suggested that information on the sex of the fetus should be withheld;
- prenatal diagnosis should be put under the control of public health authorities. No private activity in this field should be allowed. A few respondents from the right-wing political scene as well as from some regional health authorities felt that prenatal diagnosis should also be extended to private medical practice;

346

- there is no need for a new law regulating the practice of prenatal diagnosis, but guidelines should be provided by the National Board of Health and Welfare;
- prenatal screening involving all pregnant women was almost universally rejected (see also 2.15.4.1).

## Ethics Committees and Councils

During 1965–1967, ethics committees were appointed at each medical school in Sweden to review research projects. Today the activities of these committees are coordinated by the Ethics Board of the Swedish Medical Research Council, thus contributing to a more unified policy of judgment and action in the area of medical research.

In 1969, the Swedish Medical Society established a Delegation for Medical Ethics, and in 1985 the National Board of Health and Welfare appointed a Council of Ethics. In addition, in 1985, the Swedish government appointed the National Medical Ethics Council, comprising 17 members (7 politicians and 10 experts). This latter council received its guidelines from the Department of Health and Social Services to function as a bridge between the scientific community and the political decision-makers. Its task is to acquire an overall view and to evaluate the long-term effects of research and technical development within the biomedical field.

## Non-official Publications

The Swedish Medical Society published the document, "Ethical Aspects of Prenatal Diagnosis" [1979], in which the ethical aspects of prenatal diagnosis were discussed in detail. In contrast to the preparatory work to the abortion law of 1975 (see 2.15.4.4), the Society emphasized the importance of the right to life of the fetus over the autonomy of the mother. This document has had a great influence on ethical discussion during subsequent years.

On behalf of the Bishops' Conference of the Swedish Church, an ecumenical group of experts (Fagerberg et al. 1980) concluded that prenatal diagnosis could be morally accepted in principle, because,

- in most cases it preserved human life;
- it paved the way for future treatment;
- it helps the fetus to be viewed and treated in its own right.

Despite the apparent advantages of prenatal diagnosis, the group called for restrictions on its use, because one aim is to abort defective fetuses. In addition, authors of several books have debated the problem of prenatal diagnosis (Gustafson 1980, 1984, 1986; Fagerberg et al. 1985; Bischofberger and Seiler 1986). In addition, a prize-winning film ("The Trial," Prövningen, 1986 by Margaret Garpe), which described a young couple considering the pros and cons of prenatal diagnosis while awaiting the result of amniocentesis, has effectively brought the debate to public attention.

## Teaching of Medical Ethics

There are no permanent teaching positions in medical ethics in Sweden, but rather each medical school has its own limited teaching program. The students are taught the elements of ethics in lectures and seminars, often using actual cases as an illustration of ethical problems. In this program, which is mostly interdisciplinary, ethical implications of medical genetics attract special attention.

## 2.15.4.1 Sources of Challenge and Support for Medical Genetics

In their answers to the 1982 report on prenatal diagnosis by the group of experts (Socialstyrelsen 1982) the *Archbishop of the Swedish Church and the Council of Free Churches* supported those aspects of medical genetics which emphasize research on treatment, and not only diagnosis of fetal defects. The idea that modern clinical genetics might negatively affect society's view of handicapped people was also put forward. This debate is continuously followed up and critically commented upon by two monthly Christian magazines, "Vår Lösen" (Lutheran) and "Signum" (Catholic). The Christian vision of man is emphasized by these magazines and underlines the humanistic position, i. e., that the value of the person is not bound to a certain bodily constitution. The mere existence of a human being accords her or him uniqueness, genetic integrity, and right to life.

The *women's organizations of the political parties* represented in the national parliament are strong supporters of the autonomy of women with respect to all abortion decisions. On the other hand, the Christian Democrats, a small party represented in the regional and local assemblies only, have a much more restrictive view. They fear that weak members of society might be defenseless in a system that promotes "genetic quality control."

*Physicians in general* are opposed to prenatal screening of all pregnant women but favor the program suggested in the 1982 report by the group of experts described above (Socialstyrelsen 1982). The general attitude was expressed in the following way by a professor of gynecology: "The interest of the pregnant woman is decisive. The interest of the fetus and of society are subordinated to that of the woman. Her feelings decide what to do. Society must offer her its help – not take command over her."

The various *associations of handicapped persons* constitute a powerful movement in Sweden in a cultural as well as in a political and social sense. From the beginning, they had a positive attitude towards prenatal diagnosis because they thought it was an instrument for the prevention of handicaps. After the debate that has taken place during the last few years, however, these associations have, on the whole, taken a more critical stand. Some, e.g., the Association of Handicapped with Visual Defects, developed a hostile attitude towards prenatal diagnosis, with no wish to compromise, because they felt that it was an existential threat to themselves. On the other hand, the National Association of Handicapped Children and Adults – an association dominated by handicapped children's parents – proposed to expand genetic counseling and prenatal diagnosis: "We think that each woman who wishes it should get prenatal diagnosis."

In his three books previously mentioned, Sture Gustafson, a journalist and radio reporter, was critical about what he felt was the premature introduction of prenatal diagnosis before society had a chance to debate its moral implications.

He summarized the debate between 1978–1984 by arguing that the main reason for genetic screening and prenatal diagnosis was economic. He also felt that the humanitarian argument, which is usually put forward, is not valid since it only obscures the underlying economic reasons. In a society where competition and profit are given preference and unemployment is accepted, he felt that handicapped people run a greater risk of being stigmatized.

## 2.15.4.2 Major Controversies

The most pronounced attitudes in the current ethical discussion on prenatal diagnosis can be summarized as follows:

The *non-compromising attitude* against all prenatal diagnosis is mainly represented by some associations of handicapped persons.

The *economic attitude* is openly represented by very few persons but is covertly represented – under the camouflage of a humanitarian attitude – by some politicians confronted with growing expenses and forced to cut the budget. They plead for an expansion of prenatal diagnosis.

The *emancipatory attitude* is mainly represented by some political women's organizations. They too advocate an expansion of prenatal diagnosis, but from a different ideological base than those who support the economic attitude.

The *humanitarian attitude*, which is rather non-restrictive, is represented by the medical profession, most political groups, most religious groups, and many mainstream interest groups.

## 2.15.4.3 National Expenditures for Medical Genetics in Sweden

See Table 2.15.4.

## 2.15.4.4 Abortion Law in Sweden

The present Swedish abortion law was instituted on January 1, 1975. According to this law, abortion is permitted within the first 18 weeks of gestation (a social worker has to be consulted after the 12th week). The decision is formally made by the pregnant woman alone. Later abortions are allowed, provided that there are "special reasons," and in such cases approval has to be obtained from the National Board of Health and Welfare. The upper time limit is determined by viability. Hence, abortions after the 22nd week of pregnancy are extremely rare.

### 2.15.4.5  Studies of the Effectiveness of Genetic Services

Studies on the effectiveness of the different genetic services in Sweden are very few indeed and limited to prenatal cytogenetic diagnosis (Jonsson 1980) and AFP screening (Schnittger 1983).

### 2.15.4.6  Is There a Need for New Laws to Protect Against Possible Abuse of New Genetic Technologies?

The present Swedish laws that regulate medical services are comprehensive and should protect society from misuse of new genetic technologies. Moreover, the professional organizations as well as the Department of Health and Social Services have, as mentioned previously, their own ethical committees. These institutions function well and have brought important issues to medical and public attention. Thus, we do not foresee a need for new laws at present.

## 2.15.5  Ethical Issues and Future Trends in Medical Genetics

Looking ahead 10–15 years, we expect that ethical issues related to medical genetics will attract even more attention than they do today, because more sophisticated techniques will allow a detailed understanding of the function of, and possibilities to interfere with, the genetic material. The mapping of the human genome – whatever the scope of this research may be – does not seem, however, to satisfy our thirst and yearning for the unknown. Medical genetics will not give the ultimate answer to our self-understanding and identity. Instead, it has opened new areas for anguish and inescapable choices, and in this respect it accentuates our existential condition. The questions will then be whether the choices are made with the moral maturity that the advanced technology requires.

Thus, the fact that medical genetics, like many other fields of human activity, seems to be guided by its own technical possibilities and promises raises the question whether we are capable of handling and governing our own technical creations with reason and conscience. Increasing refinement of our technological ability, whether genetic or not, to elucidate structures and functions could give rise to a view of the human being as a mosaic of traits rather than as an integrated unity. This possibility could, but need not necessarily, lead to devaluing of the individual on the basis of one or a few unwanted, but not seriously threatening, traits.

Today, it is difficult to evaluate the long-term impact of the fact that prenatal diagnosis has emphasized that the fetus has unique traits. This might very well lead to an earlier parental bonding with the fetus, which in turn could strengthen the moral position of the fetus. On the other hand, because prenatal diagnosis can also identify unwanted traits, the moral position and rights of the fetus could be weakened. Whereas prenatal diagnosis is rather abortion-oriented at present, it is hopeful to note that research in the field is more treatment-oriented.

350

There is growing risk that the psychological and ethical uneasiness created by prenatal diagnosis and other applications of recent technological developments might be transferred to other areas of the biomedical field, such as fertilization techniques and neurobiology. The desire to find out and to control with even more precise instruments is likely to create requests for further knowledge. New ethical problems are therefore likely to arise. The sensitivity to ethical problems that has developed in recent years must therefore be nurtured, and the awareness of such problems broadened in the society.

The ethical resources in Sweden, as presented in 2.15.4, seem to be sufficient to meet moral conflict today as well as in the near future. The variation in moral opinions and positions is likely to widen, but also, in some aspects, to diminish. In this context, we would like to make a distinction between, on the one hand, *basic moral principles* (such as personal integrity, each person's human dignity and equal value, equality of opportunity and equal access to public health services) all of which are widely accepted, and, on the other hand, *application of such principles* in the balancing of values where there is much controversy and diversity of opinion. The conflict arises when there is no consensus about which value should have priority over the others. For example, in a clash of interests and values, does the right of the woman to obtain information about the genetic constitution of the fetus, and thus to abort the fetus with an unwanted defect, take priority over the right to life of the fetus? In Sweden, a pragmatic solution to this problem has been reached. Each woman has, as already mentioned, the exclusive right to decide whether she wants to continue or to terminate her pregnancy. She can receive significant information about her fetus, and she retains the right to abortion, although within certain limits. If, for the time being, the consensus in Sweden is not to limit the right of the woman, the question is then how society can deepen its moral responsibility.

The common and generally accepted values mentioned above are not theoretically questioned, but are often violated in practice. Thus, in the debate the question has been asked whether there exists one official, public moral standard and another, covert moral standard, which is widely practiced under the shield of public declarations of the official moral standard. The public, official values are humanitarian and idealistic, while the covert values sometimes are destructive but real. Now and then a gap may exist between the official humanitarian and the covert values. There is concern that the latter could be adopted by a future economy-minded political elite, which under the disguise of democratic and humanitarian intentions ("the defective child must not suffer") might introduce compulsory genetic screening combined with pressure to abort.

Despite the potential conflicts and seriousness of the problems discussed, Sweden can, in our opinion, be considered an ethically oriented and morally engaged society with many common values and institutionalized forms of dealing with new ethical challenges. This constitutes our basis for taking the optimistic view that Swedish society will be able to cope successfully with the ethical issues raised by medical genetics.

# Acknowledgement

The authors are grateful to Dr. Shirley Bach for valuable discussions.

# References

Alm J, Larsson A, Rosenqvist U [1982] Health Economic Analysis of the Swedish Neonatal Metabolic Screening Programme. A method of optimizing routines. J Med Decision Making 2: 33–45

Bischofberger E, Seiler H (eds) [1986] Etiska riktmärken vid livets gränser II. Katolska bokförlaget, Uppsala

Ds U 1978: 11 Hybrid-DNA tekniken under kontroll. Liber förlag, Stockholm

Ericsson A, Källén B, Winberg J [1977] Surveillance of Malformations at Birth: A Comparison of Two Record Systems Run in Parallel. Int J Epidemiol 5 [1]: 35–41

Fagerberg H (ed) [1980] Foster Familj Samhälle. Liber läromedel, Lund

Fagerberg H, Bischofberger E, Jacobsson L, Lindmark G [1985] Medicinsk etik och människosyn, 2nd ed. Liber förlag, Stockholm

Giertz G [1984] Etik i läkarens vardag. Svenska Läkaresällskapets förlag, band 93, häfte 1

Giertz G (ed) [1976] Etiska värderingar – medicinskt handlande. Svenska Läkaresällskapets handlingar, Band 85, häfte 1

Gustafson S [1980] Fosterdiagnostik – för vem? LTs förlag, Stockholm

Gustafson S [1984] Vem har rätt att födas? LTs förlag, Stockholm

Gustafson S [1986] Kunskapens frukter och livets träd. Verbum förlag, Stockholm

Jonsson M [1980] Fosterdiagnostik inom Stockholmsregionen. En kartläggning av patientinformationen. Rapport från projektet för patientinformation Karolinska sjukhuset, Stockholm

Källén B [1987] Search for Teratogenic Risks with Aid of Malformation Registries Teratol 35: 47

Schnittger A [1983] Alpha-fetoprotein screening in obstetric practice. Thesis, Linköping University, Linköping

Socialstyrelsen Hälso – och sjukvård inför 80- talet [1976] Klinisk genetik. Supplement till Medicinsk service. Stockholm

Socialstyrelsen [1982] Fosterdiagnostik. Stockholm

SOU 1983: 42 Barn genom insemination. Liber förlag, Stockholm

SOU 1984: 88 Genetisk integritet. Liber förlag, Stockholm

SOU 1984: 5 Befruktning utanför kroppen mm. Liber förlag, Stockholm

Svenska Läkaresällskapets Delegation för medicinsk etik [1979] Etiska synpunkter på fosterdiagnostik. Läkartidningen 76: 2540–2542

# 2.16 Ethics and Medical Genetics in Switzerland

E. Engel and C. D. DeLozier-Blanchet

## 2.16.1 Medical Genetics in Switzerland

Switzerland is a small country, in which the limited area (41,000 km$^2$) and number of inhabitants (6.5 million) contrast sharply with a number of demographic features that render Switzerland unique. The 23 states, or "cantons," employ three different languages and several dozen dialects; the cultural and economic differences between them are often significant. Of the five principal schools of medicine, two (Geneva and Lausanne) are situated in French-speaking Switzerland, whereas three (Bern, Zurich, and Basel) are in German-speaking regions. Genetics centers developed within the preexisting medical faculties, which had their germination in ancient times within the walled cities. Given the disparity of languages and mentalities within our country, generalizations concerning the practice of medical genetics – except to say that the common goal of Swiss geneticists is to serve their patients and their regions well – would be misleading.

Historically speaking, the first genetics center in Switzerland was created by Dr. A. Franceschetti who, in 1947, opened a human genetics service within his ophthalmology clinic, with the goal of studying the frequency and the distribution of hereditary diseases in our country [11]. The intellectual climate had of course been prepared by such pioneers as Bleuler, Brugger, Hanhart, Lehmann, and Schinz. The establishment of parochial and communal registries, the stable population, which was little modified by two World Wars, and a people generally educated and open to research in the domains of genealogy and genetics, all contributed to create a favorable terrain for the geneticist. Nonetheless, only in the past ten years have the five medical schools come together to create the Swiss Society of Medical Genetics [14]. Although this society is an important link between physicians interested in hereditary diseases, it does not include all of those involved in clinical genetics, for certain laboratory activities are performed outside the university domain. Switzerland has two private cytogenetics laboratories, and a regional hospital in Italian Switzerland is involved in several aspects of reproductive genetics.

It would thus be futile to try to represent Switzerland as a homogeneous country as far as the practice of medical genetics is concerned.

### 2.16.1.1 Scope of the Problem

*a) Number of Births per Year (1975–1985).* Over the past ten years the number of births in Switzerland has fluctuated little; the lowest was in 1978, with 71,373 births, whereas the peak occurred in 1982, with 74,916.

*b) Incidence of Genetic Disease and Congenital Malformation.* The exact incidence of congenital anomalies in Switzerland is unknown, due to the federalistic structure of the government and to important gaps in documentation of congenital problems. However, it can be assumed that some 2-3% of liveborn infants (1500-2200 babies per year) in Switzerland, as elsewhere, have congenital malformations or important genetic problems.

*c) Childhood Mortality and Congenital Malformations.* The incidence of infant mortality from congenital anomalies, measured from the day of birth until the end of the first year, can be summarized as follows: between 1976-1980, the figure oscillated between 0.37-0.41%, but began a steady decline as of 1981, from 0.36% to 0.28% in 1985. If we examine the breakdown of congenital malformations resulting in infant death in 1985, we see that nearly one-third of the deaths were secondary to congenital heart malformations (although the proportion was even higher several years ago); given the high frequency of such anomalies, this figure is less than surprising. We might, in a second group, include those malformations which were responsible for 5-10% of deaths from congenital problems; these were chromosomal syndromes (9.1%), multisystem malformations (7.7%), anomalies of the digestive (6.7%) and respiratory (6.3%) systems, as well as neural tube defects (7.6%) and hydrocephalus (5.8%). Ocular, urinary, neurologic, skeletal or muscular anomalies, along with metabolic causes, each accounted for between 2-5% of the deaths from congenital malformations. Among those accounting for less than 2% of this mortality, cystic fibrosis was responsible for 1.4% of deaths (Office Fédéral Suisse de la Statistique, Service de la Statistique Fédérale Sanitaire, Bern, personal communication, 1986).

We can thus observe that, whereas chromosomal aberrations are the cause of nearly 10% of deaths from congenital malformations (which points out the need for more widespread use of prenatal diagnosis), mortality from Mendelian disorders is relatively rare. It is striking that, among the genetic or partially-genetic causes of neonatal death, anomalies of multifactorial etiology account by far for the greatest proportion.

## 2.16.1.2 Organization of Clinical Genetics Services in Switzerland

*a) Description of the Centers, the Geneticists, and the Services Offered.* The five university medical genetics centers each offer the principal services required for diagnosis and counseling in medical genetics. Included are, of course, clinical genetics consultations, cytogenetic studies, and biochemical analyses (direct analysis of DNA is a recent addition). An important proportion of the laboratory work is devoted to prenatal diagnosis. In addition to the clinical and laboratory aspects, each genetics center is involved in the teaching of medical and paramedical personnel, and, to diverse degrees, in clinical research. Each genetics center is headed by an M. D., generally a university professor. This person is aided by several senior collaborators and a variable number of interns and residents. The team is completed by technical and clerical personnel.

Clinical geneticists from Switzerland, as from other countries participating in the current survey, provided, in response to a written questionnaire, professional and demographic data, which allow comparisons between clinical geneticists in Switzerland and those from the other countries. In fact, there were few differences between Swiss geneticists and the average profile of medical geneticists world-wide. The average age, sex, marital status, type of professional training and years of experience (as revealed by the questionnaire) were remarkably close to the overall means. In regard to professional background, this may reflect the fact that most medical geneticists practicing in Switzerland trained for at least part of their careers in other countries, notably the United States.

The organization of the week's work in medical genetics in Switzerland was also very similar to that in other countries (total number of hours, number of patients per week, number of hours in the laboratory). However, the number of hours spent in administrative genetic tasks was extremely variable among Swiss geneticists, which may well reflect the varying hierarchical ranks of the respondents (in a university system which is itself hierarchical).

The five university genetics centers compose the nucleus of the Swiss Medical Genetics Society, which includes a small number of active members (about two per genetics center) and a much larger body of associate members. The active members are generally professional full-time geneticists, whereas any member of the medical community (including Ph. D. geneticists, nurses, etc.) may be an associate member. The Society publishes a biannual bulletin of medical genetics, which informs the medical community of the essential developments within our specialty [14]. Each issue includes a list of genetic counseling and laboratory facilities, a schedule of courses and seminars held in the university genetics departments, and a bibliography of recent publications from each center. In addition, review articles on selected subjects and a reference list for general use are provided. The Society also holds an annual meeting, often in conjunction with colleagues from related branches, such as pediatrics or obstetrics. The Society and its publication are the most obvious aspects of the cooperation, actually rather poorly developed, between the different medical schools in our country and genetics departments.

*b) Postnatal Chromosome Studies.* Although the number of postnatal chromosome studies performed in Switzerland each year is unknown, the figure would be of little importance in our opinion; in our liberal system, requests for cytogenetic studies are often accepted even in the absence of a strong clinical indication. This is not to say that there is no selection of cases, but rather that such an "open-door" policy encourages the very individualistic doctors in our country, particularly those in private practice, to more often consider cytogenetic explanations for their patients' difficulties, and thus leads to diagnosis in a certain number of cases that would not otherwise come to study. This apparent availability of laboratories, which are nonetheless overworked, is probably greater in the French-speaking regions of Switzerland, which are generally considered to be less structured and disciplined. To be effective, such a policy must of course be accompanied by the dispersion of information fostering improved knowledge of medical genetics to the public and to the medical community.

Over the 7-year period from 1980–1986, nearly 2,000 postnatal chromosomal studies were completed at the University Medical Genetics Institute in Geneva; 188 (nearly 10%) resulted in detection of a chromosome aberration. Even this information concerning Geneva is somewhat fragmentary, however, for the nonnegligible proportion of postnatal studies done by the private cytogenetics laboratory here is unknown to us. Although we have the impression that relatively few individuals with clinically obvious cytogenetic anomalies remain undiagnosed, any geneticist knows that Klinefelter syndrome and other anomalies of the sex chromosomes may, because of their clinical subtlety, elude diagnosis. Although the number of postnatal cytogenetic studies done in Geneva has increased considerably over the past few years, a calculation makes it obvious that a proportion of cytogenetic aberrations remain undiagnosed: in a population of 300,000–400,000 individuals, some 1,500–2,000 should carry a cytogenetic abnormality; only about 10% of this number have been diagnosed in our laboratory over the past 7 years (and the number of cytogenetic studies done prior to that time in Geneva was quite limited). A similar situation probably exists in other parts of Switzerland, although some centers perform a greater number of postnatal cytogenetic studies, of which more give a positive diagnosis, since such laboratories must apply stricter criteria for the acceptance of samples.

*c) Investigation of Genetic Diseases.* Once again, Switzerland, with its diversity and its federalist system, has as yet no national registry for congenital malformations and genetic diseases, although an infrastructure is slowly being put into place to provide such statistics. Efforts toward centralization in the past have encountered conceptual divergences. Thus, certain regions of Switzerland, divided between two linguistic influences, have turned towards Gallic or Germanic countries for collaboration. The "Club Européen de Conseil Génétique," a French-speaking group, has such a registry; efforts at documentation on a multi-nation level are also undertaken by EUROCAT [4].

*d) Genetic Counseling.* An effort is made to provide genetic counseling to the parents of each infant in whom a chromosomal anomaly or other genetic problem is diagnosed, at least as far as the genetics institutes are informed of these cases. In Geneva, for example, over a period of 7 years, 2,013 consultations (either at the Institute or in various hospital units) were given, at a rate of 300 consultations per year. Not all of these consultations were for parents of children with congenital malformations, however; the total includes both genetic counseling for adults, and a sizeable number of counseling sessions organized prior to amniocentesis or chorion villus sampling.

In Geneva, it is our impression that we see the parents of most infants born with chromosomal anomalies, as well as the majority of those with multiple malformations. In the case of isolated malformations, however, particularly those which are well-known to the medical community (heart malformations, neural tube defects, clefts, etc.), counseling for the parents often seems to come from the family doctor, the pediatrician, or the obstetrician.

Although similar figures could be given for the other university hospitals with genetics services, the total number of genetics consultations is certainly less than the number of families suffering from congenital or hereditary anomalies. And it is even more difficult to estimate counseling in the cases born in private or district hospitals that have no geneticist available.

## 2.16.1.3 Prenatal Diagnosis

*a) Description of Services.* Each of the five universities with a department, institute, or division of genetics is involved in prenatal diagnosis. Aside from these five, as mentioned earlier, a regional hospital in the Italian part of Switzerland offers cytogenetic services, as do private laboratories in Geneva and Zurich. Most efforts are, of course, mobilized to detect chromosomal anomalies. An indication of the growing demand for prenatal diagnosis is that, whereas some 8,000 amniocenteses were performed in Switzerland from 1971–1980, in the most recent three-year period (1984–1986) the corresponding figure was nearly 17,500 [16].

*b) Breakdown of Cases by Indication and Results. Main Indications.* A review of the years 1981–1983 [15] reveals that almost two-thirds of the approximately 12,000 prenatal tests were performed for a maternal age of 35 or greater (Table 2.16.1). Slightly more than one-fourth of women choosing amniocentesis were under 35 and came for medically non-specific reasons, such as maternal anxiety or cytogenetic control of a pregnancy achieved by artificial insemination. Considerably less frequent were other genetic indications, such as a chromosomal anomaly in a previous infant (2.5% of amniocenteses were performed for previous trisomy 21), a previous neural tube defect in a parent or sibling (1.7% of tests), or the presence in one parent of a chromosomal variation, usually a balanced translocation (0.5% of cases). In addition to these diverse categories, summarized in Table 2.16.1, amniocentesis was also performed because of serially-elevated AFP levels in the maternal blood or for the detection of metabolic disorders.

*Abnormal Results.* Of 7816 analyses of amniotic fluid done for maternal age, 132 (1.7%) were abnormal (Table 2.16.1), including 127 (1.6%) that were aneuploid. In the case of tests done because of a cytogenetic anomaly in a previous infant, the incidence of aberration was 1.9%. More surprising is the fact that no case of unbalanced translocation was documented among the 56 pregnancies tested because one of the parents carried a balanced translocation.

Table 2.16.2 gives additional information concerning the aberrations diagnosed during the years 1981–1983. Aside from the analyses of amniotic fluid done for maternal age that were aneuploid (1.6%), studies without a specific medical indication done on women under 35 (such as parental anxiety) revealed a chromosomal aberration in 10 (0.3%) of 3,175 amniocenteses, and a non-chromosomal anomaly in 3 others (total abnormal = 0.4%, Table 2.16.1). This incidence, although five times lower than that found in women over 35, is far from negligible.

A new method of prenatal diagnosis, the first trimester sampling of chorionic villi (which we call choriocentesis), has recently become available. The application of this technique implies the same ethical problems as does amniocentesis, but

357

**Table 2.16.1.** Prenatal Diagnosis in Switzerland

| Indications | 1981–1983 | | | | 1984–1986 | | | |
|---|---|---|---|---|---|---|---|---|
| | Number of tests | | Pathologic result | | Number of tests | | Pathologic result | |
| | n | % | n | % | n | % | n | % |
| Maternal age (35 and over) | 7,816 | 64.9 | 132 | 1.7 | 10,548 | 60.4 | 207 | 1.9 |
| Maternal anxiety, artificial inseminations by donors, etc. (Mostly women under 35) | 3,175 | 26.4 | 13 | 0.4 | 5,204 | 29.8 | 35 | 0.7 |
| Previous aneuploid pregnancy (i.e., child with trisomy 21) | 297 | 2.5 | 5 | 1.9 | 325 | 1.86 | 8 | 2.5 |
| Abnormal maternal alphafetoprotein levels | 251 | 2.1 | 30 | 11.9 | 533 | 3.03 | 33 | 6.2 |
| Open neural tube defects in family (usually in earlier pregnancy) | 200 | 1.7 | 3 | 1.5 | 229 | 1.31 | 5 | 2.2 |
| "Obstetrical indication." Post-20th week amniocentesis for abnormal echography, hydramnios, etc. | 173 | 1.4 | 37 | 21.4 | 419 | 2.4 | 63 | 15.0 |
| Chromosomal aberration in one parent (mostly balanced translocation) | 56 | 0.5 | 0 | 0 | 82 | 0.47 | 6 | 7.4 |
| X-linked recessive disorders (carrier mother for hemophilia, muscular dystrophy, etc.) | 42 | 0.3 | 10 | 23.8 | 54 | 0.3 | 15 | 27.8 |
| Metabolic disorder (usually parental heterozygosity for an autosomal recessive disease) | 28 | 0.2 | 3 | 10.7 | 58 | 0.33 | 14 | 25.8 |
| Total | 12,038 | 100.0 | 233 | 1.93 | 17,452 | 100.0 | 386 | 2.2 |

**Table 2.16.2.** Details of Pathologic Results

| Results | Indications | | | | | | | | | | | | | | | | | | | |
| --- | --- | --- | --- | --- | --- | --- | --- | --- | --- | --- | --- | --- | --- | --- | --- | --- | --- | --- | --- | --- |
| | Maternal Age >35 | | Obstetrical Indication | | Maternal Alphafetoprotein | | Maternal Anxiety | | X-linked recessive | | Aneuploid offspring | | Spina Bifida in family | | Metabolic | | Parental translocation | | Total | |
| | 1981–3 | 1984–6 | 1981–3 | 1984–6 | 1981–3 | 1984–6 | 1981–3 | 1984–6 | 1981–3 | 1984–6 | 1981–3 | 1984–6 | 1981–3 | 1984–6 | 1981–3 | 1984–6 | 1981–3 | 1984–6 | 1981–3 | 1984–6 |
| Trisomy 21 | 72 | 92 | 1 | 10 | – | 1 | 5 | 4 | – | – | 1 | 3 | – | 1 | – | – | – | 1 | 79 | 112 |
| Trisomy 18 | 18 | 21 | 3 | 9 | 2 | 2 | – | 1 | – | – | 1 | 1 | – | – | – | – | – | – | 24 | 34 |
| Meningomyelocele | 4 | 6 | 3 | 3 | 8 | 11 | 1 | 2 | – | – | 2 | – | 1 | 1 | – | 1 | – | – | 19 | 24 |
| Anencephaly | – | – | 10 | 11 | 6 | 3 | – | 1 | – | – | – | – | 2 | 1 | – | – | – | – | 18 | 16 |
| 47, XXY | 15 | 17 | – | – | – | – | – | 3 | – | – | – | – | – | – | – | – | – | – | 15 | 20 |
| Malformation, hydrops | – | 2 | 8 | 9 | 4 | 7 | 2 | 2 | – | – | – | – | – | 2 | – | – | – | – | 14 | 22 |
| Turner | 5 | 13 | 4 | 5 | – | 1 | 1 | 3 | – | – | – | 2 | – | – | – | – | – | 1 | 10 | 25 |
| X-linked recessive disorder | – | – | – | – | – | – | – | – | 10 | 14 | – | – | – | – | – | – | – | – | 10 | 14 |
| Unbalanced karyotype | 5 | 20 | 1 | 4 | 2 | 2 | 1 | 4 | – | – | – | 1 | – | – | – | – | – | 4 | 9 | 35 |
| Abdomen wall defect | 1 | 2 | 3 | 3 | 5 | 5 | – | 1 | – | – | – | – | – | – | – | – | – | – | 9 | 11 |
| Trisomy 13 | 5 | 6 | 2 | 3 | – | – | 1 | – | – | – | – | 1 | – | – | – | – | – | – | 8 | 10 |
| De novo balanced translocation | 3 | 11 | – | – | 1 | 1 | 1 | 8 | – | – | 1 | – | – | – | – | – | – | – | 6 | 20 |
| Triploidy | 2 | 2 | 2 | 6 | 2 | – | – | – | – | – | – | – | – | – | – | – | – | – | 6 | 8 |
| 47, XXX | 2 | 10 | – | – | – | – | 1 | 1 | – | – | – | – | – | – | – | – | – | – | 3 | 11 |
| Autosomal recessive metabolic disorder | – | – | – | – | – | – | – | – | – | – | – | – | – | – | 3 | 13 | – | – | 3 | 13 |
| 47, XYY | – | 5 | – | – | – | – | – | 5 | – | 1 | – | – | – | – | – | – | – | – | – | 11 |
| Total | 132 | 207 | 37 | 63 | 30 | 33 | 13 | 35 | 10 | 15 | 5 | 8 | 3 | 5 | 3 | 14 | 0 | 6 | 233 | 386 |

with an added dimension. While choriocentesis has the advantage of being performed earlier in pregnancy than amniocentesis, it generally carries a higher risk of spontaneous abortion than does the latter test. An additional problem is that, in some 2% of cases, the cytogenetic results obtained from the study of this material seem to reflect principally the situation in the chorionic villi, without being truly characteristic of the fetal genotype. Such a situation can lead to an abortion that is probably unnecessary, but which the knowledgeable geneticist can sometimes avoid, particularly by suggesting an amniocentesis to investigate the karyotype in fetal, rather than extrafetal cells [6].

In a country as conservative as Switzerland, it is interesting to mention that the testing of this method, now available in the five university medical centers, began rather early here, as compared to the introduction of the technique elsewhere. Development of the necessary obstetrical and cytogenetic methodology began, for example, in our center in 1983 [3], the same year in which the meetings of the American Society of Human Genetics included several memorable presentations on the subject.

As we were completing this chapter additional information on prenatal diagnosis in Switzerland, for the years 1984–1986, became available [16]. These data are summarized in the right hand columns of Tables 2.16.1 and 2.16.2. In comparing the figures for the two periods, several trends become evident:

1) The total number of tests, nearly 17,500 for the latter three-year period, increased by nearly 40%. These data include prenatal diagnosis by chorionic villus biopsy, which accounts for a growing percentage of the total. In 1981–1983 trials were underway, but clinical application of choriocentesis had not begun. The 1984–1986 figures, on the other hand, include over 1,000 diagnoses achieved by this newer technique.

2) When we consider the indications for testing, a smaller proportion of analyses were done in 1984–1986 for advanced maternal age (60.4% vs. 64.9%) or because of a previous aneuploid child (1.86% vs. 2.5%) than in the three preceding years. An important increase, on the other hand, was observed in the category "obstetrical indication" (2.4% vs. 1.4%) and in a "new" group, i.e., low maternal alpha-fetoprotein (now the indication for 1.1% of tests).

3) Although the overall proportion of prenatal evaluations performed to detect hereditary (often metabolic) autosomal and X-linked recessive disorders changed little from 1981–1983 to 1984–1986, in an increasing proportion of situations the question could be specifically addressed by DNA analysis, rather than by the conventional methods of fetal sex determination or of enzymatic determinations.

4) As far as abnormal results are concerned, these represented 2.2% of the total (compared to 1.93% for 1981–1983). For the indications of maternal age and previous aneuploid child the figures were 1.9% and 2.5% respectively. Concerning the tests done because of a chromosomal alteration in one parent, 6 of 82 pregnancies monitored (7.4%) were cytogenetically abnormal, whereas no such unbalanced fetuses had been detected in the 1981–1983 tests. Of the cases submitted to prenatal diagnosis because of maternal anxiety (and various other indications), 0.7% were found to be abnormal, once again a surprisingly high figure.

5) The percentage of pathological results observed in the category of abnormal maternal alphafetoprotein decreased in the second period; this is primarily be-

cause low AFP levels, a recent indication for testing, are associated with a lower relative risk of fetal abnormality than are high AFP levels, a classic indication. Fewer pathological results (15.0% vs. 21.4%) were observed when sampling was done for obstetrical reasons, presumably reflecting the growing use of amniocentesis for evaluating late stages of pregnancy, even if only moderately abnormal.

*c) Policy on Indications for Prenatal Diagnosis.* Although there is currently neither legislation nor formally-accepted guidelines on the criteria for prenatal diagnosis in Switzerland, the medical indications are well-enough defined that a tacit consensus on who should receive prenatal diagnosis exists between the various services. To the classical indications of advanced maternal age, a previous chromosomal anomaly, and the risk of recurrence of a neural tube defect, the finding of low AFP levels in maternal blood can now be added as an indication for prenatal diagnosis. Amniocentesis for metabolic studies or to allow direct analysis of the DNA is, of course, becoming more frequent. The prenatal diagnostic policies of the five Swiss centers are not fundamentally different concerning the indication of parental desire/anxiety. Such requests are accepted, on the condition that the person(s) involved have been counseled concerning the benefits and risks of prenatal diagnostic procedures. At the Geneva Institute we frequently have such counseling sessions, in which we attempt to counsel nondirectively by putting into perspective the advantages of the test versus the risks that it carries. In certain instances, however, the reimbursement of the test may be refused, if the indication for prenatal diagnosis is judged insufficient. There are some differences in attitude concerning another category of motivation for amniocentesis, i.e., pregnancy following multiple spontaneous abortions or subsequent to the birth of a handicapped but chromosomally normal child. In Geneva, we mention to these couples the existence of prenatal diagnostic tests, while explaining that they would not serve to detect such a problem as was present in the previous infant. The choice is then left to the informed parents. All genetics centers in Switzerland abhor the application of prenatal diagnosis to the selection of fetal sex for reasons of parental desire; when such a motive is known, prenatal diagnosis is refused.

In spite of the relative philosophic harmony among the various genetic centers in Switzerland concerning prenatal diagnosis, there are, for geographic and religious reasons, important differences concerning access of the population to genetic services. Since Switzerland is composed of a mosaic of 23 states, only five of which have a medical faculty, the result is that most cantons (states) do not have easy access to a genetics center. In practical terms, prenatal testing is often available to only a part of the population, since the possibility of study depends on a laboratory in another region. This problem is aggravated by the fact that many cantons lacking laboratories for prenatal diagnosis are located in conservative, primarily agricultural regions, in which the religious environment is often unfavorable or even hostile to prenatal diagnosis.

## 2.16.1.4 Cost-benefit of Early Diagnosis and Genetic Counseling

Economically speaking, it is difficult to discern the relationship between the costs of genetic counseling activities, on the one hand, and the financial impact of the results, on the other. For any such consideration of the subject, we must, in any case, distinguish between the process of genetic counseling and prenatal laboratory activities.

Very little information is available about the budgets of the various departments and institutions that are involved in such reproductive services. Even with such figures in hand, however, it would be necessary to compare them with an estimate of the expenses that were avoided as a result of genetic counseling and prenatal diagnosis. Each birth of a child handicapped by trisomy 21 or other viable chromosomal anomaly involves an annual economic cost of several thousand dollars for physical care alone. The moral obligation to assure not only adequate physical care, but educational and recreational facilities for these individuals further increases these expenses. It is the opinion of the authors that the cost of thousands of prenatal tests, of which fewer than 2% will result in the detection of abnormalities, is only a fraction of the money that would necessarily be spent if these methods of prenatal detection were not available. It is easier to count what is spent by the taxpayers than to keep a registry of what would have been spent if certain situations had occurred (such as the case of a trisomic infant, who was never born because the parents, aware of the defect through prenatal testing, decided to end development before the 20th week of pregnancy). Putting aside notions of quality of life, as well as considerations of the emotional problems raised by these tragic situations, the material cost of the care of an aneuploid infant is considerable. The bill for institutionalization of a child in Switzerland is about $4,000 per month, which represents an annual sum of some $48,000; if this figure is multiplied over 30 years (a common lifespan figure in Down syndrome), it easily reaches one-and-a-half million dollars for each institutionalized individual. In economic terms, then, the sums of money invested to permit this type of prenatal testing are quite justified. It would be beside the point to detail the amount spent in our Institute to accomplish this task of prevention; it probably represents close to a million dollars per year. Even if more were to be spent, the material benefit of the work performed is obvious.

The problem becomes even more abstract if the financial benefits of genetic counseling are considered; savings cannot be calculated in situations where giving concrete information has allowed parents to avoid, before conception, the birth of individuals whose diverse problems would have financial, social, and psychological consequences for both parents and society.

We have concentrated on the financial benefits of early diagnosis and genetic counseling because, even though difficult to calculate, they are perhaps more easily quantified than are the social and psychological benefits to individuals and thus to society.

## 2.16.1.5 Abortions

*a) Incidence of Elective Abortions (1975–1985).* As will be explained later, in spite of the laws regulating the practice of elective abortions, pregnancy termination before 12 weeks is frequently performed in some cantons, including Geneva. Although figures for the number of abortions per year at the maternity hospital in Geneva can be cited, these statistics tell us very little. On the one hand, a certain percentage of women come from other Swiss cantons, as well as from neighboring France or even more distant countries. On the other hand, abortions performed in private clinics are not reflected in these figures. It should also be kept in mind that the indications for these abortions are extremely variable, ranging from termination because of a maternal infection or disease with a high risk to the fetus, to pregnancies with abnormal progression, to abortion for purely social or economic reasons. Keeping these reservations in mind, however, the statistics show that each year from 1978–1986 some 750–1150 abortions were performed at the University Maternity Hospital.

In our personal experience, if we consider the biased group of women who come to us for genetic counseling, we note in taking family histories that an important proportion of women have had at least one elective abortion. This fact, and its relative acceptance by a part of the population, paradoxically reflects the high standard of living in this country, for once people have control over all of the basic needs and desires in their lives, control over reproduction and reproductive options is also considered a right.

*b) Elective Abortion/Livebirth Ratio.* An exact ratio cannot be calculated but must be relatively high in view of what has just been stated under a), namely a cultural acceptance of early pregnancy interruption for social reasons. The progress of contraceptive methods, however, particularly hormonal contraception, should decrease the number of situations where interruption becomes a necessary, even though avoidable, evil.

*c) Incidence of Abortion Following Genetic Diagnosis.* The frequency of such terminations is almost negligible, if compared with the incidence of abortions performed for other reasons. In our liberal genetic counseling system, we note that, whereas all parents who learned of a trisomic fetus chose to abort, this was not the case for those whose fetuses were found to have an anomaly of the sex chromosomes or a structural modification of the karyotype [6, 2]. Of 49 cases of cytogenetic anomaly detected in our series of nearly 3,000 amniocenteses, we have observed three of 14 cases of sex chromosome aneuploidy in which the parents decided to continue the pregnancy; in each case a child with a normal physical appearance was born. In several other situations, the detection of an apparently balanced translocation or of a structural rearrangement of benign aspect resulted in continuation of pregnancy, the parents having had in each case a counseling session regarding the risks of abnormalities as well as the chances that the child would be normal. In comparison with the nearly 3,000 pregnancies tested in our series, in which less than 2% had a chromosomal anomaly, the level of abortion is even less than that of abnormality; the ratio of interruptions to pregnancy continuations for the total group tested is truly quite low.

*d) Social Abortion/Genetic Abortion Ratio.* Once it has been shown that the proportion of abortions performed for genetic aberrations is quite low as compared to those requested for social or psychological reasons, it becomes unnecessary to attempt to establish a ratio between the two groups in Switzerland.


## 2.16.2 Ethical Problems Faced by Medical Geneticists in Switzerland

Switzerland is a country of contrasts in which, although technical and scientific developments are similar to those of neighboring countries, prosperity is much more widespread. This enviable situation is partly the result of historical circumstances, since, with Sweden, Switzerland is one of the countries that has suffered least from the natural and man-induced catastrophes of recent centuries. It is a country of material abundance, in which relatively few forces have intervened to modify traditional values. In Switzerland unemployment is nearly nonexistent, virtually no one goes hungry, and social programs enjoy a priority. Nonetheless, anxiety is widespread, and often accompanied by an ill-defined feeling of guilt. These attitudes and emotions, we feel, play a major role in all aspects of medical genetics activities.


### 2.16.2.1 Genetic Counseling

To some extent, ethical problems result from the relationship between information given to a patient, and the nature and degree of the effect that this information may have on the individual. Several years ago, certain members of the medical community were more concerned about the effects that genetic counseling might have on the patient's psychological balance than about the consequences of the hereditary problem itself. It was common to warn geneticists of the anxiety that the familial clan would suffer following revelatory counseling. This concealing attitude often had the opposite effect, resulting in patients exaggerating the severity of their genetic problems. Over the past decade, however, belief in sincere but nondirective genetic counseling has grown by leaps and bounds, and with the intervention of the media to spread knowledge about means of dealing with once hopeless situations, the public is increasingly better informed. It thus seems to us that genetic counseling – the provision of information concerning a hereditary problem, and the presentation of the options that the family has – is acquiring greater acceptance. In our opinion, the major forces at work in ethical genetic counseling should be: knowledge, conscientiousness, and compassion. Ideally, these should help the patients to replace the guilt, sorrow, and anger from which they suffer with more positive emotions.

## 2.16.2.2  Prenatal Diagnosis

The most prominent ethical considerations in prenatal diagnosis involve problems of adequate access to the tests, and of quality control [10]. When sampling involves human life, there is little place for negligence or ineptitude. In addition, public access to such tests should be diminished neither by limited resources nor by lack of crucial information that would enable couples to decide whether they want to use prenatal testing. Additionally, counseling prior to prenatal diagnosis should be nondirective, leaving to the couple both the choice of its use and the liberty to act upon the results. Although prenatal diagnostic tests are admittedly, and hopefully for a time only, the privilege of technologically well-developed societies, we maintain that they are essential to ensure a certain quality of life for those who, after being adequately informed, request them.

In a country of several religious confessions, in which Protestants and Catholics are nearly equal numerically, it is obvious that attitudes concerning the morality of prenatal diagnosis vary. Thus, in the case of detection of a serious anomaly, the choice of action is influenced both by prevailing religious dogma, and by the individual's or the family's acceptance of such religious concepts. The conflict that sometimes exists between the overall outlook of a social group and the situational pragmatism of the individual is nowhere more obvious than in the following letter, received from a husband whose wife had prenatal diagnosis:

"Subject: The amniocentesis test questionnaire sent to my wife, Mrs. ...
To the attention of Dr. X., Resident
Madam:

The answers given by my wife comply with the facts. I was indeed very well informed, both by our doctor and my wife herself. I gave my consent to the test without any outside pressure. What then would have been my line of conduct if I had been told: "Your child is mongoloid?" I truly do not know. I hope that I would have had the strength to decide that the life of the child be spared, that is to say that I would have accepted him as he was. I believe that my wife would have had this strength of character. As a matter of fact my thoughts, which I set forth to you and about which you might have something to say or write, are as follows:

I have accepted knowingly, willingly, against my religious beliefs, against my mere conscience as an honest, straightforward man to put at risk the life of a human being, the odds being, I believe, in the range of 1/200 (as a matter of fact the probability is without bearing on the ethical nature of the problem).

By doing so my conduct was personally and socially plainly immoral, since the life of someone else was at stake. I am not passing judgment on the behavior of anyone else. But it seems clear that any person who engages in an action does not carry out a morally neutral act; this act is no less neutral than that of the last soldier of the Third German Reich, who was standing guard at the gate in a camp where Jews were on their way to the gas chamber.

It is always Mozart who is assassinated, even if he was mongoloid (Down syndrome).

The geneticists would do well to reread the writings of J. Rostand, *Inquié-tudes d'un biologiste* (The worries of a biologist), and reflect upon the following sentence, among others: 'Perhaps our temporary powerlessness to intervene is in itself a richness.' [Authors' note: What is meant here, we think, is that our inability to intervene in certain medical/biological situations carries its own values since, in spite of its harshness, it demands and teaches valor, courage, and resiliance.]

The ethical side of your inquiry – if it has such a dimension, which I hope it does – is of interest to me not so much from the standpoint of the parents but from that of the practitioner who in my view is, in fact, a potential 'murderer through deception' as much as I was one, to my great shame. Please let me know the results of this inquiry."

On the back of the letter there was an addendum which is as follows:

"This is the innocent potential victim (if she gives me some problems and worries when grown up I will always think that she is giving me change for my money!)"

And then there was a picture showing a lovely normal little girl – the one tested – whose eyes and facial expression were interpreted as follows:

"My life belongs neither to my mother nor my father, nor to society, nor to the medical community, nor to sociologists, nor to social security and insurances,

even though I have slanted eyes,

even though I am idiotic,

even though I am costly,

even though I am a nuisance,

even though I am an object of shame."                                    Véronique

By giving the users of prenatal tests the chance to express themselves, as in this remarkable letter, we can discover the psychological sensitivities, the moral problems and the practical difficulties which give its ethical dimensions to prenatal diagnosis. We thus contacted, by means of a written questionnaire, nearly 1,500 women having opted for amniocentesis, of whom 82% responded [2]. This questionnaire, which will be the object of a later publication, also offered to couples the occasion to comment. The following are some consistent responses from this questionnaire:

- many women underlined their feeling that the information given to couples concerning the goals, limitations, procedures, and difficulties of the prenatal test could never be too complete. Those who had received pre-amniocentesis professional counseling considered it adequate, but only a small percentage of these women had been so counseled;
- the majority of the women, both in their comments and in answer to a specific question, cited their anxiety during the period of waiting for the results, which were often not available before the 20th week of pregnancy;
- many persons, in regard to this same delay, expressed qualms concerning the decision that they would have taken if, instead of reassuring them, as is generally the case, the results would have required a decision concerning the continuation or interruption of the pregnancy.

## 2.16.2.3  Genetic Screening

As mass genetic screening has not yet entered the practice of medical genetics in Switzerland, the ethical problems that could result are still theoretical. Switzerland has no systematic screening programs for specific genetic diseases, since the population, although including 15% foreigners and immigrants, is not under the menace of a particularly frequent and detectable disease, such as sickle cell anemia, the thalassemias and glucose-6-phosphate dehydrogenase or hexosaminidase deficiencies.

There is nonetheless a voluntary program of perinatal screening in Switzerland, which includes the Guthrie test, to detect certain metabolic diseases, as well as congenital hypothyroidism. This perinatal testing is well accepted, perhaps because it occurs almost without notice, and also because there are practical steps to take in the case of abnormal results. The positive attitude of the population toward screening when there is therapy available is of course different from what one could expect in screening for diseases for which there is less adequate therapy.

## 2.16.3  Consensus and Variation in Switzerland

**Results of the Questionnaire**

The ideas relative to consensus and differences of opinion among medical geneticists in Switzerland were drawn from answers to the written questionnaire developed by Drs. Fletcher and Wertz. Situations presented in the questionnaire were divided into five categorical situations; full disclosure of genetic information, confidentiality and duties to third parties; directive versus nondirective counseling; indications for prenatal diagnosis; and screening. The reasons for the responses given by Swiss geneticists to situations posed in the questionnaire, however, as well as the degree of consensus, will become clearer if we first review the goals of genetic counseling stated by these individuals. Swiss geneticists agreed unanimously that the most essential goal of the geneticist is "to help couples understand their options and the present state of medical knowledge so that they can make informed decisions." Opinions on the methods by which this should be done differed, although there was strong consensus that "telling patients what they ought to do" is rarely, or never, appropriate, and that "informing patients what most people would do in their situation" is only sometimes appropriate. In fact, it can be reasonably stated that nondirective counseling, for reasons of patient autonomy and beneficence, is the guiding principle among Swiss geneticists, as among the geneticists of other countries participating in the study.

*a) Full Disclosure of Genetic Information.* Responses related to the five questions treating full disclosure of genetic information revealed strong agreement among Swiss medical geneticists in almost every case. In four of the five situations there was a strong consensus for *disclosing* all information to the patient; only in the case concerning disclosure to parents of who was the carrier of a balanced translocation leading to trisomy 21 was there some divergence in attitude (moderate consensus). On all of these questions the responses of Swiss geneticists, as well as the degree of consensus achieved, were similar to those of other countries in the study. Autonomy of the patients was the dominant reason cited in each example.

In only one of the hypothetical situations would Swiss geneticists, with a strong consensus, choose *not* to disclose information to the patient: this was the case of the phenotypic female with an XY genotype. The reasons involved nonmaleficence. We feel in fact that this is one of the rare exceptions to the "rule" of full disclosure in genetic counseling. It is of interest that there was strong consensus on the decision to disclose or not in less than half of the countries reported, and the overall tally shows (worldwide) that about half of geneticists would disclose the information and half would not. We wonder whether legal questions play a role in that decision in countries where malpractice suits are frequent, unlike Switzerland.

*b) Confidentiality and Duties to Third Parties.* For the questions related to confidentiality and disclosure of information to relatives, there was no consensus among Swiss geneticists concerning disclosure of either Huntington disease (HD) testing or hemophilia A diagnosis, although the decision would be more difficult in the case of Huntington disease. The tendency would be not to disclose the information to relatives, unless asked, but both Swiss geneticists and those of most nations surveyed demonstrated that there is as yet little agreement on this question. This may relate to the fact that at least for HD, sure diagnostic tests have not been available prior to the onset of clinical disease, so that the issues are only now being concretely addressed.

In the third situation presented, concerning the mother's confidentiality versus full disclosure of false paternity, both Swiss geneticists and geneticists from *all* countries demonstrated a strong consensus of opinion: protection of the mother's confidentiality overrides disclosure of true paternity, and this for reasons embracing autonomy and nonmaleficence. In our opinion, this is one situation where the potential *harmful* effects of disclosing that information to persons other than the mother are so strong that the course of action is clear to geneticists.

*c) Directive vs. Nondirective Counseling.* As far as counseling after detection of a 45, X or 47, XYY fetus was concerned, Swiss geneticists, like those in the great majority of countries studied, would give nondirective counseling, with reasons being autonomy or beneficence. In spite of the fact that the 45, X syndrome is medically more severe than the 47, XYY, the approach and the consensus were almost identical in these two cases. There was also a strong consensus, in Switzerland as elsewhere, to give full information to patients when there are conflicting results about a possible neural tube defect; autonomy is again the most important consideration.

In counseling a couple, one member of which has tuberous sclerosis, most Swiss geneticists preferred to inform them of all reproductive options, with the possible exception of surrogate motherhood (no consensus, some would discuss only if asked). The fact that the strongest consensus, both in Switzerland and in other countries, was to inform the parents about adoption and about artificial insemination by donor (A. I. D.) if the father is affected, probably reflects the high chance of "success" (i.e., an unaffected child) that these options carry. Switzerland differed from other countries only in that there was a strong consensus here (moderate or none elsewhere) to discuss the option of IVF with a donor egg when the affected person is the mother.

*d) Indications for Prenatal Diagnosis.* Swiss geneticists were in almost total agreement concerning the course to take in all three questionnaire situations related to prenatal diagnosis. We would perform prenatal diagnosis for reasons of parental anxiety, and for parents who would refuse abortion in the case of anomaly, but would refuse prenatal diagnosis for fetal sexing. The acceptance of the first and second cases in Switzerland, whereas there was little or no consensus among geneticists in many other countries, may well stem from the fact that Switzerland is a privileged country both economically and socially, in which the resources for prenatal diagnosis are not yet fully saturated; it is considered "normal" that parents choose the timing and the conditions of their reproductive life.

The *refusal* of prenatal diagnosis for sex selection, while posing an ethical dilemma for both Swiss geneticists and those of other countries, was agreed upon with a strong consensus. This question was seen by some in Switzerland as presenting the *most* difficult ethical conflict presented in the questionnaire, but by others as the *least* difficult, although all of us would refuse the request. The reasons given were of nonmaleficence and justice. This attitude may change somewhat with the liberalization of abortion laws and the wider availability of first trimester prenatal diagnosis, but Swiss geneticists all feel that abortion because of undesired fetal sex is ethically and morally wrong.

*e) Screening.* For most questions relative to screening tests there was a strong consensus among Swiss geneticists, as among those of other countries. Autonomy and nonmaleficence guide the approaches: screening in the workplace should be voluntary, with access to results of testing for workers only; the results should not be available to employers or insurance companies. Opinion was divided in Switzerland, as elsewhere, about giving this information to the worker's doctor or the government health department even *after* worker consent.

In Switzerland, as in the majority of countries polled, there was a strong consensus that cystic fibrosis testing should be voluntary (only 3 of 19 countries would prefer that it be mandatory). Switzerland, however, favored a newborn screening program, whereas geneticists from other countries were divided as to the appropriate ages for testing.

There was a strong consensus in our country that the *patient* should have access to the results of presymptomatic testing for Huntington disease if he or she desires, and that relatives, school, insurance companies, and employer should *not* have access unless the patient permits it. For Swiss geneticists, as for others, the difficult question was whether the spouse should be informed – there was no consensus on this question. Answers to these questions may well change as we gain personal experience in Huntington testing.

## Dominant Approach to Ethical Problems and Genetic Counseling

Thus, in spite of cultural differences among different regions of Switzerland, which make the practice of medical genetics in this country heterogeneous, those of us who work as clinical geneticists apparently have rather similar ethical guidelines in our practice of genetic diagnosis and counseling. In fact, the main features of the "dominant moral approach to medical genetics" among Swiss geneticists are as follows: 1) respect for parental autonomy (non-directive counseling, full disclosure), 2) fear of inflicting harm on individuals and families, and 3) voluntary programs of screening. In addition, Swiss geneticists strive for an optimal availability of genetic services for all, so that couples have several options in making reproductive decisions.

In the domain of prenatal diagnosis, we previously set down in writing [5, 7] our personal ethical approach and guidelines, which are summarized here:

- Being confronted each day with the grief and suffering resulting from congenital malformations, we recognize that the chances of having normal children are not equal for all couples.
- We firmly believe that the goal of procreation is the birth of healthy children, who enrich their families and their society as a result of the natural physical and intellectual differences characterizing the familial and racial groups of which they are a part.
- The spectrum of congenital malformation begins at the extremes of this natural variation. The former can be distinguished from the latter by the fact, generally evident, that malformations prevent or seriously alter the functions which they affect.
- We recognize the principle that the moral and practical judgments and consequences resulting from the presence of a malformation vary according to the individual, the couple, and the society in which it occurs.
- We confirm that ongoing and evolving medical techniques permit, between the time of conception and birth, the detection of anomalies of development for which there exist absolutely no treatments at present.
- It is the moral responsibility of the specialists involved in these analyses to assure that prenatal diagnostic techniques be well-tested, safe, and accessible to all. It must be the needs of the potential beneficiaries, themselves carefully informed, which dictate the usage of tests.
- Modern science imparts, therefore, knowledge which can no longer be ignored by those possessing it, even if they would so prefer it. Because the parents are, with their children, directly concerned by the events that will so deeply affect their future, we must leave to them the choice of measures that may actually determine their reproductive success.
- The choices offered by prenatal diagnosis must be exercised only in regard to a fetal organism still totally dependent for its existence on the physiology of the mother.

## 2.16.4  Cultural Context of Medical Genetics in Switzerland

### 2.16.4.1  Sources of Challenge and Support

The media, religious assemblies, university and public debates constitute some of the forums in which the various schools of thought concerning genetic intervention meet. We find on this subject, as in all other human conflicts, the customary intellectual bias of those who possess (or think that they possess) the "truth" of the matter, vis-à-vis others who are searching for the answers. Whatever the potential benefits and consequences, certain religious currents will always be categorically opposed to scientific and technical advances that can be applied to procreation and the giving of life. At the opposite extreme, we may fear that if certain interventions and manipulations by laboratory technocrats are not closely monitored, they could exceed the ethical limits of research by seeking to modify our genetic constitution. Some of the major challenges to those involved in medically-inspired genetic intervention result from such absolute doctrines or uncontrolled fantasies. At one extreme are those persons who fear even the simplest genetic intervention and who prefer that nothing be attempted in this area, and at the other extreme are those exalted individuals who see no limit to the list of genetic functions that could be thus modified. When the latter expose their excessive ideas, reinforced by their conviction and the fascination of a credulous public, that public is given a false impression of the existing technical possibilities.

To us, the most reasonable and fertile ethical approach to genetic intervention is one inspired by three basic virtues: conscientiousness, knowledge, and compassion. All three must be present for this ethical approach to function correctly, however; the application of conscientiousness without knowledge and compassion can produce insurmountable dogmatic barriers. This is the case with certain religious inspirations, which we respect, but which, by an excess of zeal, tend to proclaim any intervention as against the will of God. Surmounting this type of attitude seems to be one of the principal challenges to the development of the new human genetics. An opposite danger is posed by those individuals and institutions that are imbued with knowledge, but lack conscientiousness and compassion; such persons or institutions may be infatuated by the power of new techniques, a situation which, in practical terms, could translate into an abusive interventionism with questionable goals. Such excesses are currently kept in check by limitations of our knowledge, the latter being actually insufficient to permit the fundamental correction of even single-gene defects. The dangers of rapidly-developing technology are nonetheless present, if conscientiousness and compassion do not guide their application. Finally, compassion itself, without the reflections and modifications provided by conscientiousness and knowledge, may lead to infractions of medical ethics. The fact that we deplore an incurable genetic fatality for the victims – parents or children – does not justify the use of measures that are poorly tested or poorly directed, as the use of such techniques may produce consequences for which we are guilty and liable. The role that conscientiousness must play in these situations requiring compassion should escape the temperate reflection of none of us.

*a) Religious Influences.* In Switzerland, as elsewhere, certain religious groups fight against any interruption of pregnancy, without considering the individual situation. This is not surprising, since the most radical of these groups are anti-contraception. Militant anti-abortion groups, linking themselves to parochial or ad hoc organizations, are found in all regions of Switzerland. These are not restricted to particular religious denominations, but are rather organized around the nature of the arguments cited. For example, one dogmatic group speaks of the sacred nature of any germ of life, since God formed it in His own image. Others emphasize the inevitable stigma that elective abortions must have on the conscience and the psychological balance of those who, spontaneously or under pressure, will consent to abortion for genetic, material, or emotional reasons.

*b) Legal Authorities.* As far as law is concerned, and aside from the general medical codes, there are very few texts that specifically treat the problems of medical genetics. Intense legal activity is currently underway in this area, but is primarily directed at deciding whether existing clauses of jurisprudence can be applied to new techniques and knowledge. The Swiss law regulating elective abortion is in our opinion an example of the important gap that exists between recent medical innovations and the necessary legal modifications.

*c) Political Parties.* Political parties reflect the same division that exists in other countries, i.e., liberalism vs. conservatism. These varying ideologies, which spring from human nature and will always exist, serve as a separating line in these matters.

*d) Parent Groups and Other Medical Interest Groups.* As in many other conservative societies, the various groups concerned with specific medical disorders are relatively isolated and poorly known. Parental associations have a definite, but somewhat limited, impact on the practice of preventive medicine, with which the new genetics is associated. This is not to say that such groups do not exist; as compared to other nations, however, there is perhaps less coordination between groups, so that the social environment is characterized more by multiple microcosms than by groups with widespread cultural objectives.

Nonetheless, among associations for the handicapped that are active and respected, there is a myopathy association which is very efficient in helping and supporting victims of such diseases. Such organizations also exist for hearing problems, blindness, and cystic fibrosis. These disorders, along with trisomy 21, are the genetic problems with which the general public is most familiar. However, we are not aware of a national parents' group of children with chromosomal anomalies.


## 2.16.4.2 Major Controversies

Major controversies include long-standing issues – selective abortion – as well as recent ones, such as in vitro fertilization and genetic manipulations. With respect to abortion, as already indicated, a recently proposed overhaul of obsolete legislation in this domain was flatly denied by the Swiss Parliament.

The treatment of sterility by in-vitro fertilization and embryo transfer was the object of stringent recommendations by the Swiss Academy of Medical Sciences [1] and the "Bioethics Committee" of the Swiss Federation of Protestant Churches (April 1987). The technologies involved, for which the neologism "procreatic" has been coined, were condemned, but not without dissent, by some other religious wings, as can be read in the "Instructions of the Congregation for the Doctrine of the Faith" delivered on February 22, 1987, and commented upon by Father Gérard Mathon [13]. Thus, these new and irreversible avenues of progress raise and will continue to evoke extreme resistance and criticism in times to come. Finally, great fear and reluctance toward attempts at modifying the human genome – an endeavor which, even though encouraging to us, is still in limbo – are obvious. Unfortunately, even at the least ambitious therapeutic level, not even simple enzymatic defects can be corrected by gene transfer. Yet, genetic engineering in man, severely limited as it is, raises anxieties about the safety, not to mention the morality of tampering with the basic heredity of living beings.

## 2.16.4.3 National Expenditures for Medical Genetics

The sources and the types of funds available to medical geneticists are diverse, but generally rather modest. The five universities with medical genetics centers are the principal financial backers, providing some six to ten million dollars of hard currency annually. The "Fonds National Suisse de la Recherche Scientifique," our equivalent of the United States National Institutes of Health, provides financial support for a certain number of research projects in genetics, although these rarely have immediate practical implications for medicine and genetic counseling. In addition, there exist a certain number of private foundations that contribute to studies of the physiopathogenesis, as well as towards the prevention of certain problems, the origins of which are often genetic or influenced by genetics. For example, the Swiss Foundation for the Encouragement of Research in Mental Retardation, as well as diverse societies interested in muscular dystrophy, cystic fibrosis, blindness, and deafness, allocate funds – on a rather modest scale – to diverse institutions. The major pharmaceutical companies sometimes contribute to research projects involving genetics, particularly when studies have potential in the domain of public health.

Recently a ruling of considerable practical importance, which will set a legal precedent, was handed down by the Federal Tribunal of Insurance in Lucerne, the highest judicial authority ruling on medical expenses covered by insurance companies. The ruling makes it mandatory that health insurance covers the cost of tests involving the preventive, particularly prenatal, detection of genetic disorders.

As far as the country's social security system is concerned, there exists, for the benefit of a certain class of unfortunate citizens obliged to spend large sums because of a congenital malformation or an hereditary disease, a branch called Invalidity Insurance; when strict criteria for inclusion are met, this agency covers a proportion of the expenses involved in the diagnosis and treatment of chronic and debilitating afflictions of genetic or congenital origin.

*a) What proportion of the health care outlay goes to medical genetics?* From the above discussion it should be clear that the proportion of material resources invested in medical genetics in Switzerland is minimal. This is partially the result of the relative lack of attention currently given to this area of public health, but also reflects the fact that some genetic problems are treated with resources allocated to other services or institutions. The public schools, for example, have health services that monitor and follow some such handicaps. Numerous malformative disorders of cardiovascular, orthopedic, and even metabolic or chromosomal origins are supported by budgets that are obviously not under the direct control of medical geneticists. In spite of all of these resources, there is no doubt that a complete view – which is nonetheless impossible to obtain – of the financial support accorded to medical genetics would surprise us by the modesty of the sum involved.

*b) How much of the Gross National Product in Switzerland is spent on health care itself?* According to the Swiss Federal Office of Social Insurances, the total cost covered by insurance companies, including their administrative expenses, amounted in 1985 to some 8,416,000,000 Swiss francs (about 5,500,000,000 of today's dollars). In addition, in the public sector the total sum covered by the federal, county and city governments, essentially to dispense health care, was computed at 7,131,000,000 francs. Thus, a total of some 15 billion, 547 million Swiss francs (about 10 billion dollars) was devoted to health care, to which should be added the expenses covered by citizens themselves or contributed by health care workers. The GNP of Switzerland was, in 1985, some 241,400,000,000 francs (over 160,000,000,000 dollars); the expenditures in the domain of health (both public and covered by insurance companies) thus represent about 6.4% of the GNP. If we try to estimate the sums that private expenses add to this financial mass, we might go even further and conclude that approximately 10% of the GNP is invested in expenses related to health. There is no doubt that health care expenses have, as elsewhere, exploded, given the increased cost of hospital care and the impressive proliferation of the medical corps. Switzerland is a country that boasts, on the average, at least one doctor for each 400 inhabitants. Nonetheless, it is certain that the money spent for medical genetics in Switzerland represents only a fraction of 1% of the total financial expenditure for health.

## 2.16.4.4 Abortion Laws in Switzerland

Article 120 of the Swiss penal code explains, in a detailed manner, under what conditions an abortion may be allowed. A legal interruption can be performed only if the following conditions are fulfilled:

- the pregnant woman, or in special cases her guardian or legal representative, must give written consent; that of the husband is not necessary;
- the abortion cannot be performed except to avoid a danger otherwise inevitable, and which menaces the life of the pregnant woman or endangers her health in a serious and permanent manner. In addition, this danger must not be amenable to change by other means besides an abortion;

374

– the reality of the conditions cited must be confirmed by a second medical doctor. The physician allowed to give this second opinion must practice a specialty that is related to the medical conditions cited as the reason for the abortion.

One can see that, in the strictest sense, the dispositions of the penal code should not allow an interruption of pregnancy even for major genetic risk. For example, imagine the following situation: after having learned by amniocentesis or choriocentesis that she is carrying a fetus affected by trisomy 21, a woman could not abort unless she could convince her doctor and a second medical expert of the imminence of her suicide in the case of refusal. In practical terms, however, a doctor can proceed with an abortion because of other states of serious (i.e., psychological) distress affecting the pregnant woman; if a judge accepts the reasons, although he has no obligation to do so, he can waive the normally required punishment (Chapter 3, Article 120 of the Swiss Penal Code). Falling in this category are, for example, abortions for social indications (material distress), eugenic concerns (transmission of an hereditary disorder), and legal indications (pregnancy following a punishable act such as rape).

The role of social opinion towards the practice of abortion naturally complicates the application of this outdated abortion law. Health officials and those doctors opposed to abortion might use the law to refuse, with a clear conscience, the much-needed role of compassionate physician helping future parents who have learned of an irreversible genetic defect in the developing fetus. Less well-defined situations are, of course, even more difficult to resolve. Some physicians or centers place a time limit on abortion; generally, interruption for genetic reasons, and without legal pursuit, can be performed until the 22nd week of pregnancy. Certain university centers, however, refuse such abortions after the 20th week of pregnancy. This attitude creates further stress for laboratories, which must obtain prenatal results as rapidly as possible so that abortions can be performed under minimally traumatic conditions.

It must be admitted, however, that in practical terms, elective termination before the 12th week of pregnancy is rather liberally performed in some states, such as Geneva; the definition of a "serious physical or psychological state" is often interpreted quite liberally. Given this situation, which leads to a marked inegality among cantons, a revision of the law concerning abortion was recently proposed to our national governing body. This revision would have decriminalized pregnancy interruption and would have left up to each of the 23 states the option to adopt the 12-week limit for abortion. Unfortunately, however, during the very moment of our writing this chapter, in early March 1987, the National Parliament refused this revision of the Swiss penal code, by a vote of 85 to 74. The power of the conservative groups that opposed such decriminalization is shown by the fact that even a proposition that the federal counsel reexamine the conditions under which pregnancy termination would be allowed was defeated easily.

## 2.16.4.5  Studies of the Effectiveness of Genetic Services

Such evaluations have not been undertaken and would be nearly impossible except at the level of the 23 local governments. Nonetheless, for the University of
Geneva, the following statistics give some insight into the situation. From September 1979 (at which time the authors assumed the responsibility for prenatal diagnosis) until the end of December 1986, 2,851 amniocenteses and 181 analyses of
chorionic villi were performed [6]. If we consider only chromosomal anomalies
(nonchromosomal aberrations account for only about 10 cases), 51 were revealed
from 3,032 tests; 18 of these were autosomal trisomies and 19 were anomalies of
the sex chromosomes. Of these chromosomal anomalies, 34 were followed by terminations of pregnancy, according to parental decision.

As far as the utilization of prenatal diagnostic tests is concerned, we are again
unaware of any systematic evaluation having been done in Switzerland. We
would, however, estimate that, at least in an urban setting such as Geneva, some
50–70% of pregnant women over 35 opt for amniocentesis or choriocentesis.

## 2.16.4.6  Need for New Laws

In Switzerland, a conservative country composed of a mosaic of autonomous
powers under a confederate structure, as we have just seen, it is difficult to obtain
a consensus for the development of new laws. Undoubtedly, it will be the pressure
of frequent situations that will most rapidly produce legal modifications and will
force legal considerations of the current perspectives offered by genetics (in-vitro
fertilization, genetic engineering for gene therapy). We definitely need a new law
concerning abortion, as well as one covering tests such as amniocentesis and choriocentesis. Access by all economic groups appears to us indispensable. A proposition has recently been submitted to parliament by a group of deputies who would
like to see the costs of prenatal diagnosis covered by the federal government, and
we await with great interest the results of their intervention.

## 2.16.5  Ethical Issues and Trends in Medical Genetics

*a) What trends or changes will have the greatest impact on ethical issues?* One portion of the questionnaire asked that we rate goals and priorities for the next ten
years, both in our countries and worldwide. The answers showed us that Switzerland is in agreement with the majority of countries, both for priorities within the
country and worldwide. For within-country priorities, as with all other nations, the
first task in Switzerland is to cope with increased demand. The development of
tests for carrier status is seen as nearly as important. Eugenic concerns and sex
preselection, for Swiss geneticists and others, are of the lowest priority. The only
notable difference between Swiss priorities and those of other countries is that
screening for cancer and heart disease is given higher priority in Switzerland

(a country with one of the world's highest life expectancies) than in most other countries.

Priorities for the world were essentially the same as those cited for Switzerland, with the exception that allocation of limited resources was given a higher priority on a worldwide scale than in our own country.

During the next few years in Switzerland, the major problem of clinical geneticists will be to obtain the funds to cover the enormous increase in demand for existing tests. Over the past two years in Geneva the number of prenatal diagnostic tests performed has increased each year by 10–20%, whereas the increase in technical personnel has in no way kept pace with this growth. Current prenatal tests, particularly amniocentesis, have reached a degree of safety which, by reducing the number of miscarriages and other complications caused by the tests, renders their utilization suitable by increasingly large numbers of couples. Although 30% of trisomic births occur to women over 35 years of age, it is among the younger couples that the majority of aneuploidies occur. These young couples are increasingly better informed and more interested in prenatal diagnosis, and if we are to offer it to them reasonably and ethically, they must have the opportunity for counseling. The need for such prenatal testing and for adequate counseling will increase rapidly with the further development of chorionic villi sampling.

*b) What will be the most serious ethical issues in the near future?* If we consider the practical problems of the diffusion of genetic services as well as the impact of new techniques on ethical views, we can analyze this question at two levels. Multiple problems will result from the availability of methods for investigating the anatomy of the gene, techniques that are currently under development. The term "reverse genetics," by which a lesion is diagnosed even before the mechanisms of action of the gene are clear, is becoming a reality [12]. The diagnosis of gene lesions will permit more prenatal identification of diseases of varying severity. It will thus be increasingly difficult to define the situation which, in the opinion of the parents as well as the medical community, justifies termination of a pregnancy. In cases where such methods help to avoid as yet incurable miseries, they will necessarily be promoted; the distribution of and access to resources will create problems of priority and resource allocation. Various religious, geographic and socio-economic factors will play essential roles in these decisions.

The clinical geneticist is discouraged by the lack of etiological treatment for congenital anomalies. Aside from the handful of genetic deficiencies where substitutions and special diets allow partial correction of the effects of a mutant pair of genes, there is currently no treatment for genetic disorders. And for the practicing physician confronted by the difficulty of caring for patients with genetic disorders, the possibility of genetic engineering, which could transform the human genome according to human desires (or satanic plans) seems a distant utopia. Although such genetic manipulation is as yet impossible, these questions should, in the face of current therapeutic impotency, be the subject of increasing debate and study.

On the other hand, modern methods of detection will amplify problems of choice, and such revelations will weigh on certain families and individuals. The resulting dilemma, however, must be faced by a larger public. Think of the difficulties that the choice of testing for Huntington's chorea poses, and of the psychological drama that the certitude of an impending fate will create, weighing down every action. Modern man, who will acquire more and more liberty to know his destiny, will also learn of the difficulties involved in accepting that knowledge.

*c) What ethical resources will Swiss medical geneticists draw upon to face these issues?* Ethical practices are formulated and influenced at different levels. On the one hand, a certain number of directives and recommendations are diffused to the professionals concerned by various organizations involved in health and medicine. On the other hand, the universities have organized ethics committees within departments or faculties, whose responsibility it is to examine the different problems related to the rights and responsibilities of doctors and their patients. These commissions can, of course, be consulted for recommendations and clarifications in specific cases. The ethics commissions, particularly the departmental ones, are set up for examination and approval of research projects involving human subjects. On a national level, the Swiss Academy of Medical Sciences has created a central medical ethics commission, to which are assigned various tasks and recommendations. The Federation of Swiss Physicians publishes a Vademecum of Swiss Medicine, which includes an important number of recommendations helpful in the handling of numerous situations [9]. Included, for example, are directives concerning treatment of sterility, in-vitro fertilization and embryo transfer, experimental research involving humans, and numerous suggestions of a deontologic nature. Otherwise, the legal community and the parliament are also regularly concerned with some of these problems. Thus, during the general assembly of the Swiss Association of "Judiciary Magistrates," subjects linking law and problems of science and medicine are addressed. As an example, the exposé entitled "The judge and genetic engineering" was the fruit of such efforts to communicate between the different branches on which the social order depends [14].

*d) Evolution of Differences Among Swiss Geneticists.* We believe that the existing differences are an enrichment of the liberal tradition, which we support. Although we sometimes deplore the lack of uniformity and cohesion concerning certain courses of action, we notice on the whole a spirit that animates those responsible for the Swiss genetics scene, and reflects certain characteristics of the nation that could be referred to as "moderate conservatism" or "reasonable liberalism." It is clear, however, that the relatively unimportant differences in genetic counseling philosophies that are evident in the domain of classical genetics may be magnified by the development of more controversial knowledge and techniques, particularly as they relate to reproductive options.

*e) As we look ahead, are we optimistic or pessimistic about Switzerland's ability to guide medical genetics?* All factors considered, we are neither optimistic nor pessimistic about the abilities of our society to guide medical genetics in an acceptable orbit. No matter what efforts are taken to control the future, it is the possibilities and promises of future achievements that will motivate our efforts. Important discoveries and contributions are conducive to abuses. The human genome is opening up to our knowledge; once that genome is exposed, man can never hide that information again. Much as a river cannot be deviated from its course to the sea, once available, that knowledge will shape our destiny. The day will come when the techniques that dissect the genome will not only search out single genes producing incurable diseases, but will try to decipher other elements, the association of which shapes our biological destiny. It is these elements which, unless accident intervenes, drive our lives toward their individual and particular termination: cancer, arteriosclerosis, and tutti quant!. . .

## Acknowledgements

The Authors are much indebted to Mrs. Georgette Chapuis and Mrs. Marianne Fischer for their dedicated assistance in preparing this manuscript. They also express gratitude to Professor Albert Schinzel for his interest in this project.

The research and clinical activities of the Geneva University Institute of Medical Genetics, with which the authors are affiliated, are supported by the State of Geneva and grants from the Swiss National Foundation for Scientific Research (3.856 - 0.85), the Swiss Foundation for the Encouragement of Scientific Research on Mental Retardation, and the Geneva Cancer Foundation.

## References

1. Cerletti A, Courvoisier B [1985] Directives médico-éthiques pour le traitement de la stérilité par fécondation in vitro et transfert d'embryons. Acad Suisse Sci Méd, Basle
2. Crusi A [1987] Revue de 1700 amniocentèses de dépistage prénatal à Genève (1979–1984): analyse des cas, commentaires des femmes testées. Thèse, Université de Genève, Genève
3. DeLozier-Blanchet CD, Engel E, Extermann Ph, Pastori B [1988] Trisomy 7 in chorionic villi: Follow-up studies of pregnancy, normal child, and placental clonal anomalies. Prenat Diagn 8, 281–286
4. De Wals PH, Weatherall JAC, Lechat MF (eds) [1985] Registration of congenital anomalies in Eurocat centres (1979–1983). Cabay, Louvain-la-Neuve
5. Engel E [1980] Essai de définition d'un code éthique à l'usage du diagnostic prénatal. Bull Schweiz Akad Med Wiss 36: 381–388
6. Engel E [1987] Amniocentèse ou choriocentèse? Avantages, inconvénients, perspectives. Méd et Hyg 45: 1346–1350
7. Engel E, Tran TN [1981] Résultats et perspectives de l'amniocentèse et du foeto-diagnostic préventifs. In: Feingold J (ed) Génétique médicale. Acquisitions et perspectives. INSERM/Flammarion Médecine, Paris, pp 237–282
8. Engel P [1985] Le juge et le génie génétique. Communication, Association Suisse des Magistrats de l'Ordre Judiciaire, Morges, 5. 10. 1985
9. Fédération des Médecins Suisses (ed) [1986] Vademecum du médecin suisse. Secrétariat général des Institutions du Corps Médical Suisse, Berne
10. Fletcher J [1979] Prenatal diagnosis, selective abortion, and the ethics of withholding treatment from the defective newborn. Birth Defects: Original Article Series XV: 2: 239–254
11. Franceschetti A, Klein D [1951] Au sujet de la création, à Genève, d'un service de Génétique Humaine rattaché à la Clinique Ophtalmologique. Bull Schweiz Akad Med Wiss 7: 351–357
12. Goodfellow PN [1987] Classical and reverse genetics. Nature 326: 824
13. Mathon G (ed) [1987] Le don de la vie. Le respect de la vie humaine naissante et la dignité de la procréation. Réponses à quelques questions d'actualité (Instructions de la Congrégation pour la Doctrine de la Foi, 22. 2. 1987) Editions du Cerf, Paris
14. Swiss Society for Medical Genetics (ed) (1978–1987) Génétique Médicale. Feuille d'Information, No. 1–18
15. Swiss Society for Medical Genetics (ed) [1984] Le diagnostic génétique prénatal. Tableau des résultats des examens effectués en Suisse de 1981 à 1983. Génétique Médicale 12: 9–12
16. Swiss Society for Medical Genetics (ed) [1987] Le diagnostic génétique prénatal. Tableaux des résultats des examens effectués en Suisse de 1984 à 1986, inclus biopsies choriales du placenta. Génétique Médicale 19: 15–20

# 2.17  Ethics and Medical Genetics in Turkey

I. Bökesoy and F. Göksel

Turkey is a country situated at the junction of Asia, Europe and Africa, like a bridge with an area of 774,815 km². This position and the fertility of the soil have attracted a wide variety of populations and made the land rich in culture through-out the ages. The people presently living in Turkey are mainly Caucasian (white) Moslems with an admixture of Jews, Catholics and those of Greek Orthodox faith. Since 1923 there has been a republic with secular rule; according to our legal code a man can marry only one woman.

## 2.17.1.1  Medical Genetics in Turkey

Nothing is known about the incidence of genetic disease in Turkey. However, with a figure for consanguineous marriages of 20.9% and for first cousin marriages of 16.9% (Institute of Population Studies, Hacettepe University, 1986) the ratios for recessive and multifactorial diseases are probably higher here than in other countries.

Statistics give a high ratio for infectious diseases in infant mortality. Considering the high ratio of unknowns, the reported low figure for congenital malformations should be taken with a grain of salt (Table 2.17.1). According to the 1985 census, the population of Turkey is 50,664,458. From this figure, expected births per year are about 1.5 million and infant deaths occurring in a year are about 128,988

**Table 2.17.1.**  Causes of infant mortality in Turkey (Yener 1981)

|  | %<br>Congenital malformations | Infections | Unknown | Others |
|---|---|---|---|---|
| Rural area | 1.08 | 36.57 | 44.32 | 17.73 |
| Urban area | 4.16 | 35.99 | 37.68 | 22.17 |
| Mean | 2.62 | 36.28 | 41.00 | 19.95 |

**Table 2.17.2.**  Vital Statistics of Turkey in 1980–1985 (Planning Organization of the State 1985)

|  | % |
|---|---|
| Crude birth rate | 3.06 |
| Crude death rate | 0.9 |
| Infant mortality rate | 8.32 |

**Table 2.17.3.** Incidence of Congenital Malformations in Turkey per 1,000 Newborns (Say et al. 1971)

| | |
|---|---|
| Neural tube defects | 2.5 |
| Cleft lip and/or palate | 1.1 |
| Cardiovascular defects | 1.7 |
| Malformation of extremities | 7.5 |
| Urogenital anomalies | 3.3 |
| Down syndrome | 0.7 |
| Trisomy 13 | 0.2 |

(Table 2.17.2). The ratio of congenital malformations in 10,000 newborns (Table 2.17.3) gives a projected figure of 25,500 congenital malformations per year, although a recent study with a smaller group gave a 10.85% ratio for congenital malformations [1].

### 2.17.1.2 *Organization of Clinical Genetic Services in Turkey*

Universities with medical schools provide genetic services for education, patient care and research. Courses in genetics were started at medical schools in the late 1960 s. Now there are genetics-related lectures at all medical schools, but with divergent content and duration, depending on the lecturers and their range of interests.

Genetics services are offered at 7 out of 19 medical faculties. Most of them work within pediatrics departments, but at Ankara University, Eskişehir and Sivas they are part of the Medical Biology departments, while at Istanbul University genetics services are dispensed by the Internal Medicine Department as well. These services tend to progress rather slowly, and the methods used are those of the 1970 s. This is mainly a question of funding, the interests of the academic staff, and the time at their disposal. Academic staff also are responsible for giving lectures in their own faculties as well as at other faculties such as science and/or social science. As an example, at the Ankara University Medical Faculty, there is an enrollment of 460 and a teaching load of 60 hours per year. These are some of the restrictions other than those related to lack of resources. We believe education has been promoting genetics, because every year more and more people study the subject, and in this way they will constitute a better-informed public while at the same time the doctors of the future will be more inclined to refer patients to genetics departments.

In the 7 centers (located in the largest cities) the main service offered is postnatal chromosome analysis. In one of them, however, some metabolic screening is also carried out. Every service tries to give genetic counseling and diagnose genetic diseases. There is a growing interest in genetics, but there is a lack of close collaboration between clinicians and geneticists. Table 2.17.4 documents two years of chromosome analysis at Ankara University [2]. Retrospective analysis (1980–85) of parents with reproductive failure gave a 1.5% rate of abnormalities, which is lower than that reported abroad [2]. Indications for chromosome analysis are mainly sex-

381

**Table 2.17.4.** Chromosome Analyses at Ankara University Medical School Cytogenetic Laboratory (unpublished results of Department)

|      | Chromosome analyses | Abnormal findings | % |
|------|---------------------|-------------------|---|
| 1985 | 633                 | 52                | 9 |
| 1986 | 718                 | 41                | 6 |

**Table 2.17.5.** Rates of Population Increase in the World and Turkey (Kocaman and Özaltın 1986)

|        | 1975–1980 % | Projected to 2000 % |
|--------|-------------|---------------------|
| World  | 1.72        | 1.50                |
| Turkey | 2.06        | 1.76                |

ual ambiguities, physical abnormalities, mental retardation, and reproductive failures. In Turkey, where the birth rate is high (Table 2.17.5), there is over-emphasis and even exploitation of this last indication, stemming from the generally great desire of the populace to have children.

After the diagnosis of genetic disorders (Mendelian, non-Mendelian, or chromosomal) genetic counseling is usually given to parents seeking a risk estimate for a future child. In recent years there has been growing interest, in cases of consanguineous marriage, in counseling before having a child or even before the marriage takes place. It is also gratifying to see such requests from workers abroad coming home for marriage with relatives. There is also a demand from intellectually trained people for information on the hazards of pharmaceuticals. Counseling is also carried out by academic persons without the help of clinicians, and by social workers trained for this purpose.

There is nobody in Turkey trained in clinical genetics. Usually patients are treated at other clinics (endocrinology, gynecology, pediatrics, etc.). One problem in Turkey is a lack of collaboration, even among geneticists. This became more apparent with the low response rate to the questionnaire (38%). Most of the subjects did not wish to expose themselves in terms of education, training, or business practice. But we need to collaborate to improve our knowledge and services; otherwise, even well into the future, we will not have advanced centers, considering our already restricted resources.

## 2.17.1.3 Prenatal Diagnosis

In spite of the presence of trained academicians, there is no established service for prenatal diagnosis in Turkey. As mentioned before, it is a matter of money, equipment and collaboration. With some patients of advanced age, or carriers of chromosomal translocations, advice is merely given that the patient seek help from abroad or send the material to centers abroad. But this is only possible for people who can afford it and otherwise find the means. We believe that prenatal diagnosis should be started in Turkey, but only after new techniques are established for precise diagnosis.

## 2.17.1.5 Abortion

In 1983, an act making elective abortion legal was passed by our parliament, for gestations prior to 10 weeks. Before the passing of this law, some illegal abortions were carried out clandestinely, and this practice continues, especially where unwanted pregnancies have advanced beyond the 10th week. The Institute of Population Studies, Hacettepe University, gives a figure of 25.6 abortions per 100 live-births registered, of which 15 are induced. We have no records for genetic indications or related statistics for abortions.

## 2.17.2 Ethical Problems Confronting Medical Geneticists in Turkey

### 2.17.2.1 Genetic Counseling

Our traditional, conservative way of life makes child-bearing the core of marriage. This is especially important in rural areas where a child is taken as a guarantee for survival of parents and families. It is also a factor promoting a high birth rate. That is why the unity of the family needs to be respected, and counseling should be given very carefully when there is no way to help in the absence of prenatal diagnosis and care of abnormal children; otherwise disclosure of a diagnosis may cause harm. The dominance of the male in Turkish society makes a woman more vulnerable when the genetic problem resides in her, but when it is a question of the male, the family makes a greater effort to manage the situation. For some problems adoption is a rare alternative, carried out secretly among close relatives. If somebody adopts an orphan, no help is asked from geneticists. Another alternative, artificial insemination by a donor (AID), is not sanctioned, and we have no legal service for it in practice.

In the case of false paternity, according to the questionnaire the majority is in favor of telling the truth to the mother alone; however, this is not easy to realize in practice because of the cultural background and position of women in the country. It is usually next to impossible to interview the mother alone.

Although a duty to divulge information to third parties appears to emerge from the results of the survey, in actual practice the patient's confidentiality is respected because of the cultural context, which tends to exclude third parties from the proceedings.

383

## 2.17.2.2 Prenatal Diagnosis

There is no religious constraint on prenatal diagnosis, which is in great demand among those with specific motivation and might easily be accepted by people at large. Providing such a service in outmoded laboratories is not practical. Logically, there is a need for up-to-date laboratories and technicians.

## 2.17.2.3 Genetic Screening

In this country there is no experience with mass screening for carrier status of common diseases, but neonatal screening for metabolic disorders has been carried out in a faculty in Ankara. Neither the results nor any ethical conflict related to screening have been revealed by said faculty to date. The consensus appears to be in favor of mandatory screening for workers, but this choice may be due to simple lack of experience.

## 2.17.3 Consensus and Variation in Turkey

In Turkey respondents displayed 100% consensus about some questions in the survey: the disclosure of XY genotype in a female and of conflicting diagnostic findings; regulations prohibiting commercial laboratories from sex selection and from operating without a medical genetics unit to interpret results; access to screening results by the worker and the worker's physician or government health department; and disclosure of pre-symptomatic test results for Huntington disease (HD) to the patient and the spouse. There was also agreement that essential counseling goals are to prevent disease and to reduce the number of carriers.

Other issues where there was strong or moderate consensus: disclosure of results to the mother alone in the case of false paternity; nondirective counseling for XYY; disclosure of ambiguous laboratory results; refusal of prenatal diagnosis for sex selection; presenting reproductive options of "taking their chances" to male and female carriers of tuberous sclerosis (TS) and contraception to female carriers; duties toward third parties in the case of HD patients, hemophilia A patients and carriers of balanced translocations; mandatory screening for workers and newborns; access to pre-symptomatic test results of HD patients by medical and life insurance companies only if the patient approves; and access without such approval for relatives. There was also consensus that patients' decisions are theirs alone, the goal of counseling being to help patients achieve parenting goals and understand their options.

Cases without consensus were as follows: Options for TS carriers (except "taking their chances" for both sexes and contraception for females); counseling about XO genotype in a fetus; performance of prenatal diagnosis for maternal anxiety and for parents who will not abort. For the last two it seems that, considering our limited resources, the desire to give help to patients who really need it makes a consensus difficult. There was no consensus concerning accessibility of genetic screening results by employer, worker's insurer, employer's insurer for worker's compensation, and worker's and employer's insurers for health insurance. This variation stems from the lack of social security in Turkey. Directive counseling was equally approved and disapproved. Those who approved had less experience in practice.

The greatest ethical conflicts among Turkish respondents were on false paternity and disclosure of an HD diagnosis to third parties. These conflicts revolve around the issues of keeping the truth from the legal father and the physician's duty to third parties overriding the wish to shelter the patient from social stigma.

The least disturbing questions for two of us concerned sex selection. We think the respondents were predecided against unnatural sex selection. The other cases of least conflict were prenatal diagnosis for maternal anxiety, counseling about XO or XYY genotypes and disclosure of a hemophilia A diagnosis.

## 2.17.4  Cultural Context of Medical Genetics in Turkey

The Talmudic form of "incest taboo" is reflected in the religious codes of both Christianity and Islam. Until 1926 Islamic legislation (sheria) regulated marriage in Turkey. According to this "law-system," marriages between progeny and parents, siblings or half-siblings were forbidden. Similarly, a person could not marry with siblings or half-siblings of parents. The Turkish Civil Code [1926] preserved these rules. Marriage between the children of siblings was permissible under Islamic law and is also permissible in modern Turkish law. This form of marriage is quite common, especially along the eastern Black Sea coast and in the south-east of Turkey.

Biological experts' reports, especially those concerning blood groups, are taken into account by Turkish courts as valid proof in cases of disputed parentage.

For eugenic reasons, the Turkish Law of Public Hygiene forbids the marriage of a person who has a mental illness or syphilis.

Until recent times, the rules regulating therapeutic abortion took into account only the life and health of the mother. Causes related to the health of the child did not have a place in law. Amniocentesis and its genetic and other indications are little known in legal codes and even in many medical circles in Turkey. For this reason, genetic diagnosis in embryo or fetus has not been reflected in abortion legislation.

In some universities, there are research fellows of the younger generation who have learned something of the techniques of "genetic engineering" abroad, and have initiated certain scientific experiments. To our knowledge there are as yet no official guidelines to restrict these experiments.

At the medical school, ethical issues are given in a 30-hour course, where the content is mainly the history of medicine.

## 2.17.4.1 Sources of Challenge and Support

Parents' organizations are very recent. However, it is gratifying to see that some intellectual parents are trying to organize such groups to share their problems and exchange their experiences with others. We believe it is very helpful, because parents learn to reveal their problems by sharing with others, and this lessens the burden on the family. When the impetus comes from the top they hesitate to join, but if it comes from among themselves it is accepted instinctively. One leader of such a group (the mother of a Down child) told me (I. B.) this year that if I desired funding for a prenatal diagnosis laboratory they would try to supply it in the future. It was an invaluable suggestion.

Among clinicians, pediatricians and hematologists are also acting as a source of challenge vis-a-vis the need for diagnosis of abnormal children.

The lack of proper knowledge about genetics causes some disagreement even between clinicians and geneticists. When a disease is hereditary in origin, some clinicians send their patients for "blood analysis" (chromosome analysis). This seems reasonable to the patient, due to popular belief that such diseases are inherited via the blood.

## 2.17.4.3 Resources Expended by Turkey in Support of Medical Genetics

Turkey is one of the developing countries of the world, with an annual per capita income of $1130. Only 2.53% of the national budget is spent on health, social security and welfare, with less than 4.5% spent for each year in the period 1980–85 [3]. These figures indicate how far we are from being well-organized in health matters and how difficult it is to obtain precise information concerning incidence of congenital malformation and genetic disease in Turkey.

## 2.17.4.4 Abortion Laws

(See 2.17.1.5 above)

## 2.17.4.5 Studies of Effectiveness of Genetic Services

There are no established studies on the effectiveness of genetic services in Turkey, but it is clear that there is a great need for such services, with more experienced staff and soundly established centers to act as reference centers for different branches of genetics. These centers should be provided with research and training activities for students, graduates and the public.

## 2.17.4.6 Need for New Laws

There is a need for legislation to protect against abuses in human genetics. One of the problems might be sex selection, which attracts many because of the preference for male children in families. In the near future AID, surrogate mothers, persons undergoing operations for sex reversal, and perhaps XX males and XY women may also require new laws.

## 2.17.5 Ethical Issues and Future Trends

We believe that the diagnosis of carrier status with refined techniques will have the greatest impact on ethical issues, because it will present new problems regarding the disclosure of diagnoses to third parties and the prevention of misuse of results. On the other hand, sex selection might be the greatest ethical issue when sex diagnosis becomes easier in the near future. That is why we need to develop strict principles regarding it now. The only way to solve problems of ethics in genetics is by educating the medical profession and the public.

In conclusion, we are optimistic for the future. Geneticists will find a society open to advances in genetics only if they themselves collaborate and agree on equity, beneficence, avoidance of harm, and respect for the integrity of the patient. Resources for new techniques should be provided in Turkey as in any other country of the world.

## Acknowledgements

The authors are indebted to Professor Nusret Fisek for his valuable discussion and Mr. Fred Stark for his kind stylistic review of this manuscript.

## References

1. Akşit MA, Sönmez B, Başaran N, Solak M [1986] The results of chromosome analysis selected from 1229 live-born newborn infants that showed multiple and major abnormalities. In: Vogel F, Sperling K (eds) Human Genetics: Proceedings of the 7th International Congress of Human Genetics. Springer-Verlag, Heidelberg, 1988
2. Bökesoy I, Karaman B, Özcengiz D [1986] Chromosome analysis in parents with reproductive failures. Proceedings of 8th pediatrics days. University of Istanbul (Turkish)
3. Fifth program of progress for five years 1985-1989 [1985] Planning organization of the state (DPT) no 1974 (Turkish)
4. Kocaman T, Özaltın I [1986] Trends of popluation growth in Turkey and comparison with other countries. DPT yayin no DPT 2054-SPD 396-Nisan (Turkish)
5. Say B, Tunçbilek E, Balcı S, Yalçın Z [1971] Incidences of congenital malformations in the Turkish population. Hacettepe Universitesi yayınları. No C-12 (Turkish)
6. Yener S [1981] Causes of deaths in Turkey. DPT yayin no DPT 1751-SPD 330-Mart (Turkish)

## 2.18 Ethics and Medical Genetics in the United Kingdom

R. Harris and D. C. Wertz

## 2.18.1 Development of the Field

Some believe, with reason, that Britain is where modern medical genetics began. Until 1935, the focus of human genetics was on research rather than clinical work. R. A. Fisher, J. B. S. Haldane, and L. S. Penrose were pioneers in applying genetic analysis to both normal human variation and disease states, although clinical genetics was not then part of medical training. In the late 1930s, J. A. Fraser Roberts developed the first course in medical genetics for medical students, followed by his textbook, *An Introduction to Medical Genetics*, in 1940. For many years this remained the only text in the field. The 1940 edition already contained a section on genetic counselling, in which Fraser Roberts stressed the role of counselling in dispelling unfounded fears as well as explaining genetic risks. Shortly after the Second World War, Fraser Roberts established the first genetic clinic in Europe, at The Hospital for Sick Children in London. The clinic was based on the belief that paediatrics should embrace both the welfare of the unborn child and the welfare of the prospective or future child. Genetic counselling was not to be left solely to the paediatricians involved in patient care. Instead, the new genetic clinic created a referral structure for anxious relatives who were seeking genetic rather than medical advice. The clinic linked The Hospital for Sick Children with the research facilities of the Institute of Child Health, University of London. This link led to important family studies of congenital malformations and to the establishment in 1957 of the first research unit in clinical genetics, headed by Fraser Roberts under the auspices of the Medical Research Council (MRC). By 1959, Fraser Roberts' textbook predicted, almost exactly, the components of modern genetic counselling. The chapter sections included: Psychological Factors, Patients Accept Advice in Terms of Odds, Answers in Terms of Odds, Demand Yardsticks, Complete Reassurance is Unwise, Diagnosis, The Family History, Alternative Modes of Transmission, and Empirical Chances. The principles of composite risk, multifactorial causation, and genetic influences in common diseases, all major research issues of the 1950s, were included in the discussion of counselling (Pembrey 1987).

It is probably fair to say that clinical genetics and genetic counselling, in its modern form of answering to patients' personal concerns without giving directive advice, began in Britain and subsequently spread to other nations such as Canada and the United States. From the outset, clinical genetics departed from the general tradition of paternalistic medicine. Instead of advising patients about what they should or should not do, geneticists saw themselves as counsellors, one of whose main tasks was to communicate empathically and accurately. In any case, it appears that clinical genetics has assumed a leadership role in the development of greater equality between doctor and patient in medicine generally.

388

As early as 1940, Fraser Roberts predicted the development of chromosome mapping and screening for genetic susceptibility (Pembrey 1987). Research expenditures in Britain, however, did not keep pace with expenditures in the United States after World War II. According to Hollingsworth [1986], an American medical sociologist and historian, by 1960 the United States had become the world leader in quantity of scientific and medical research, spending between 1.7 and 1.9 times more of its GNP on medical research than did Britain. The same author also noted that the overall quality of scientific medical work has been somewhat higher in Britain than in the United States. This may be because fewer people with marginal ability have been able to engage in medical research, given the limitations of funds (Brooks 1973). On a per-person basis, British scientists have generally been more productive and have received more awards than American scientists (Hollingsworth 1986).

## 2.18.1.1 Scope of the Problem

The numbers of births per year and the perinatal and neonatal mortality rates between 1978 and 1982 are shown in Tables 2.18.1 and 2.18.2 (Great Britain, Parliamentary Papers [Commons] 1984). Mortality rates were higher among the lower social classes, culminating in a two-fold difference between the highest and the lowest, a possible reflection of the greater number of low birthweight infants born to mothers in Social Classes IV and V. Fetal malformation was the underlying cause of 27% of perinatal and neonatal deaths, including 23% of infants ≤ 2,500 grams and 33% of those over 2,500 grams in 1977 (Great Britain, Parliamentary Papers [Commons], 1980). As elsewhere, congenital abnormalities were responsible for a great proportion of perinatal mortality overall (1,818 of 8,317 deaths, or 22%) in 1980 (Great Britain, Parliamentary Papers [Commons], 1984). The incidence and burden of common important genetic disorders in the U.K. are shown in Table 2.18.3 (Great Britain, Department of Health and Social Security [DHSS] 1987). The incidence and recurrence risk of important congenital malformations are shown in Table 2.18.4 (Great Britain, DHSS 1987). Anencephaly ± spina bifida, cardiac malformations, cleft lip/palate, Down syndrome, fragile X syndrome, hydrocephaly, and adult polycystic kidney disease have the greatest

**Table 2.18.1.** Perinatal Mortality in England

|  | 1978 | 1979 | 1980 | 1981 | 1982* |
|---|---|---|---|---|---|
| Total number of births (live and still) | 567,380 | 606,127 | 622,894 | 602,063 | 593,442 |
| Number of perinatal deaths | 8,766 | 8,839 | 8,316 | 7,047 | 6,670 |
| Perinatal mortality rate per 1,000 total births | 15.4 | 14.6 | 13.4 | 11.7 | 11.2 |

\* provisional

Great Britain, Parliamentary Papers (Commons) (1984) Third Report from the Social Services Committee, Session 1983-84: Perinatal and Neonatal Mortality Report: Follow-up. London: HMSO, p. 99

**Table 2.18.2.** Perinatal Mortality* by Social Class, England

| Social class | Perinatal Mortality per 1,000 total births | | | | | | | | | |
|---|---|---|---|---|---|---|---|---|---|---|
| | 1978 | | 1979** | | 1979*** | | 1980 | | 1981 | |
| | Number | Rate | Number | Rate | Number | Rate | Number | Rate | Number | Rate |
| I | 520 | 12.0 | 461 | 10.6 | 378 | 10.3 | 379 | 9.7 | 323 | 8.3 |
| II | 1,225 | 12.2 | 1,260 | 11.8 | 1,376 | 11.9 | 1,308 | 11.1 | 1,122 | 9.4 |
| III | 3,602 | 14.8 | 3,623 | 14.0 | 3,569 | 14.0 | 3,319 | 12.8 | 2,713 | 11.1 |
| IV | 1,368 | 16.7 | 1,414 | 16.3 | 1,379 | 16.3 | 1,252 | 15.0 | 996 | 13.1 |
| V | 468 | 20.1 | 486 | 18.6 | 543 | 18.2 | 516 | 17.5 | 446 | 15.6 |
| All legitimate births**** | 7,509 | 14.7 | 7,527 | 14.0 | 7,527 | 14.0 | 7,064 | 12.9 | 5,844 | 11.1 |
| Gap between highest and lowest rate | | 8.1 | | 8.0 | | 8.0 | | 7.8 | | 7.3 |
| Ratio of rate in Class V to rate in Class I | | 1.68 | | 1.75 | | 1.78 | | 1.80 | | 1.88 |

* Legitimate births only ** Classified using 1970 Classification of Occupations *** Classified using 1980 Classification of Occupations
**** Includes births not assigned to the above classes (unstated, Armed Forces, etc.)
Great Britain, Parliamentary Papers (Commons) (1984) Third Report from the Social Services Committee, Session 1983–84: Perinatal and Neonatal Mortality Report: Followup. London: HMSO, p. 100

**Table 2.18.3.** Incidence and Burden of Common Important Genetic Disorders in the U.K.

| Condition | Birth incidence per 10,000 | Average years of | | Lost life years |
|---|---|---|---|---|
| | | Unimpaired life | Impaired life (& degree of impairment) | |
| **Autosomal dominants** | | | | |
| *Adult polycystic kidney disease | 8 | 30 | 30 (30%) | 10 |
| *Huntington's chorea** | 5 | 40 | 10 (50%) | 20 |
| *Neurofibromatosis | 4 | 20 | 30 (50%) | 20 |
| *Retinoblastoma (treated) | 3 | 3 | ? (20%) | ? |
| *Myotonic dystrophy** | 2 | 40 | 10 (50%) | 20 |
| Tuberous sclerosis** | 1 | 5 | 45 (80%) | 20 |
| *Multiple polyposis (Familial Adenomatous Polyposis) | 1 | 20 | 30 (20%) | 20 |
| **Autosomal recessives** | | | | |
| *Cystic fibrosis | 5 | 2 | 10 (50%) | 30 |
| *Phenylketonuria (treated) | 1 | 60 | 10 (10%) | 0 |
| Neurogenic muscle atrophy | 1 | 1 | 4 (90%) | 65 |
| Early onset blindness | 1 | 5 | 70 (50%) | 0 |
| Non-specific mental retardation**[1] | 5 | 0 | 50 (90%) | 20 |
| *Sickle cell disease | 0.5[2] | 30 | 20 (20%) | 20 |
| *Thalassaemia major | 1[2] | 0 | 35 (20%) | 35 |
| Tay-Sachs disease** | 0.4[3] | 0 | 3 (90%) | 67 |
| **X-linked recessives** | | | | |
| *Duchenne muscular dystrophy | 2 | 4 | 16 (60%) | 50 |
| *Haemophilia A | 1 | 0 | 60 (20%) | 10 |
| X-linked mental retardation** | 10 | 0 | 50 (80%) | 20 |
| **Chromosomal abnormalities** | | | | |
| Down syndrome ** | 12 | 0 | 35 (80%) | 35 |
| Autosomal structural aneuploidy | 5 | 0 | 20 (95%) | 50 |

Note: [1] Includes polygenic forms
[2] 50 per 10,000 in the ethnic groups most affected.
[3] 4 per 10,000 in the Jewish population
* DNA markers available    ** Indicates a cause of mental handicap
Great Britain, Department of Health and Social Security (1987) On the State of the Public Health for the Year 1986. London: HMSO, p. 112

**Table 2.18.4.** Important Common Congenital Malformations. Incidence and Risk

| Condition | Incidence/ 10,000 births | % | Recurrence risk % siblings |
|---|---|---|---|
| *Anencephaly ± spina bifida ** | 20–300 | 0.2–3.0 | 5 |
| Cardiac malformations | 60–80 | 0.6–0.8 | 3 |
| Spina bifida (without anencephaly) | 3 | 0.03 | 5 |
| Hydrocephaly (without spina bifida) | 5–14 | 0.05–0.14 | 5 |
| Talipes equinovarus | 10 | 0.1 | 3 |
| Cleft lip/palate | 10–20 | 0.1–0.2 | 4 |
| Cleft palate | 5 | 0.05 | 2 |

* Not compatible with life ** Wide geographical variation
Great Britain, Department of Health and Social Security (1987) On the State of the Public Health for the Year 1986. London: HMSO, p.112

incidence. Thus at least one in 50 children is born with a congenitally handicapping disorder.

## 2.18.1.2 Organisation of Clinical Genetic Services in the United Kingdom

All but two of the National Health Service (NHS) regions have at least one consultant clinical geneticist, and the remaining two have recently been funded (Table 2.18.5). These individuals provide the essential link between cytogenetic, DNA, and biochemical laboratories, consultants in other specialities, general practitioners, and patients. In these centres, the genetically trained clinician has the special responsibility for confirming clinical diagnoses, recognising genetic heterogeneity, and assessing risks (Harris et al. 1983). In order to reach and counsel extended families, the clinical geneticist must work with a team of medically trained assistants, genetic nurses, and nonmedical counsellors to follow up patients in their own homes, where far more relaxed communication is possible than in the hospital clinic. The accumulation, maintenance, and analysis of genetic information on whole families requires that members of the team must be computer literate, understand risk estimation, and be sensitive to the requirements of confidentiality (Harris 1988).

There are approximately 35 consultant clinical geneticists, but some are university-funded or part-time, so that there are the equivalent of only 27 whole-time posts (Table 2.18.5). Of these, all new consultants have been accredited by the Specialty Advisory Committee (SAC) of the Joint Committee on Higher Medical Training of the four Royal Colleges of Physicians (London, Dublin, Edinburgh, and Glasgow). In order to receive accreditation, a fully qualified clinical geneticist must have a total of at least seven years training beyond medical school and house jobs (internship). The first three years constitute General Professional Training (GPT), which must include at least one year of paediatrics, general internal medicine, and may include other specialty areas. At an early stage, usually after 18 months of GPT, the trainee takes the demanding examination for membership in the Royal College of Physicians, which is the "entrance examination" necessary before enrollment for the four years of Higher Specialty Training (HST) as a senior registrar in clinical genetics. HST is obtained in posts approved by the SAC and located in regional genetics centres. The equivalent of one of the four years is spent on basic genetics, including laboratory work and trainees are expected to undertake research and are encouraged to spend some time in another centre, preferably abroad. Accreditation is not a prerequisite for practise, however, and many senior geneticists, who began to practise before the existence of formal training programs, are not formally accredited.

The training of medical school undergraduates has not generally been adequate to encompass the projected increase in demands for counselling and new diagnostic techniques (Harris 1987a). According to a survey by RH in 1986, 21 of 29 medical schools were not connected with a human or medical genetics department,

**Table 2.18.5.** Consultant Clinical Geneticists and Senior Registrars in UK (Whole Time Equivalents)

| NHS Region/Health Board | | Senior Registrars | Consultants | | |
|---|---|---|---|---|---|
| | | | 1982 | 1986 | Shortfall* |
| | Pop x 1,000 | | | | |
| Highland | 191 | 0 | 0 | 0 | 0 |
| Tayside | 400 | 0 | 0 | 0 | 1 |
| Grampian | 523 | 0 | 0 | 0 | 1 |
| Lothian | 1,195 | 0 | 0.6 | 0.6 | 1 |
| N Ireland | 1,547 | SR | 0.6 | 0.6 | 1 |
| East Anglia | 1,916 | 0 | 0.6 | 0.6 | 1 |
| Oxford | 2,355 | 0 | 1.6 | 1.6 | 1 |
| Mersey | 2,435 | 0 | 0 | 0 | 2–3 |
| Wessex | 2,724 | 0 | 0.6 | 0.6 | 2 |
| Wales | 2,786 | SR | 1.2 | 2.2 | 1 |
| Strathclyde | 2,829 | SR | 2.2 | 2.2 | 1 |
| SW Thames | 2,859 | 0 | 0 | 1 | 2 |
| Northern | 3,070 | 0 | 0.6 | 1.6 | 2 |
| S Western | 3,249 | 0 | 0.6 | 0.6 | 3 |
| NW Thames | 3,431 | SR | 1.2 | 1.2 | 2 |
| SE Thames | 3,530 | SR | 1.6 | 1.6 | 2 |
| Yorkshire | 3,580 | 0 | 0 | 1 | 3 |
| NE Thames | 3,670 | SR, HSRx2 | 2.2 | 2.2 | 1 |
| N Western | 3,985 | SR | 2.6 | 3.6 | 0 |
| Trent | 4,557 | 0 | 2.2 | 2.2 | 2 |
| W Midlands | 5,153 | 0 | 1.2 | 3.2 | 2 |
| Totals, whole–time equivalents (WTE) | | | | | |
| UK | | SRx7**,HSRx2 19.6 | 26.6 | 31–32 | |
| Engl & Wales | | SRx5#,HSRx2 16.2 | 23.2 | 26–27 | |
| Planned Total (WTE) | UK | SRx20, HSR ad hoc | 58–59 | | |
| | E&W | | 50–51 | | |

Key. SR = NHS/Univ Senior Registrar Posts
   HSR = Honorary (Charities) Senior Registrar Posts
(*) *Shortfall* calculated from the very conservative *Projection* of 1 WTE consultant per region then at the rate of 1 per million population. This shortfall does not adequately take into account the workloads associated with the clinical genetic applications of *DNA*, and the increasing expectations of the professions and public.
SR soon to be increased to **14 and #12 respectively
Source: Harris R, personal communication

and 13 offered no clinical courses in genetics. Students received a mean of 23.5 hours of pre-clinical teaching and 8.1 hours of clinical training in genetics at the 8 schools associated with genetics departments, and 14.4 and 1.8 hours respectively at the other 21 schools. It is feared that many general practitioners (GPs) and non-genetic specialists do not have sufficient training or experience to counsel patients about the implications of genetic tests. Publicity about the availability of DNA probes for Huntington disease, cystic fibrosis, and Duchenne muscular dystrophy, amongst others, has made both clinicians and the public aware of the need for more education.

There is a total of 44 chromosome laboratories (Association of Clinical Cytogeneticists [ACC] 1986), most of which are associated with regional clinical genetic centres. The origins of some of the chromosome laboratories go back to the late 1950s, when diagnostic chromosome analysis began. Until 1965, the majority of laboratories were funded by research bodies such as the Medical Research Council (MRC) or by university departments of Child Health or Genetics. With the advent of effective prenatal diagnostic techniques, an increasing number of NHS laboratories were set up, either independently or within departments of Pathology, Clinical Genetics, or Obstetrics and Gynaecology. By 1984, almost 80% of laboratories were NHS-funded and almost half were units administered under departments of Pathology or Laboratory Medicine. Most of those not funded by the NHS were supported by universities (ACC 1986). There are, however, two private cytogenetics laboratories that perform fee-for-service work, and unmet demands for prenatal diagnosis may lead to the establishment of more such laboratories in the future. A small number of private analyses are performed at the request of obstetricians in NHS laboratories, but these must meet the same criteria as NHS patients.

With the exception of a few private laboratories, genetics services are completely dependent on the NHS, with important contributions from the universities and medical charities. Consultants are salaried employees. Every individual in Britain should be registered with a GP, who will refer them to hospital specialist services as necessary. All services are "free at the point of delivery" but consultants aim to perform services which are considered medically necessary. However, such services are limited by available resources. The most common example of a service which is not freely available is prenatal diagnosis for anxious young women with no medical indications. If a genetic centre does provide this service, however, it is performed without direct cost to the patient.

At present, it is almost impossible for patients to obtain genetics services on a fee-for-service basis, even at private laboratories. In the future, however, it is possible that the role of private services will increase, as they are doing in other areas of medicine. Private costs to patients, however, are relatively low in comparison to the United States (£100 for CVS as compared to $1,000 in the U.S.), because the basic costs of training, capital investment, and services are in effect partly underwritten by the NHS.

## 2.18.1.3 Prenatal Diagnosis

As elsewhere, over the past few years it has become increasingly possible to detect many congenital abnormalities during pregnancy. The Royal College of Obstetricians and Gynaecologists (RCOG) has recommended a routine ultrasound scan at 16–18 weeks of pregnancy to assess gestational age and identify multiple pregnancies or abnormalities (RCOG 1984). The RCOG stresses, however, that women should not be persuaded to have routine ultrasound against their will. When there is an increased risk of fetal structural abnormality (head, spine, heart, kidneys, abdominal wall, and skeleton) additional diagnostic ultrasound scans are routinely available during the second trimester. Most pregnant women now receive at least one ultrasound scan, usually at about 18 weeks (Oakley 1983).

It is now generally accepted that all women aged 35 and over and all women with a family history of, or previous child with, a chromosome aberration should be offered amniocentesis. In 1980, the recommended age cut-off was 40 (Great Britain, Parliamentary Papers [Commons] 1980), but subsequent cost-benefit analyses led to its reduction (see Section 2.18.1.4 below). At present, facilities available in the U.K. fall short of those necessary to provide services to all women over 35. In 1984, there were 24,222 known prenatal diagnostic chromosome analyses for 705,456 live and still births, or 34.3 per 1,000. Of these, 66% were performed on the basis of maternal age over 35, 13% were done on amniotic fluid obtained for raised MSAFP, 10% were done on the basis of family history, 3% were done because of a previous child with a chromosome defect, and 3% were for maternal anxiety in the absence of medical indications (ACC 1986). Table 2.18.6 shows the percents of uptake for women in each group. The highest uptake, 44%, was for mothers over 40, but this varied by region, ranging from 27% in Yorkshire to 63% in Wessex. In the 35–39 age group, 27% had prenatal diagnosis, ranging from 16% in the West Midlands to 40% in Mersey. Below age 35, only 1% had prenatal diagnosis (ACC 1986). The geographical differences stem largely from availability of laboratory services. Most geneticists would like to provide prenatal diagnosis to all women aged 35 and over, and also to very anxious women of any age, especially when anxiety is founded on personal experience with handicapped children, for

**Table 2.18.6.** Uptake of the Prenatal Diagnostic Service – 1984 Percentage Tested – Women in Different Age Groups

| Region | Age 35–39 Years | | | Age >40 Years | | | Age ≤34 Years | | |
|---|---|---|---|---|---|---|---|---|---|
|  | B* | T* | % | B | T | % | B | T | % |
| Northern | 2,079 | 420 | 20.20 | 286 | 109 | 38.11 | 37,133 | 256 | 0.69 |
| Yorkshire | 2,634 | 653* | 24.79* | 532 | 142* | 26.69* | 43,821 | 461* | 1.05* |
| Trent | 3,332 | 1,104* | 33.13* | 538 | 231* | 42.94* | 54,097 | 1,223* | 2.26* |
| East Anglia | 1,542 | 513* | 33.27* | 232 | 127* | 54.74* | 22,045 | 279* | 1.26* |
| NW Thames | 4,011 | 958 | 23.88 | 676 | 325 | 48.08 | 41,747 | 312 | 0.75 |
| NE Thames | 3,950 | 960 | 24.30 | 749 | 381 | 50.87 | 46,828 | 394 | 0.84 |
| SE Thames | 3,374 | 1,043 | 30.91 | 500 | 277 | 55.40 | 41,030 | 422 | 1.03 |
| SW Thames | 3,471 | 735 | 21.18 | 502 | 184 | 36.65 | 31,117 | 171 | 0.55 |
| Wessex | 2,248 | 736* | 32.74* | 320 | 200* | 62.50* | 31,399 | 596* | 1.90* |
| Oxford | 2,449 | 666 | 27.19 | 363 | 197 | 54.27 | 29,149 | 473 | 1.62 |
| S Western | 2,367 | 690 | 29.15 | 341 | 179 | 52.49 | 33,685 | 392 | 1.16 |
| W Midlands | 4,325 | 681 | 15.75 | 892 | 284 | 31.84 | 63,940 | 418 | 0.65 |
| Mersey | 2,102 | 850* | 40.44* | 317 | 126* | 39.75* | 29,363 | 284* | 0.97* |
| N Western | 3,192 | 898 | 28.13 | 590 | 267 | 45.25 | 50,730 | 676 | 1.33 |
| England | 41,076 | 11,070 | 26.95 | 6,838 | 3,105 | 45.41 | 556,084 | 6,390 | 1.15 |
| Wales | 2,131 | 542* | 25.43* | 371 | 205* | 55.26* | 33,568 | 397* | 1.18* |
| Scotland | 3,536 | 1,153 | 32.61 | 573 | 226 | 39.44 | 61,279 | 1,406 | 2.29 |
| Total | 46,743 | 12,602 | 26.96 | 7,782 | 3,460 | 44.46 | 650,931 | 8,160 | 1.25 |

*B = Number of live and still births to women in each age group. Figures extracted from OPCS tables and from the General Register Office for Scotland.
*T = Number of patients tested in each age group
% = Patients tested, expressed as percentage of births to mothers in each age group. Where figures in the body of the Table are starred, known crossregional flow has been taken into account.
Association of Clinical Cytogeneticists (1986) Review of Clinical Cytogenetics Services 1984: England, Scotland, and Wales

**Table 2.18.7.** Mean Age of Women at First Legitimate Live Birth, According to Social Class* of Husband: 1976 and 1986, England and Wales

| Social class of husband | Mean age of woman at first legitimate birth | |
|---|---|---|
| | 1976 | 1986 (est) |
| All Social Classes (including 'other') | 24.9 | 26.2 |
| I and II | 26.9 | 28.1 |
| III Non-manual | 25.7 | 26.9 |
| III Manual | 24.1 | 25.5 |
| IV and V | 23.1 | 24.2 |

* Definition of Registrar General's Social Classes:

| | | |
|---|---|---|
| Non-manual: | I | Professional occupations |
| | II | Intermediate occupations (including most managerial and senior administrative occupations) |
| | IIIN | Skilled occupations (non-manual) |
| Manual: | IIIM | Skilled occupations (manual) |
| | IV | Partly-skilled occupations |
| | V | Unskilled occupations |
| Other: | | Residual groups (including for example Armed Forces, students and those whose occupations were inadequately described) |

Great Britain, Department of Health and Social Security (1987) On the State of the Public Health for the Year 1986. London: HMSO, p.13

example in a worker in a school for the retarded or a hospital nurse. In some regions, there appear to be sufficient laboratory facilities to provide services for all those with medical indications and to serve the anxious as well. In 1984, 786 diagnoses (3% of the total) were done for anxiety (ACC 1986). In other regions, prenatal diagnosis must be carefully rationed to those age 37 or above, and women of 35 or 36 cannot be served. In fact, there are not enough services anywhere to cover all the prenatal diagnoses that are medically indicated. This explains in part the low uptake rates. In order to conserve scarce laboratory facilities, many clinicians are probably not offering the service unless patients ask for it. Another reason why uptake is lower than optimal is that about 16% of women receive antenatal care too late to have amniocentesis and another 7% refuse amniocentesis on moral grounds (Ferguson-Smith 1983a). A recent survey suggests that 88% of women aged 35–39 and 98% of women 40 or over would wish to have prenatal diagnosis available (ACC 1986).

The problem of unmet need is likely to become more acute because of demographic changes. During the past ten years, increases in the average age at which women marry and in the interval between marriage and first birth have raised the average age at which women have children. Table 2.18.7 shows that between 1976 and 1986 the average age at first legitimate birth increased from 24.9 to 26.2 years, a pattern evident in all social classes (Great Britain, DHSS 1987). In 1986, 39% of all legitimate first births were to women aged 30 or above, compared to 29% in 1966. As these women have subsequent children, an increasing proportion of pregnancies will occur to women over 35, and more prenatal diagnoses will be needed.

**New Techniques**

Chorionic villus sampling (CVS) at 8–10 weeks of gestation now makes chromosomal and DNA analysis possible at an earlier age. If the technique is proven acceptably safe, most women and doctors would presumably prefer it, because an abortion can be performed in the first trimester. At present, few centres use CVS routinely for chromosome analysis, partly because of expense, and it is generally reserved for DNA analysis, where it is technically superior. Clinicians have been reluctant to use CVS until its safety has been adequately demonstrated. Consequently, in 1986 the MRC launched a trial, now underway, of the safety and effectiveness of CVS. If CVS is to replace amniocentesis for suitable chromosome tests, this will require a massive effort at patient education. At present, almost half receive antenatal care too late to have CVS (Ferguson-Smith 1983 a).

MSAFP screening for neural tube defects has had greater uptake than amniocentesis or CVS. In practice, about 59% of mothers use the test. Only 7% decline it on moral grounds, and the remainder receive antenatal care too late in pregnancy (Cuckle and Wald 1987).

The application of advances in molecular biology, most recently of recombinant DNA technology, has given clinical genetics fresh impetus. it has already improved the potential precision of detection in individuals at risk for common single gene disorders, including adult polycystic kidney disease, Huntington's chorea, retinoblastoma, myotonic dystrophy, cystic fibrosis, sickle cell disease, thalassaemias, Duchenne muscular dystrophy, and haemophilia. In 1985 the DHSS funded a Special Medical Development (SMD) to evaluate the introduction of molecular genetics in the clinical genetic services in Manchester, Cardiff, and London (see below). Although these tests have become available only very recently, in some regions with well organised services many families at risk have already requested testing for Huntington's chorea, cystic fibrosis, Duchenne muscular dystrophy or adult polycystic kidney disease. A study of the psychosocial effects of presymptomatic testing for Huntington's is currently underway in Manchester, Cardiff, and several other centres (Craufurd and Harris 1986). Demand for these tests will place a greater burden on an already overburdened laboratory and counselling system.

Some fetal abnormalities, e.g., fragile X, are detectable by CVS but may require confirmation by examining fetal blood. Recognition of the need that then existed for a national facility for detecting fetal haematological disorders led in 1983 to the funding of a service at King's College Hospital, London (Great Britain, DHSS 1987).

## 2.18.1.4 Cost-benefit of early diagnosis

The DHSS has accepted that in a high-risk area for neural tube defects, the savings from providing resources for severely handicapped survivors exceeds the total costs of the screening programme. For example, the saving per spina bifida birth avoided has been calculated at £16,200 to £21,600 in 1979 prices (Hibbard et al. 1985; Glass and Cove 1978; Haggard, Carter and Milne 1976). For a programme of prenatal diagnosis and termination of pregnancy in Down syndrome, the estimated cost of caring for the affected children was greater than the cost of prenatal diagnosis in mothers of 36 years or older, at which age the risk of having a Down baby is about 1 in 200 (Haggard and Carter 1976). Economic calculations, however, are based on the assumptions that most women will receive early diagnosis and that all affected fetuses will be terminated. This is not necessarily the case. At least 6,000 (almost 1 in 100) babies born alive each year are seriously impaired, in spite of nearly 2,000 planned terminations for fetal and genetic abnormalities (King's Fund 1987). In the West of Scotland, 30% of Down syndrome children are born to mothers over 35, only 30–40% of *these* women have prenatal diagnosis, and, as a consequence, in 1985 only 12% of total affected fetuses were terminated (Ferguson-Smith 1983a).

MSAFP screening has fared better (Ferguson-Smith 1983b). Over a ten-year period, the overall rate of neural tube defects in the West of Scotland has fallen from 5 per 1,000 to 2 per 1,000 (Ferguson-Smith 1983b, and personal communication). In England and Wales, the birth prevalence of spina bifida and anencephaly declined from 31.5 to 6.2 per 10,000 between 1964–72 and 1985.

Economic cost-benefit analyses fail to include the important intangible aspects of early diagnosis and counselling, which include reassurance to the majority of prospective parents that their baby is not going to be handicapped, or, for the minority with an affected fetus, the opportunity to make choices. Intangible costs include anxiety, discomfort, and possible complications of prenatal diagnosis for mother or fetus.

At present, the principal justification for providing screening and early diagnosis programmes lies in unquantified, rather than quantified, effects. Examples of benefits are the provision of authoritative information, relief from uncertainty, support during a period of crisis, and the expansion of an individual's scope for exercising choice. Examples of potential harms are the introduction of worrying delays while confirmatory tests are conducted, the distress that may result from false positive results, and the illusory reassurance given by false negative results. Another set of considerations concerns long-term social effects, such as changes in the status and social integration of the handicapped. The King's Fund, an independent philanthropic foundation established by Edward VII to improve health care, influence standards of professional practise, and help clarify health policy, has recently investigated these problems through a Forum on Screening for Fetal and Genetic Abnormality. According to the December 1987 King's Fund Forum Consensus Statement,

> If only monetary information is considered, there is a danger that the quantified may drive out the important in a kind of Gresham's law of screening. This is a particular danger when the quantified costs of a service exceed the subsequent financial savings. A further difficulty occurs when the costs of the tests are borne by one sector of the community and the savings are found in another (King's Fund 1987).

Frequently the costs of testing are borne by the NHS, while savings accrue to individual families or to the Social Services Department. The King's Fund consensus suggests that it is unfair to 1) judge testing primarily on monetary grounds, and 2) to limit testing because it does not save money for the NHS itself.

The NHS might be expected not to favor programmes without discernible monetary savings or where these do not accrue to the NHS. However, three years ago DHSS asked the Departments of Medical Genetics in Manchester, Institute of Child Health (London) and Cardiff to assess the remarkable advances which have been made in recombinant DNA technology in relation to NHS Clinical Services (Great Britain, DHSS, Medical Division CDPNM 1987). DHSS attaches such importance to these developments that it has taken the unusual step of an interim report. This report is extremely favourable and it is noteworthy that it stresses the importance of information allowing reproductive decisions and the clinical geneticist-genetic register-laboratory team arrangements in the centres. The report concludes:

"From the information provided by the directors of the three centres of the Special Medical Development ..... and work elsewhere, we are satisfied that
i. recombinant-DNA techniques can be applied effectively to increase the precision of diagnosis and risk assessment of carrier status in single-gene disorders
ii. these applications allow important decisions of individuals and families at risk to be better informed, enabling them to achieve more favoured birth outcomes
iii. the effectiveness of services now introduced in the SMD centres testifies the soundness of arrangements made for their delivery. These arrangements therefore provide a base from which more comprehensive services may evolve."

## 2.18.1.5 Abortion

Under the Abortion Act of 1967, abortions are permitted up to 28 weeks gestation to preserve the mother's life or physical or mental health, to protect the physical or mental health of the mother's other children, or if "there is a substantial risk that if the child were born, it would suffer from such physical or mental abnormalities as to be seriously handicapped" (see Section 2.18.4.4 for more detail about grounds for legal abortion). In 1967, 28 weeks was considered the limit of fetal viability. Viable fetuses at any gestational age are still protected under the Infant Life (Preservation) Act of 1929. The Abortion Act of 1967 made no specific provision for abortions on social or economic grounds or for abortions on demand. Nevertheless, it was the first Act to decriminalize a substantial number of abortions in Britain. In practise, the Abortion Act of 1967 has been interpreted very liberally. "Mental health" has been construed so as to cover most conditions that would be considered "social" or "on demand" in other countries, even though two doctors must attest that the abortion is necessary on the grounds of health.

In 1984, approximately one-third of conceptions to women under 20 (including about 40% of conceptions outside marriage) ended in abortion (Great Britain, DHSS 1987). "Genetic" abortions were a very small percentage of the total. In England and Wales in 1986 there were 147,619 legal abortions to resident women, or 22 for every 100 live births (Great Britain, Office of Population Census and Surveys [OPCS] 1987). Of these, 1,987 (1.34%) were on the grounds that "there is a substantial risk that ... the child ... [would] be seriously handicapped"(Great Britain, OPCS 1987; Ian Leck, personal communication 1988).

The incidence of abortion after genetic diagnosis varies with the disorder. The number of terminations for central nervous system abnormalities more than doubled between 1971 and 1977 (Turnbull and MacKenzie 1983). In the West of Scotland, the percent of women electing abortion for fetal neural tube defects rose steadily, from 21% in 1976 to 74% in 1985, as the procedure gained acceptance (Ferguson-Smith 1983b and personal communication). In England and Wales, abortions for suspected neural tube defects increased from less than 1% in 1972 to 56% in 1985, and accounted for 31% of the decline in births of affected infants (Cuckle and Wald 1987). Personal experience suggests that most women known to be carrying fetuses with Down syndrome or cystic fibrosis have elected abortion. On the other hand, with sympathetic and well-informed counselling, our experience is that the proportion electing abortion is far lower for low-burden disorders such as Turner, XXY, XXX or XYY.

## 2.18.2  Ethical Problems

### 2.18.2.1  Ethical Problems in Genetic Counselling

A major ethical problem in genetic counselling lies in the sheer quantity of information provided by testing. How much of this information should be given to the patient? How much *can* be told to the patient without causing needless confusion and potential psychological harm? In the past five years there has been a major shift in clinician and student attitudes, in the direction of providing all relevant information revealed by testing, including information that the patient had not originally sought. For example, only a few years ago, it is likely that many doctors would not have revealed the accidental discovery of a sex chromosome abnormality such as Turner or XYY to a patient undergoing prenatal diagnosis for Down syndrome. Now many more would tell the patient. It is likely, however, that in many cases communication is not as good as it should be, especially in counselling before screening or before prenatal diagnosis. For example, how many women understand that when blood is drawn for MSAFP testing this is a first step in a process that may lead to the termination of pregnancy? A significant minority probably do not understand. Although all women should receive counselling before routine testing, the shortage of trained personnel makes it impossible to guarantee that this is always done effectively. There is a danger that as tests proliferate, more will be done on patients who do not understand their future implications for the pregnancy. In order to prevent this, there is a need for widespread training in genetic counselling for health professionals, including obstetric and community services.

400

## Non-directive genetic counselling

Because patients vary greatly in their responses to genetic risk and wish to make their own reproductive decisions, genetic counselling should not be directive and should concentrate on the presentation of accurate facts and options with such empathy as to facilitate decision-making by the consultand. Non-directive genetic counselling has much in common with informed consent, and its features are amplified in Table 2.18.8.

Genetic counselling must be preceded by an accurate diagnosis or a clear understanding that this is not possible. There is much genetic heterogeneity, and apparently similar disorders may be Mendelian, chromosomal, environmental or multifactorial, each with different implications for recurrence risk and for outcome.

Counselling must be timely with insight into the recipients' ability to comprehend. For example, counselling immediately after a stillbirth or the birth of a handicapped infant will usually be inappropriate because consultands will be too emotionally drained to be receptive.

Genetic counselling in ethnic minority communities frequently requires the assistance of a knowledgeable member of the same community with whom both counsellor and consultand can achieve good rapport.

Genetic counselling is a partnership between consultand and counsellor, the latter offering information, investigation, options and support, while the consultand makes the decisions.

**Table 2.18.8.** The Non-directive Paradigm

The essential features of genetic counselling are:

*Underlying principles*
* Freedom of reproductive choice
* Assisting the client to make decisions that the *client* believes appropriate
* Counsellor's opinions should generally not intrude
* Prevention important but secondary
* Eugenics as an aim rejected

*Scientific basis*
Accurate facts, diagnosis and interpretation including information on:
* Risk hereditary disease will develop/be transmitted
* Prognosis, explanation of e.g., severity if the disease does occur
* Options: contraception, abortion, treatment, etc.

*Presentation*
Empathic, taking into account the client's:
* Knowledge
* Emotional state
* Religious or ethnic beliefs
* Rapport with counsellor

*Mobilization of Support*
* Other medical specialties for treatment, etc.
* Social services
Harris R (1988) Genetic Counselling and the New Genetics. Trends in Genetics, 4:52-56

## Origin of Non-directive Genetic Counselling

In most western cultures there is a strong belief in the worth and autonomy of the individual. This applies in disease as in health and most of all in reproductive decision-making. Non-directive genetic counselling was generated (Fraser 1979) against this background and encouraged by other powerful forces. It is in part a reaction to the misapplication of eugenics (Kevles 1986) earlier this century in some parts of the United States and in Nazi Germany, an experience that has left a legacy of profound distrust for any reproductive coercion.

Clinical geneticists are generally anxious to be seen to be non-directive, but the manner of presenting the same set of facts may vary greatly. Few counsellors are so dispassionate in their views that they are always neutral when describing risk or expected degree of disability. Non-genetic clinicians who deal frequently with patients with genetic diseases are sometimes convinced that the specialist with long experience of the disease is better able than the patient to judge between reproductive options.

## Sources of Bias in Counselling: Severe X-linked Disorders

The interplay of patients' attitudes, genetic counselling and new discoveries is illustrated by the way carriers of severe haemophilia have varied in their wish for prenatal diagnosis (Markova et al. 1984). A woman's appreciation of the *pros* and *cons* of prenatal diagnosis for haemophilia (and other serious X-linked diseases) is most powerfully influenced by personal experience of the lives of her close male relatives (Beeson and Golbus 1985). In the absence of such formative experience of the disease she will be more responsive to the haematologist's explicit or more subtle messages about the quality of life of haemophiliacs. Until recently, prenatal diagnosis using reliable RFLP has not been widely used, perhaps because treatment with pooled Factor VIII was judged successful by haematologists, particularly compared with the unpleasantness of late abortion. However, the knowledge that many haemophiliacs have become HIV positive following treatment with pooled human Factor VIII has apparently resulted in a marked increase in requests for prenatal diagnosis (Tuddenham, personal communication), which by means of CVS has become possible in the first trimester. This trend may be reversed yet again when safe cloned human Factor VIII becomes freely available.

## Directive Counselling

There are suggestions from time to time that some individuals are unable to make sound reproductive decisions because of mental handicap, lack of social responsibility, or other limitations. Some commentators advocate positive direction because they believe that this would provide the least unhappiness in the long run for the individual and family, and perhaps for society. Difficult ethical issues are raised, but experience suggests that attempts at direction will be resisted (Anonymous 1982) and reproductive decisions the counsellor might regard as "sensible" appear to be no more common when patients are told what the counsellor believes to be the best option.

## Psychological Aspects

It is important that counsellors above all be sensitive to the psychological needs of anxious families awaiting test results, and to the grief of those who choose to ter-

minate a much-wanted pregnancy on genetic grounds. Some parents of handicapped children complain that, although counsellors were personally sensitive as
individuals, the hospital's system of presenting results did not take into account
the needs of families, particularly the mother's need for support from her spouse
or other family members.

As one parent of a Hunter disease child put it, many parents

... felt that the sequence of events followed too quickly for the couple to feel in
control and there is a need for all hospitals to allow participation by the father
at the antenatal level including being present during a scanning and prenatal
diagnosis.

A large majority of couples learn the results of their amniocentesis or chorion
biopsy over the telephone from the hospital. Although always dealt with sensitively, is it not possible for the news to be broken by the primary health care
Team or family GP? Often mum was alone at the time the news was broken and
faced the added burden of giving bad news to her partner. In my sample of 70
mums who have undergone at least one termination, hindsight suggests that details on groups of parents offering support would have helped enormously and
given [parents] the opportunity to share experiences with someone who had
been in a similar situation, helping to ease the emotional pain and guilt of terminating a much wanted baby. In almost all cases parents were ignorant of
what an induced labour involved and were resentful that husbands in many
cases were not welcome (Lavery, paper presented at Kings' Fund Forum 1987).

Follow-up studies of the psychological sequelae of abortion for genetic reasons
(Donnai, Charles, and Harris 1983; Forrest, Standish, and Baum 1982; Lloyd and
Laurence 1985) have led the King's Fund [1987] to recommend that a bereavement
counselling service be available to every such mother.

## 2.18.2.2  Ethical Problems in Prenatal Diagnosis

The major ethical problems associated with prenatal diagnosis are those of fairness of access for those who could benefit from the service. At present, there are
inequalities between regions. A woman of 36 might be able to have tests in one region but not another. A more ethically distressing situation is when prenatal diagnosis is provided mainly to those who are sufficiently well informed to request it
rather than to all who have the appropriate indications. Thus, the burden of making the request falls on the patient. Many doctors do not routinely offer prenatal
diagnosis to all women over 35, because they know the laboratories are already
overburdened. This means that educated women of the higher social classes, who
are more likely to know about it and request it, will receive a greater proportion
of prenatal diagnostic services, unless the NHS makes an intensive effort at educating patients. It is ironic that the limitation and rationing of services has led
to some inequalities that contravene the ethic of fairness on which the NHS is
based.

Another problem of inequality is posed by those who do not fall into risk-referral groups but are nevertheless anxious. Most British geneticists (88% in our survey) would gladly perform prenatal diagnosis for an anxious woman of 25, if there were an open system with plenty of facilities. Some perform it anyway, but in so doing they recognise that they may be depriving some women over 35 of the service, and they often tell this to the anxious patient in order to dissuade her. The geneticist feels a conflict between two widely-accepted ethical principles: to alleviate suffering (in this case mental anguish) and to be fair to all. Those who perform the service are aware that this may not be standard practise, except when the anxiety appears psychiatrically convincing.

In Britain, prenatal diagnosis for selecting the sex of the child is generally considered inappropriate, both as a misuse of health services and for ethical reasons. In the survey, most British geneticists (91%) would not perform it for this purpose, although 15% would offer a referral to a practitioner who might do so. Nevertheless, the clinical situation in the survey describing a request for sex selection was the one that gave the most British geneticists (30%) greatest ethical conflict. The conflict arises in part from the British liberal tradition of toleration towards ethnic minorities, as most couples who request sex selection in Britain are from ethnic minorities whose tradition requires them to have at least one son. As cultural differences fade with prospective assimilation, requests for sex selection will presumably disappear. There is no generally accepted policy in Britain amongst chromosome laboratories about withholding the gender of some fetuses.

Another ethical problem is whether to provide prenatal diagnosis for potentially treatable disorders such as PKU or "borderline" disorders with low burden. If a disorder is treatable, the NHS should presumably assess the cost-effectiveness, as has been done for Down syndrome and neural tube defects (see Section 2.18.1.4). On the other hand, successful treatment of individuals may pose problems for the next generation. The woman with PKU, whose treatment has enabled her to mature normally and to marry, is at higher risk of having severely retarded offspring unless she reinstates dietary therapy, which is usually very difficult to accept and has not been truly proven.

## 2.18.2.3 Ethical Problems in Genetic Screening

The scientific and ethical requirements for a successful screening programme are outlined in Table 2.18.9. The major ethical problem is that a *de facto* programme of crude eugenics might be introduced, and that resources will be spent on screening rather than services for handicapped people. Screening of ethnic minorities who are at high risk of recessive disorders because of consanguinity may foster racist attitudes.

Some fear that screening is changing the entire character of pregnancy, which is ceasing to be a natural family event and is becoming a technological activity. Increasingly, screening (MSAFP and routine ultrasound) affects the pregnancies of women who are not at increased risk. Before screening tests became available, most of these women did not suspect that they might be carrying a malformed fe-

**Table 2.18.9.** Requirements for a Worthwhile Screening Programme

| Aspect | Requirement |
| --- | --- |
| 1. Disorder | Well defined |
| 2. Prevalence | Known |
| 3. Natural history | Medically important disorder for which there is an effective remedy available |
| 4. Financial | Cost effective |
| 5. Facilities | Available or easily installed |
| 6. Ethical | Procedures following a positive result are generally agreed and acceptable both to the screening authorities and the patients |
| 7. Test | Simple, and safe |
| 8. Test performance | Distributions of test values in affected and unaffected individuals known, extent of overlap sufficiently small, and a suitable cut-off level defined |

Cuckle HS, Wald NJ (1984) Principles of Screening. In: Wald NJ (ed) Antenatal and Neonatal Screening. Oxford: Oxford University Press

tus. One effect of screening has been to raise people's levels of expectation about perfection. Many women now believe that screening can guarantee them a perfect baby. The anguish for those who have passed all the tests and nevertheless produce a malformed infant is perhaps greater than before.

A considerable potential ethical problem is that in the future being handicapped could become a mark of the underprivileged, who are less likely to receive antenatal care early enough for screening or prenatal diagnosis. They are also less likely to request these techniques from their doctors. It will be the educated, articulate, vocal, and economically privileged who will use the system most effectively and for whom there will be the most marked fall in births of affected children. Further, the burden of caring for handicapped children might increasingly fall on those who can least afford it and are least able to press for better services.

According to the King's Fund Consensus,

> Screening is only one possible approach to reducing disability. The primary prevention of environmentally determined congenital impairments and improving the facilities and attitudes of society to physically or mentally impaired people must be components of a comprehensive approach – the success of a screening programme should be judged not only by its effect on the prevalence of impairments at birth, but by its total effect on the wellbeing of women and their families (King's Fund 1987).

Screening for genetic susceptibility to occupationally-related diseases is virtually unknown in the United Kingdom. If such screening is ever introduced, most geneticists would oppose mandatory screening or unauthorized release of information to employers.

## 2.18.2.4 Ethical Problems in Other Contexts

**Confidentiality**

Confidentiality of patient records is considered by British geneticists to be of paramount importance. Genetic information has a uniquely private quality, and it frequently provides knowledge about other family members who may not know that such knowledge exists. In the future, great emphasis will be given to keeping genetic information confidential, as genetic registers are established in most regions for families with Huntington disease, Duchenne muscular dystrophy, adult polycystic kidney disease, cystic fibrosis, and other disorders amenable to DNA testing for carrier state and prenatal diagnosis. Most staff must become aware of the potential seriousness of confidentiality problems associated with computerized record-keeping. The Government is taking these problems seriously and the Data Protection Act [1985], now the law of the land, requires that all computer lists containing identifiable information must be registered, and access is restricted to qualified persons. Subjects will have the right to see, and if necessary correct, data about themselves.

**Embryo research**

At present, research on the human embryo is being conducted without legal regulation, but with a voluntary limit of embryos up to 14 days of age. Responses to the Warnock Report (Great Britain, DHSS 1984) focussed on research on human embryos and led the Government to postpone introduction of comprehensive legislation on embryo research until there was more consultation (see 2.18.4.2).

## 2.18.3 Consensus and Variation Among Medical Geneticists in Britain: Survey Results

British geneticists were in ≥ 75% agreement about the resolution of 62% of the 14 clinical cases, 68% of the screening situations and questions of access to results, and 75% of the 12 counselling goals and approaches (Part 1, Table 1.23). There was virtually no "moderate" (67–74%) consensus. Wherever agreement existed, it was strong agreement. The percent of strong consensus was similar to that in the United States, though there was not always consensus about the same questions. British geneticists had a strong consensus that the mother's confidentiality should be maintained in cases of false paternity (97%); conflicting test results (94%) and new or controversial interpretations of test results (84%) should be disclosed; prenatal diagnosis should be provided for patients who refuse abortion (91%) or in cases of maternal anxiety without medical indications (88%); prenatal diagnosis should *not* be performed for sex selection in the absence of X-linked disease (91%); regulations should prohibit private commercial laboratories from performing prenatal diagnosis solely for sex selection (83%) or from operating without being associated with a medical genetics unit to interpret results (79%); full information should be presented about XYY (91%), Turner (97%), or a possible small neural tube defect (84%) without giving advice about termination or carrying to term; adoption (93%), A.I.D. (94%), taking their chances (94%), contraception (90%), vasectomy (90%) or tubal ligation (90%) should be presented as reproductive options, without being asked and without giving directive advice, to carriers of disorders not diagnosable prenatally; mass screening for genetic susceptibility to occupationally-related disease should be voluntary (87%) and employers (84%), insurers (88%), and the Government health department (81%) should *not* have access to the results without the patient's consent; mass screening for carriers of cystic fibrosis, when and if this becomes available, should be voluntary (94%), but there was no consensus about the age group that should be screened.

With regard to counselling, there was 100% consensus that it was important to 1) help individuals/couples understand their options so that they can make informed decisions; 2) help individuals/couples cope with their genetic problems; 3) remove or lessen guilt or anxiety; and 4) help individuals/couples achieve their parenting goals (Part 1, Table 1.17). There was 100% consensus that it was appropriate to suggest that while you will not make decisions for patients you will support any they make. There was 94% consensus that it was appropriate to 1) tell patients that decisions are theirs alone and refuse to make any for them; and 2) inform patients what most other people in their situation have done. The latter approach is seen as responding to patients' requests for guidance, without being directive. There was 100% consensus that it is inappropriate to advise patients what they ought to do (Part 1, Table 1.18).

There was no consensus about disclosure, against the patient's wishes, of a diagnosis of Huntington disease or haemophilia A to relatives at risk. The Huntington case was the one that gave the greatest ethical conflict to the greatest number (23%) after sex selection (30%). There was also no consensus about whether to disclose which parent carried a balanced translocation, whether to disclose XY genotype in a female, or whether to disclose colleague disagreement about the meaning of test results. British geneticists differed significantly ($p < 0.05$) from their colleagues in the United States and Canada about the latter two types of disclosure (see Part 1, section 1.4.2). Significantly fewer British geneticists would disclose XY genotype or colleague disagreement. There are several possible reasons for these differences. There is in British medicine a tradition against providing gratuitous information or information that may only serve to confuse or distress the patient. Also, the word "disagreement" may imply "dispute" to the British; had the words been "difference of opinion," more might have been willing to disclose. In 1985, when the survey questionnaires were distributed, the British, in common with their U.S. or Canadian counterparts, would have disclosed the existence of the new, and then controversial, interpretation of low MSAFP, but the British would have been less likely to have advocated it. At that time, British geneticists appeared to have preferred to wait until there was more confirmation of results (Cuckle, Wald, and Thompson 1987).

One very important question where British geneticists differed significantly ($p < 0.05$) from their U.S. or Canadian colleagues was in favouring regulations for private commercial laboratories. In Britain, 83% favoured regulations prohibiting private commercial laboratories from performing prenatal diagnosis for sex selection and 43% favoured regulations prohibiting performance for maternal anxiety.

There is amongst British geneticists a strong feeling that patients should not be able to buy services when the objective criteria are not met. Free health care is regarded as a right that should be equally accessible to all.

## 2.18.4 Cultural Context of Medical Genetics in Britain

The most outstanding cultural aspect of British medical genetics is its belief in fairness and access to free health care, exemplified by the National Health Service (NHS). Britain had already had a National Health Insurance system by 1911. Lower-income consumers have had a much stronger tradition of shaping the structures and policies of the British medical system than they have in the United States. For this reason, the medical needs of lower-income consumers have received more attention in Britain than in the United States. From the beginning, workers' movements were influential in the establishment of National Health Insurance. The working class was influential in the creation of general public hospitals in 1929 and in the development of maternity and home visiting services. With the Great Depression of the 1930s, it became evident that National Health Insurance needed to be extended. Labour Party militants agitated for extension to cover 90% of the population. What finally crystallized reform, however, was the experiences of World War II, which alerted the overwhelming majority of people to serious inadequacies in the medical delivery system. During the War, of necessity many middle and upper-class people received care in types of hospitals different from those to which they were accustomed. As these middle- and upper-income people entered public hospitals for the first time, they saw firsthand the relics of old workhouses and the conditions under which the poor and elderly received medical care. As the well-to-do mingled with the less fortunate, they became more sensitive to the problems of poverty, old age, and chronic disease. The War did much to soften the class rigidities of British society and to generate a collective conscience that focussed on reshaping the delivery of medical care. As a result of a national consensus that the health system needed reform, Aneurin Bevan, the new Labour Minister of Health, was able to bring about postwar cooperation between disparate sections of society. After careful consultation with all interested groups, Bevan submitted to Parliament the Government's plan for a National Health Service. The plan was approved without difficulty in 1946 and implemented in 1948. Under the new NHS, doctors received salaries from the Government and patients received all medical care "free at the point of delivery." The organisation of care included some structural features inherited from the earlier National Health Insurance. In 1911, when the NHI came into existence, hospital-based technology was relatively unimportant and the administrative-financial structure encouraged most doctors into general practise. By 1948, when the NHS came into existence, a large proportion of doctors were still engaged in general practise. Patients gain access to a hospital specialist primarily by referral from GPs, who account for about two-thirds or more of clinical doctors.

The consuming public still exerts considerable influence on the NHS. The NHS is committed to providing an adequate minimum level of care for *all* rather than optimum care for a few. Minimum care is historically defined as the services that most people use most of the time or the services necessary to treat diseases that are common for certain age groups (Hollingsworth 1986). Genetic services are included as part of basic health care. Ideally, any innovation of proven value should be available to all patients without cost.

The centralisation of services under the NHS gave hospital-based specialists and consultants greater power and influence than they had formerly. The British medical elite became increasingly successful at influencing government policy (Klein 1983), although the trend is reversing under the present administration.

The British tradition of medical research differs somewhat from the American. The British attitude is that the most creative scientific work is performed by small groups who have the time to think about the meaning of findings. The large groups of scientists and vast accumulation of publications favoured in the U.S. appear to the British as both wasteful and scientifically confusing, although secretly envied.

In both countries, however, medicine has emphasised the curative over the preventive, with the result that education of patients about health matters remains poorly developed, although its importance is now recognised. In both countries, biomedical research has favoured the study of underlying physical processes of specific diseases rather that the role of environment or society. In common with Western medicine generally, the microcausal approach, which emphasises microorganisms or genetic causes, has been preferred over a macrocausal approach that would study how the social and economic environment both defines what is considered a "disease" and also shapes its distribution among social classes (Hollingsworth 1986). It has been suggested that the renewed interest in genetics might intensify the emphasis on microcauses rather than macrocauses of disease. However, clinical genetics training emphasises the pervasive influence of environmental factors on genetic expression.

In the past, British clinicians have tended to be more paternalistic than their counterparts in the United States. British patients went to the doctor expecting to be told what to do and rarely questioned the doctor's authority. Now the entire social scene is changing, as consumers are beginning to question the judgement of professionals of all kinds, including lawyers and doctors. Clients are developing a healthy iconoclasm about professional experts and no longer accept advice without questioning. Increasingly, clinicians are being sued for malpractice. Monetary awards are much smaller than in the United States, however, perhaps because British lawyers do not take a percentage of the settlement as their fee. The media have had a powerful influence in leading consumers to question the advice of medical as well as other experts. In response, medical schools are training their students to respect patients' autonomy and doctors are treating patients more as equals.

Medical genetics has assumed a leadership role in the turn away from medical paternalism, because the centerpiece of medical genetics is counselling rather than surgery or drugs. Counselling requires dialogue; its therapy is through communication. The field of genetics has a uniquely well-developed sense of multidisciplinary partnership in which clinical doctors, laboratory scientists, and others work in harmony as a team. The consultant clinical geneticist regards him/herself as *pri-*

*mus inter pares* in clinical matters, rather than as an autocratic leader, a view that is accepted by the majority of laboratory colleagues.

There are no major cultural barriers to public acceptance of medical genetics. Many Britons have no strong religious loyalties, and congregations in churches are smaller than previously. Religious fundamentalism is uncommon, and the British appear generally to be more open about sexual matters than Americans. Cultural minorities – largely from the Indian Subcontinent and the West Indies – may have different beliefs from the majority about abortion or the value of female children, and sometimes have special problems in counselling, which is best performed by trained individuals of the same ethnic group.

## 2.18.4.1 Sources of Challenge and Support

The major challenge to medical genetics comes from religious groups opposed to abortion. Believing that it is politically impossible to repeal the Abortion Act of 1967, attempts are made periodically (about once every two years) to chip away at legal abortion by severely restricting, for example, the maximum age of gestation beyond which abortion would be illegal (see 2.18.4.4 below). As a result, obstetricians may become increasingly cautious about performing abortions on "mental health" grounds. The anti-abortionists also oppose all research on human embryos (see 2.18.4.2). The most recent attempts to introduce restrictive legislation were Enoch Powell's bill for the Protection of the Unborn child [sic.], which would have made embryo research illegal, and David Alton's bill prohibiting abortion after 18 weeks (see 2.18.4.4 below).

## 2.18.4.2 Major Controversies

At present the most intrusive problem is the alleged underfunding of the NHS. If the new genetics of diagnosis by DNA probes, establishment of family registers, and services for members of the extended family is to become accessible to most in Britain, NHS funding for these purposes must be increased. Only in this way can the tradition of equal access be maintained, a principle that is clearly understood by DHSS (see 2.18.1.4 above). If additional NHS funding were not to be provided, there might well be an increasing privatisation of genetic services. Not only would private laboratories be established to meet unmet needs, but there would be increasing pressure on existing NHS-supported laboratories to become commercially orientated so as to contract with the NHS and with private obstetricians. This will mean that genetic services could become a fee-for-service enterprise, available mostly to those who are able to pay. Such an arrangement would appear to many to violate the basic principles of fairness that established the NHS, and would perpetuate social inequality.

Embryo research is another major controversy. At present, a White Paper on the Warnock Report seeks to give the House of Commons a free vote on whether re-

410

search on the human embryo should be abolished completely, except for tests on its normality that would be used as precursors to its implantation (for example, after IVF), *or* whether all research on embryos up to 14 days should be permitted, provided that it takes place in licensed facilities.

A third major controversy is the current attempt of antiabortionists to change the legal limit from 28 to 18 weeks (see 2.18.4.4 below).

## 2.18.4.3  National Expenditures for Medical Genetics

There are no definitive estimates of NHS expenditures on genetics services. The estimated cost of setting up a basic recombinant DNA laboratory as part of a Regional Genetic Service is £80,000 or less for basic equipment and £117,000 for annual operating expenses, including salaries. This does not take into account clinical salaries or the knock-on costs for other services such as obstetrics, ultrasound, etc.

## 2.18.4.4  Abortion Laws in Britain

Under the Abortion Act of 1967, abortions are permitted up to the presumed limit of fetal viability on the following grounds:

"1. The continuance of the pregnancy would involve risk to the life of the pregnant woman greater than if the pregnancy were terminated.
 2. The continuance of the pregnancy would involve risk of injury to the physical or mental health of the pregnant woman greater than if the pregnancy were terminated.
 3. The continuance of the pregnancy would involve risk of injury to the physical or mental health of the existing child(ren) of the family of the pregnant woman greater than if the pregnancy were terminated.
 4. There is a substantial risk that if the child were born, it would suffer from such physical or mental abnormalities as to be seriously handicapped."

Ground # 2 has been interpreted very broadly in practise. There is no specific provision for abortion for social or economic reasons.

In 1967, 28 weeks was set as the presumed lower limit of fetal viability. Before 28 weeks, the burden of proof of viability falls on the prosecution, though since 1967 no criminal charges have been brought against a clinician for performing an abortion under 28 weeks. After 28 weeks, the fetus is presumed viable and is protected under the Infant Life (Preservation) Act of 1929. The burden of proving nonviability falls on the defense.

A bill recently before Parliament would have reduced the limit of presumed viability to 18 weeks and received a majority vote at the second reading. Introduced by David Alton, Liberal Party MP from Liverpool Mossley Hill, the bill was supported by the anti-abortion lobby and by members of the public who believe that the Abortion Act of 1967 has been interpreted too liberally. It is believed that much of the Parliamentary support was from MPs who would seek modification to 24 weeks and/or exceptions for fetal abnormality before the bill became law. However, Parliamentary procedures, as anticipated, actually prevented the bill from becoming law.

The Royal College of Obstetricians and Gynaecologists (RCOG), Royal College of Midwives, Royal College of General Practitioners, British Medical Association, British Paediatric Association, and Clinical Genetics Society, in opposing the Alton Bill, gave many details (RCOG 1987). In 1986, 314 (15.5%) of 2,019 abortions performed at 20 weeks and over for residents of England and Wales were solely on Ground # 4, "substantial risk that the child would be seriously handicapped" (Ian Leck, personal communication 1988). Approximately 25.5% of all abortions done for fetal abnormality in 1986 were performed after 19 weeks gestation (Ian Leck, personal communication 1988) because of the time required to report amniocentesis results. In 1982, for 17,878 amniocenteses at 26 laboratories, results were reported at 22–23 weeks for 11.5% and at 24 weeks or later for an additional 3% (RCOG 1985). Women found to have an abnormal fetus need time to consider whether to have an abortion. Consequently, such terminations tend to be performed several days or even longer after a diagnosis of fetal malformation has been made. Replacing amniocentesis with CVS, which would make possible earlier reports and first-trimester abortions, would not solve the problem, for several reasons. First, many women book for antenatal care after the 12th week. Second, the estimated miscarriage rate for CVS is 4%, compared with 0.5–1% for amniocentesis. Finally, CVS does not diagnose many disorders detectable by maternal serum alpha-fetoprotein, ultrasound and/or amniocentesis, notably neural tube defects and Down syndrome.

The RCOG and collaborating medical associations have proposed that the presumed limit of fetal viability be reduced to 24 weeks, because even with intensive neonatal care babies of this age do not survive. Before 24 weeks the fetal lungs are not sufficiently developed to sustain life. Only about 4.7% of legal abortions for fetal malformations are done after 24 weeks (RCOG 1985), and earlier reporting of amniocentesis results could reduce this percentage. The RCOG proposal represents a balance between conflicting interests and is consistent with the recently published Report of the Select Committee on the Infant Life (Preservation) Bill of the House of Lords (Great Britain, Parlimentary Papers [Lords] 1988). The great majority of viable fetuses would be protected, while, with few exceptions, women with currently accepted reasons for a legal abortion would still be able to obtain one.

## 2.18.4.5 Studies of Effectiveness of Genetic Services

Effectiveness may be interpreted in several ways: as patient (or clinician) satisfaction, as a reduction in the numbers of births of affected children, as monetary savings, or as a reduction in the anxiety or guilt felt by patients. Surveys of patient satisfaction are generally not informative, because most patients say that they are satisfied, not only in surveys of genetic counselling, but with virtually any medical service surveyed (Sorenson et al. 1981). The same is true of clinicians, who reported satisfaction after 95% of 1069 genetic counselling sessions in a U.S. survey (Wertz, Sorenson, and Heeren 1988). Clinician satisfaction was not related to successful communication with patients nor to patient learning of genetic information.

A reduction in the number of children born with neural tube defects has been described earlier (Section 2.18.1.4). Carter [1971] and others have shown that reproductive decisions made after counselling were pretty much related to the magnitude of risk the consultand was given.

Some "genetic" screening programmes, referred to earlier in section 2.18.1.4, have been shown to pay for themselves in the sense that the cost of screening is more than offset by the savings in lifetime care (Wald 1984). These include screening and prenatal diagnosis for Down syndrome, neural tube defects and Tay-Sachs disease, screening and treatment of phenylketonuria and congenital hypothyroidism, and the reduction in the frequency of erythroblastosis fetalis by maternal immunization. Old et al. [1986] provide a particularly relevant example in the successful application of recombinant DNA technology in the first trimester diagnosis of haemoglobinopathies following screening for carriers.

Evaluation of genetic services in cost-benefit terms overlooks the most important aspects, which include providing people with opportunities to choose, helping them to cope with genetic risks or disorders, and alleviating anxiety, guilt, and fear. Success in these aspects of counselling cannot be measured in economic terms.

Follow-up evaluations of the psychological and support aspects of counselling have concentrated on the psychological sequelae of abortion for genetic reasons (Donnai et al. 1981; Forrest et al. 1982; Lloyd and Laurence 1985). The results led to a King's Fund Forum [1987] recommendation that bereavement counselling be provided for such patients.

More recently, psychosocial research has focussed on presymptomatic testing for Huntington's chorea and other disorders detectable through DNA probes. Before such tests were available, surveys indicated that 75% of those at risk would accept a predictive test for Huntington's (Tyler and Harper 1983). Actual uptake of the DNA predictive test, which requires the cooperation of key family members, has thus far been far less.

There is a need for more research into the factors that underlie decisions about testing (Craufurd and Harris 1986), and some information is now becoming available on how subjects actually behave when they are offered predictive tests (Mastromauro et al. 1986). Some procrastinate, while others are convinced that their test will prove negative. There is a strong desire for relief from uncertainty and this is frequently generated by the need to be able to make informed decisions about reproduction. We must not overlook the altruistic concern of many couples for the future welfare of their putative offspring. One of the rewards of caring for families with severe hereditary disease is to witness the remarkable common sense, resilience, and mutual concern that their members often demonstrate (Wexler 1984).

413

## 2.18.4.6 Need for New Laws

The development of computerized family registries for genetic disorders has led to a need for new laws to protect confidentiality. The doctor's ability to safeguard confidential information is endangered by the increasing involvement of large health care teams, including those associated with genetic registers. The more people with access, the more difficult it becomes to guarantee confidentiality. Recent legislation (Data Protection Act 1985) has provided some protection against the possible misuse of computerized health data. Similarly the Code on Confidentiality of Personal Health Information now being prepared by DHSS should provide additional safeguards. At a recent conference on medical ethics, Sir Douglas Black echoed the general feeling that confidentiality must be jealously guarded, except only for cases of truly *overriding* public health concern and for things that one would be prepared to justify in a court of law (Harris 1987b).

There is a likelihood of new laws concerning donor eggs or sperm and the legal status of children born following egg or embryo donation. A Consultation Paper on the Warnock Report (Great Britain, DHSS 1986) invited comments on a proposed licensing authority for infertility treatments such as IVF, donor insemination, and egg or embryo donation; proposed statutory requirements for counselling of couples prior to such treatments; and on ways in which a system of registering and recording children born as a result of donor insemination or egg/embryo donation might be set up. The Consultation Paper sought views on how best such a registration system might a) meet the child's need for access to the truth about his or her genetic origins and some information about the genetic father or mother; b) satisfy the family's need for privacy; and c) take account of the donor's wish for anonymity. Comments were also invited on the legal status of such children, and on surrogacy.

As discussed above in 2.18.4.4, there is a recommendation to reduce the lower limit of presumed fetal viability from 28 to 24 weeks (RCOG 1985), in order to reflect advances in neonatal care.

## 2.18.5 Ethical Issues and Future Trends

The "New Genetics" using recombinant DNA technology represents arguably the greatest challenge that clinical medicine has yet faced (Harris 1988). At the present rate, all genetic disorders will probably be mapped to their chromosomal location by the year 2000 (Cooper and Schmidtke 1987), and most important genes will eventually be sequenced and their products identified. It is not known to what extent the active use of recombinant DNA technology for prevention will alter the balance of favourable genetic polymorphisms (Rotter and Diamond 1987). The ethical issues of counselling, consent and confidentiality are of more immediate concern. It is not clear who will look after the interests of families and undertake the explanation and counselling that must precede tests designed to probe the most intimate and socially sensitive genetic secrets. Who will insure that informed consent is obtained, arrange the family studies, keep the confidential records and computerized family registers, and store the banks of DNA spanning whole families and several generations? Who will be responsible for contacting each family regularly to update the registers and to inform them of any new tests or treatments? These are dangerous topics for amateurs, and if they have received little genetic training doctors may have difficulty recognising genetic risk. Genetic specialists are already overburdened; those in the survey saw more patients per week than geneticists in any other country except France. The number of clinical geneticists falls far short of the minimum required. There are only about 35 consultants and 7 training posts for senior registrars for the UK as a whole. Although the number of training posts has been increased to 14, plans to increase the number of consultants to 60 were developed before the New Genetics. One clinical geneticist per million population will be hard pressed indeed (Harris 1987a).

Some foresee the privatisation of NHS genetics laboratories, which would then do contract work for both NHS and private clinicians, and in addition, the establishment of private laboratories. This would mean that an increased proportion of genetics patients would be those who can pay for testing. The two-income family that has postponed child-raising until their mid-thirties would become the primary customers for chromosome analyses. This prospect challenges the British sense of fairness and the belief that health care is a right rather than a privilege. If there is indeed increasing privatisation, there may eventually be a need for a national policy about revelation of fetal sex, in order to prevent misuse of services. At present this misuse, deprecated by DHSS, is in large part prevented by the effective rationing of amniocentesis under the NHS.

Other ethical problems of the future include the possible social effects of DNA carrier testing (for example on choice of marital partners) and the possibility that when the human genome is mapped and DNA testing becomes automated there will be a push to make CVS routine for every pregnancy. If CVS is offered for each of an annual 700,000 pregnancies, it will be essential to counsel women adequately about its risks and to obtain informed consent. It appears likely that, whatever happens, pregnancy will be subjected to increased technological intervention and that people's expectations about perfection in their children will also increase. The New Genetics has the potential to change our definition of health and disease, and we should be prepared for its social impact.

# Acknowledgements

The authors would like to thank Tony Andrews, David Craufurd, and Lauren Kerzen Storer, Department of Medical Genetics, St. Mary's Hospital, Manchester, for useful discussion. Dr. M. A. Ferguson-Smith of Cambridge University was responsible for distributing and collecting the survey questionnaires.

415

# Abbreviations

ACC   Association of Clinical Cytogeneticists
DHSS  Department of Health and Social Security
HMSO  Her Majesty's Stationery Office
NHS   National Health Service
OPCS  Office of Population Censuses and Surveys
RCOG  Royal College of Obstetricians and Gynaecologists

# References

Anonymous [1982] Directive counselling. Lancet i: 368–369

Association of Clinical Cytogeneticists [1986] Review of clinical cytogenetics services 1984: England, Scotland, and Wales

Beeson D, Golbus MS [1985] Decisionmaking: whether or not to have prenatal diagnosis and abortion for X-linked conditions. Am J Med Genet 20: 107–114

Brooks H [1973] The physical sciences: bellwether of science policy. In: Shannon JA (ed) Science and the evolution of public policy. Rockefeller University Press, New York

Carter CO, Fraser Roberts JA, Evans KA, Buck AR [1971] Genetic clinic: a follow-up. Lancet i: 281–285

Cooper DN, Schmidtke J [1987] Human gene cloning and disease analysis. Lancet i: 273

Craufurd DIO, Harris R [1986] Ethics of predictive testing for Huntington's chorea: the need for more information. Br Med J 293: 249–251

Crawfurd M d'A [1983] Ethical and legal aspects of early prenatal diagnosis. Br Med Bull 39 [4]: 310–314

Cuckle HS, Wald NJ [1984] Principles of screening. In: Wald NJ (ed) Antenatal and neonatal screening. Oxford University Press, Oxford

Cuckle HS, Wald NJ [1987] Impact of screening for open neural tube defects in England and Wales. Prenat Diagn 7: 91–99

Cuckle HS, Wald NJ, Thompson SG [1987] Estimating a woman's risk of having a pregnancy associated with Down's syndrome using her age and serum alpha-fetoprotein level. Br J Obstet Gyn 94: 387–402

Donnai P, Charles N, Harris R [1981] Attitudes of patients after "genetic" termination of pregnancy. Br Med J 282: 621–622

Emery AEH, Pullen I (eds) [1984] Psychological aspects of genetic counselling. Academic Press, London

Evers-Kiebooms G, van den Berghe H [1979] Impact of genetic counselling: a review of published follow-up studies. Clin Genet 15: 465–474

Ferguson-Smith MA (1983a) Prenatal chromosome analysis and its impact on the birth incidence of chromosome disorders. Br Med Bull 39 [4]: 355–364

Ferguson-Smith MA (1983b) The reduction of anencephalic and spina bifida births by Maternal Serum Alpha-fetoprotein screening. Br Med Bull 39 [4]: 365–372

Forrest GC, Standish E, Baum JD [1982] Support after perinatal death: a study of support and counselling after perinatal bereavement. Br Med J 285: 1475–1479

Fraser FC [1979] The development of genetic counselling. In: Capron AM, Lappe M, Murray RF, Powledge TM, Twiss SB, Bergsma D (eds) Birth defects: Original article series XV: 5–15. Alan R Liss for the National Foundation – March of Dimes, New York

Fraser Roberts JA [1940] An introduction to medical genetics. Oxford University Press, London

Glass NJ, Cove AR [1978] Cost effectiveness of screening for neural tube defects. In: Scrimgeour JB (ed) Towards the prevention of fetal malformation. Edinburgh University Press, Edinburgh

416

Great Britain, Department of Health and Social Security [1984] Report of the Committee of Enquiry into Human Fertilisation and Embryology. HMSO (Cmnd 9314). Chair: Dame Mary Warnock, London

Great Britain, Department of Health and Social Security [1986] Legislation on human infertility services and embryo research: a consultation paper. HMSO (Cmnd 46), London

Great Britain, Department of Health and Social Security [1987] On the state of the public health for the year 1986. HMSO, London

Great Britain, Department of Health and Social Security, Medical Division CDPNM [1987] Special Medical Development in Clinical Genetics; Interim Report: Clinical Effectiveness in the Service Context. HMSO, London

Great Britain, Office of Population Censuses and Surveys [1987] Monitor AB 87/3

Great Britain, Parliamentary Papers (Commons) [1980] Second report from the Social Services Committee, Session 1979-80: Perinatal and neonatal mortality. HMSO, London

Great Britain, Parliamentary Papers (Commons) [1984] Third report from the Social Services Committee, Session 1983-84: Perinatal and neonatal mortality report: follow-up. HMSO, London

Great Britain, Parliamentary Papers (Lords) [1988] Report of the Select Committee on the Infant Life (Preservation) Bill, Session 1987-88. HMSO, London

Haggard S, Carter FA [1976] Preventing the births of infants with Down's syndrome: cost-benefit analysis. Br Med J i: 735-36

Haggard S, Carter FA, Milne RG [1976] Screening for spina bifida cystica. Br J Prevent Soc Med 30: 40-53

Ham C [1985] Health policy in Britain: the politics and organisation of the National Health Service, second edition. Macmillan Publishers, London

Harper PS [1983] Genetic counselling and prenatal diagnosis. Br Med Bull 39 [4]: 302-309

Harris R (1987a) Make way for the new genetics. Br Med J 295: 349-350

Harris R (1987b) Royal College of Physicians Conference on Medical Ethics, 23 Oct 1986. J Med Genet 24: 251-253

Harris R [1988] Genetic counselling and the new genetics. Trends in Genetics, 4: 52-56

Harris R, Emery AEH, Johnston AW, Pembrey ME, Winter R, Insley J [1983] Role and training of clinical geneticists. Report of the Clinical Genetics Society Working Party. Eugenics Society, London

Hibbard BM, Roberts CJ, Elder GH, Evans KT, Laurence KM [1985] Can we afford screening for neural tube defects? The South Wales experience. Br Med J [Clin Res] 290 [6464]: 293-295

Hollingsworth JR [1986] A political economy of medicine: Great Britain and the United States. Johns Hopkins University Press, Baltimore and London

Kevles DJ [1986] In the name of eugenics: genetics and the uses of human heredity. Penguin, New York

King's Fund Forum [1987] King's Fund Forum consensus statement: screening for fetal and genetic abnormality. Br Med J 295: 1551-1553

Klein R [1983] The politics of the National Health Service. Longman, London

Lavery C [1987] Impact on the family. Paper presented at King's Fund Forum, London, Nov 30-Dec 1, 1987, and personal communication

Lloyd J, Laurence KM [1985] Sequelae and support after termination of pregnancy for fetal malformation. Br Med J 290: 967-969

Markova I, Forbes CD, Inwood M [1984] The consumers' views of genetic counseling of hemophilia. Am J Med Genet 17: 741-752

Mastromauro C, Myers RH, Berkman B [1986] Letter to the editor: change in attitudes toward presymptomatic testing in Huntington disease. Am J Med Genet 24: 369-371

Oakley A [1984] The captured womb: a history of the medical care of pregnant women. Basil Blackwell, Oxford

Old JM, Heath C, Fitches A, Thein SL, Weatherall DJ, Warren R, McKenzie C, Rodeck CH, Modell B, Petrou M, Ward RHT [1986] First-trimester fetal diagnosis for haemoglobinopathies: report on 200 cases, Lancet ii: 763-769

Pembrey ME [1987] Obituary for Dr. John Alexander Fraser Roberts. J Med Genet 24: 442-444

Rotter JI, Diamond JM [1987] What maintains the frequency of human genetic diseases? Nature 329: 289-290

417

Royal College of Obstetricians and Gynaecologists [1984] Report of the RCOG Working Party on routine ultrasound in pregnancy. RCOG, London

Royal College of Obstetricians and Gynaecologists [1985] Report on fetal viability and clinical practise. RCOG, London

Royal College of Obstetricians and Gynaecologists [1987] Fetal viability; a report by a committee representing medical bodies as listed below (RCOG, Royal College of Midwives, Royal College of General Practitioners, British Medical Association, British Paediatric Association, Clinical Genetics Society) RCOG, London

Sorenson JR, Swazey JP, Scotch NA [1981] Reproductive pasts, reproductive futures: genetic counselling and its effectiveness. Alan R Liss, New York

Super M, Schwarz M, Elles RG, Harris R, Ivinson A, Giles L, Read AP [1987] Clinic experience of prenatal diagnosis of cystic fibrosis by use of linked DNA probes. Lancet ii: 782–784

Turnbull AC, MacKenzie IZ [1983] Second-trimester amniocentesis and termination of pregnancy. Br Med Bull 39: 315–321

Tyler A, Harper PS [1983] Attitudes of subjects at risk and their relatives towards genetic counselling in Huntingon's chorea. J Med Genet 20: 179–188

Wald NJ [1984] Antenatal and neonatal screening. Oxford University Press, Oxford

Wertz DC, Sorenson JR, Heeren TC [1988] "Can't get no (dis)satisfaction": professional satisfaction with professional-client encounters. Work and Occupations 15: 36–54

Wexler N [1984] Huntington's disease and other late-onset genetic disorders. In Emery AEH, Pullen I (eds) Psychological aspects of genetic counselling. Academic Press, London, pp 125–146

# Important Publications on Ethics and Human Genetics in Britain

Brazier M [1987] Medicine, patients and the law. Penguin Books, Harmondsworth

Byrne P (ed) [1986] Rights and wrongs in medicine. King's College Studies 1985–1986, King Edward's Hospital Fund for London

Campbell AV [1975] Moral dilemmas in medicine. Churchill Livingstone, Edinburgh

Downie RS, Calman KC [1987] Healthy respect: ethics in health care. Faber & Faber, London

Gillon R [1985, 1986] Philosophical medical ethics. John Wiley & Sons for British Medical Journal, London

Harris J [1985] The value of life: an introduction to medical ethics. Routledge & Kegan Paul, London

Kennedy I [1983] The unmasking of medicine. Paladin, London

Lockwood M (ed) [1985] Moral dilemmas in modern medicine. Oxford University Press, London

## 2.19 The United States of America

J. J. Mulvihill, L. Walters, and D. C. Wertz

### 2.19.1.1 Scope of the Problem

The population of the United States was estimated at 241,078,000 in 1986. Some 114,880,000 were between the ages of 15 and 44 years, considered the age of likely reproduction. The racial distribution of the population was 85% white, 12% black, and 3% other. There were about 18,091,000 persons of Hispanic origin, who may be of any race. The religious preferences of the population were 59% Protestant, 27% Catholic, 2% Jewish, 4% other, and 8% none (U.S., Department of Commerce 1988a, pp 16, 17, 52).

On average from 1976–1986, there have been 3.5 million births, 2 million deaths, 2.4 million marriages and 1.2 million divorces annually. The birth rate has fallen from 18.4 per 1,000 population in 1970 to 15.9 in 1980 and 15.5 in 1986. In 1986 there were 3,731,000 live births. The 1985 infant mortality rate, higher than many other nations at 10.6 per 1,000 live births, is attributed largely to poor access to prenatal services, especially for poor and minority women, and not to any excess of genetic disorders. There is a large difference in infant mortality by race: 9.3 per 1,000 for whites and 18.2 per 1,000 for blacks (U.S., Department of Commerce 1988a, pp 59, 75).

The relative contribution of genetic conditions to the infant mortality rate has increased dramatically as infant deaths from infections and other causes have been reduced by advances in medicine and improved maternal nutrition. The percent of infant deaths due to congenital malformations rose from an estimated 6.4% in 1915 to 17.3% in 1976 (U.S., Dept. of Health, Education and Welfare 1979).

Genetic disorders are also important causes of childhood mortality. Of 40,030 deaths under one year of age, the major causes in 1985 were perinatal problems (48%, including respiratory illness, prematurity, and low birthweight), congenital anomalies (21%), sudden infant death syndrome (13%), and accidents (2%). The three most common birth defects were heart, respiratory, and chromosomal anomalies (U.S., National Center for Health Statistics 1987). Of 16,272 deaths of children age one to 14 years in 1985, the major causes were accidents (44%), malignant neoplasms (11%), congenital anomalies (8%), homicide (5%) and acquired heart disease (4%).

It is estimated that at least 40% of all persons with an I.Q. of less than 50 in the United States have genetic disorders or severe developmental malformation syndromes (Stein et al. 1978). In the 1960s, approximately 25% to 30% of admissions to major acute care hospitals of persons 1 day to 18 years of age were for conditions of genetic origin (Childs 1972).

**Table 2.19.1.** Estimated Frequency of Selected Genetic Abnormalities in the Newborn

| Disorder | Incidence |
|---|---|
| Chromosomal Abnormalities[a] | |
| Trisomy 21 | 1 in 800 – 1,000 births |
| Trisomy 18 | 1 in 8,000 births |
| Trisomy 13 | 1 in 20,000 births |
| XXY | 1 in 1,000 male births |
| XYY | 1 in 1,000 male births |
| XXX | 1 in 950 female births |
| 45, X | 1 in 10,000 female births |
| Inborn Errors of Metabolism[b] | |
| Sickle-cell anemia[c] | 1 in 400 American Blacks |
| Cystic fibrosis | 1 in 1,600–2,500 Caucasians |
| Tay-Sachs disease | 1 in 3,600 Ashkenazi Jews |
| Phenylketonuria | 1 in 14,000 of the general population |
| Neural Tube Defects[d] | |
| Anencephaly | 1 in 1,000 live births |
| Spina bifida | 1 in 1,000 live births |

[a] Hook 1977
[b] U.S., President's Commission 1983, p 13
[c] In addition to those of African heritage, persons of Greek or Italian background are also at increased risk
[d] U.S., President's Commission, p 27

In contrast, the incidence of genetic disease is not well documented. There are several systems that monitor congenital malformations, some of which have major genetic determinants. One system, known as the Birth Defects Monitoring Program of the Centers for Disease Control, keeps track of malformations occurring in the first thirty days of life for about one third of the births in the United States (Edmonds 1981).

In addition, there are regional malformation registries, the best being in Metropolitan Atlanta, Georgia, with a population base of 2 million persons with 32,439 births in 1986. At least 12 states register birth defects (Andrews 1985, p 187), but they often count only what is written by the obstetrician on the birth certificate in the first three days of life; they are very imperfect for estimating the frequency of genetic diseases. Special surveys of genetic diseases have been undertaken for research purposes that established the prevalence rates for various disorders (Table 2.19.1) but do not provide systematic monitoring for trends over time.

## 2.19.1.2  Organization of Clinical Genetics Services

Like other aspects of life in the United States, genetics services are very much a pluralistic, capitalistic activity. There is great diversity in types of clinics, services offered, and methods of payment. Free-standing commercial laboratories for prenatal diagnosis co-exist with private hospitals, university hospitals, and public, state-supported clinics that serve lower-income people. Payment is on a fee-for-service basis, on the model of business enterprises. Patients may be insured by a variety of private insurance companies, by a health maintenance organization (HMO) that provides most of their medical care, by Medicaid, a federal program that covers some low-income persons, or they may have no insurance at all. Geneticists may have private practices, essentially run as businesses, but most work for salaries in private university or public hospitals. The Federal Government does not regulate medical practice or fees, although it does regulate drugs through the Food and Drug Administration (FDA), medical devices, and government-sponsored research (but not privately sponsored research).

The licensing and disciplining of physicians, including geneticists, is done mainly by professional organizations in cooperation with licensing boards in individual states. Lawsuits initiated by patients are also a powerful force in setting standards of practice.

Most clinical geneticists belong to the American Society of Human Genetics (as do many researchers who do not see patients). As of 1988, the Society had some 2,968 members whose addresses were in the United States. In 1981, the American Board of Medical Genetics was founded for the purposes of certifying individuals as experts in medical genetics and accrediting training programs in medical genetics. The Board has given three examinations and has certified 1,292 individuals with U.S. addresses and accredited 67 training programs. Candidates have been certified in five subspecialties: clinical genetics [509], biochemical genetics [106], cytogenetics [293], genetic counseling [486], and Ph.D. medical genetics [113]. Some members are certified in more than one subspecialty, so the total of all subspecialists exceeds the actual number of members.

Most of the 127 U.S. medical schools have divisions of clinical genetics within departments of pediatrics, obstetrics-gynecology or sometimes other specialties. Genetics is not emphasized in medical education, however. In 1983–84, more than 50 schools did not require courses in genetics and in the remainder, an average of 27 hours was devoted to genetics (Rothstein 1987, p 298). Most tertiary care centers provide some genetics services as indicated in directories of genetics services (U.S., National Center for Education in Maternal and Child Health 1985; March of Dimes Birth Defects Foundation 1986).

The local laboratory for genetics services is often limited to cytogenetics. Comprehensive biochemical genetics assays are found in just a few centers. Many specimens are shipped to large laboratories that centralize cytogenetics and biochemical genetics. The quality of genetics laboratory services is monitored by the American College of Pathology for Cytogenetics and plans are underway for assuring quality in the provision of DNA genetics services.

A typical genetics clinic service has one senior physician, one or two additional physicians, and one or two fellows who are subspecializing in genetics, having achieved primary specialization in pediatrics, obstetrics-gynecology, or internal medicine. In addition, there are laboratory geneticists and technicians, as well as a type of clinician peculiar to the provision of genetics services in North America: a genetics associate who is trained to the level of a Master's degree in genetics and psychology and who performs many of the tasks of genetic counseling beyond the single session with a doctorate level clinician. These tasks include exploring the patient's concerns, eliciting and documenting family medical history, reiterating the primary counseling session and following up to reinforce the information. Special training for counselors was formalized in 1969 with the establishment of the first master's degree program in genetic counseling at Sarah Lawrence College in Bronxville, New York. There are now 12 training programs for genetic associates in the United States and one in Canada.

The counselors often join the National Society of Genetic Counselors, which registers some 639 members, including 507 Master's level members. Almost 400 Master's level counselors are certified by the American Board of Medical Genetics. Most are women.

Holtzman [1988] has estimated that approximately 100 clinical geneticists at the doctoral level and 75 masters-level genetic counselors enter the field each year, while approximately 25 persons retire or leave the field. At this rate it will take at least ten years to double the number of geneticists. Holtzman thinks that genetic centers now serve 500,000 persons annually at most.

The Federal Government provides some support for genetics services through the Genetics Services Branch of the Health Services Administration of the Department of Health and Human Services. Apart from limited Federal Government support, families and patients with genetic disorders must meet expenses by their own resources, either directly or through private insurance (see 2.19.4.3 below). The Sickle Cell Anemia Control Act, passed in 1972, was the first Federal legislation providing support for genetic disease. The law provided for research and treatment, for the establishment of voluntary sickle cell screening and counseling, and for disseminating educational materials to health care providers and the general public. By 1975, 26 such clinics were in operation in 20 states. In 1976, the National Genetic Disease Act (Title XI of the Public Health Service Act) established "a national program to provide for basic and applied research, research training, testing, counseling, information and education programs with respect to genetic diseases (University of Colorado 1987; Forsman 1983)."

Under this law and its successors, 85% of the funds went to states to set up genetic services, but only for a period of four years for each state, after which funding was withdrawn. By 1986, all states except Texas had been incorporated into 1 of 9 regional genetics networks (University of Colorado 1987).

Genetics services are typically provided on referral by a primary physician or self-referral of the proband or family. In addition, some families and individuals enter a genetics clinic through statewide screening programs. There is no mandatory screening for genetic disease at the national level, but most state governments require routine screening of newborns for PKU and congenital hypothyroidism, and several states also screen for galactosemia, maple syrup urine disease, tyrosinemia, homocystinuria, and sickle cell anemia. Screening tests are performed only with parental consent. The adequacy of medical genetics services has never been documented, but is felt to be limited for some segments of the population, especially those of modest means, but not poor enough to require total government assistance.

## 2.19.1.3 Prenatal Diagnosis

Most practicing obstetricians probably alert appropriate patients to the availability of prenatal diagnosis. Sometimes, however, prenatal diagnosis is not offered. In a study of 520 women who had had amniocentesis, only 36% had learned of the procedure from their obstetricians; another 36% had learned of it from the media (McGovern et al. 1986). Physicians who neglect to offer the tests to patients when medically indicated are legally liable. In 1985, a West Virginia court ordered a physician to pay the special cost of raising a child with Down syndrome, for the child's lifetime (even after reaching adulthood), because the physician had neglected to offer amniocentesis to the parent (Andrews 1987, pp 140-141). Judgments of this magnitude have undoubtedly led most to offer the service, but this has not been documented. Many pregnant women who may merit prenatal genetic services do not use them, some perhaps because they present too late in pregnancy. In 1985, 24% of mothers did not seek prenatal care in the first trimester; 21% of white mothers, 38% of black mothers, and 39% of Hispanic mothers did not receive prenatal care in the first trimester (U.S., National Center for Health Statistics 1987). In many inner-city public hospitals that serve poor women, over half do not seek prenatal care until after the 25th week. This is one reason why diagnoses for disorders prevalent in this group – such as sickle cell – are performed less often than diagnoses for other types of disorders.

Utilization of prenatal diagnosis is increasing, however. For example, 35% of pregnant women age 35 or over in New York State underwent the procedure in 1980, as compared to 29% in 1979 (Hook and Schreinemachers 1983). In New York City, the rates increased from 34% in 1979 to 44% in 1982, largely because of a publicly-funded program to provide services to the indigent (Schreinemachers and Hook 1984). The proportion utilizing the tests increased sharply from age 34 on, reached a peak at age 39 or 40, but then declined sharply at older ages. The decline in utilization after age 40 may be because there is a growing proportion with age who would not elect abortion under any circumstances. The most important variables influencing rate of utilization were the knowledge, interest, and attitudes of obstetricians (Bernhardt and Bannerman 1983). There are wide regional and racial variations. For example, in a Georgia study of women aged 40 years and over, 15% used prenatal diagnosis, ranging from 60% among whites in urban areas to 0.5% of blacks in rural areas (Sokal et al. 1980). There are unfortunately no national data on utilization.

The number of pregnancies for which prenatal diagnosis is appropriate because of advanced maternal age has steadily grown, as women postpone childbearing. Births to women aged 35 to 39 increased from 115,000 in 1975 to 141,000 in 1980, and to 214,000 in 1985. Births to women aged 40 or more held relatively steady (28,000 in 1975 and 29,000 in 1985). Births to women aged 30 to 34, however, also increased, from 376,000 in 1975 to 550,000 in 1980 and 696,000 in 1985. Providing prenatal diagnosis to all women 35 and over would therefore mean 243,000 procedures annually. Including women 30-34, which some studies suggest might be cost-beneficial (Hook 1977), would mean 939,000 procedures annually, which is far beyond present capacity.

If a completely safe procedure (such as obtaining fetal cells from the maternal circulation) becomes available, about 1,985,000 procedures would be needed annually. This is a conservative estimate, based on data that about 76% of pregnant women receive prenatal care in the first trimester and approximately 70% of these will accept prenatal diagnoses (Faden et al. 1987; Holtzman 1989). Approximately 3,573 affected fetuses would be diagnosed.

**Indications**

In 1979, a Consensus Development Conference on Antenatal Diagnosis sponsored by the National Institute of Child Health and Human Development recommended the following as indications for amniocentesis: pregnancies in women 35 years of age or more; a previous pregnancy that has resulted in the birth of a chromosomally abnormal offspring; a chromosome abnormality in either parent; history of Down syndrome or other chromosome abnormality in a family; history of multiple (three or more) spontaneous abortions in this marriage or in a previous mating of either spouse; previous birth of a child with multiple major malformations; women with male relatives with X-linked disorders; couples at risk for detectable inborn errors of metabolism; and pregnancies at increased risk for neural tube defects (U.S., Department of Health, Education, and Welfare 1979, pp 201–203). The conference suggested that the 35-year age limit should be interpreted flexibly. The Consensus Development Conference recommendations were not mandatory in the sense of law or government policy, but were purely advisory.

Studies have subsequently shown that there are wide variations between clinics and changes over time. Data from three surveys were compared: one from Boston in the late 1960s and early 1970s (Milunsky 1975), another from 1978 through July 1, 1984, in Ohio (Naber 1987), and a third from a large private clinic in suburban Washington, D.C. from 1985 to 1986 (Green 1988). The first two relate to amniocentesis, the third to chorionic villus biopsy. The percentages of procedures done for advanced maternal age (generally 35 or more) increased from 52%, to 71% and 90%; the percent of procedures done for family history of or previous child with genetic defect fell from 34%, to 10% and 7%. Additionally, the Ohio study reported that 15% of amniocenteses were performed for anxiety due to increased maternal age (30–34 years of age.) The indications for prenatal diagnoses have likely changed over the years with physician and public education, and improved techniques. No firm policy is established by any single organization; rather, practices are defined by consensus among the general public, pregnant women, doctors, hospitals, and to a lesser extent, government and insurance companies. For example, some Catholic hospitals prohibit abortions. Also the early declarations by the Federal Government that chorionic villus sampling was considered a research procedure delayed the widespread use of the technique in the U.S.

## 2.19.1.4  Cost-benefit of Early Diagnosis

A recent cost-benefit analysis of prenatal screening for neural tube defects (NTDs) illustrates the ethical problems involved both in such analyses and in mass screening itself (Meister et al. 1987). In the United States, NTDs affect 1 to 2 per 1,000 live births. Almost half (46%) are anencephalics, who will die shortly after birth. Many of the rest will live normal lifespans; some will be mildly disabled, but some will require lifetime care estimated at $40,000 to $50,000 a year. The monetary costs of screening per woman come to $39 (Table 2.19.2), including abortions for those with positive findings. The cost per NTD detected would be $87,274, which is far less than the projected costs of lifetime care for an affected child. The problem lies in the sensitivity and specificity of the tests, and the fact that after each stage of testing, some women decline further tests. Table 2.19.3 shows the diagnoses that would result from screening 1 million women with a cutoff at the 95th percentile for the first test (that is, a positive result means the woman showed a maternal serum alpha fetoprotein value above that of 95% of women found to be unaffected). The program would identify 52% (424 out of 819) of the fetuses with

**Table 2.19.2.** Monetary Costs of Screening for Neural Tube Defects[a]

| Test | | Unit Cost | Utilization per Woman in Cohort | Cost per woman in Cohort |
|---|---|---|---|---|
| First maternal serum alpha fetoprotein | $ | 25 | 1.0000 | $25.00 |
| Second maternal serum alpha fetoprotein | | 25 | 0.0571 | 1.43 |
| Ultrasonography | | 180 | 0.0398 | 7.17 |
| Alpha fetoprotein (amniocentesis) | | 225 | 0.0195 | 4.39 |
| Abortion | | 1,200 | 0.0009 | 1.10 |
| Total | | | 1.1174 | $39.10 |

[a] Meister et al. 1987

**Table 2.19.3.** Projected Outcomes of Screening 1,000,000 Women for Neural Tube Defects[a]

| | Anen-cephaly | Spina Bifida | Unaffected | Multiple Gestation | Total |
|---|---|---|---|---|---|
| Total Number in Cohort | 747[b] | 870[b] | 988,933 | 9,450[c] | 1,000,000 |
| Alive at End of Testing | 699 | 819 | 986,645 | 8,986 | 997,149 |
| °No Neural Tube Defect Diagnosed | 141 | 245 | 979,503 | 8,346 | 988,235 |
| °Incomplete Testing | 146 | 150 | 7,053 | 640 | 7,989 |
| °Neural Tube Defect Diagnosed | 412 | 424 | 89 | 0 | 925 |
| Spontaneous Fetal Death | 49 | 50 | 2,287 | 465 | 2,851 |
| Cases Found by Screening | 412 | 424 | −89[d] | 0 | 747 |

[a] Meister et al. 1987, p 80
"Alive at end of testing" and "spontaneous fetal death" sum to total number in cohort. The three rows with bullets sum to "alive at end of testing." "Cases found by screening" are the number of pregnancies diagnosed with neural tube defects. Elements may not sum exactly due to rounding.
[b] Population incidence, from Goldberg and Oakley 1979
[c] Population incidence from National Center for Health Statistics 1982
[d] The negative number of unaffected pregnancies indicates that these pregnancies are misdiagnosed as affected by neural tube defects.

spina bifida and 59% (412 out of 699) of those with anencephaly. It would mistakenly identify as abnormal 89 with unaffected pregnancies. It would also leave 7,989 women who received positive results on an interim screening test and who discontinued testing with the thought that their fetuses might have an NTD. Of these, 296 would actually be affected and 7,693 would be normal. The number of false positives could be reduced by setting the cutoff in the first test at the 99th percentile, but this would lower the NTD detection rate (Goldberg and Oakley 1979). Monetary cost-benefit analyses do not take into account the anxiety suffered by women who leave the testing program under a cloud of uncertainty or the loss of normal fetuses aborted after false positive diagnoses. Nor can cost-benefit analyses find a monetary justification for providing prenatal NTD screening for women who would not abort but wish to prepare for the birth of an affected child. Cost-benefit analyses can only find value in prenatal screening if affected fetuses are aborted.

Cost-benefit analyses have in fact been used by policy-makers in setting the age limits for prenatal diagnosis of Down syndrome. The incidence of Down syndrome varies from 1/885 to 1/32 as maternal age increases from 30 to 45. If the diagnostic sensitivity and specificity of testing were both 99.5%, the probability that the fetus is affected, given a trisomy 21 karyotype, would vary from 0.18 for a 30-year-old woman to 0.87 for a 45-year-old woman. For a 30-year-old woman, the risk is 1/885. Thus, of 1,000,000 pregnancies, 1,130 fetuses would have Down syndrome and 99.5% of these, or 1,124, would have trisomy 21 karyotypes (true positives). Of the 998,870 unaffected pregnancies, 0.5%, or 4,994, would have trisomy 21 karyotypes (false positives). Thus, only 1,124 of the 6,118 trisomy 21 karyotypes or 18% of the total positives, would have Down syndrome. For a 45-year-old woman, the risk is 1/32, or 31,250 Down syndrome fetuses per 1,000,000 pregnancies. Of those, 99.5% or 31,094 would have trisomy 21 karyotypes (true positives). Of the 968,750 unaffected pregnancies, 0.5%, or 4,844 would also have trisomy 21 karyotypes (false positives). Of the 35,938 total positives, 31,094 or 87% would be affected. Sensitivities and specificities of 99.9% would give probabilities of 0.53 that the fetus of a 30-year-old woman with a trisomy 21 has Down syndrome, and 0.97 for the fetus of a 45-year-old (Pauker and Pauker 1979).

If one looks at these probabilities in terms of potential cost-savings, however, it seems, at first glance, fairly easy to justify prenatal diagnosis (Hook 1977). Studies of prospective parents suggest that even if the probability of Down syndrome is as low as 20%, half would abort (Pauker et al. 1981). One study found a benefit/cost ratio of 1.9 for amniocentesis and abortion of Down syndrome or trisomy 18 fetuses, a ratio that increased to 219 if the affected fetus was subsequently replaced by a normal child (Conley and Milunsky 1975).

The President's Commission for the Study of Ethical Problems in Medicine and Biomedical and Behavioral Research [1983] has pointed to the significant limitations of cost-benefit analysis as a method of determining public policy.

"Cost-benefit analysis is most useful when the cost and benefits of the action under consideration are tangible, can be measured by a common unit of measurement, and can be known with certainty. These conditions are rarely satisfied in public policy situations and they can be particularly elusive in genetic screening and counseling programs. For example, cost-benefit calculations can accurately evaluate the worth of a projected prenatal screening program if the only costs measured are the financial outlays (that is, administering a screening and counseling program and performing abortions when defects are detected) and the benefits measured are the dollars that would have been spent on care of affected children. But the calculations become both much more complex and much less accurate if an attempt is made to quantify the psychological 'cost' and 'benefits' to screenees, their families, and society.

"A more fundamental limitation on cost-benefit analysis is that in its simplest form it assumes that the governing moral value is to maximize the general welfare (utilitarianism). Simply aggregating gains and losses across all the individuals affected omits conditions of equity or fairness. Indeed, cost-benefit methodology itself does not distinguish as to *whose* costs and benefits are to be considered. But in the case at hand, it is an ethical question as to whether the costs and benefits to the fetus are to be considered, and, if so, whether they are to be given the same weight as those of the mother and family....

"In any case, *cost-benefit analysis must be regarded as a technical instrument to be used within an ethical framework (whether utilitarian or otherwise), rather than as a method of avoiding difficult ethical judgments.*"

The Commission concluded that cost-benefit analysis "performs the useful function of forcing policy-makers to envision as clearly as possible the consequences of a decision (President's Commission 1983, p 85)."

## 2.19.1.5 Abortion

In 1985, an estimated 1,588,600 legal abortions were performed, or 425 for each 1,000 live births (Henshaw et al. 1987). Only 1% were performed after 20 weeks. Induced abortions that follow abnormal results of prenatal diagnosis comprise less than 1% of all induced abortions.

Most women who have positive findings for severe abnormalities choose abortion. In a study of 3,000 amniocenteses, 113 chromosomal abnormalities were discovered, and 93.8% of women with affected fetuses chose abortion (Golbus et al. 1979). In a study of 7,000 amniocenteses with 149 chromosomal abnormalities, 97% of women whose fetuses had autosomal abnormalities (trisomy 13, 18, 21), but only 62% of those whose fetuses had sex chromosome abnormalities, chose abortion (Benn et al. 1985).

## 2.19.2 Ethical Problems

**Introduction**
Many ethical questions raised by the survey instrument were discussed by an interdisciplinary, public committee appointed by the President of the United States. This body was called the President's Commission for the Study of Ethical Problems in Medicine and Biomedical and Behavioral Research (often abbreviated to

427

President's Commission). The Commission, which existed from 1980 to 1983, produced a major report on genetic counseling and screening in February 1983 (U.S., President's Commission 1983). In the paragraphs that follow, the Commission's conclusions and recommendations are cited when they pertain to the issues under discussion.

## 2.19.2.1 Genetic Counseling

Genetic counseling in its modern form began in the United States. The term was coined by Sheldon Reed in 1947. Reed was concerned that the then-prevailing names for the service, "genetic advice" or "genetic hygiene", were too eugenically oriented (Reed 1947). In their place he suggested "genetic counseling" to emphasize the individual, more egalitarian relationships he thought should exist between client and counselor. Reed had reason to be sensitive about eugenics, because earlier in this century negative eugenics played a role in public policy. Between 1907 and 1928, 21 states enacted eugenic sterilization laws aimed at controlling the reproductive behavior of socially deviant individuals, including, as a New Jersey law of 1911 stated, "criminals, rapists, idiots, feeble-minded, imbeciles, lunatics, drunkards, drug fiends, epileptics, syphilitics, moral and sexual perverts, and diseased and degenerate persons." Some of these laws were never enforced, and most others were only enforced sporadically. Nevertheless, an estimated 8,500 eugenic sterilizations were performed before 1929, and the Nazis pointed to United States laws when advocating their own eugenic legislation in the early 1930s (Chorover 1979, p 42). Negative eugenics fit well with Americans' fear of being inundated by waves of immigration from southern and eastern Europe, a fear that led Congress to restrict immigration severely after 1921, except for immigrants from northern and western Europe. Once the flow of new immigrants was shut off, negative eugenics fell out of favor with lawmakers. The Nazis' eugenic policies in Germany further discredited eugenics in the United States. Most of the scientists who had espoused eugenics were either zoologists or psychologists who developed early I.Q. tests, not human geneticists. There was no historical continuity between the eugenics movement of the 1880s to 1920s and the new fields of human genetics and genetic counseling that began to develop after World War II. Genetic counseling, as Reed described it, set out to be non-directive from the very beginning. Counselors were to provide information, never advice. Patients were to make their own decisions.

In order to formulate guidelines for optimal genetic counseling, a Workshop on Genetic Counseling was held in Washington in 1972, sponsored by the National Genetics Foundation. Several members of the Committee on Genetic Counseling of the American Society of Human Genetics participated. The workshop agreed that "genetic counseling is a communication process which deals with the human problems associated with occurrence, or risk of occurrence, of a genetic disorder in a family. This process involves an attempt by one or more appropriately trained persons to help the individual or the family to [1] comprehend the medical facts, including the diagnosis, the probable course of the disorder and the available management; [2] appreciate the way heredity contributes to the disorder and the risk of recurrence in specified relatives; [3] understand the options for dealing with the risk of recurrence; [4] choose the course of action which seems appropriate to them in view of their risk and their family goals and act in accordance with that decision; and [5] make the best possible adjustment to the disorder in an affected family member and/or to the risk of recurrence of that disorder (Fraser 1974, p 637)."

There was substantial agreement among U.S. respondents to the survey that the informing of individuals and the enhancement of their capacity for autonomous choice should be the principal goal of genetic counseling (Wertz and Fletcher 1988). The President's Commission also supported the ideals of nondirectiveness in counseling (U.S., President's Commission 1983, pp 37–38, 47–56).

The United States has always been a leader in the development of counseling. Personal interaction, communication with clients, and counseling psychology are important parts of a counselor's training. The training of Master's-level genetic associates, found in few other countries, emphasizes the psycho-social aspects of counseling, but also has a major scientific component. The philosophy of nondirectiveness as a paradigm for counseling is probably greater in the United States than elsewhere in the world. Nevertheless, there remain unresolved problems, such as the disclosure of potentially embarrassing findings to clients and third parties. The President's Commission presented five alternative approaches to disclosure in cases of non-paternity, none of which the Commission regarded as entirely satisfactory. An alternative approach, apparently favored by the Commission, would be to warn all counselees in advance that incidental findings of nonpaternity will be disclosed (U.S., President's Commission 1983, pp 60–61). On the matter of disclosing an XY karyotype to a person who has been socialized as a woman, the Commission argued that the surprising and probably unwelcome information should be disclosed but that the disclosure should be made with great tact and sensitivity in a context that provides maximum psychological support to the patient. For example, the Commission suggested that "the person needs to be told that she did not develop uterus and ovaries (and hence cannot bear children) and has nonfunctioning reproductive tissue that must be surgically removed in order to avoid a risk of cancer" (U.S., President's Commission 1983, pp 62–63).

The question of disclosing to third parties information acquired in the genetic counseling context is, of course, highly controversial. On this difficult issue, the President's Commission elaborated a kind of ethical algorithm, a set of necessary and sufficient conditions for overriding the *prima facie* duty to protect patient confidentiality.

"A professional's ethical duty of confidentiality to an immediate patient or client can be overridden only if several conditions are satisfied: [1] Reasonable efforts to elicit voluntary consent to disclosure have failed; [2] there is a high probability both that harm will occur if the information is withheld and that the disclosed information will actually be used to prevent the harm; [3] the harm that identifiable individuals would suffer would be serious; and [4] appropriate precautions are taken to ensure that only the genetic information needed for diagnosis and/or treatment of the disease in question is disclosed (U.S., President's Commission 1983, p 44)."

## 2.19.2.2 Prenatal Diagnosis

From the viewpoint of an ethicist, prenatal diagnosis is likely to be more controversial than simple genetic counseling because prenatal diagnosis occurs after the initiation of a pregnancy and involves the willingness at least to *consider* the termination of the pregnancy. U.S. respondents to the survey indicated a very strong commitment to disclosing all relevant information – including information about uncertainties in laboratory findings – to the parents faced with making a decision about abortion. U.S. respondents also overwhelmingly indicated their deference to parental decisions about the hard choices described in several of these cases – the response to diagnosis of a 45, X or XYY karyotype, to a borderline result in testing for neural tube defects, and to an abnormally low maternal serum alpha-fetoprotein value when the interpretation of low values was still a matter of dispute among professionals.

On the matter of preconditions for prenatal diagnosis, U.S. respondents agreed that parental opposition in principle to abortion should not disqualify the pregnant woman from receiving prenatal diagnosis. On indications for prenatal diagnosis, there was both agreement and disagreement among U.S. respondents. They were agreed that anxiety in a 25-year-old pregnant woman was a sufficient reason for performing prenatal diagnosis at her request, despite her relatively low risk of carrying a fetus afflicted with a chromosomal abnormality. On the other hand, U.S. respondents were deeply divided on the question of prenatal diagnosis for sex determination.

The President's Commission report on genetic counseling and screening commented on two issues discussed in this section. The Commission's commitment to the fullest possible disclosure of test findings and to the protection of familial autonomy against both professional and social pressures is clear throughout its report (U.S., President's Commission 1983, pp 54–56). However, the limiting case for the President's Commission was prenatal diagnosis and selective abortion on the grounds of fetal gender alone. Here a higher principle than individual and familial autonomy, namely the principle of justice, prevails, with its implication that discrimination on the basis of gender is to be avoided and indeed actively opposed. Therefore the Commission argued for the moral proposition that "although individual physicians are free to follow the dictates of conscience, public policy should discourage the use of amniocentesis [and, by implication, other modes of prenatal diagnosis] for sex selection" (U.S., President's Commission 1983, p 58). The Commission simultaneously recognized that any attempt to translate this moral advice into a legal prohibition of prenatal diagnosis for sex selection would be likely to fail.

As more commercial laboratories are established, some of them on a frankly for-profit basis, questions of regulation will arise once again. Such laboratories may further increase existing inequalities in medical care by offering prenatal diagnosis to all who can pay for it, regardless of indications.

## 2.19.2.3  Genetic Screening

The use of genetic testing on large populations raises ethical questions that differ from those encountered in the clinical relationship. Until now, mass screening in the U.S. has been employed primarily with newborns and for conditions where early intervention is likely to improve the quality of life for the genetically afflicted. Genetic screening has also been performed on a voluntary basis in ethnic groups at special risk for a particular condition – for example, among Ashkenazi Jews for Tay-Sachs carrier status. More recently, the State of California has begun offering maternal serum alpha-fetoprotein testing to all pregnant women (Steinbrook 1986).

Mass screening can produce more false positives than true positives, unless the population to be screened is carefully selected for incidence of the disorder (see 2.19.1.4 above, and Table 2.19.4). Ethical questions to be considered before offering a test include what lower limits to set on its predictive value (% of those who test positive who actually develop the disorder) and whether it should be used only on those whose social-ethnic backgrounds place them at higher risk (Holtzman 1988, 1989).

The issue of potential stigmatization is also important. Experience with sickle-cell screening programs in the early 1970s demonstrated the importance of adequate genetic counseling and public education (U.S., President's Commission 1987, p 23). Sickle-cell programs "evolved in a rapid, haphazard, often poorly planned fashion, generated in large measure by public clamor and political pressure" (National Academy of Sciences 1975). In a few states, laws were even passed requiring sickle-cell tests for newborns, school-children, marriage license appli-

**Table 2.19.4.**  Parameters of the Validity of Genetic Tests[a]

| Test Result | Disease Status | |
|---|---|---|
| | Present | Absent |
| Positive (+) ............... | A | B |
| Negative (–) ............... | C | D |

Note: A = True positives, i.e., those with positive test results who *will* manifest the disease; B = false positives, i.e., those with positive test results who *may* or *may not* have the genetic defect but who *will never* manifest the disease; C = false negatives, i.e., those with negative test results who *will* manifest the disease; and D = true negatives, i.e., those with negative test results who will never manifest the disease. Sensitivity: the probability that the test will be positive in someone who has the condition in question (A/A + C). Specificity: the probability that the test will be negative in someone without the condition (D/B + D). Predictive value positive: the probability that a person with a positive result will manifest the disease (A/A + B). Predictive value negative: the probability that a person with a negative result will not manifest the disease (D/C + D).

[a] Holtzman 1988

cants, and inmates of penal institutions. The public confused carrier status with having sickle-cell disease, and some carriers were denied employment. When screening programs were initiated, prenatal diagnosis was not available, and the only way carrier couples could avoid the risk of having a child with sickle-cell was to avoid childbearing altogether. In a time of rising racial tension, the implication that some blacks should not have children was seen by some as a racist agenda. Thus, early sickle-cell anemia screening programs, although largely voluntary, had a largely negative impact: instead of enhancing choices, they stigmatized carriers (Andrews 1985, pp 149–155; Reilly 1977, pp 62–86).

Today these programs are conducted without incident, as a result of involvement by the black community, more adequate counseling for carriers, and public education. All agree that screening school-children, who would make little use of the information, is counterproductive.

By contrast, Tay-Sachs screening was generally successful from the beginning. The Jewish community was actively involved in planning, personnel development, and public education. Furthermore, in contrast to sickle-cell, Tay-Sachs was diagnosable prenatally when screening programs began. This meant that those carrier couples whose beliefs premitted abortion could proceed to have children. As a result of screening, the incidence of Tay-Sachs in newborns was reduced from 50–100 per year prior to 1970 to about 13 in 1980 (U.S., President's Commission 1983, pp 18–20).

Screening in the workplace and potential discrimination in employment are major future issues. A U.S. Congress Office of Technology Assessment (OTA) survey of 336 major U.S. corporations showed that 17 had already used genetic testing and 59 were planning to do so within 5 years (U.S. Congress, OTA 1983, pp 33–61). Tests used or contemplated had little or no predictive value. The test most frequently used was for sickle-cell carrier status, which causes no disability except under extremely rare conditions (planes that accidentally become depressurized at high altitudes). The second most commonly used test – for alpha-1-antitrypsin deficiency – has no proven benefits.

An OTA survey of 12 companies interested in developing genetic screening tests showed that 9 thought that employers are likely to use genetic tests to exclude workers from occupational hazards by the year 2000, and 5 thought that employers would use genetic tests to screen job applicants (U.S. Congress, Office of Technology Assessment 1988). They did not expect occupational screening to occur immediately, however. Most thought that the first applications (by 1990) would occur in the insurance industry. Most representatives of the genetic testing industry thought that by the year 2000, individuals would benefit from genetic testing because those identified as susceptible to common disorders would likely alter their lifestyles to reduce their risk of disease. Few biotechnology companies (3 of 12) thought that individuals carrying deleterious genes would be stigmatized, and only 2 thought that eugenic applications (infringement on reproductive rights) were likely by the year 2000.

Most testing will be developed and marketed by private companies on a commercial basis. Company decisions whether to develop particular tests will be made on economic grounds (development costs, size of market, competition from other companies) as well as medical grounds (disease incidence, prevalence, availability

**Table 2.19.5.** DNA Probe Tests for Inherited Diseases – Estimated U.S. Market, 1992[a]

| Disease | Number of Tests/yr | Value ($ million) |
|---|---|---|
| *Purely genetic diseases* | | |
| Adult polycystic kidney | 250,000 | 7.5 |
| Cystic fibrosis | 333,000 | 10.0 |
| Duchenne muscular dystrophy | 333,000 | 10.0 |
| Familial hypercholesterolemia | 250,000 | 7.5 |
| Familial polyposis | 165,000 | 5.0 |
| Huntington disease | 20,000 | 0.6 |
| Neurofibromatosis | 250,000 | 7.5 |
| Retinoblastoma | 250,000 | 7.5 |
| Sickle cell anemia | 250,000 | 7.5 |
| Other | 500,000 | 15.0 |
| Subtotal | 2,500,000 | 75.0 |
| *Common diseases with a genetic component* | | |
| Alzheimer's | 1,000,000 | 30.0 |
| Cancer | 12,000,000 | 360.0 |
| Diabetes | 5,000,000 | 150.0 |
| Heart disease | 12,000,000 | 360.0 |
| Subtotal | 30,000,000 | 900.0 |
| Total | 32,500,000 | $950–1,000 |

[a] Genetic Technology News (1986) Market for DNA Probe Tests for Genetic Diseases pp 6–7, November

of treatment, severity of disorder). According to market researchers, U.S. sales of tests to identify genetic diseases and genetic predispositions will reach several hundred million dollars within the next five to ten years (Table 2.19.5). The table assumes that population-wide testing will become available for cystic fibrosis and other disorders that can at present be diagnosed only for families that already have an affected member. If new technologies develop as projected, in the next five to ten years the number of people screened for just a few common predispositions, such as insulin-dependent diabetes, coronary artery disease, and predisposition to lung cancer from smoking, could exceed 10 million/year, entailing 18 million tests, of which 1.2 million would be positive (Holtzman 1988). This far exceeds the capacity of present genetic centers.

The President's Commission devoted substantial attention to the question of voluntary versus mandatory screening. Its conclusion represents a balancing of the sometimes conflicting principles of beneficence and respect for autonomy:

> Although a strong presumption prevails in favor of voluntary screening programs, the Commission concludes that programs requiring the performance of low-risk minimally intrusive procedures may be justified if voluntary testing would fail to prevent an avoidable, serious injury to people – such as children – who are unable to protect themselves (U.S., President's Commission 1983, p 51).

On the matter of disclosing test results to unrelated third parties, the Commission argued that no such results should be provided to insurers or employers without

433

the explicit consent of the person screened (U.S., President's Commission 1983, p 42). Non-consensual disclosure of test results to spouses and to at-risk relatives was advocated by the Commission under carefully specified conditions, as noted above (2.19.2.1). The Commission also devoted substantial attention to the future possibility of cystic fibrosis screening in an extended case study. Newborn screening, obstetrics-based screening, and mass screening for cystic fibrosis among all adults, or all Caucasian adults, were among the policy options considered by the Commission. The ethical issues raised by such a potential program were thought to be quantitatively but not qualitatively different from those raised by existing technologies (U.S., President's Commission 1983, pp 93–102).

In practical terms, voluntary testing and protection of results from institutional third parties may be difficult to maintain. Insurance companies can effectively coerce consent by denying coverage to all who refuse testing or refuse to disclose the results. Companies can argue that genetic screening is no different from other kinds of medical tests that applicants for life or health insurance are required to undergo. Genetic testing would allow some persons who are now refused insurance, such as the children or grandchildren of Huntington disease patients, to purchase coverage if their test results are negative. For many people, however, genetic testing is likely to mean exclusion from coverage or higher premiums. Insurance companies are regulated by the states, and if a company demonstrated that the disease predicted by a test increased the number of claims, state insurance commissioners would probably grant company requests for higher rates for individuals with positive test results. In the early 1970s, some insurance companies charged blacks with sickle-cell trait higher rates, even though they were not at higher risk for disease or reduced life span (National Academy of Sciences 1975).

In the past, insurance companies have tried to exclude birth defects from coverage. Prior to the late 1960s, newborns were excluded from health insurance coverage for the first 14 to 30 days of life and for subsequent coverage of medical conditions existing during this period. In the mid-1960s, the American Academy of Pediatrics (AAP) made a nationwide effort to change this policy, in order to protect young families from catastrophic financial losses. In 1973, the AAP developed model legislation mandating insurance coverage for sick or impaired newborns. By 1980, almost all states required that newborns be covered for the first 30 days of life under the mother's policy, after which they are included in "family coverage" (Matlin S, American Academy of Pediatrics, private communication).

Testing for insurance purposes could also affect employment. Although most life insurance is covered through individual policies, most health and disability insurance is through group policies partly paid for by employers. Medical information is not usually a condition for group policies, but the rates paid by employers are determined by the amount of medical care required by the group. Employers could reduce their insurance costs by denying employment to workers found, by genetic tests, to be at greater risk of future disease (Holtzman 1988, 1989). Although it is illegal for employers covered by federal ERISA (Employees Retirement and Income Security Act) legislation to fire employees because their use of medical care raises the company's insurance premiums, it is legal to refuse to hire on medical or genetic grounds. Genetic testing and subsequent refusal to hire could increase the number of people who are unemployed and therefore without medical insurance. About 11 states have attempted to provide coverage by establishing "high-risk pools" for those not otherwise eligible for health insurance, but the premiums, which cost a minimum of $4,000 to $7,000 a year, are beyond the means of many people (Weigle 1988). For some families this is a bargain when compared to the cost of the child's medical care. A national or state-based health system that guarantees care to all would be another solution.


## 2.19.2.4 Other Contexts

**Research on the Human Embryo and Fetus**

Since 1974, the Federal Government has forbidden federal conduct or funding of research on viable fetuses *ex utero*, with the exception of research that is therapeutic or will pose no added risk of harm. For living fetuses *in utero*, starting with implantation, federal regulations require that the "minimal risk" standard be applied equally in nontherapeutic research in fetuses that will be aborted and fetuses that will be carried to term (Andrews 1987, pp 68-70). Also, there has been a *de facto* moratorium since 1975 on all federally supported research on the pre-implantation human embryo. This moratorium is all the more remarkable because an Ethics Advisory Board (1979), appointed by Federal law to study the IVF research question, did recommend that Federal funds to study the safety and efficacy of clinical activities with IVF should be used. The Ethics Advisory Board also stated that research with embryos that are not used for transfer could be done up to 14 days after fertilization. These events in the history of embryo and fetal research show how fears of political and social reaction by anti-abortion and conservative groups affect ethical considerations of new reproductive and genetic technologies.

These regulations and the moratorium have in effect stopped federally funded research on the fetus prior to elective abortion as well as any embryo research at all to study the causes of infertility or genetic questions. The regulations effectively cover all federally funded institutions, regardless of the source of funds the institution may be using for fetal research (Baron 1985). Also, 24 states have laws regulating research on the fetus or conceptus.

However, research on CVS was widely done, except in some states with laws forbidding any fetal research. In 1982-83, researchers obtained villi, after the woman's choice of an elective abortion, to study the feasibility and complications of CVS in its early research stage. Such research received approval of local Institutional Review Boards (IRBs), required by the same federal regulations that would likely restrict this research, because it is nontherapeutic and higher than "minimal risk." Institutional or private funds supported CVS research. Although this activity technically violated the risk standard for fetuses to be aborted, no official complaints were made to the Federal Government about the IRB approvals or the CVS research itself.

Research on the technology of prenatal diagnosis in the U.S. has been totally supported by private or institutional means. Federal funding has been limited to data collection only in a case-controlled study of the safety and efficacy of amniocentesis (National Institute of Child Health and Development 1976). Similarly, the

Federal Government funded only data collection but not procedures in a later seven-center comparative study, without randomization, of the safety and accuracy of CVS and amniocentesis (Cowart 1984).

Research on infertility, including IVF, has been totally pushed into the private or commercial sector, except for one National Institute of Child Health and Development contract for a detailed follow-up study of children born after IVF. We are aware of no diagnostic or interventionist research on the pre-implantation embryo, even with private support. Infertility researchers in the U.S. are reluctant to initiate any embryo research in the light of an existing Federal ban on support. An Ethics Committee (1986) of the American Fertility Society noted the serious negative consequences of federal nonsupport.

The consequences of the bifurcation of Federal and private funding of fetal and infertility research have seriously inhibited these scientific activities, restricted the National Institutes of Health from its vital role in scientific peer review, and deprived families at higher genetic risk and infertile persons of the benefits of research (Fletcher and Ryan 1987). Review of the fetal research regulations and the ban on Federal support of IVF research will be the concern of a new Congressional Biomedical Ethics Board, created by legislation in 1985 and comprised of 12 members of Congress with an outside Advisory Committee (U.S. Congress, Legislative History 1985).

## 2.19.3 Consensus and Variation in the United States

The primary goal of medical geneticists in the United States is to provide information to individuals or families which those individuals or families can then employ in making major life-decisions. There is a strong bias against mandatory programs, except in the case of newborn screening, where there is also overwhelming public support for voluntary screening programs. This commitment to providing information directly to patients or clients also means that U.S. medical geneticists are hesitant to reveal genetic information to third parties – whether to members of the extended family or to employers, insurers, or government agencies. However, when the stakes are sufficiently high and the relationship to the prevention of harm sufficiently close and direct, a minority of geneticists are willing to make exceptions to the general rule in favor of preserving confidentiality. (The parallels between the genetic context and the context of HIV infection are perhaps instructive.)

### Results of the Survey
Of the 490 United States geneticists asked to participate in the study, 295 (60%) returned completed questionnaires by the close of the study in January, 1986. Seventy-four percent held M.D.s, 22% Ph.D.s, and 4% held other degrees. They had a median of 14 years in the practice of genetics; 86% were members of the American Society of Human Genetics, and 83% were board certified. Respondents spent a median of 45 hours a week in genetics. Sixty-seven percent were male, and 81% were married with a median of 1.5 children. Religious backgrounds were 46% Protestant, 28% Jewish, 14% Catholic, 6% other, and 6% none. As a whole, they were

nonpracticing, attending a median of three religious observances a year, although 39% attended once a month or more. Fifty-one percent characterized themselves as politically liberal, 18% as conservative, and 31% as both equally. Sociodemographically, United States geneticists differed from respondents in most other nations in only one variable: attendance at religious services. In the United States, 39% attended more than once a month. The two other countries with more than 25% were France (63%) and India (35%). A comparison between 274 respondents and 208 nonrespondents listed in the 1986 combined *Membership Directory* of the Genetics Society of America, American Society of Human Genetics, and American Board of Medical Genetics revealed no statistically significant differences between respondents and nonrespondents in type of degree, gender, geographical area, or subspecialty.

In order to see whether geneticists' responses were related to factors in their professional or personal backgrounds, we entered all socio-demographic data, including degree, age, gender, years of experience, patients per week, subspecialty, political inclination, religious background, and religiosity into a stepwise logistic regression for each question, using their responses to that question as the dependent variable. This method orders each background variable in terms of its strength of association with the dependent variable, while controlling for other statistically significant ($p < 0.05$) variables. In addition, this analysis provides an estimate of the odds ratio, e.g., the odds that a geneticist with a particular background variable will choose a particular response.

**Total Consensus**

There was $\geq 75$ consensus on nine (64%) of the 14 clinical cases: [1] non-disclosure of false paternity; [2] disclosure of conflicting test results; [3] disclosure of new/controversial interpretations; [4] disclosure of ambiguous/artifactual results, including colleague disagreements; [5] and [6] presenting reproductive options to carriers of disorders not diagnosable prenatally (except surrogacy, 67%); [7] performance of prenatal diagnosis for parents who refuse abortion; [8] performance of prenatal diagnosis for maternal anxiety; [9] nondirective counseling about fetuses with low-burden disorders. There was $\geq 75\%$ consensus on one of three screening situations, screening in the workplace and access to results.

**Cases with Consensus**

Ninety-four percent would *not* disclose false paternity to the husband. Most (84%) thought that they had fulfilled their duties as geneticists by telling the mother alone, without the husband present. By so doing, they have informed her that she is a carrier and that the disorder will not occur in offspring sired by her husband. Ten percent would lie (tell the couple that they are both genetically responsible or that there is a new mutation) in order to protect the mother's privacy. The major reasons given for protecting confidentiality were preserving the family unit (53%) and the mother's right to decide what to do with the information (34%). Only 11% thought that she ought to tell her husband. The odds that women geneticists would preserve the mother's confidentiality were 6.6 times those for men geneticists, and the odds that women geneticists would mention marital conflict in their comments on the questionnaires were 2.7 times those of men.

437

There was widespread agreement that conflicting, new/controversial, or ambiguous/artifactual test results should be disclosed without giving directive advice. The only exception was disclosure of colleague disagreement in the case of ambiguous/artifactual results. Although 99% would disclose the possibility of an abnormality, 24% would not tell the patient that their colleagues disagreed.

There was strong consensus that all reproductive options except surrogacy should be presented to carriers of disorders not diagnosable prenatally. There was broad acceptance of AID: 96% would present AID as an option for male carriers. Counseling of male and female carriers was the same with regard to four options available to both: 95% would present adoption, 88% taking their chances, 85% contraception, and 84% sterilization. IVF with donor eggs has thus far produced about a dozen live births around the world, but 83% would present this as an option. Sixty-seven percent (72% of men and 57% of women) would present surrogacy as an option; 22% would discuss it if asked, and only 9% would refuse to discuss it at all. Many respondents said that they regarded IVF with a donor egg as ultimately less complicated than surrogacy and less likely to cause harm.

Ninety-six percent of respondents would perform prenatal diagnosis for those who refuse abortion. In their reasoning, 69% stated that performance of prenatal diagnosis should not depend on the use that patients intend to make of the information. Thirty-four percent stated that such patients may change their minds about termination and thereby justified performing prenatal diagnosis. Refusals were based on lack of resources.

Seventy-eight percent would perform prenatal diagnosis for maternal anxiety in the absence of other indications and 11% would refer the patient to someone who would perform it. Of those in favor, 52% mentioned patient autonomy and 32% mentioned the removal of anxiety. Only 14% cited possible harm to the fetus from the procedure. The odds that women would perform prenatal diagnosis for an anxious woman were 2.8 times the odds for men; 51% of women and 33% of men cited patient autonomy in their reasoning.

For fetuses with low burden disorders like 45, X and XYY, 92% and 95%, respectively, would counsel nondirectively; 24% would also include a discussion of the emotional difficulties associated with terminating the pregnancy. Women were 4.4 times more likely than men to say that they would counsel nondirectively about XYY fetuses, and 3.6 times more likely than men to counsel nondirectively about 45, X fetuses.

**Cases without Consensus**

There was no consensus on five of the 14 cases: [1] disclosure to relatives at risk for Huntington disease (HD); [2] disclosure to relatives at risk for hemophilia A; [3] disclosure of parental translocation; [4] disclosure of XY genotype in a female; and [5] prenatal diagnosis for sex selection.

In all, 53% would tell the relatives of the Huntington patient, and 54% would tell the relatives of the hemophilia A patient. These percentages include 34% and 29% respectively, who would seek out and tell the relatives even if they did not ask for information. Thirty-nine percent would preserve the confidentiality of the Huntington patient, and 8% would refer the matter to the patient's family physician for decision; 36% would respect the confidentiality of the hemophilia A patient, and 10% would refer to the family physician. In both cases those who would disclose were significantly more likely (p < 0.00001) to envision and discuss the consequences of their action in their comments on the questionnaires than were those who would preserve patient confidentiality.

In their reasoning about the hemophilia A case, 37% cited the relatives' right to know, 34% the patient's right to privacy, 22% the duty to warn third parties of harm, 23% preserving the doctor-patient relationship, 19% reproductive planning, and 8% the prevention of birth defects. Reasoning in the HD case followed a similar pattern, but fewer (2%) mentioned preventing birth defects and 6% said that disclosure might cause psychological harm to the relatives. The older the geneticist, the more likely she/he would disclose the HD diagnosis to relatives of the patient; the odds of disclosure increased by 1.9 for each ten years of age.

In all, 62% would disclose, unasked, which parent carried a balanced translocation. This included 14% who would also attempt to locate and disclose to all relatives at risk of being carriers. Thirty-seven percent would tell the couple that test results revealed which one was a carrier, and let them decide whether they wished to know; this included 25% who would tell them before the test that carrier status would be revealed. Only 1% would wait for them to ask, and none would conceal the results. In their reasoning, 42% said that the couple had a right not to know, and 16% said that they had a duty to know and to use the information. Women were 1.9 times more likely than men to cite the welfare of relatives at risk.

Sixty-four percent would disclose an XY genotype in a female, while 36% would give other reasons for infertility. Thirty-three percent believed that they could tell the truth in such a way as to minimize harm, by providing supportive counseling, 32% saw the truth as a source of harm, and 29% would tell the truth in order to avoid the harm that would result from the patient's learning the truth from someone less skilled in counseling. In both this and the parental translocation case, those who would not disclose were significantly more likely (p < 0.00001) to envision and discuss the consequences of their actions than those who would disclose.

Thirty-four percent would perform prenatal diagnosis for sex selection, 28% would refer the couple to another medical geneticist or genetics unit offering the service, and 38% would refuse. Of those who would perform prenatal diagnosis, 68% said that they would do so out of respect for parental autonomy; and 19% would do so to prevent the otherwise certain abortion of a normal fetus. Those who would actually perform prenatal diagnosis were more likely (p < 0.0001) to cite the consequences of their actions, whereas those who would refuse or refer did not give their rationale. Stated consequences related to the fetus or parents, and not to society. Only 3.4% mentioned the position of women in society, 3.3% mentioned maintaining a balanced sex ratio, and 4% mentioned setting a precedent that would harm the moral order. Women were twice as likely as men to say that they would perform prenatal diagnosis; women would do so on the basis of respect for patient autonomy.

In all, 90% favored no regulations prohibiting commercial laboratories from performing prenatal diagnosis for parents who refuse abortion, 80% favored no regulations prohibiting performance for maternal anxiety in the absence of medical indications, and 50% favored no regulations about sex selection. Twelve percent said that ethics should not be established through regulations; only 2% cited the "Relman Rule" that "medicine should not be a business" (put forward by Arthur Relman, Editor of the *New England Journal of Medicine*).

## Most and Least Difficult Cases

The cases that respondents found most difficult to resolve were sex selection (28%), confidentiality of an HD patient (18%), and false paternity (13%). In all, 50% said that these cases were the most difficult because of conflicting responsibilities to different parties, and 43% described conflicts between ethical principles. The least difficult cases were prenatal diagnosis for parents who refuse abortions (26%), prenatal diagnosis for maternal anxiety (14%), and disclosure of parental translocation (13%).

## Screening

Seventy-seven percent thought that screening in the workplace should be voluntary; 34% cited potential conflicts between workers and employers, and 29% mentioned stigmatization. All thought that the worker should be told the results of any such screening; only 24% thought employers should have access without consent, and less that 12% thought that insurance companies should have such access.

There was no consensus about the best approach to a hypothetical test that would detect both cystic fibrosis carriers and homozygotes; 23% said the test should be given to newborns by law; 23% to newborns with parental consent, 13% to adolescents ages 13–17, by consent, 35% preferred persons over 18, by consent, and 6% mentioned other ages by law. Only 16% thought that screening should be restricted to Caucasians; most considered such a limitation racially discriminatory.

Respondents were more willing to respect patient confidentiality for presymptomatic tests for Huntington disease than they were for an actual diagnosis; 67% would not disclose results to patients against their wishes, 65% would not disclose to the spouse, and 56% would not disclose to relatives at risk. In their reasoning, 62% said that patients had a "right not to know" their test results if they so chose. Many of those who would preserve patient confidentiality argued that in the event that accurate tests become available, the relatives could be tested themselves without needing access to anyone else's results.

## Future Priorities

Issues that should be of most concern to medical geneticists in the United States in the next 10 to 15 years were ranked as follows: [1] development of new treatments for genetic disorders including treatment in utero, organ transplantation, and molecular genetic manipulation; [2] carrier screening for common genetic disorders; [3] increased demand for genetic services; [4] environmental damage to the unborn; [5] allocation of limited resources; [6] screening for genetic susceptibility to cancer and heart disease; [7] research on the human embryo, zygote, and fetus; [8] genetic screening in the workplace; [9] long-range eugenic concerns; and [10] sex preselection for sex desired by parents.

**How the United States Differs from Other Nations**

There were four questions on which the United States stood virtually alone among nations: surrogate motherhood, sex selection, disclosure of an XY genotype in a female, and regulations for commercial laboratories. The United States was the only nation where a majority of geneticists (67%) would present surrogate mother-hood as an option in counseling. The United States was one of three nations where a majority (62%) would either perform prenatal diagnosis for sex selection or refer to someone who would. In the United States, those who would perform would do so out of respect for parental autonomy. In the other two nations, Hungary and India, the reasons were different. Sixty percent of Hungarian geneti-cists would perform prenatal diagnosis to prevent the abortion of a normal fetus, and 52% of Indian geneticists would perform or refer for social reasons, such as limiting the population or preventing harm to an unwanted girl. The United States and Canada were the two nations where more that 62% would disclose an XY genotype in a female. Willingness to disclose in these nations was based on confi-dence that, with proper counseling methods, the truth could be told in a manner that would not destroy the woman's self-image. This approach reflects increases in the numbers of geneticists who have undergone clinical training in counseling. Fi-nally, the United States stood alone in regard to commercial laboratories' perfor-mance of prenatal diagnosis for sex selection, with 50% favoring *no* regulations. Among the other nations, Canada came closest to this laissez faire approach, with 34% favoring no regulations; elsewhere, $\geq 82\%$ said that regulations should pro-hibit performance.

## 2.19.4 Cultural Context of Medical Genetics

Six features of United States culture affect the ethics of medical genetics: these are [1] popular acceptance of science and technology; [2] belief in individual autono-my and individual responsibility; [3] a medical profession that developed in an en-trepreneurial, commercial climate; [4] the fee-for-service system of medical care; [5] the consumer movement; and [6] the desire for "perfect" children.

Our belief in science goes back to seventeenth-century Protestantism, which taught that nature must be conquered by "art." The history of the transformation of childbirth from natural to technological event illustrates our belief that the road to perfection lies in high technology (Wertz and Wertz 1989). Today we use more technical and surgical intervention in birth than any other country; 24% of births are by Cesarean section. Historically, the emphasis of U.S. medicine has always been on the heroic rather than the preventative. Doctors have seen themselves as engaged in a battle with death.

A recent survey of public perceptions of biotechnology showed that most resi-dents of the United States think that they will benefit "a lot" (41%) or "some" (39%) from developments in science and technology in the next 20 years. The ma-jority (62%) think that the benefits to society resulting from continued technologi-cal and scientific innovation outweigh the related risks to society (U.S. Congress, Office of Technology Assessment 1987, pp 26, 29).

Individual liberty and responsibility have always been part of our tradition. Writing in 1835, de Toqueville noted Americans' refusal to be bound by traditions, their innovativeness in politics, and seemingly boundless optimism, which paralleled their belief in science.

"The settlers of New England were at the same time ardent sectarians and daring innovators. Narrow as the limits of some of their religious opinions were, they were free from all political prejudices.

"Under their hand, political principles, laws, and human institutions seem malleable, capable of being shaped and combined at will. As they go forward, the barriers which imprisoned society and behind which they were born are lowered; old opinions, which for centuries had been controlling the world, vanish; a course almost without limits, a field without horizon, is revealed; the human spirit rushes forward and traverses them in every direction (de Toqueville 1951, p 43)."

A parallel belief is that individuals should have control over their own interests and that society cannot, and should not, try to interpret the interests of individuals. De Toqueville wrote,

"Every individual, private person, society, community, or nation, is the only lawful judge of its own interest, and, provided it does not harm the interests of others, nobody has the right to interfere. I think that one must never lose sight of this point."

"Another principle of American society of which one must never lose sight [is that] every individual being the most competent judge of his own interest, society must not carry its solicitude on his behalf too far, for fear that in the end he might come to count on society, and so a duty might be laid on society which it is incapable of performing... (Schleifer 1980, pp 124–125)."

In keeping with this tradition of individualism, Americans have always maintained independence in the doctor-patient relationship, partly because during our history qualified doctors were extremely scarce or geographically distant, and people had to be their own doctors. Self-help is an old tradition in the United States. Government responsibility for health care is not.

Many immigrants came to the United States seeking freedom to practice their own religion (rather than a state religion) and to publicize their own social or political beliefs. Some felt that orthodox medicine was as oppressive as the orthodox religion from which they had fled. Freedom of choice in health care, by which we mean the right to choose one's own doctor and one's own treatment (including treatments that are rejected by orthodox medicine) and the right to reject orthodox medical care entirely are analogous to freedom of religion and freedom of speech in many people's minds. These beliefs crystallized into a social movement in the 1830s, the era of "Jacksonian Democracy", when the "Common Man," particularly in the South and West, rejected the aristocracy that had developed in the urban East, along with "expertise" of all kinds, including "priest-craft, lawyer-craft, and doctor-craft" (Shryock 1962). Individuals saw health as their own responsibility. Frequently they were right, for it was not until about 1900 that more patients were helped than harmed by medicine.

Today this individualism persists. Patients in the United States enjoy more personal autonomy and more choice in medical care (if they can pay for it) than patients in most other countries. The United States has been a leader in developing policies for informed consent. Doctors, including geneticists, regard patients first as individuals and only secondarily as members of family units. Social agencies are reluctant to intervene in individual or family choices about medical care, even if harm results from these choices.

One reason for our individualistic approach to health care is that medicine developed into a profession much later in the United States than in Europe. Licensing laws were largely ignored until the end of the nineteenth century, because those who called themselves doctors demanded the right to freedom of practice, just as their patients demanded freedom of choice. There was no guild system for American medicine and no tradition of government responsibility to oversee standards or to guarantee access to health care. In fact, most doctors were either outright quacks or minimally educated, and medicine held a low social status compared to law or theology. Medicine developed in an entrepreneurial, commercial climate. Most doctors were really small businessmen. It was not until almost 1900 that better educated doctors were able to convince states to enforce their licensing laws and drive out the quacks and most of the unorthodox practitioners. Full professionalization, with specialty boards and standards for medical education, was not completed until the 1930s.

The fee-for-service system – modeled on the billing system used by small businesses or skilled tradesmen – is the legacy of this historical development. As early as 1917, many of the better-educated doctors and hospital-based specialists supported legislation for national health insurance, because they saw that many patients were not receiving adequate care; in contrast, general practitioners, who had less education and saw fewer patients who could not pay, rejected such insurance as a threat to freedom of competition (Hirshfield 1970). When health insurance came in the early 1940s, it was through private companies and was modeled on life insurance. The result was a two-class system of medical care. Private patients paid private physicians and private hospitals either from their own funds or, increasingly often, through insurance policies that they or their employers had purchased, even though such policies usually reimbursed only 80% of charges. Private patients could choose their own physicians or hospitals. They were rarely, if ever, subjects for research, but they were usually the first to benefit from the findings of research. Clinic patients, on the other hand, were those who could not pay for their own care or had no private insurance. They received care at the clinics of public hospitals. In return for their care, they were expected to serve as "teaching material" for doctors-in-training or as research subjects. They had no choice of physician and usually no access to elective surgical operations.

After 1971, hospitals were reimbursed for some of their care by Medicaid, a federally supported system in which states participate and which covers many, but not all, persons whose incomes fall below designated levels. Medicaid does not cover all procedures adequately, especially in genetics (see 2.19.4.3 below). Therefore, clinic patients, many of whom belong to minority groups, do not have access

443

to many services available to private patients. Many individuals, perhaps 12% of all individuals under age 65 years in the United States, have no health insurance of any kind; another 8% are probably underinsured (Davis and Rowland 1983). Further, even people who are insured often find that their policies cover operative procedures rather than cognitive services. Amniocentesis is readily reimbursed, but health insurance seems reluctant to pay for the hours of history-taking and discussion often involved in thorough genetic counseling. A state like California, with its provision of maternal serum alpha-fetoprotein screening to all women and its offer of amniocentesis to all pregnant women over the age of 35, provides a clear illustration that broad access to genetic services is possible if policy makers make such access a matter of priority (Steinbrook 1986).

The consumer movement in medicine, and, more recently, the Women's Health Movement, are part of the tradition of American individualism. Both appeared, as the Popular Health Movement, in the Jacksonian Era of the 1830s. The goal of the movements is to enable individuals to control their own lives and physiological processes through education. These movements stress prevention rather than treatment. Books, manuals, periodicals, conferences, classes, all teach people how to care for themselves and also how to get the most out of their doctors. Traditionally, women were responsible for the family's health care, so women constituted a large part of early consumer movements. In the late nineteenth and early twentieth centuries, women were leaders of the Birth Control Movement, an attempt to gain freedom in reproductive choices (Kennedy 1974; Reed 1978). In the late 1960s, women's health groups gained new power with the renewal of the Feminist Movement (Boston Women's Health Book Collective 1985). In addition, people became more ready to sue their doctors, especially after prenatal testing and legal abortion made possible suits for "wrongful births."

Most people desire perfect children, or at least children who are as nearly perfect as possible. The paradigm of industrial production seems to represent most people's view of gestation and birth, with prenatal diagnosis serving as quality control. The desire for perfect children is the result of many converging social trends: medicine's ability to save or lengthen the lives of severely handicapped infants, the absence of financial and social support for such infants and their families, and the trend toward small families of one or two children. Perhaps most important are the changes in the roles of women and children. The majority of mothers now work outside the home, including over half the mothers (with husbands in the home) of infants under one year of age, in spite of the absence of national programs for child care. Many women regard themselves primarily as workers, rather than mothers, and families expect to pay considerable sums (at least $160,000, plus college expenses) to see each child reach adulthood. In return, they expect children to give love and affection and to benefit from their expensive educations (Zelizer 1985), things severely handicapped children may be unable to do.

Given the large number of mothers in the workforce, the extended longevity of handicapped children, and the erosion of social supports for their care, the birth of a severely handicapped child may be perceived as a proportionately greater burden than ever before. Women, especially, may perceive the burden as greater, because they are the ones who most frequently give up their jobs to stay home and care for handicapped children.

## 2.19.4.1 Sources of Challenge and Support

Political, social, and psychological support for medical genetics in the United States is provided chiefly by three groups: individuals afflicted with genetic disease and their families, non-professional voluntary associations interested in genetic disease, and professional organizations. In addition, geneticists can turn to the reports of several expert panels.

There are approximately 150 national voluntary organizations for those with genetic disorders, or their parents (National Center for Education in Maternal and Child Health 1987). In addition, there are almost 250 national voluntary organizations for maternal and child health (National Center for Education in Maternal and Child Health 1988). There is an active movement for rights for the handicapped. People who are afflicted with genetic disorders that are diagnosable before birth, but who have led productive lives, are ambivalent about prenatal diagnosis and abortion (Saxton 1984). They are concerned that counselors may not provide a complete picture of the disorder. They fear that in the future being malformed or congenitally diseased or handicapped will become a mark of social class. To be physically or mentally abnormal or imperfect will mean that one's parents did not have the education or financial means to seek genetic counseling and prenatal diagnosis, or that they were too ignorant or deviant to use the information properly. Abnormality will be seen as the product not of fate but of bad choices, though still perhaps deserving sympathy. But funds may be diverted from services for the handicapped to services that will prevent their replication.

Two important documents for those who wish to study ethical issues in U.S. medical genetics were published in 1975 and 1983. *Genetic Screening: Programs, Principles, and Research* was prepared by health professionals who were members of the Committee for the Study of Inborn Errors of Metabolism of the National Academy of Sciences (National Academy of Sciences 1975). This report was drafted in an effort to counter the rush toward mandatory screening programs by some professionals and legislators who had not adequately considered the reliability of the screening tests or the problem of stigmatizing screenees. As noted above, in 1983, the President's Commission produced *Screening and Counseling for Genetic Conditions*, a mature, well-balanced consideration of a wide range of issues based on the medical, ethical, and legal literature of the preceding decade and a half (U.S., President's Commission 1983). This newer report was compiled in the context of rapidly developing techniques for genetic diagnosis; the technological advances were discussed at greater length in the Commission's companion report entitled *Splicing Life* (U.S., President's Commission 1982).

Medical geneticists in the United States may consult these pivotal reports, as well as a substantial literature on ethical and legal questions in human genetics, which is contained in books, legislative hearings, government reports (especially from the Congressional Office of Technology Assessment), and articles. Relevant articles appear in the specialty journals for medical genetics, in general journals of science or medicine, in ethics journals, and in law journals. Immediate access to the medical literature is provided by MEDLINE; access to the cross-disciplinary literature appearing in journals and other types of documents is provided by

445

BIOETHICSLINE. Both databases are included in the MEDLARS information network of the U.S. National Library of Medicine, available worldwide.

Nevertheless, papers that deal with technical or analytical questions rarely deal with ethical concerns. A review of 143 articles on screening for neural tube defects showed that 45% made no mention of social or ethical issues, 32% mentioned "nonmedical" factors but did not discuss them, while 23% made ethical or legal matters their major focus (Nightingale 1987).

## 2.19.4.2 Major Controversies, Including Abortion

The two major controversies that have arisen in connection with medical genetics in the United States have been the discussion of mandatory genetic screening and the debate about abortion. In the early 1970s, genetic screening laws for sickle-cell anemia were enacted quickly by 12 states and the District Columbia. Some of the laws made screening mandatory; some did not distinguish between carrier status and affected status; and some made no provision for counseling in connection with screening (Reilly 1977, pp 62–86; Andrews 1985, pp 147–178). As a result of further public discussion and, in part, the 1975 National Academy of Sciences report, most of these laws have since been repealed or modified, and sickle-cell anemia screening is voluntary (Andrews 1985, pp 149–155). Mandatory genetic screening of newborns for at least some conditions is currently required in 45 states. Only three jurisdictions – the District of Columbia, Maryland, and North Carolina – clearly stipulate that all newborn screening is voluntary (Andrews 1987, p 238).

The abortion controversy has implications for decisions by couples concerning prenatal diagnosis and selective termination of pregnancy. The right of women to secure abortions until the end of the second trimester – the presumed stage of fetal viability – is clearly guaranteed by the 1973 U.S. Supreme Court decision in *Roe v. Wade*. The ruling effectively made it impossible for state legislatures to interfere with the legal right to first- or second-trimester abortion, though some states do not fund abortions for those who cannot pay. The abortion issue definitely decreases the willingness of the U.S. Congress and at least some state legislatures to provide funding for genetic programs that may include prenatal diagnosis and selective abortion as components.

U.S. public opinion strongly supports the legal right to abortion in cases of fetal defect. One question that has been asked of national samples of U.S. adults on 13 occasions from 1972 through 1987 is the following: "Please tell me whether or not *you* think it should be possible for a pregnant woman to obtain a *legal* abortion if there is a strong chance of a serious defect in the baby?" The percentage of respondents who answered this question with a "yes" was consistently between 75% and 78% (National Opinion Research Center 1987).

## 2.19.4.3  National Expenditures for Medical Genetics

The Genetic Diseases Services Branch of the Health Services Resource Administration has a budget of approximately 12 million U.S. dollars for 1988, part of which is granted to networks of genetics services in the various states. These networks in turn allow the states to provide genetic services to people who could not otherwise afford them, and to fund education and small research projects concerning the delivery of genetic services. (In contrast, it is estimated that the National Institutes of Health spent some 90 million dollars in 1986 on research directly related to human genetics, and the Howard Hughes Medical Institution an additional 10 to 15 million for medical genetics research).

In addition to Genetic Diseases Services Branch funds, the Federal Government spends approximately 6.9 million dollars annually on genetics services, including 4.8 million through Medicaid (the program for those below the federal poverty line) and 2.1 million through grants for Children's Medical Services and Special Projects of Regional and National Significance (SPRANS). Federal *per capita* expenditures for genetics services range from $0.00 to $0.58, depending on region (Table 2.19.6). For persons on Medicaid, the average genetic services funding is $0.32. Medicaid reimbursement is far below levels of reimbursement by private insurance companies for the same services (Table 2.19.7) and may be far less than the cost of services to the provider (e. g., $15 for amniocentesis or chorionic villus sampling, $1.00 for Level 2 ultrasound) (Greenstein et al. 1988, p 189). This means

**Table 2.19.6.**  Per Capita Expenditures for Genetics Services by Genetic Disease Services Branch[a]

| Region | Total Payments for Genetics Services | % of Total | Population by Region | % of Total | Per Capita Expenditures[c] |
|---|---|---|---|---|---|
| Great Plains Genetic Services Network (GPGSN) | 1,570,840 | 7.5 | 9,242,459 | 7.9 | 0.17 |
| Middle Atlantic Regional Human Genetics Network (MARHGN) | 3,835,000[b] | 18.2 | 16,063,117 | 13.7 | 0.24 |
| Great Lakes Regional Genetics Group (GLaRGG) | 2,356,700 | 11.2 | 24,150,445 | 20.6 | 0.10 |
| Mountain States Regional Genetics Services Network (MSRGSN) | 0 | 0 | 5,245,282 | 4.5 | 0 |
| New England Regional Genetics Group (NERGG) | 384,650 | 1.8 | 6,200,306 | 5.3 | 0.06 |
| Genetic Network of the Empire State [New York] (GENES) | 5,035,783 | 24.1 | 8,647,803 | 7.4 | 0.58 |
| Pacific Northwest Regional Genetics Group (PacNoRGG) | 1,514,410 | 7.2 | 4,366,821 | 3.7 | 0.35 |
| Southeastern Regional Genetics Group (SERGG) | 4,749,756 | 22.6 | 22,439,857 | 19.2 | 0.21 |
| Pacific Southwest Regional Genetics Network (PSRGN) | 1,500,000[b] | 7.1 | 13,082,176 | 11.2 | 0.11 |
| Texas | 74,000 | 0.3 | 7,634,875 | 6.5 | 0.01 |
| Total | 21,021,139 | 100.0 | 117,073,141 | 100.0 | |

[a] Greenstein 1988, p 185
[b] Major contribution and coverage based on a single state's data
[c] Mean $0.18 (range $0.00–0.58)

**Table 2.19.7.** Medicaid and Private Insurance Reimbursement for Genetics Services 1985–86[a] (U.S. dollars)

| | Medicaid | | Private Companies | |
|---|---|---|---|---|
| | Mean | Range | Mean | Range |
| A. Professional Reimbursement for Procedures | | | | |
| 1. Amniocentesis | 64.42 | 15.00–450.00 | 173 | 130–250 |
| 2. Ultrasound Level 1 | 44.25 | 12.00–112.40 | 185 | 140–268 |
| 3. Ultrasound Level 2 | 47.81 | 1.00–115.70 | 128 | 67–168 |
| 4. Chorionic villus sampling | 120.37 | 15.00–431.90 | 130 | 130 |
| B. Laboratory Tests | | | | |
| 1. Amniotic fluid cell culture (with karyotype) | 205.40 | 21.00–450.00 | 506 | 420–625 |
| 2. Peripheral blood karyotype | 116.15 | 4.50–350.00 | 415 | 305–525 |
| 3. Amniotic fluid alpha fetoprotein | 26.00 | 6.50–136.32 | 47 | 36–65 |
| 4. Maternal serum alpha fetoprotein | 28.04 | 6.20–113.60 | 45 | 37–56 |
| 5. Chorionic villus sampling | 145.84 | 15.00–311.14 | 232 | 232 |

[a] Greenstein 1988, pp 48ff, 189

that patients on Medicaid do not have equal access to services, except in some cases where a state or city health department has provided funds to fill the gap, as California and New York City have done with amniocentesis and maternal serum alpha-fetoprotein screening.

Medicaid does not cover all poor people in the U.S. Two-parent families are generally ineligible, and single adults are covered only if they are aged or disabled. Many states have set income limits for eligibility that are far below the official poverty level. In 1983, approximately 35.6 million persons, mostly workers in low-wage industries, were uninsured, either by Medicaid or private insurance (Freedman 1988).

## 2.19.4.4 Abortion Laws

See 2.19.4.2 above.

## 2.19.4.5 Studies of Effectiveness of Genetic Services

Evaluation of genetic counseling has been a concern ever since prenatal diagnosis presented prospective parents with difficult choices (Evers-Kieboom and Van den Berghe 1979; Leonard et al. 1972). The effectiveness of counseling is usually evaluated in terms of the counselee's comprehension of genetic facts, such as risk, diagnosis and recurrence, or in terms of changes in their reproductive plans or behavior. Patients' interpretation of genetic risks and uncertainties are central to their making decisions. Early studies, using interviews with small numbers of patients at individual centers, showed that most interpreted risks as binary (either/or), what-ever their numeric risk. The majority of patients interpreted their risks as lower af-ter counseling than before, which explains in part why more expressed an inten-tion to have children after counseling than before counseling (Pauker and Pauker 1979; Lippman-Hand and Fraser 1979; Black 1979; Lubs 1979). These studies also suggest that effective counseling results in "rational" reproductive behavior, mean-ing that patients at high risk for serious, untreatable disorders are less likely to plan to have children than those at low risk or those at risk for treatable disorders (Bobrow 1977).

Evaluators have usually viewed genetic counseling as "preventive medicine" (Sorenson et al. 1981, p 9). However, they have also looked at effects of counseling on parental self-concepts (Antley et al. 1973; Corgan 1979) and on the family and at the psychological impact of abortion for genetic defects (Beeson and Golbus 1979). Most studies have been retrospective.

The major study of counseling's effectiveness – a study not duplicated in size or rigor anywhere in the world – was conducted by Sorenson et al. in 1977–79 (Soren-son et al. 1981). This prospective study comprised 1,369 genetic counseling cases (77% of those asked to participate) seen by 205 counselors at 47 clinics. Almost all the counselors were M.D.s or Ph.D.s. Patients and their spouses filled out de-tailed anonymous questionnaires before counseling, within 7–10 days after coun-seling, and at 6 months. Counselors also completed a questionnaire after each counseling session.

On average, 55% of patients' genetic/medical concerns and only 16% of their sociomedical concerns (financial costs, education, effect of an affected child on the marriage or family life) were actually discussed in counseling. Forty-six per-cent of patients were given a numeric risk of having a child with a birth defect. Im-mediately after counseling, 54% of those who were given a numeric risk were un-able to report it. Forty percent of those who were given a diagnosis were unable to name the genetic disorder diagnosed (Sorenson et al. 1981, p 135). These figures point to difficulties in doctor-patient communication.

The Sorenson study was the first social-scientific effort to compare doctor and patient awareness of what the other had wanted to discuss during an encounter. Awareness was judged after counseling sessions that typically lasted 45 to 60 mi-nutes. It seems reasonable to assume that after a session of this length, devoted al-most entirely to education (not diagnosis or treatment), doctors and patients should have been aware of the topic that the other party had most wanted to dis-cuss. This was not the case: *both* parties were aware in only 26% of sessions, nei-ther party was aware in 47% of sessions, counselors only were aware in 16% of sessions and clients only in 11%. Joint awareness was most likely if patients were college-educated and well paid and had a risk of under 10% for having a child with a birth defect (Wertz et al. 1988a). Women patients who sought counseling alone, without their husbands, were more likely to have their concerns addressed if the counselor were a woman (Zare 1984). Yet, counselors said they were satis-fied with 95% of counseling sessions (Wertz et al. 1988b). Their level of satisfac-tion was based on their own inaccurate perceptions that they had effectively com-municated risk, etiology and prognosis. They were most likely to be satisfied if patients were well-educated.

Communication is probably less effective with low-income minority group patients than with white middle-class patients (Naranjo and Lockhart 1979; Rapp 1988). A recent study in New York City showed that 50% of patients at publicly-supported clinics break their appointments for genetic counseling, and 20% to 50% of those counseled decide not to have amniocentesis, largely because their cultural beliefs differ from those of counselors (Rapp 1988). In contrast, only about 10% of private patients break their appointments for counseling.

In about 70% of genetic counseling sessions, the counselees are members of a couple, seen together. In 55% of cases, each partner has sought counseling for different reasons, and about half the time they disagree about the seriousness of potential social and financial problems that might result from the birth of an affected child (Sorenson and Wertz 1986). About 75% agree about their reproductive plans for the next two years, and 60% agree about their ideal number of children. Counseling does not significantly increase agreement between spouses on these issues.

The only area where counseling increases spousal agreement significantly is in regard to the interpretation of recurrence risk. Couples agree about risk interpretation 44% of the time before counseling and 52% afterwards. Patients' interpretation of risk is central to their subsequent reproductive behavior. Patients almost invariably interpret a given numeric risk as lower than do doctors. Doctors interpret risks of 7–19% as moderate, 20–24% as high, and 25% or more as high to very high (Wertz et al. 1986). Patients interpret risks under 10% as low, 10–14% as low to moderate, and 15–50% as moderate. As numeric risk increases, certainty about the normalcy of the next child decreases. At risks below 10%, most patients say that the next child will "probably" be normal; at 25% the mode of expectation becomes "not sure." What counselors see as a high risk, patients see as at most a moderate risk, one that may be worth taking in view of the value of the desired outcome, a normal child. On the other hand, discussion of future problems associated with raising an affected child in the home increases the perception of risk. Genetic counseling does not always resolve uncertainties about reproductive plans: approximately one-third of patients complete counseling uncertain in this regard (Wertz et al. 1984). They are less likely to use contraceptives effectively than are patients who leave counseling with definite plans (Wertz and Sorenson 1983).

As regards reproductive plans, patients take an independent attitude toward what counselors say. Those who reported, six months later, that their reproductive plans had been influenced by counseling (about 44% of all counselees) had similar reproductive plans to the 56% who said that they had not been influenced (Wertz and Sorenson 1986). Furthermore, more than half of those who said they were influenced maintained the same plans that they had had before counseling. The influenced group had more education than the uninfluenced. It appears that educated patients may pick and choose from the information provided and utilize some portion of it (accurately or inaccurately) to support a decision made for other reasons, or, in many cases, to reinforce a preexisting decision.

Patients at all levels of numeric risk were more likely to plan to have a child after counseling than they were before, regardless of the seriousness or treatability of the disorder. This was true even among those at risk for disorders not diagnosable prenatally: Among those facing risks of 10% or less, 52% intended to have a child before and 60% intended to have a child after counseling. Among those with risks of 11% or higher, 27% planned a child before and 42% after counseling. Both of these increases are significant at the $p < 0.001$ level (McNemar's chi-square). The most significant predictors of patients' plans to have children after counseling were the plans that they had had before counseling (Sorenson et al. 1987). The magnitude of risk was not significantly related to reproductive plans at six months after counseling.

In sum, it appears that the benefits of counseling, if judged in terms of successful communication and informed decision-making, are most likely to accrue to middle-class, well-educated patients, but overall there is much room for improvement.

### 2.19.4.6 Need for New Laws

Because of a still-pervasive suspicion of government in the United States, it seems likely that any government effort to secure detailed information about individuals would be vigorously resisted by the citizenry. Much less clear is the probable public response to efforts by the so-called "private sector" - especially insurance companies and employers - to secure genetic information that would be rationally related to the companies' efforts to reduce their exposure and control their costs. Critics of such efforts use the notion of *discrimination* in employment or access to health insurance and clearly view people afflicted with genetic disease, or carrying recessive genetic traits, as people who are, to a greater or lesser degree, *handicapped*. At last report only three states in the United States - Florida, Louisiana, and New Jersey - had enacted statutes prohibiting discrimination in educational admission, insurance, or employment on the basis of genetic diagnosis. The only conditions covered by these statutes are sickle-cell trait and sickle-cell disease (Andrews 1987, pp 19-20). If the current controversies about screening for antibody to the human immunodeficiency virus among applicants for insurance are in any sense relevant to the issue of genetic screening, then one can expect a vigorous debate on required screening and on access to screening results in the U.S. in the years ahead.

## 2.19.5 Ethical Issues and Future Trends

The human genome mapping and sequencing effort is well under way in the United States, Japan, the United Kingdom and the Federal Republic of Germany. In the long run, this effort will provide important new information for both genetic diagnosis and human gene therapy. In the short run, however, it seems likely that the diagnostic information produced by scientists will far outstrip medicine's therapeutic capabilities (Walters 1986). We will shortly know, or at least be able to know, about presymptomatic conditions, as well as about predispositions to complex conditions like heart disease and cancer. In this uncomfortable interim - between the time when we will know what ails us and the time when effective preventive or therapeutic strategies can be developed – we will need to develop an increased tolerance for living with ambiguity and for accepting ourselves and our neighbors despite newly-discovered susceptibilities and disabilities. In short, we will probably need to construct an interim ethic, if we are to be able to cope with new genetic knowledge.

# References

Andrews LB [1987] Medical genetics: a legal frontier. American Bar Foundation, Chicago

Andrews LB (comp) [1985] State laws and regulations governing newborn screening. American Bar Foundation, Chicago

Antley M, Antley RM, Hartlage LC [1973] Effects of genetic counseling on parental self-concepts. J Psychol 83: 335-338

Baron CH [1985] Legislative regulation of fetal experimentation. In: Milunsky A, Annas G (eds) Genetics and the law III. Plenum Press, New York, pp 431-435

Beeson D, Golbus MS [1979] Anxiety engendered by amniocentesis. In: Epstein CJ, Curry CJR, Packman S, Sherman S, Hall BD (eds) Risk, communication, and decision making in genetic counseling. Ann Rev Birth Defects C. Alan R Liss, New York, pp 191-198

Benn PA, Hsu LYF, Carlson A, Tannenbaum HL [1985] The centralized prenatal genetics screening program of New York City III: the first 7,000 cases. Am J Med Genet 20 [2]: 369-384

Bernhardt BA, Bannerman RM [1984] The influence of obstetricians on the utilization of amniocentesis. Prenat Diagn 4: 43-49

Black RB [1979] Effects of diagnostic uncertainty and available options on perceptions of risk. In: Epstein CJ, Curry CJR, Packman S, Sherman S, Hall BD (eds) Risk, communication, and decision making in genetic counseling. Ann Rev Birth Defects C. Alan R Liss, New York, pp 341-354

Bobrow M (1977) Genetic counseling: a tool for the prevention of some abnormal pregnancies. J Clin Pathol 20 (Suppl 10): 145

Boston Women's Health Book Collective [1985] The new our bodies, ourselves. Simon & Schuster, New York

Chorover SL [1979] From genesis to genocide: the meaning of human nature and the power of behavior control. Massachusetts Institute of Technology Press, Cambridge, MA and London, pp 57-76

Conley R, Milunsky A [1975] The economics of prenatal genetic diagnosis. In: Milunsky A (ed) The prevention of genetic disease and mental retardation. WB Saunders, Philadelphia

Corgan RL [1979] Genetic counseling and parental self-concept change. In: Epstein CJ, Curry CJR, Packman S, Sherman S, Hall BD (eds) Risk, communication, and decision making in genetic counseling. Ann Rev Birth Defects C. Alan R Liss, New York, pp 233-244

Cowart V [1984] NIH considers large-scale study to evaluate chorionic villi sampling. JAMA 252: 11-15

Davis K, Rowland D [1983] Uninsured and underserved: inequities in health care in the United States. Milbank Mem Fund Q/Health and Society 61: 149-176

Edmonds LD, Layde PM, James LM, Flynt JW Jr, Erickson JD, Oakley GP Jr [1981] Congenital malformations surveillance: two American systems. Int J Epidemiol 10: 247-52

Ethics Advisory Board of the U.S. Department of Health, Education, and Welfare [1979] Report and conclusions: DHEW support of research involving in vitro fertilization and embryo transfer. May 4, 1979; also Federal Register 1979, 44: 35.

Ethics Committee of the American Fertility Society [1986] Ethical consideration of the new reproductive technologies. Fert & Steril 46 (Supp 1): 74

Evers-Kieboom G, Van den Berghe L [1979] Impact of genetic counseling: a review of published follow-up studies. Clin Genet 15: 465-474

Faden R, Chwalow JA, Quaid K, Chase GA, Lopes C, Leonard CO, Holtzman NA [1987] Prenatal screening and pregnant women's attitudes toward the abortion of defective fetuses. Am J Publ Hlth 77 [3]: 288-290

Fletcher JC, Ryan KJ [1987] Federal regulations for fetal research: a case for reform. Law, Medicine & Health Care 15 [3]: 126-138

Forsman I [1983] Clinical genetics: an overview. Occ Hlth Nurs, Oct: 11-13

Fraser FC [1974] Genetic counseling. Am J Hum Genet 26: 636-659

Freedman L [1988] Health and social consequences of the uninsured: a challenge to third party payment systems. In: Greenstein RM, Gardiner GB, Young DL (eds) The challenge to provide genetics services: reimbursement for medical genetics services. Division of Human Genetics, University of Connecticut School of Medicine, Farmington CT, pp 190-194

Golbus MS, Loughman WD, Epstein CJ, Halbasch G, Stephens JD, Hall BD [1979] Prenatal diagnosis in 3,000 amniocenteses. N Engl J Med 300 [4]: 157-163

Goldberg MF, Oakley GP [1979] Prenatal screening for anencephaly - spina bifida: some epidemiological projections for a national program. In: Porter IH, Hook EB (eds) Service and education in medical genetics. New York, Academic Press

Green JE, Dorfmann A, Jones SL, Bender S, Patton L, Schulman JD [1988] Chorionic villus sampling: Experience with an initial 940 cases. Obstet Gynecol 71: 208-212

Greenstein RM, Gardiner GB [1988] Assessment of reimbursement for genetic diseases. In: Greenstein RM, Gardiner GB, Young DL (eds) The challenge to provide genetics services: reimbursement for medical genetics services. Division of Human Genetics, University of Connecticut School of Medicine, Farmington CT, pp 36-48

Greenstein RM, Gardiner GB, Young DL [1988] A fifty-state analysis of Medicaid reimbursement for genetics services. In: Greenstein RM, Gardiner GB, Young DL (eds) The challenge to provide genetics services: reimbursement for medical genetics services. Division of Human Genetics, University of Connecticut School of Medicine, Farmington CT, pp 175-189

Henshaw SK, Forrest JD, Van Vort J [1987] Abortion services in the United States, 1984 and 1985. Family Planning Perspectives 19 [2]. Alan Guttmacher Institute, New York

Hirschfield DS [1970] The lost reform: the campaign for compulsory health insurance in the United States from 1932 to 1943. Harvard University Press, Cambridge, MA

Holtzman NA [1988] Recombinant DNA technology, genetic tests, and public policy. Am J Hum Genet 42 [4]: 624-630

Holtzman NA [1989] Proceed with caution: predicting genetic risks in the recombinant DNA era. Johns Hopkins University Press, Baltimore

Hook EB, Chambers GM [1977] Estimated rates of Down syndrome in live births by one year maternal age intervals for mothers aged 20-49 in a New York State study - implications of the risk figures for genetic counseling and cost benefit analysis of prenatal diagnosis programs. In: Bergsma D, Lowry RB (eds) Numerical taxonomy of birth defects and polygenic disorders. Alan R Liss, New York

Hook EB, Schreinemachers DM [1983] Trends in utilization of prenatal cytogenetic diagnosis by New York State residents in 1979 and 1980. Am J Publ Hlth 73 [2]: 198-202

Kennedy DM [1970] Birth control in America: the career of Margaret Sanger. Yale University Press, New Haven

Kevles DJ [1985] In the name of eugenics: genetics and the uses of human heredity. Knopf, New York

Layde PM, von Allmen SD, Oakley GP [1979] Maternal serum alpha-fetoprotein screening: a cost-benefit analysis. Am J Publ Hlth 69: 566-573

Leonard CO, Chase G, Childs B [1972] Genetic counseling: a consumer's view. N Engl J Med 287: 433-439

Lippman-Hand A, Fraser FC [1979] Genetic counseling - the postcounseling period. I. Parents' perceptions of uncertainty. Am J Med Genet 4: 51-71

Lubs ML [1979] Does genetic counseling influence risk attitudes and decision making? In: Epstein CJ, Curry CJR, Packman S, Sherman S, Hall BD (eds) Risk, communication, and decision making in genetic counseling. Ann Rev Birth Defects C. Alan R Liss, New York, pp 355-366

Ludmerer KM [1972] Genetics and American society. Johns Hopkins University Press, Baltimore

March of Dimes Birth Defects Foundation [1986] International Directory of Genetic Services, Eighth Edition. March of Dimes, White Plains, NY

McGovern MM, Goldberg JD, and Disnick RJ [1986] Acceptability of chorionic villi sampling for prenatal diagnosis. Am J Obstet Gyn 155 [1]: 25-29

Meister SB, Shepard D, Zeckhauser R [1987] cost-effectiveness of prenatal screening for neural tube defects. In: Nightingale EO, Meister SB (eds) Prenatal screening, policies, and values: the example of neural tube defects. Division of Health Policy Research and Education, Harvard University, Cambridge, MA

Milunsky A, Atkins L [1975] Prenatal diagnosis of genetic disorders. In: Milunsky A (ed) The prevention of genetic diseases and mental retardation. Saunders, Philadelphia, pp 221-263

Naber JM, Huether CA, Goodwin BA [1987] Temporal changes in Ohio amniocentesis utilization during the first twelve years (1972-1983), and frequency of chromosome abnormalities observed. Prenat Diagn 7: 51-65

Naranjo MSF, Lockhart LH [1979] Quantitative analysis and discussion of Mexican- and Anglo-Americans' response to intervention in genetic disease. In: Epstein CJ, Curry CJR, Packman S, Sherman S, Hall BD (eds) Risk, communication, and decision making in genetic counseling. Ann Rev Birth Defects C. Alan R Liss, New York, pp 267-280

National Academy of Sciences, Committee for the Study of Inborn Errors of Metabolism [1975] Genetic screening: programs, principles, and research. National Academy of Sciences, Washington, D.C.

National Center for Education in Maternal and Child Health [1985] Comprehensive clinical genetic services centers: a national directory. DHHS Pub. No. HRS-D-MC 86-1. U.S. Government Printing Office, Washington, DC

National Center for Education in Maternal and Child Health [1987] A guide to selected national genetic voluntary organizations. NCEMCH, 3520 Prospect St. NW, Washington DC

National Center for Education in Maternal and Child Health [1988] Reaching out – a directory of voluntary organizations in maternal and child health. NCEMCH, 3520 Prospect St. NW, Washington DC

National Institute of Child Health and Development National Registry for Amniocentesis Study Group [1976] Midtrimester amniocentesis for prenatal diagnosis: safety and accuracy. JAMA 236: 1471-1476

National Opinion Research Center (University of Chicago) [1987] General social surveys, 1972-1987: cumulative codebook. National Opinion Research Center, Chicago, July

Nightingale EO, Meister SB (eds) [1987] Prenatal screening, policies, and values: the example of neural tube defects. Division of Health Policy Research and Education, Harvard University, Cambridge, MA

Pauker SG, Pauker SP, McNeil BJ [1981] The effect of private attitudes on public policy: prenatal screening for neural tube defects as a prototype. Medical Decision Making 1: 103-114

Pauker SP, Pauker SG [1979] The amniocentesis decision: an explicit guide for parents. In: Epstein CJ, Curry CJR, Packman S, Sherman S, Hall BD (eds) Risk, communication, and decision making in genetic counseling. Ann Rev Birth Defects C. Alan R Liss, New York, pp 289-324

Rapp R [1988] Chromosomes and communication: the discourse of genetic counseling. Med Anthropology 2 [2]: 143-157

Reed J [1978] From private vice to public virtue: the birth control movement and American society, 1830-1975. Basic Books, New York

Reed S [1974] A short history of genetic counseling. Soc Biol 21: 332-339

Reilly P [1977] Genetics, law and social policy. Harvard University Press, Cambridge, MA

Rothstein WG [1987] American medical schools and the practice of medicine: a history. Oxford University Press, New York and Oxford

Saxton M [1984] Born and unborn: the implications of reproductive technologies for people with disabilities. In: Arditti R, Klein RD, Minden S (eds) Test-tube women: what future motherhood? Methuen, New York, pp 298-312

Schleifer JT [1980] The making of Tocqueville's *Democracy in America.* University of North Carolina Press, Chapel Hill, NC

Schreinemachers DM, Hook EB [1984] Prenatal cytogenetic utilization in New York State, 1979-82 by county and HSA region. Report from the New York State Chromosome Registry, Albany, NY

Shryock RH [1962] Medicine and society in America: 1660-1860. Cornell University Press, Ithaca, NY

Sokal DC, Byrd JR, Chen ATL, Goldberg MF, Oakley GP [1980] Prenatal chromosome diagnosis: racial and geographic variation for older women in Georgia. JAMA 244 [12]: 1355-1357

454

Sorenson JR, Scotch NA, Swazey JP, Wertz DC, Heeren TC [1987] Reproductive plans of genetic counseling clients not eligible for prenatal diagnosis. Am J Med Genet 28: 345-352

Sorenson JR, Swazey JP, Scotch NA [1981] Reproductive pasts, reproductive futures: genetic counselling and its effectiveness. Alan R Liss, New York

Sorenson JR, Wertz DC [1986] Couple agreement before and after genetic counseling. Am J Med Genet 25 [3]: 549-555

Stein Z, Susser M [1978] Epidemiologic and genetic issues in mental retardation. In: Morton N (ed) Genetic epidemiology. Academic Press, New York

Steinbrook R [1986] In California, voluntary mass prenatal screening. Hastings Center Rep 16 (Oct): 5-7

Tocqueville A de (1951; orig ed 1835) Democracy in America, vol I. Bradley P (ed) Alfred A Knopf, New York

U.S. Congress (1985) Health Research Extension Act of 1985, Legislative History, Public Law 99-158, pp 718-719

U.S. Congress, Office of Technology Assessment [1983] The role of genetic testing in the prevention of occupational disease. OTA-BA-194. U.S. Government Printing Office, Washington, DC

U.S. Congress, Office of Technology Assessment [1987] New developments in biotechnology 2: public perceptions of biotechnology. U.S. Government Printing Office, Washington, DC

U.S. Congress, Office of Technology Assessment (1988a) The commercial development of tests for human genetic disorders, prepared by Hewitt M, Holtzman NA. OTA, Washington DC

U.S. Congress, Office of Technology Assessment (1988b) Mapping our genes: genome projects: how big, how fast? Office of Technology Assessment, Washington DC, April

U.S., Department of Commerce, Bureau of the Census (1988a) Statistical Abstract of the United States 1987. U.S. Government Printing Office, Washington, DC

U.S. Department of Commerce, Bureau of the Census (1988b) Current population reports, series P-25, No. 1022, United States population estimates, by age, sex, and race: 1980 to 1987. U.S. Government Printing Office, Washington, DC

U.S., Department of Health, Education, and Welfare, Public Health Service, National Institutes of Health [1979] Antenatal diagnosis: report of a consensus conference. NIH Publication No. 79-1973, Bethesda, MD

U.S., National Center for Health Statistics: Advance report of final mortality statistics, 1985 [1987] Monthly Vital Statistics Report Vol. 36, No. 5, Suppl. DHHS Pub. No. (PHS) 87-1120. Public Health Service, Hyattsville, MD, August

U.S., President's Commission for the Study of Ethical Problems in Medicine and Biomedical and Behavioral Research [1982] Splicing life. U.S. Government Printing Office, Washington, DC, November

U.S., President's Commission for the Study of Ethical Problems in Medicine and Biomedical and Behavioral Research [1983] Screening and counseling for genetic conditions. U.S. Government Printing Office, Washington, DC, February

University of Colorado School of Nursing [1987] Genetics applications for health professionals (prepared by Forsman I) Lerner Managed Designs, Lawrence, KS

Walters L [1986] The ethics of human gene therapy. Nature 320: 225-227

Weigle G [1988] Are the medically uninsurable really uninsurable? In: Greenstein RM, Gardiner GB, Young DL (eds) The challenge to provide genetics services. Division of Human Genetics. University of Connecticut School of Medicine, Farmington, CT pp 148-154

Wertz DC, Fletcher JC [1988] Ethics and medical genetics in the United States: a national survey. Am J Med Genet 29: 815-827

Wertz DC, Sorenson JR [1983] Contraceptive use and efficacy in a genetically counseled population. Soc Biol 30 [3]: 328-334

Wertz DC, Sorenson JR [1986] Client reactions to genetic counseling: self-reports of influence. Clin Genet 30: 494-502

Wertz DC, Sorenson JR [1989] Sociologic implications. In: Evans MI, Fletcher JC, Dixler AO, Schulman JD (eds) Fetal diagnosis and therapy: science, ethics, and the law. JB Lippincott, Philadelphia, pp 554-565

Wertz DC, Sorenson JR, Heeren TC [1984] Genetic counseling and reproductive uncertainty. Am J Med Genet 18 [1]: 79-88

Wertz DC, Sorenson JR, Heeren TC [1986] Clients' interpretations of risks provided in genetic counseling. Am J Hum Genet 39: 253–264

Wertz DC, Sorenson JR, Heeren TC (1988a) Communication in health professional-lay encounters. In Ruben BD (ed) Information and Behavior 2. Transaction Books, New Brunswick, NJ, pp 329–342

Wertz DC, Sorenson JR, Heeren TC (1988b) 'Can't get no (dis)satisfaction': professional satisfaction with professional-client encounters. Work and Occupations 15 [1]: 36–54

Wertz RW, Wertz DC [1989] Lying-in: a history of childbirth in America, enlarged edition. Yale University Press, New Haven [First ed 1977, Free Press, New York]

Zare N, Sorenson JR, Heeren TC [1984] Sex of provider as a variable in effective genetic counseling. Soc Sci Med 19: 671–675

Zelizer VA [1985] Pricing the priceless child: the changing social value of children. Basic Books, New York

# 3. Ethics and Human Genetics: A Cross-Cultural Perspective

J. C. Fletcher

This final chapter will discuss these questions:

1) As viewed cross-culturally, what are the major ethical problems in the practice of human genetics today? What are the major social-ethical and policy issues presented to societies and their leaders today and in the near future?
2) What will happen if ethically adequate, unified, and teachable approaches to these issues are not developed?
3) How can the results of this study help to develop such approaches?
4) Is there a viable cross-cultural perspective in *ethics* for evaluating different cultural and personal approaches to ethical problems in human genetics? Is there a constructive "middle ground" between ethical relativism and ethical absolutism?
5) If so, what evaluations can we make from this perspective about the prevailing approaches to difficult ethical problems in medical genetics today and in the near future?
6) What priority should human genetics and genetic services have in society's overall medical expenditures? What are geneticists' responsibilities towards formulating public policies affecting human genetics and reproductive choices?
7) What steps can medical geneticists, policy makers, and public and parent groups take, nationally and internationally, to study social-ethical issues in this field?

These questions belong to the domain of applied ethics. The primary task of applied ethics is to evaluate the adequacy of the prevailing set of approaches to ethical problems in a particular field of human endeavor. A four-step evaluation of approaches in medical genetics appears later in this chapter.

"Approaches" are bridges between a general level of ethical concepts and principles – the domain of general normative ethics – and the concrete level of decision making about problems in actual cases. Approaches in an area like medical genetics are needed for each major problem frequently faced by practitioners. The approaches should be responsive on the one hand to the responsibilities and evolving experience of the patient-physician relationship, and on the other hand, to the claims of ethical principles widely respected in a society. Thus, applied ethics in medical genetics ought to be a dialogue between good studies of actual approaches to ethical problems in practice and critical reflection on the adequacy of these approaches. Critical reflection ought to draw upon resources from significant traditions of ethical thought and discourse for its work.

A set of approaches needs to be unified in the sense that each approach can be consistently explained and taught, in terms of principle and practice, without significant contradictions with other approaches in the set. Also, the practitioners and patients who learn these approaches in one generation need to be able to teach them clearly to those who follow them in the next generation. Well-reasoned approaches that have been effectively applied to ethical problems do not, however, provide an exact formula for exactly what ought to be done in each case. An approach bridges principle and practice and links them, predisposing but not dictating to persons exactly what they ought to do. Approaches, like other dimensions of moral experience, must be learned and internalized. Then the approach helps decision makers prepare for difficult cases. Once learned, the approach takes decision makers to the doorway of a case but does not dictate the final judgment, since the situational factors of the case will not be apparent until the case begins. We undertook the study reported in Part 1 primarily to learn how geneticists would approach ethical problems in practice and how much variation exists in their approaches.

Geneticists and their societies face an enormous task in developing clear and unified approaches to ethical problems. The set of problems consists of three tiers: a) ethical problems in the practice of human genetics, b) additional ethical concerns created by developments in allied fields, and c) social-ethical problems of human genetics.

## 3.1 Major Ethical Problems in the Practice of Human Genetics

To discuss ethics and human genetics in a cross-cultural perspective, I distinguish between ethical problems *in* the practice of human genetics and social-ethical issues *of* human genetics. This distinction conveys the difference between recurring areas of conflict of interests and duties within professional practice, and new social alternatives and policy choices stemming from the impacts of basic and applied research in human genetics on societies.

There are two types of situations commonly identified as "ethical problems." The first is when a person or group is perceived by others to be in fundamental violation of responsibilities to the welfare of a significant human community (Parsons 1951). The ethical problem is how the community ought to respond. The second situation finds persons, like the geneticists in this study or their patients, confronting sharply conflicting duties, making a decision that expresses the conflict. And, of course, these two situations can and often do coalesce into one. Every ethical problem arises in a situation that has elements of 1) collectively defined loyalty, and 2) individuals or groups confronting decisions that express conflicts. These conflicts may be among ethical principles, among responsibilities transmitted in roles like "physician" and "patient," or among loyalties owed to communities beyond the medical situation, e.g., familial, legal, or religious.

Part 2 shows that geneticists and their patients, even in nations as culturally different as those in this study, tend to face a similar set of ethical problems. These problems are: access to and adequacy of genetic services, abortion choices, confidentiality conflicts, disclosure dilemmas, indications for prenatal diagnosis, and exceptions to the practice of nondirective counseling. I rank these problems using three criteria: 1) the study's results, 2) frequency of discussion in Part 2, and 3) by numbers of persons whose welfare is adversely affected by the problem.

1. A two-sided problem – unfairness in access to genetic services (i.e., counseling, screening, prenatal diagnosis) and insufficient services to meet needs – is the most ubiquitous ethical problem in human genetics, cross-culturally considered. This problem is especially acute for individuals, families and pregnant women who are not referred to genetic services by physicians, who suffer from poverty or lack of education, or who live far from a genetic center.

2. Abortion choices for genetic reasons present difficult conflicts and concerns in every society due to several causes:

a) beliefs about the higher moral status of the fetus at midtrimester; b) the wide spectrum of severity in some disorders; c) the treatability of some disorders; d) concern that a practice of selective abortion creates a precedent for neglect of genetically affected persons who survive, including precedent for a practice of pediatric euthanasia; and e) the possibility to diagnose twins where one is healthy and the other affected. A decision not to abort after a positive genetic finding can also be an ethical problem if the woman or couple involved are pressured to abort or threatened with loss of medical care.

3. The duty to protect patients' privacy and to maintain the confidentiality of the patient-geneticist relationship is a problem in every nation. Geneticists have a duty to prevent unconsenting disclosures of their patients' genetic diagnoses and health prognoses. This duty can sometimes conflict with the interests of relatives at risk and especially with the collective interests of institutional third parties, e.g., insurers, employers, or government health authorities.

4. Disclosure dilemmas in medical genetics exist in every society. They arise largely from the geneticist's access to psychologically sensitive information, e.g., when the geneticist knows, but a married couple does not yet know which one has transmitted a disorder to a child; when tests reveal that a phenotypical female has an XY genotype; when tests show false paternity; when a woman has had previous elective abortions and her husband does not know; when scientific conflicts occur about the interpretation of findings and an abortion might ensue; when disclosure of a genetic diagnosis to a vulnerable or fragile individual may carry a risk of harm.

5. Some patient requests or preconditions for prenatal diagnosis, e.g., maternal anxiety, refusal of abortion, and sex selection are ethically controversial, especially the latter. However, ethical problems in indications for prenatal diagnosis affect the welfare of far fewer persons than the four problems introduced above.

6. This study shows that nondirectiveness is the most widely ingrained approach to genetic counseling, when viewed cross-culturally. However, ethical problems do arise in choices to be nondirective, especially in counseling patients whose capacity to participate in counseling and decision making is impaired. These patients may be mentally ill, significantly retarded, or abusers of alcohol or drugs. Some patients may be disadvantaged in terms of communication because they lack adequate education. Further, some patients from a different culture may hold different views about science and nature than the geneticist. For such reasons all of the patients above may be functionally unable to appreciate the significance of genetic risks. These cases are infrequently mentioned in Part 2, except in the

discussion of a directive counseling strategy in Hungary that is applicable to cases of severe retardation and substance abuse.

These six ethical problems *in* medical genetics have been present since the introduction of amniocentesis and carrier screening in the late 1960s, but the problems magnify in complexity and frequency as genetic technologies improve and the numbers of persons seen in genetic clinics grow. This magnification is especially obvious in the context of the "new genetics."

## 3.1.1 The "New Genetics"

This international study began when the "new genetics," a term coined by Comings [1980], was first applied very widely in practice (Weatherall 1985). Before the development of DNA technology and its first use in prenatal diagnosis (Kan and Dozy 1978), geneticists tested for harmful genetic mutations in two main ways: 1) tests applied to proteins assumed to be defective due to an inherited gene, and 2) measurements of the molecular weight of compounds assumed to be abnormal due to inheritance. Observation of infants and children with genetic abnormalities and abnormal chromosomal findings were two additional methods of confirming hereditary disorders (U.S. Congress, Office of Technology Assessment 1986). In short, the older method was to test or observe the *expression* of the harmful gene(s). The new genetics exactly reverses this method and uses a direct test of DNA obtained from nucleated cells of any tissue. The methodologies to develop, validate, and apply DNA tests clinically need not be reviewed here. Holtzman (1988) raised the most relevant public policy considerations for use of DNA technology in the U.S., and these also apply to other nations. According to his assessment, the most important ethical aspects of the new DNA era are:

- potentially, DNA tests for affected persons and carriers of all major genetic disorders will become available as the human genome is mapped, although the validation of these tests will be extraordinarily difficult because of genetic heterogeneity.
- DNA tests will also become available to detect genotypes that result in higher susceptibility to common diseases (e.g., familial cancers, heart disease, diabetes). The same consideration about difficulty of validation also applies.
- the number of persons to be screened will be extremely large (Holtzman 1988).
- the number of interested third parties, besides family members, family physicians, and health authorities, will multiply, e.g., insurers and employers, and thus increase the chances for genetic discrimination; privacy and confidentiality issues will proliferate.
- because DNA must often be collected from members of whole families, and in some cases, from generations of family members, their awareness of the ethical implications of testing will be deeper; secrets will be virtually impossible to keep.
- disclosure dilemmas will multiply, especially because harmful genes will be detected presymptomatically in persons at high risk for disorders of late onset (Harris 1988).

● earlier prenatal diagnosis (9–11 weeks) is now possible and will see greater demand if chorionic villus sampling (CVS) proves to be as safe and accurate as
amniocentesis; because information about gender will be more available earlier in pregnancy, the opportunities for sex choice abortions unrelated to genetic disease will greatly increase.

The six ethical problems in the practice of human genetics identified in the previous section preexisted the "new genetics." The new genetics does not create *new*
ethical problems but magnifies each problem. DNA approaches to genetic diagnosis will intensify and complicate the ethical problems that emerged in the late
1960s and 1970s. In effect, the set of six continuing ethical problems will confront
more persons in a more complex technological situation that will interact with
older traditions of human reproduction and parenthood and will pose alternatives
for radical change. Trends in human genetics will interact with trends in fetal and
reproductive medicine to create a complex, interrelated set of technological possibilities with important ethical concerns:

1) Earlier methods of prenatal diagnosis, including the potential for diagnosis in
the preimplantation human embryo (McLaren 1985)
2) Potential for general pregnancy screening in a population
3) Potential for fetal therapy, including attempts on the molecular level (Harrison,
Golbus and Filly 1988)
4) The potential for using fetal cells and tissues after induced abortion for treatment of disorders, including genetic disorders, in older persons and children
(Sladek and Shoulson 1988)
5) Screening for genotypes that render individuals more susceptible to common
diseases such as cancer and heart disease (White and Caskey 1988)
6) Screening in the workplace for genotypes that render individuals more susceptible to harms from toxins and other industrial hazards (Murray 1984)
7) Opportunities for clinical treatment of DNA-diagnosed genetic disorders
(White and Caskey 1988) and for somatic cell human gene therapy (Anderson
1984)
8) *In vitro* fertilization and the potential it creates for:
   a) genetic research on the preimplantation human embryo (West et al. 1987)
   b) future attempts at human germline gene therapy (Anderson 1985; Fletcher
      1985)
   c) eugenically-inspired genetic engineering (Glover 1984).

These technical possibilities in human genetics and related fields raise significant
concerns at the societal level that require study and guidance by policy councils at
the highest level of government. In the interests of space, I have merely listed these
possibilities, choosing to concentrate instead on the six major ethical problems below.

## 3.1.2 Social-Ethical Issues of Human Genetics

Any adequate estimate of the social significance of ethical problems in the practice of human genetics must account for the impacts *of* these six ethical problems on societies and their members. These consequences flow beyond the practice setting to wider medical, political, legal and religious communities which interpret, guide and regulate the limits of medical progress. The cumulative impacts of advances in human genetics on these communities create social-ethical issues. This term describes: 1) an ethical dispute with some social causes that requires consideration on a societal level, and 2) a matter requiring deliberation by a society's leaders and policy makers. The major social-ethical issues of human genetics today and in the near future are:

1. *Whether to provide fairer access to existing genetic services and increase services to meet the need*

Many natural injustices and grievous physical burdens originate in the randomness of the "natural lottery" of reproduction. No child enjoys freedom of choice as to genetic inheritance and the destiny to which genes contribute. But now genetic dangers can be foreseen and prevented by using genetic knowledge, diagnosis, and intervention in pregnancy to abort or prepare for the birth of an affected child. Rawls [1971], in a noted treatise on justice, regarded the use of genetic knowledge to prevent the most serious genetic defects as a matter of intergenerational justice, or what the present generation, whose genetic inheritance is fixed, owes to later generations. Confronted by the injustices of the natural lottery, yet facing a future in which the most harmful burdens can be avoided, the policy issue facing nations desirous of avoiding eugenic policies is how to provide the fairest and most voluntary approach. Can every individual who needs genetic services learn about them and make an informed decision whether to use them or not?

A reading of the first sections of each chapter in Part 2 shows wide variability in data to document utilization of services. Comparison between the extensive documentation from the Federal Republic of Germany and the meager data from the U.S. not only reflects the differences between the health care systems of the two nations but basic problems of fairness in access to genetic and other medical services. The U.S. has no national mandate or mechanism to gather utilization and birth defects data. Only 14 of 50 states provide for recordkeeping in newborn screening programs. Only 12 states in the U.S. have birth defects registries (Andrews 1987, p 187). Modell and others (WHO/Serono 1985) point out that in most developed nations less than 50% of women over 35 years of age have prenatal diagnosis, although 80% request it when informed. The best current estimate (University of Colorado School of Nursing 1987) for the U.S. is that about 25% of women in the over-35 age group are served.

Each chapter in Part 2 reported problems of unfair access and insufficient genetic services. The gap between need and supply will increase in every nation as improvements occur in genetic technology. When the human genome is mapped it will be possible to diagnose virtually every single-gene disorder. Unfairness of limited access and insufficient genetic services will be dramatically heightened.

The two-sided problem of access and inadequate services is the most significant social-ethical issue in human genetics today. The issue is basic and distributive justice, especially when a society can provide fairer access for those at genetic risk and can increase services to meet the need but does not act to do so. In ethics "ought implies can." Ladd (1973, p 127) argued that this maxim points to a presupposition of moral discourse itself. If persons, a group, or a society "ought" to do something but "cannot," then the "moral proposition containing the ought is void and pointless." For example, if a person is drowning five feet from a bank and a person on the bank has a fifteen-foot rope, the person on the bank is clearly blameworthy not to try to save the one in danger. If no rope exists and the one on the bank cannot swim, no blame should be assigned, provided the non-swimmer goes for help. If the nonswimmer is too weak, or is ill, paralyzed, or without sight or hearing, he or she cannot respond, even to seek help, and no moral blame can by definition be assigned if the one in danger drowns. In this third case, another coming on the scene who states "you ought to have helped" smuggles a false premise into moral discourse and violates the maxim "ought implies can."

Societies around the world are, by analogy, in one of the three positions of the person on the bank in relation to their capacity to respond to problems of access to and the supply of genetic services. Some societies have a capacity to respond equivalent to a fifteen-foot rope but do not use it. The United States and Norway, for example, are in this position. Other societies are in the second position. Not having the present capacity to respond to the need, these societies can, in effect, "go for help" by making plans, seeking to bring individuals most affected and at higher risk in contact with the modest services that do exist, and investing in the training of geneticists who will eventually deliver wider services. Brazil, India, Greece, and Turkey are probably in this position.

Some societies, but none in the present study, are in the third position, so beset by conditions like war, famine, poverty, and geographical isolation that little capacity to respond to basic health problems, including human genetics, now exists. No moral judgment should be assigned in these instances to the lack of genetic services, because the capacity to act is not present. If a person, a group, or a society "cannot," the "ought" is not binding, although the incapacity to act is not permanently frozen in time.

2. *Whether to protect the choice of abortion for genetic reasons or the choice not to abort, where either of these choices is under attack, whether to establish the choice to abort for genetic reasons where it does not exist, and whether to reduce the need for abortion by increasing research and development of effective treatments for genetic disorders.*

The abortion issue, viewed cross-culturally, is exceedingly complex and difficult. Here, I address only the practice of selective abortion to prevent genetic disorders, which raises at least two social-ethical issues: 1) every society able to offer genetic services must confront the question of whether compelling moral reasons exist to permit abortions for genetic indications, i.e., for serious and untreatable genetic disorders, and 2) each society that permits selective abortion in the context of genetic services must determine whether treatment for genetic disorders, including fetal therapy, is a better alternative and social policy in the long run than prevention by abortion.

The main arguments for selective abortion arise from: 1) the obligation to reduce suffering for the affected family and the fetus when a serious and untreatable genetic disorder has been diagnosed, and 2) the obligation to prevent genetic disease and its impact on present society and future generations, in the absence of effective genetic therapies. The major arguments against selective abortion have two main thrusts: 1) a basic purpose of medicine – to save life – is violated, and 2) while some abortions might be justified, the use of prenatal diagnosis tends to set apart certain fetuses as deserving of abortion and thus treats fetuses unequally and unjustly. I have compared these arguments extensively elsewhere (Fletcher 1978, p 1,337).

In my view, the most crucial element in a choice about selective abortion is how to weigh the seriousness and untreatability of a particular genetic disease. What criteria of seriousness and treatability should be used? And who should decide? A leading U.S. Catholic moral theologian, McCormick [1981], advocates a public policy permitting abortion for "tragic" pregnancies, including those diagnosed with serious genetic problems. He argues that the policy ought to permit genetic abortions only for "fetal deformity of such magnitude that life-supporting efforts would not be considered obligatory after birth." To embody this view in public policy would require the same strict standards for selective non-treatment of handicapped newborns used in today's neonatal intensive care. These standards of decision making largely exclude parental participation. McCormick's position is based on a view of the moral status of the fetus as equal to that of the newborn. His view contrasts sharply with the prevailing practice in medical genetics confirmed by this study, which leaves the final decision about selective abortion with parents, after counseling about the seriousness and treatability of the disorder. The study's finding on counseling for fetal diagnosis of XYY and 45, X (Turner syndrome) are good examples of this practice (Table 1.13). Thus, as a policy matter, society's leaders face a choice about whether to leave the present standard as it stands, i.e., letting parents decide how much suffering they wish to accept or prevent by the choice of abortion, or authorizing a list of untreatable fetal disorders for which abortion would be permitted.

The prevailing approach is based on respect for parental autonomy, to be sure, but it also draws upon a "graded" view of the moral status of fetal life, governing how much protection society owes to the fetus. The prevailing view accords a lower moral status to the fetus in the first and second trimesters than to the viable fetus, and says that the newborn should be protected apart from the interests of the woman and family (Dunstan 1984).

The ethical principle most relevant to the choice for abortion is respect for persons' self-determination and autonomy. The legal grounding of protection of the choice of genetic abortions varies widely, as a review of the abortion laws in the nations reporting in Part 2 (Figure 1.1) shows. However, access to genetic abortion is possible in all these nations, despite ambiguity of some laws (Japan) or very restrictive abortion laws in one (Brazil).

The issue of a better approach to prevention than abortion arises from the ethical principle of nonmaleficence, which requires that harm to persons not be inflicted, if at all possible. Abortion carries harm, in that it kills the fetus and carries some risks of complications to the woman, especially in the second trimester. Also, the emotional trauma of mid-trimester genetic abortion for the couple is well-documented by research in several nations (Blumberg et al. 1975; Donnai et al. 1981; Leschot et al. 1982; Adler and Kusnick 1982; Jones et al. 1984). Where there is little or no societal investment in research on therapies for genetic disease, the use of selective abortion as prevention will become entrenched. With DNA technologies, the numbers of pregnancies to be screened will increase sharply, and more abortions will occur. Effective treatment for genetic disorders is the only strategy that will reduce the incidence of abortions for genetic reasons, assuming that legal protection of the abortion choice will be secured and extended where it did not previously exist. However, societies that place a high priority on treatment for genetic disorders need to face the required imperatives in research with the human embryo and fetus.

The final four social-ethical issues will be discussed below in Section 3.5. Here I simply list the issues for the reader.

3. Whether access to information about persons at higher genetic risk needs to be legally protected from institutional third parties, e. g., employers or insurers, to prevent genetic discrimination.

4. Whether resolution of disclosure dilemmas will be left entirely to professional judgment, with consultation, or whether the patient's right to know everything materially relevant to his or her genetic condition should be protected by law.

5. Whether an indications policy for prenatal diagnosis (who shall be served when all who need it cannot have it?) should be a matter of law or public policy, due to the considerations of justice involved, and whether an indications policy should rule out use of prenatal diagnosis for sex selection alone.

6. Whether directive genetic counseling should be encouraged by public policy in exceptional cases of extremely high genetic risk and parental incapacity.

## 3.2 What Could Happen in the Future? Need for a Unified Approach

If approaches to these problems remain variable, many unfortunate results could occur. The first result may be that the beneficial potential of genetic services will be lost. The public and policy makers could become disaffected and distrustful of human genetics services due to multiple unresolved ethical and social conflicts. The greatest loss would be that those who need them most would not receive the benefits of genetic services.

If geneticists cannot successfully fashion their own practice-based approaches to ethical problems, more powerful forces in their societies may fill the vacuum. In nations with a predominantly capitalistic and free market approach to health care, commercial firms with a profit motive could eventually dominate the genetic service system. In a fee-for-service system, moral lines are harder to maintain and physicians are more easily mistaken for mere technicians. Only the already well-off can now afford access to genetic services. This trend further harms the health, in the long run, of the children of the least well-off and leads to more social conflict. In nations with health care systems under state control and where geneticists'

465

approaches to ethical problems are undeveloped, state interests could elevate cost-benefit considerations as the dominant theme in the provision of genetic services. These interests might result in compulsory genetic screening, including population and pregnancy screening.

## 3.2.1 Research Ethics: A Historical Analogy

The evolution of the ethics of human experimentation presents a historical analogy to the ill-defined ethical situation of human genetics today. In human genetics today, the stakes for practitioners and societies are very high. Yet there is little basic agreement on approaches to fundamental ethical problems. The same situation prevailed in the ethics of research involving human subjects just after World War II (Berg and Tranøy 1983; Fletcher 1983). In research, the oldest resource for protection of human subjects was the conscience of the individual investigator. In genetics, there is a similar situation today in many nations, where the individual geneticist is the main guardian of the welfare of the patient. Is this enough? It was not sufficient protection in the practice of clinical research. History shows that reliance on the good intentions and consciences of investigators was sadly insufficient for an adequate ethics of research. No widely shared, clearly delineated approaches to the ethical problems of research and protection of especially vulnerable subjects were worked out among scientists until the 1960s. Tranøy (1983) reviewed the achievements of the post-war Nuremberg trials, where a Code (U.S. Government 1948) was promulgated based on three ethical premises: 1) the obligations of the researcher to the subject are higher than the obligations of the researcher to the state, 2) the distinction between therapeutic and nontherapeutic research has ethical significance, and 3) the informed consent of the prospective research subject is morally essential. Even with this new guidance from Nuremberg by the mid-1960s, a number of ethical crises and disasters occurred due to the lack of impartial consideration of whether research ought to be done at all (Beecher 1966; Pappworth 1967). These dire events sensitized leaders in science and political life to take action, not only within nations but internationally. Tranøy (1983) discusses two important international documents, the Declaration of Helsinki adopted by the World Medical Assembly (1964, revised 1975) and the Declaration of Hawaii adopted by the World Psychiatric Association [1977]. These international bodies applied and elaborated the Nuremberg principles for their members. However, the single most important reform in approaches to ethical problems of research with human subjects, in my view, was to require prior group review – in a group that includes public members – of the risks and benefits of each proposed study. By analogy, public participation in the process of finding ethically acceptable approaches in human genetics may be required, especially in the context of the new genetics, to give assurance that progress in human genetics ought to be sustained. It is reasonable to ask whether publics will continue to support and cooperate with advances in human genetics when so large an agenda of ethical problems and concerns remain unresolved. The essence of the problem in research ethics was that those with the greatest self-interest in the research were permitted to decide when it was ethical to do research with human subjects at all. This occurred at a time when funds for research were greatly increasing in every developed nation. This problem in partiality had to be remedied by group review. Today, we find a situation strikingly similar. A crucial field of human endeavor is poised on the brink of remarkable technical achievements, yet this field has a number of crucial, unsettling ethical problems about which practitioners themselves are strongly divided. Society's interests in human genetics will need to be expressed and protected for the field to progress with strong public support.

## 3.3  How Can the Results of This Study Help to Develop an Approach?

Ladd [1978] writes that a method of argument used (in the West) is "appeal to *consensus hominem*, that is, the citing of the alleged agreement of people in general or of particular groups of people concerning an issue to establish a particular ethical contention." (p 403) This study shows more than "alleged" agreement on some ethical issues. For the first time we know what a sizable group of medical geneticists could likely agree upon in the ethics of their practice. More to the point, because we found more variation than consensus, the study shows where the greatest ethical differences of opinion lie. The findings create opportunities for more careful argument and discussion of proposals for approaches to the most unsettled problems.

Ladd also notes two additional questions about this method of argument, which mark the limits of such a study in drawing confident ethical conclusions. Are the people cited *especially* wise and ethically competent? Secondly, do they *in fact* actually subscribe to the beliefs attributed to them? (italics added) The answer to the first question is that medical geneticists, and their patients, are probably the best sources of information about ethical problems in practice. But experience with problems does not equate to wisdom or competence in dealing with ethical questions. Some geneticists who responded had difficulty distinguishing between technical and ethical issues. Patients were not included in this study. No claims for ethical competence can be attributed to medical geneticists as a group. However, if improvements in applied ethics ought to be made in medical genetics, these ought to follow a careful study of the approaches that medical geneticists claim to take. The second question was not addressed, since the study asked respondents what they would do in clinical cases and for their reasons for such choices, but it did not ask them about their ethical beliefs or if they would subscribe to a set of ethical guidelines. This latter step should be taken, if at all, by professional and scientific societies of medical geneticists themselves.

Are geneticists ready to shape unified codes of ethics on a national or international basis, as represented by the Helsinki declaration for research ethics? Some clues arise from this study. Table 1.23 shows the degree of internal consensus within each of the 19 nations. It would appear that some nations have a trend towards internal consensus. In our study there were ten nations with more than a 50% participation rate (Table 1.3) that also had an internal consensus on more than 60% of the clinical cases (Table 1.23). These nations were Australia, Brazil, Canada, Denmark, Federal Republic of Germany, Israel, Norway, Sweden, United Kingdom, and the United States. Japan could very well be included, because of a good participation rate (69%) and an internal consensus on 59% of cases. There may be more internal consensus in some of the other nations than was revealed by the survey, especially in those nations with lower participation rates. At any rate, in view of the difficulty of the ethical problems in this field, it is time for geneticists to discuss adoption of unified ethical codes in their professional societies. From the evidence of the study, it appears that a nation-by-nation approach to ethical codes could result in very different approaches to ethical problems.

Discussion of ethical codes ought to consider the merits of seeking consensus, whether by nation or internationally. Also, geneticists and policy makers in each nation and internationally need to face the issues of ethical relativism and absolutism. Why pursue consensus in ethics if no middle ground truly exists between these positions?

## 3.3.1 Strengths and Weaknesses of Appeals to Consensus in Ethics

Attempts to gain consensus about approaches to ethical problems have strengths and weaknesses. On the positive side, consensus-seeking helps to consolidate experience and enable older practitioners to transmit what they have learned to younger ones. Findings about consensus are useful in conveying clear positions to the public and to policy makers. Also, formulating consensus on older problems releases valuable energy to focus on new, unfamiliar problems.

On the negative side, the mere fact that consensus exists about an approach to an ethical problem is not the primary source of ethical grounding of the approach. As Mareno [1988] correctly points out, consensus should be primarily regarded as a condition of ethical inquiry rather than its goal. The goal of ethical inquiry is a well-reasoned conclusion of an argument, based on a premise which soundly appeals to ethical principles, and which takes into account all sides of a question and all rational approaches. The conclusion, with the accompanying argument, should be within the ethical reach of many and also teachable. That many, perhaps most, persons will be persuaded by the argument is an important condition but does not by itself win the day for the argument.

Appeal to consensus can also mask cultural dominance. Preference for individual over societal interests, a U.S.-Western cultural bias, is clearly evident in the study findings. Also, excessive attempts at consensus could suppress vital minority positions, which often are the most creative and critical. Finally, some geneticists objected to an effort at consensus because it could lead to "written guidelines" that invite legal vulnerability for those who act differently. Others pointed out that the field of medical genetics is too technologically fluid to find strong consensus on some issues.

## 3.3.2 State of Ethical Guidance in Medical Genetics Today

The main lesson of the study is that the central thrust of the moral reasoning of medical geneticists in these 19 nations is to protect the autonomy of the individual patient (or parents) and exercise responsibility to meet the needs of the patient. The centrality of autonomy to moral reasoning appears in the dominance of the principle of autonomy (Table 1.32), the reciprocal relationships of needs and responsibilities (Table 1.34), and the primacy of the welfare of the patient (Table 1.38). The study found strongest consensus about cases in which it is relatively easy to enhance and protect the welfare of the patient, e.g., that counseling should be nondirective, that genetic information should be protected from insurers and employers, and that ambiguous test findings ought to be fully disclosed. Cases that respondents judged to be the most difficult (confidentiality vs. interests of relatives, disclosure of XY in a female, and sex selection) had conflicts between respect for the autonomy of patients and the welfare of *others*. In the new genetics, these problems involve the welfare of *many others* and the best interests of society itself. Compared with the claims of autonomy, the concerns of justice appeared less frequently in responses, except for strong recognition of problems of distributive justice in inadequate genetic services.

The major tension in health care ethics is between the interests of individuals and families and the larger interests of society. From the ethical perspective to be outlined in a later section, the major weakness of the approaches that have evolved in most nations in the West is that interests of society are too heavily outweighed in crucial cases by the interests of individuals. This international study can also be justifiably criticized along these lines, since the case problems favored problems of individuals more than larger social problems. The discussion below will consider the interests of society, especially in the three problems in the survey that medical geneticists found most difficult. A stronger balance between societal interests and individual interests can help to reshape an overly individualistic approach that could have harmful consequences to other persons (not the patient), to society's best interests, and also to medical genetics.

## 3.4 Ethics and Human Genetics: A Cross-Cultural Perspective

This section has three parts. First, I will discuss the key elements of a cross-cultural perspective in ethics. Second, I will show that this perspective offers a constructive middle ground between the extremes of "destructive" ethical relativism and ethical absolutism. Third, using the perspective I will consider the ethical problems about which geneticists were the most troubled and those on which they had strong consensus.

## 3.4.1 Ethics in a Cross-Cultural Perspective

Any viable practical approach to ethical problems in medical genetics must be able to address cross-cultural problems in ethics. Increasingly, medical geneticists in a society see patients from other cultures who have different ethical beliefs and worldviews. Also, medical geneticists from one nation who work in another nation are expected to participate in approaches to ethical problems to which they have serious objections. Most importantly, medical geneticists from a wide variety of religious, cultural, and social backgrounds must work together under the same roof, in the same national scientific and professional societies, and in the same international associations. They confront the same serious ethical problems. Can these problems be understood and resolved without adopting absolutistic ethical views, on the one hand, or on the other hand, without falling back on a view of relativism with no limits to toleration of harmful or oppressive acts, if these are considered morally right in some society? Can one accept cultural and personal differences in ethics and still have an *ethically* valid view? Does not ethics demand only one "right" approach to moral problems, rather than toleration of diversity? Is there "common ground" in ethics which lies between toleration of some cultural and personal differences and yet permits line-drawing? The discussion below will take up this problem.

## 3.4.2 The Two Tasks of Ethics

As a discipline in any culture, ethics has two purposes: i. e, knowledge-seeking and guidance-seeking. Niebuhr (1963), a theologian whose work was open to the insights of moral philosophy and the social sciences, defined the dual purpose of ethics as knowledge and guidance, that is, "to obey the ancient and perennial commandment, 'Gnothi seauton,' 'know thyself;' and to seek guidance for our activity as we decide, choose, commit ourselves, and otherwise bear the burden of our necessary human freedom." Like Niebuhr, many philosophers and religious ethicists (Gewirth 1983; Beauchamp and Childress 1983) define ethics as having two branches: nonnormative (knowledge-seeking) and normative (guidance-seeking) tasks.

The knowledge-seeking goal of this study has two dimensions. First, we posed a question in descriptive ethics about the degree of consensus and variation among geneticists in approaches to ethical problems. What approaches do practitioners prefer and how similar or variable are these preferences? Second, the self-knowledge of geneticists can benefit if they critically examine their choices and reasoning about ethical problems and *compare* them with those taken in other nations. Cross-cultural studies of moral beliefs and approaches to ethical problems have a special benefit for self-knowledge among professionals. One can clarify and criticize one's own beliefs and positions by comparing them with those of colleagues in one's own and other nations. If one's own approach is found inadequate, one should be motivated to change and improve. In this sense, this knowledge-seeking dimension of the study is compatible with the main thesis of Toulmin's (1972) project to study human understanding:

> "in science and philosophy alike, an exclusive preoccupation with logical systematicity has been destructive of both historical understanding and rational criticism. Humans demonstrate their rationality, not by ordering their concepts and beliefs in tidy formal structures, but by their preparedness to respond to novel situations with open minds – acknowledging the shortcomings of their former procedures and moving beyond them (p viii)."

We also hoped that the study would preface and inform the guidance-seeking task that must continue among medical geneticists, leaders in their societies, parents' groups, and scholars in ethics, law, and the social sciences. The guidance-seeking process should continue, first nationally and then internationally. How ought this task be approached, especially in the light of many significant differences that are traceable to political, cultural, and religious sources?

As mentioned at the outset, applied ethics lies between two levels. These are a level of "general normative ethics" (Beauchamp and Childress 1983, p 8) and a level of actual moral problems. The task of applied ethics is to evaluate the adequacy of approaches to a particular set of ethical problems in social life. Applied ethics must shape optimal "approaches" to prepare persons for concrete decisions and judgments. If the study had asked respondents a second "why" question, i.e., "Why did you choose the reason(s) that you gave for your choice about the approach to the case?" it would have pushed medical geneticists to reflect on the *sources and foundations* of their ethical beliefs. These sources are at the level of general normative ethics, composed of ethical theories that answer the question, "which action-guides are worthy of moral acceptance and for what reasons?" (Beauchamp and Childress 1983, p 8). It is true that different ethical theories, arising from religious or secular worldviews that rest on different foundations, compete and contend for dominance at the level of general normative ethics. But experience shows that there is little hope of resolving ethical problems like those discussed here by primary reliance on normative ethical theory. Jonsen's and Toulmin's account (1988) of the deliberations in the U.S. of a National Commission between 1974 and 1979 on the ethics of research with human subjects is illuminating. They stated that as long as the diverse group of commissioners focused on ways to understand and resolve specific problems in research ethics, the Commission's work progressed. However, when they stated their *reasons* why an approach was ethically acceptable or objectionable, the work resulted in philosophical "paradox." "They agreed what it was they agreed about; but the one thing they could not agree on was *why* they agreed about it ... Instead of securely established universal principles, in which they had unqualified confidence, giving them intellectual grounding for particular judgments about specific kinds of cases, it was the other way round." (p 18) Jonsen and Toulmin stress that what the commissioners shared as a "locus of certitude" for their ethical judgments was not a set of universal principles but "a shared perception of what was *specifically* at stake in particular kinds of human situations."

Likewise, geneticists and their colleagues today must increasingly choose among competing arguments in *applied* or practical ethics and must be tolerant of diverse ethical theories that support applied ethics. Having made this point, it is important to remember that the need for *critical distance* provided by ethical theory remains. All attempts to resolve ethical problems on the practical level will be historically and culturally conditioned. Bias can only be identified and criticized from a more general and impartial level. However, my point is that the *common ground* needed will not be found at the level of general theory about normative ethics. Common ground in ethics today lies in the possibility of agreement about approaches to particular cases. Why is there a possibility of agreement in applied ethics? This perhaps points to a special trait in human beings that allows experience to prevail over systematization. "Preparedness to respond to novel situations with open minds" (Toulmin 1972, p viii) is also required in the guidance-seeking task of applied ethics. Tolerance of diversity at the level of ethical theory must be combined with an unwavering commitment to draw moral lines at the level of applied ethics, especially in urgent circumstances.

### 3.4.3  Seeking Cross-Cultural Ethical Guidance for Medical Genetics

The findings of this study would not surprise anthropologists (Hatch 1983) or dismay advocates of cultural or ethical relativism. Cultural diversity in moral views is a social fact observed since Herodotus. One response to cultural diversity is to treat it as a factual datum for ethics, without drawing any conclusion about what is right or wrong. Another response is to draw conclusions by taking a position of ethical relativism. Ladd (1973), the author of an outstanding text on the subject, defines ethical relativism as "the doctrine that the moral rightness and wrongness of actions varies from society to society and that there are no absolute universal moral standards binding on all men at all times. Accordingly, it holds that whether or not it is right for an individual to act in a certain way depends on or is relative to the society to which he belongs. What is right in one society may be wrong in another society and may be neither right nor wrong in a third society" (p 1). The relativist traces concepts of right and wrong back to cultural origins and concludes on the normative level of ethics that right and wrong are relative to culture. An ethical relativist viewing this study would deny that any common ground exists for a cross-cultural perspective in ethics and would advise tolerance. At its extreme, the relativist view would permit approaches to ethical problems in human genetics that most rational persons would find intolerable. Therefore, it is necessary to go beyond the relativist view and seek ethical guidance on a cross-cultural basis.

### 3.4.4  Four Steps in Guidance-Seeking

Guidance-seeking in applied ethics involves four steps. These steps can be used whether the evaluation is about approaches to ethical problems in one, pluralistic society, or in several societies across cultures. First, the major problems of moral choice in the area under study must be accurately described. Such studies in descriptive ethics can be done if investigators enable those who have ethical problems (e. g., geneticists) to collect and describe them.

Secondly, studies must also be done to show how much consensus or variation exists in prevailing approaches to ethical problems. Such studies should be done among geneticists in many more societies and repeated in several of the nations in our study. Our study has prepared preliminary groundwork for more definitive studies in individual nations and internationally.

It 1) confirmed that there is a strong consensus about approaches to some problems (e. g., to nondirective counseling, disclosure of ambiguous laboratory results, fairness to the couple who will not use abortion, protection of the woman in false paternity, protection of genetic screening information from insurers and employers, etc.), and 2) revealed wide variation in approaches to other problems (e. g., to confidentiality vs. duties to relatives at risk, or to disclosure of clinical findings that are psychologically sensitive, or in some nations to sex selection). Some problems are so new or limited in appearance to so few nations (e. g., surrogate motherhood and egg donation to avoid genetic disease) that it is perhaps impossible to develop a cross-cultural approach at this time.

There is also a need for good studies of the consequences of prevailing approaches, as done for the nondirective approach in genetic counseling in the U.S. (Sorenson, Swazey and Scotch 1981). Such studies are vital to know the actual benefits or harms of an approach to ethical problems. Reform of prevailing practice can then follow, if indicated.

The third step is, ethically considered, the most crucial in the guidance-seeking process. It involves evaluation of the strengths and weaknesses of a prevailing set of approaches (or lack of approaches) to ethical problems for a whole field like medical genetics. Technically, the source of my evaluation arises from "rule-utilitarian" ethical theory. Utilitarianism is primarily committed to the view that the most important criterion for morality is the consequences of decisions and actions. There are two main types of utilitarianism, and both stress maximizing the general good. Beauchamp and Childress (1983, p 26) describe the differences between them. "The act-utilitarian considers the consequences of each particular act, while the rule-utilitarian considers the consequences of generally observing a rule." For example, in a sex selection case, the act-utilitarian asks, "What would be the consequences if Dr. A responded to patient B's request for sex choice in this particular situation?" The rule-utilitarian, by contrast, asks, "What moral guidance exists for cases like this and what would be the consequences if Dr. A, and other physicians in similar cases, follows it?" I equate "moral guidance" with "approaches" to problems of moral choice discussed earlier. Rule-utilitarianism is especially concerned with evaluating whether whole systems of moral rules and guidance produce more good than harm, rather than with evaluating single, independent moral rules (Beauchamp and Childress 1983, p 32). If, in a crucial social arena like medical genetics, already laden with value-conflicts, there is an inadequate and unintegrated system of ethical guidance, conflict and discord will predictably diminish benefits (utility).

This view encourages respect for the ordinary forms of moral guidance generated in society and is critical of the conventional approach of many physicians, which is "case-bound." The conventional way of thinking about ethics in medicine

473

is that since each individual case is different, ethical guidance must be found for each case. Physicians with this view get caught up in the immediacy of the case and in making a choice do not look beyond the case to the implications for society or persons in similar situations. The conventional view about case-by-case decision making is clearly inadequate for guidance in an arena like human genetics. As mentioned above, an analogous situation occurred in medical research in the years 1945-1966, until leaders in this field studied the problems and developed a more unified system of approaches. (Levine 1986; Berg and Tranøy 1983). A lesson from the evolution of the ethics of medical research is that many ethical megadisasters occurred before researchers developed comprehensive approaches and codes of ethics. Medical geneticists should take note, because it is doubtful that societies will be as tolerant of ethical disasters in human genetics as in medical research. Human genetics affects more people and mistakes are not likely to be reversible. Human genetics, like medical research, requires a unified set of approaches to its ethical problems that is responsive to basic ethical principles and to relationships of responsibility, and that is also internally consistent.

This view involves respect for the dominant moral opinion found in different cultures and also in various sectors of a pluralistic society. But this respect is not unlimited. Following MacBeath [1952], Ladd (1973, p 121) states that culturally variable moral opinions ought to be seen as "experiments in living" which provide data for ethics, and which ethicists should not neglect. In this sense, giving respect to the differing moral opinions of geneticists is the equivalent of what Ladd calls "constructive relativism." This position elevates popular moral opinion (such as the moral views held by geneticists in this study) to the moral level. Ladd adopts this position, likens popular moral opinion in a society to the legislative will, and accords it a leading, but not absolute role, in constituting morality. He notes that this view of moral opinion or custom has "affinities with the general ethical position known as voluntarism, for, by analogy, we can conceive of popular opinion as embodying the will of the people, which determines what is right and wrong" (p 123). The connection between Ladd's thought and the work here is that approaches taken by practitioners of human genetics should be viewed as voluntary and chosen by them as morally serious persons, rather than imposed upon them unwillingly. The good response rate (62%) to a questionnaire requiring several hours to complete supports an impression of moral seriousness among geneticists. Also, most respondents gave ethical reasons for their choice of approaches, although a few consistently confused technical and ethical issues.

The opposite of constructive relativism is "destructive relativism," (Ladd 1973, p 124) a view that reduces morality itself to the level of popular opinion and drains all of its moral character away. Ladd observes that this form of reductionism is commonly used to convert a moral proposition into a statement about the proposer or the society of the proposer. Thus, the normative character of moral statements is neutralized and morality is understood as not binding at all.

Alongside the voluntaristic element in morality, Ladd requires a "nonvoluntaristic element," independent of the received moral opinions. He moves between two descriptions of the nonvoluntaristic element. Ladd describes it in one place as "a principle, however formal and general, that confers authority and legitimacy" on "quasi-legislative cultural definitions of what is right and wrong." In another, he calls it a "schema for morals which is to be filled in by the culture itself as it experiments in living" (p 123). He notes that the "schema" is necessary to answer objections against ethical relativism that it would require recognition of the moral opinion that fostered Nazism and its atrocities as "equally valid." Constructive relativism is thus a form of restricted relativism, permitting variety in moral institutions, but ruling out the intolerable. Destructive relativism, i.e., reductionism, leaves room for no ethical response in the face of the intolerable, since mere opinion is seen to be the stuff of morality.

Perhaps the clearest example of a totally nonvoluntaristic element (but not what I employ) is the concept of natural law. Natural law embodies the idea that objective ethical standards are "given" in human nature itself, independent of a society's laws or religion, and that these standards can be known by all rational persons. As applied to human genetics, a natural law view would hold that certain actions, e.g., sex selection, attempts to make chimeras by human-animal hybrids, or causing harmful mutations in a population, are wrong because they are "unnatural." This judgment would be made independently of harmful consequences because of the violation of natural law. Today, moral judgments made in terms of natural law as applied to human genetics are most often made in opposition to the practice of selective abortion (Atkinson and Moraczewski, 1980).

Natural law is, of course, not the only example of a "schema" or nonvoluntaristic element. Schema-building in contemporary Western cultures mainly employs ethical principles widely recognized across religious, philosophical, and cultural boundaries. Several anthropologists, such as Hatch [1983] have evoked *prima facie* (at first view) principles to "use in evaluating cultures, including our own." (p 133) In fact, he chooses four principles but only one is recognizably "ethical." He refers to a "humanistic" principle, namely, that "the well-being of people ought to be respected." (p 134) He uses well-being to make moral judgments on starvation and violence wherever these occur. Contemporary moral philosophers have used other terms to describe what Ladd calls the "schema," e.g., a "second tier of the moral life" (Engelhardt 1986), "the critical level of basic ethical principles" (Hare 1981), "the ethical level *per se*" (Aiken 1962). All of these terms describe a move from a level of popular, intuitive morality in particular communities to a more general and impartial level of principles.

Instead of using the term "schema," I prefer to use "a cross-cultural perspective" in ethics. Just as Ladd requires that "popular moral opinion" be limited by a "schema" or nonvoluntaristic element, I would require that geneticists' approaches to ethical problems be limited by a cross-cultural perspective in ethics. Ordinarily, the term "cross-cultural" conveys a relativistic approach. I hold, with Ladd, that constructive relativism is the correct view of cultural diversity in morality. Therefore, in my thinking a cross-cultural perspective is a schema both to prevent the intolerable and to encourage cross-cultural "experiments in living" that would help geneticists be open to change. A cross-cultural perspective would encourage experimentation in breaking out of old moral molds, drawing new lines where none existed before, or in redrawing moral lines that have been allowed to blur.

I agree with Ladd that the "schema" or (in my terms) the "perspective" is culture-dependent, or "must be filled in by the culture." No view in ethics is entirely free from its cultural origins and dependency. Ethical absolutism will always founder on this historical reality as well as on the coercion and dislocation required to impose it on those with different views. The perspective that I take (basic ethical principles and relationships) is characteristic of some contemporary Western ethical reasoning, as will be obvious. However, the middle way between ethical relativism and absolutism lies precisely in the claim that ethical principles make demands on everyone alike and that the responsibilities inherent in certain relationships (e.g., physician-patient) make demands on all who are in these relationships. Basic ethical principles are universal and objective in just this sense, namely, that everyone ought to do what the principles say, assuming that persons 1) know the principles and 2) "can" do what they require (Ladd 1973, pp 127–129). In ethics, "ought implies can." If it is impossible to respond to the ought, allowances must be made. This principle, "ought implies can" is the antidote for ethical absolutism. Below, I make no recommendations that geneticists in most nations are incapable of following.

To repeat, in my view the answer to destructive ethical relativism and absolutism is found in a cross-cultural perspective. This perspective is composed of a set of basic ethical principles and relationships that have wide recognition and acceptance across religious, cultural, and political boundaries. The force of these principles and relationships is not their direct application to cases. Such an approach is wooden, abstract, and ultimately leads to ethical absolutism by a "tyranny of principles" (Toulmin 1981). The principles and moral relationships are to be applied as criteria for evaluation of the strengths and weaknesses of *approaches* to moral problems. They can also be used to evaluate wide diversity in approaches and the lack of approaches when approaches are needed. The approaches, thus evaluated, are the major resources to prepare decision makers for practice.

To recapitulate, guidance-seeking in applied ethics has involved three steps thus far: 1) to describe accurately the major problems in moral choice in the field under study, 2) to conduct accurate studies of consensus and variation in prevailing approaches to ethical problems and of the consequences of these approaches; and 3) to evaluate the prevailing set of approaches using a "schema" in ethics such as the cross-cultural perspective described above. The fourth step in guidance-seeking is to recommend reforms in the prevailing approaches to a particular field.

What appears below is our perspective, culturally dependent but the best we can offer, to limit the intolerable and to maximize the benefits that human genetics can offer to individuals, families, and societies. Others must (and will) follow this lead and present their "schemas" for the ethics of human genetics. Openness to schemas that originate either in religious or secular worldviews is indicated, the more to encourage "corrective vision" (May 1983).

## 3.4.5 Basic Ethical Principles and the Ethics of Relationships

As noted in Part 1, we organized the answers of respondents to the "why" (ethical reasoning) questions under two paradigms in ethics. The first paradigm was a set of basic ethical principles widely discussed in biomedical ethics (National Commission for the Protection of Human Subjects of Biomedical and Behavioral Research 1979; Beauchamp and Childress 1983). These principles were:

1. *Autonomy (Respect for Persons)*: the duty to respect the self-determination and choices of autonomous persons, as well as to protect persons with diminished autonomy, e.g., young children, mentally retarded persons, and those with other mental impairments.
2. *Beneficence*: the obligation to secure the well-being of persons by acting positively on their behalf, and moreover, to maximize the benefits that can be attained.
3. *Nonmaleficence*: the obligation to minimize harm to persons and wherever possible to remove the causes of harm altogether.
4. *Justice*: the obligation to distribute benefits and burdens fairly, to treat equals equally and to give reasons for differential treatment based upon widely accepted criteria for just ways to distribute benefits and burdens.

Although we had little trouble organizing the answers of respondents under these principles, we quickly noted that geneticists' own discourse about their moral reasoning did not occur within the paradigm of ethical principles. A second paradigm was needed to provide a closer fit with their discourse, and to overcome some of the abstractness and generality at the level of principles. The appeal of principles is to their general and universal significance. Also, the main force of principles is to shape approaches to ethical problems and not to provide "answers" in the context of a case.

However, the discourse of relationships more closely fits the moral experience of clinicians. We called the second paradigm "the ethics of relationships." By this we meant dyadic interactions that tend to involve reciprocity (Ladd 1982). The relationship approach emphasizes "needs" (usually patients') and "responsibilities" (usually clinicians'). Also, in describing responsibilities as a basis of ethical action, this approach incorporates elements of Gilligan's [1982] and other feminist theories of moral development, which provides balance to the paradigm of ethical principles.

According to the relationship approach, moral reasons are organized under five headings:

1) Rights and obligations       – reciprocals
2) Needs and responsibilities     – reciprocals
3) Deserts and justice           – reciprocals
4) Good of the health care system and other institutions
5) Good of society

In the interest of space, the reader is reminded that a fuller discussion of the ethics of relationships is found in Part 1.7.3. The schema that we offer requires the relationship approach to compensate for the tendency of reasoning based entirely on principles toward abstraction. The pull of relationships is always towards experience.

## 3.5 Evaluation of Approaches to Ethical Problems in Medical Genetics

Following the fieldwork preparatory to this study, Fletcher, Berg, and Tranøy (1985) made an estimate about possible areas of consensus and variation among medical geneticists. This study shows that medical geneticists in many nations have clearly delineated approaches to some ethical problems. Geneticists are also clear about their ethical reasons for following these approaches. We find strong support for these approaches based on ethical principles, especially respect for the autonomy of patients and parents, as well as responsibilities in the physician-patient relationship. Table 1.22 shows these areas of strong agreement, which are arranged below under three of the six major problems in practice (Section 3.1).

Confidentiality problems:

1. In respect for the autonomy of the individual, to protect the patient from harm, and to maintain the confidentiality of the geneticist-patient relationship, genetic information derived from screening in the workplace or from presymptomatic testing (Huntington disease) should not be given to insurers and employers without the consent of the worker or the patient.

Disclosure problems:

2. In incidental findings that strongly suggest nonpaternity, and when this fact must unavoidably be disclosed because of genetic risks, physicians should meet with the woman first, in respect for her privacy, to advise her of the finding. They should recommend special care to help her with her choice about disclosure and the process of any future genetic counseling. The choices about disclosure are the woman's and should be safeguarded.

3. When prenatal studies yield conflicting findings, these should be fully disclosed to the parents, followed by nondirective counseling.

4. New interpretations of prenatal studies in a research phase of development should be fully disclosed to parents, followed by an explanation of the unproven status of the interpretation.

5. Prenatal results of sex chromosome abnormalities with a relatively low burden (XYY and 45, X) should be fully disclosed to parents, followed by nondirective counseling with a full description of the potential and problems of individuals who live with these conditions.

Genetic counseling problems:

6. In counseling competent persons, geneticists should a) help individuals/couples understand their options and the present state of medical knowledge so they can make informed decisions, b) suggest that while they will not make decisions for patients, they will support any they make, and c) tell patients that decisions, especially about reproduction, are theirs alone to make and refuse to make any for them.

7. In counseling carriers of a genetic disorder for which prenatal diagnosis is not available, adoption ought to be presented as an option to reproduction; the option of artificial insemination can also be discussed, recognizing that some may object on religious grounds.

8. Genetic counseling should also be conducted according to goals of a) helping

couples/individuals adjust to and cope with their genetic problems, b) the removal or lessening of patient guilt or anxiety, c) helping individuals/couples achieve their parenting goals, and d) the prevention of disease and abnormality.

It appears that geneticists in many nations could conscientiously follow these approaches in cases that present such problems.

The evaluation now turns to approaches to three problems about which geneticists were troubled and divided, i. e., confidentiality in counseling when the patient forbids the geneticist from contacting relatives at risk, full disclosure of an XY genotype to a phenotypical female, and (in some nations) prenatal diagnosis for sex selection.

## 3.5.1 Confidentiality in Counseling and Risks to Relatives

The issue of whether confidentiality ought to be breached when an affected patient refuses to warn relatives of potential harm to themselves (e.g., Huntington disease) or to offspring (e.g., hemophilia A) reflects claims from the principles of justice, beneficence and nonmaleficence, as well as a claim to respect the patient's autonomy by protecting confidentiality. What line can be drawn between the tolerable and intolerable in such cases? A recent work on reproductive genetics, social policy, and the law (Elias and Annas 1987), poses the case of a mother, a carrier of Lesch-Nyhan syndrome, who has an affected son. She "adamantly" refuses to notify her sisters, each of whom has a 50% risk of being a carrier. The authors state their "bias toward a policy of strict nondisclosure" in cases of counselee refusal, because it "fosters client self-determination and confidence in the integrity of the counseling process." On the other hand, they "recognize the serious implications of genetic disorders and understand why a counselor might want to breach confidentiality under certain circumstances." This case is similar in risk to the Huntington disease case posed in the survey. In responding to that case, 58% of respondents would disclose to relatives, including 24% who would take the risk of an unsolicited disclosure, presumably after voluntary efforts at getting the patient's cooperation had failed (Table 1.7). In short, although strong consensus does not exist on this question, geneticists lean towards disclosure to prevent significant harm to others. A U.S. President's Commission's [1983] recommendation for this type of case is also for disclosure, provided four conditions are met:

"A professional's ethical duty of confidentiality to an immediate patient or client can be overridden only if several conditions are satisfied: [1] reasonable efforts to elicit voluntary consent to disclosure have failed; [2] there is a high probability both that harm will occur if the information is withheld and that the disclosed information will actually be used to avert harm; [3] the harm that identifiable individuals would suffer would be serious; and [4] appropriate precautions are taken to ensure that only the genetic information needed for diagnosis and/or treatment of the disease in question is disclosed" (p 44).

In a legal analysis, Andrews (1987, p 198) recognizes that compelling individual cases exist to override patient confidentiality in order to convey genetic information to relatives. But she warns geneticists to consider the potentially "awesome" systemic consequences of exercising a right to disclose to relatives, because it may lead to a standard of care based on a duty to disclose. Then there would be a duty to contact and inform all relatives at potential risk. She also cautions that if geneticists begin to contact relatives they may establish a standard of care in which relatives who are not contacted will sue them. Andrews' arguments are realistic. The duty to disclose to relatives compels many geneticists, because they know that disclosure can prevent serious harm. It would be unfair, at present, for society to expect more of geneticists than to act in the clearest, most compelling cases of *highest* genetic harm (e.g., cases like Lesch-Nyhan or Huntington, 25%–50% risk of serious disorder). Surely, such cases and degrees of risk are exactly what the President's Commission intended by its recommendation with its four conditions.

Any discussion of risk in human genetics must combine the probability and the severity of the disorder for which the patient is at risk. Patients place more emphasis on "what" is risked than on numerical probability. Furthermore, patients have widely varying perceptions of the severity of disorders. Thus, it is very difficult to draw guidelines for priorities in disclosure. Given adequate records and resources for locating relatives at risk, there will surely be societal and legal pressure for disclosure in virtually all cases. Anticipating this state of affairs, physicians should be protected against suits for breach of confidentiality in cases where they have satisfied the conditions to override it. Also, the resources to make ethically sensitive contacts with families at highest genetic risk must be given to medical geneticists now as society's expectations rise. If societies do not provide the resources for geneticists to locate relatives at risk, persons who are not contacted about genetic risks in the lower ranges (e.g., 1–5%) may sue physicians. But it is unlikely that any court would find negligence or award damages, in the absence of records or resources that would enable physicians to contact other family members. This defense would also be strengthened if physicians could show that existing resources were being used for contact with relatives at higher genetic risk for more serious disorders.

The ethics of disclosure of genetic risks *begin* with intrafamilial duties to warn and protect family members from harm, and these duties are not confined to the immediate family. Identified patients or parents of an affected child, according to Andrews (p 199) have an ethical duty to inform relatives in the extended family, once they are informed themselves about the condition. This duty arises from kinship bonds and the ethical principle of non-maleficence. A basic function of the family itself is protection from harm for its members. However, those at risk must first *learn* about their risks. Physicians, especially geneticists, are the primary mediators of genetic knowledge in society today. Geneticists are surely entitled to ask assertively, if not to require, that the identified patient or parents help in contacting relatives so that they may be informed about specific risks. As indicated above, DNA testing requires cooperation of family members to bank DNA. The first contact with the index patient or key family members ought to include discussion about family involvement and responsibilities to disclose findings. Also, depending upon the degree and magnitude of harm that may occur from non-disclosure, the counselor should discuss the limits of confidentiality at the outset.

Cases of outright patient refusal to contact relatives will, however, continue to occur. If geneticists have informed patients at the outset about the need and duty to inform other family members who have a reproductive or health risk, and that confidentiality is limited by this duty, geneticists have laid the groundwork for action if the patient subsequently refuses to contact relatives. Should geneticists enter into a professional relationship with a potential patient who states from the beginning that he or she will not, under any circumstances, contact relatives and that a genetic condition must be kept secret? In my view, it is ill-advised to permit patients to dictate the terms of communication, especially in problems where harm to others may well be a factor. Absolute confidentiality cannot rationally be promised in any medical relationship. A better approach is not to promise absolute confidentiality at the outset of any genetic counseling, since the duty to inform others at risk will take precedence over any presumed right of the counselee to keep the risk a secret. By what ethical argument could such a secret be justified? I cannot think of one nor has such an argument or defense appeared in the literature. Physicians can make it clear to a patient that if the patient will not carry out his or her own duty it places physicians in an intolerable position. If a history of alienation and emotional problems in the family emerges, the patient can be offered help from a mental health specialist with the task of disclosure.

Andrews' caution about the "awesomeness" of the task of contacting relatives at risk is in fact an indication of how knowledge of human genetics will vastly transform the practice of medicine in the future. Physicians had best be prepared to *use* genetic knowledge in a context of cooperation with *families* in the practice of medicine, rather than relying on an overly individualistic standard of patient communication and education. Legally, would not grounds exist for a "wrongful birth" claim (Andrews 1987, p 138) against the geneticist who withheld information from a relative who proceeded to give birth to an affected child? DNA testing requires the cooperation of several family members. The incidence of secret-keeping will decrease. It is unlikely, however, that patient refusals to disclose voluntarily will disappear. A clear policy, supported by a high ethical standard of disclosure, would protect geneticists who were justifiably paternalistic.

## 3.5.2 Full Disclosure of Clinically Relevant Information

One of the strongest findings of this study is how committed medical geneticists are, in most cases, to complete disclosure to patients of clinically relevant information, even if the information is ambiguous, or based on disputed laboratory results, or scientifically unproven (Table 1.9). The practice of full disclosure is compatible with the value of distributing genetic services fairly.

One case, the XY female, appears to be an exception to the practice of full disclosure, due to the psychologically sensitive nature of the information (Table 1.8). Such patients are genetically male but phenotypically female and infertile (McKusick 1986). Since they have been raised and socialized as females, it is ethically objectionable to refer to them as "males" in physician, patient, or family communication. Should a full, biological explanation of this condition, testicular feminization syndrome or androgen insensitivity syndrome, be given? The reasoning of those who favor nondisclosure is that psychological harm may be done to the patient. In Brazil, France, German Democratic Republic, Greece, Hungary, Norway, and Switzerland, there was a strong consensus (>75%) among respondents against full disclosure. Israel and Italy came close (73%) to a strong consensus against disclosure.

Three reasons support full disclosure. First, the infertility should be explained. A genetic explanation may actually relieve the patient, if she feels that she is personally to blame. Secondly, since the syndrome includes abdominal or inguinal testes, surgical removal is indicated to prevent cancer (President's Commission 1983, p 62). The informed consent standards for surgery will be violated if a full explanation is not given. The patient must be told the basic facts of the problem that gives rise to the need for surgery, if she can comprehend these facts, in order to give a valid consent.

The third reason that supports full disclosure is the open communication and trust that needs to mark the physician-patient relationship. If vital facts are edited out of the communication by the physician, the relationship is less than optimal and can be harmed. If the patient later discovers non-disclosure, her confidence in physicians could well be shaken or undermined and result in further harm.

Several exceptions to full disclosure of XY in a female are defensible. Examples are immaturity, mental illness, retardation, and educational barriers to understanding. Another exception is based upon an assessment of potential for psychological harm, followed by invoking the "therapeutic privilege" of delayed disclosure. This assessment is best done in consultation with a mental health professional knowledgeable about genetic disorders and their psychological consequences. The counselor should determine before disclosure if psychological help will be available. In the absence of such help, and when assessment shows that emotional harm is possible, nondisclosure or delayed disclosure of the full scientific facts about XY genotype can be justified. A genetic explanation of the cause of the syndrome is indicated, if the patient can comprehend it, namely that an X-linked gene caused her to be resistant to male hormone. Psychological help may be needed for the patient, if anxiety or gender confusion appears to be a problem.

If the patient is married, does the husband need an explanation of the cause of infertility and discomfort? Ideally, the time to have been informed was before marriage, if the information was available. After marriage, the geneticist's concern is whether disclosure might destroy a marital relationship begun under a different set of assumptions (Riskin and Reilly 1977). The approach in this case ought to follow the approach most geneticists take to findings of false paternity. The information is primarily the patient's and she should be offered help with the emotional and ethical dimensions of the decision about disclosure to her husband. The risks of her not telling her husband involve harm to a marital relationship grounded in promises of mutual support and trust. A secret of this magnitude is not likely to be kept without damage to the relationship itself. However, since there is no risk of direct *genetic or physical* harm to the husband, there is no ethical reason for geneticists to consider a breach of confidentiality. Geneticists can encourage their patient to consider the benefits of full disclosure and to seek help if there are emotional problems or a threat to the marriage by disclosure. Geneticists

482

should not be the final arbiters about what is best for a patient's marriage or family, since their expertise does not extend to these areas. However, they should seek help from others more skilled and able to give direct help with emotional and ethical problems.

## 3.5.3 Sex Selection by Prenatal Diagnosis

Table 1.15 shows that the sex selection case gave respondents the greatest ethical conflict. The number of U.S. geneticists (30%) who had the most ethical conflict about this case is the main reason why sex selection was first on this scale. The case given on the questionnaire may have been extreme. A couple requests prenatal diagnosis for sex selection who have four girls and are desperate for a boy. They say if the fetus is a girl they will abort it and keep trying until they conceive a boy. They also say that if prenatal diagnosis is refused they will abort the fetus rather than run the risk of having another girl. Would the number of geneticists willing to perform or refer (42%) have been as high if the case had described a couple with either a boy or girl as first child, who wanted to balance the gender of two and only two desired children? Subsequent studies of this issue ought to pose other cases for comparison.

The study found 34% of U.S. respondents willing to perform prenatal diagnosis and another 28% willing to refer the couple to a physician who would. Those who would refuse outright or try to dissuade the couple and refuse totalled 38%. In Canada, 30% of respondents were willing to perform, 17% willing to refer, and 53% would refuse or dissuade and refuse. These findings are surprising because studies conducted in the U.S. in 1972–73 (Sorenson 1976) and in Canada in 1975 (Fraser and Pressor 1977) found only 1% (of 448) and 21% (of 149) of genetic counselors, respectively, willing to meet this request. No empirical study of the actual incidence of requests and performance of prenatal diagnosis for sex selection exists, although sex selection has been reported as an ethical problem in prenatal diagnosis since the 1970s (Etzioni 1976, Dove and Blow 1979). Our study and the two earlier studies were of attitudes of geneticists and counselors about a hypothetical case and a simple question. It is important not to confuse what geneticists say they would do in a hypothetical case with what geneticists actually do in practice. However, the increase in openness of attitude about such requests in the U.S. and Canada, as well as the responses in Hungary, India, and Sweden, raise questions about whether medical geneticists have seriously weighed the consequences. This newer openness, based on moral reasoning about patient or parental autonomy, cuts directly against statements on the ethics and public policy of prenatal diagnosis from an interdisciplinary group (Powledge and Fletcher 1979), an international meeting of geneticists (Hamerton et al. 1980) and the President's Commission (1983, pp 56–58). Each statement recommends that prenatal diagnosis not be performed for sex selection.

Medical geneticists probably believe that sex selection is not a serious problem, even though the case gave them considerable ethical difficulty. Respondents ranked sex preselection last on the list (Table 1.25) of issues that ought to be of pri-

mary ethical concern to medical geneticists in the near future. A sign medical geneticists may take this issue lightly is shown by Elias' and Annas' (1987) omission
of this problem in an otherwise outstanding treatment of social problems in human genetics.

There are three reasons why it is important to draw a moral line on sex selection
and stay behind it. The first is that gender is *not* a genetic defect. There are no
medically valid reasons for giving prenatal diagnosis for gender choice except for
a sex-linked disease that cannot be diagnosed by DNA methods.

Second, as noted by the President's Commission (1983, p 57), sex selection violates the principle of equality between females and males and the attitude of unconditional acceptance of a new child by parents, so psychologically crucial to
parenting. A moral belief about "unconditional acceptance" of children has strong
cultural determinants, to be sure, but this belief clearly leads to great benefits to
children.

Third, sex selection is an unacceptable precedent for "genetic tinkering" at parental whim with characteristics that are unrelated to any disease. It is deeply ironic that geneticists determined not to repeat the errors of an older eugenic movement (Kevles 1985) would now make a precedent for a new eugenics. If geneticists
want to assure their societies that they are able to guide their work in a socially
beneficial direction, they must draw a moral line and take self-regulatory steps in a
code of ethics to avoid meeting any requests for sex selection. To fail to do this
much undermines the main ethical reason for society's support of medical genetics, i.e., to prevent the great suffering caused by genetic disease or to treat it effectively. In cases where parents have a genetic indication for prenatal diagnosis and
also show an excessive interest in the gender of the child, a practice of delayed disclosure of gender can be used as a last resort, assuming that the center has adopted such a policy. In my view, cases of sex selection are the most serious threat to
the moral integrity of human genetics as a profession today. These cases play directly into the hands of groups that aim to prohibit legal abortions, including genetically indicated abortions.

An important moral line about selective abortion exists in the public mind: "as
controversial as elective abortion is, the use of abortion when a woman is carrying
a fetus with a *severe* (italics added) genetic defect is very well accepted by a vast
majority of both the public and physicians" (Elias and Annas 1987, p 146). Data
collected by the National Opinion Research Center (1987) between 1972 and 1987
on trends in U.S. public opinion on genetic reasons for abortion show that between 75% and 77% support abortion for a serious genetic disease. The U.S. public's views also overwhelmingly support (89%) making genetic testing available for
serious and fatal genetic diseases (U.S. Congress, Office of Technology Assessment 1987).

My arguments in the section above were based on a conviction that there are
serious limitations to the toleration of wide cultural differences on *some* ethical
problems, despite apparently wide cultural differences.

When the claims of basic ethical principles are considered together with the
needs of patients and families and the responsibilities of geneticists, the following
guidelines should and *can* be adopted in each of the participating nations:

1) Medical geneticists should disclose all clinically relevant information to pa-

tients and family members, consistent with considerations of immaturity and psychological well-being. Psychological assessments are best done in consultation with mental health professionals.

2) Confidentiality is a strong but not absolute norm in medicine and in medical genetics. When the claim of nonmaleficence to prevent harm to others places a limit on the physician's or counselor's duty of confidentiality, the four conditions recommended by the President's Commission (1983, p 44) should be satisfied before breaching confidentiality.

3) Medical geneticists should not acquiesce to patient requests for sex selection unrelated to the diagnosis of a sex-linked disease. If patients have a genetic reason for diagnosis and also show excessive interest in the gender of the fetus, geneticists can consider delayed disclosure of gender after timely disclosure of clinical findings.

Use of these guidelines to overcome diversity strengthens the profession to meet the very complex problems immediately on the horizon. The guidance-seeking task for medical geneticists should be primarily in the hands of the profession itself in its national and international organizations.

## 3.6 What are Society's Interests in Human Genetics?

Societies around the world have at least three major interests in human genetics. First, societies have an overriding interest in relieving and preventing the suffering of their members, especially suffering that is undeserved. Those who are grievously burdened by disease or whose lives are drastically foreshortened are prevented from contribution to cultural life and continuity. Thus, it is in society's best interests to provide and distribute fairly resources that so clearly prevent great suffering and enable its citizens to make informed, voluntary choices about reproduction and the continuity of social and family life. Genetic burdens are among the most arbitrary and punishing that life imposes upon human beings. From the standpoint of ethics grounded either in religious or secular sources, remedying natural injustices and injustices that stem from lack of opportunity for education and access to health care are at the heart of the enterprise of human genetics. Many grievous burdens originate in the random results of the "natural lottery." No person has, or ever will have, an opportunity to choose his or her genetic identity. To neglect genetic knowledge and education is to be passive and neglectful in the face of blind genetic fate. The injustices of the genetic lottery can be partially remedied by distributing genetic knowledge and services. Society benefits by prevention and preparation for premature mortality and excessive morbidity. If persons and families at genetic risk *know* about their risks and options, and make their reproductive and life plans accordingly, these benefits can accrue. The goods for society are mainly in prevention of harm and injury, and in the added years of opportunity for economic and social life among persons whose lives are less dominated by disease and disability. The benefits are inarguably clear when the disease can be diagnosed and treated effectively. Benefits are also evident, but arguably so, when

485

methods of prevention include genetic abortion, artificial insemination by donor or oocyte donation, sterilization, or adoption.

However, individuals should enjoy the right to choose not to know the results of presymptomatic tests for untreatable diseases of late onset, such as Huntington disease. Coercive truth-telling in such a case can cause psychological harm and violates respect for persons.

The high ethical priority that geneticists assigned to the provision of genetic services (Tables 1.24, 1.25) could be seen as self-serving. However, if this priority is grounded in justice, and if individual and family interests are given proper social protection, the provision of genetic services to prevent human suffering of the most arbitrary kind ought to be one of the highest goals, current or projected, in any developed or developing society. It follows that serious threats to this goal, especially from the consequences of decisions of geneticists themselves, ought to be avoided if at all possible.

Policy choices about allocation of health care, including genetic services, are of significant ethical concern. What economic and social priority ought to be assigned to genetic services and biomedical research bearing upon human genetics compared with the other requirements of a society's health system? Each nation's leaders and their advisers need to confront this complex social-ethical issue. How should they consider such allocation choices? In an essay on the ethical implications of funding biomedical research, Gustafson (1984) gave four criteria to use; medical, ethical, economic, and political. The medical criteria relate to disease frequency, mortality, morbidity, age of onset, effectiveness of therapy, and the state of research on the particular problem. By each of these standards, priorities for diagnosis, treatment, counseling, and prevention of genetic diseases should be very high. Gustafson, a theologian, notes that "arguments are very strong for the support of basic biological research in...genetics...because of the potential general applicability of the new knowledge to a wide range of human diseases" (p 262). The major ethical criterion used by Gustafson is justice in distributing the benefits of the health care system, which has been discussed extensively above. The economic criterion, in the light of very high costs of health care, is efficiency, which he describes as "not an end in itself," but as a function of technical reason, the calculation of "the use of means to achieve a desired end." Gustafson refers to the revulsion shared by many in using monetary terms to weigh choices in health allocations. Yet he also points to the fact that the deferral of such consideration only postpones hard choices that must eventually be made. The political criterion refers to the stake of various interest groups in the political process that accompanies allocation choices. From these criteria, except in societies that have not yet achieved the minimal standards of preventive public health, the priority for genetic services would have to be high.

Secondly, it follows that society's best interests are served by directing scientific and medical efforts in human genetics towards prevention and treatment of genetic disorders that cause early death and/or serious, life-long morbidity, and away from eugenic goals of genetic improvement or enhancement of characteristics generally considered "normal." Thirdly, society's best interests are served by vigilant protection and public support of scientific freedom to learn about the origins and consequences of genetic disorders. In nations like the United States, where a *de facto* ban exists on research with the human embryo, the opportunity to study the chromosomal and molecular-genetic features of the earliest stage of genetic disorders is blocked (Fletcher and Ryan 1987).

The approaches recommended for the special ethical problems above are grounded in a dual social-ethical imperative. Societies that have achieved significant levels of development in health care ought to pursue two balanced goals: 1) to provide and distribute genetic services, including genetic education, sufficient for the real needs and interests of those at genetic risk and 2) to develop protections against unfair treatment or discrimination in opportunities for education, employment, insurability, and participation in social life due to a genetic diagnosis. Societies that have less developed health care systems can adopt these goals as desirable future states.

## 3.7 Proposal for an International Foundation for the Study of Ethics in Human Genetics and Reproduction

Beyond the work that medical geneticists must do to consolidate their moral experience, what can citizens and policy makers do in cooperation with geneticists and other scientists to prepare for the complex issues on the horizon? Scientific advances in understanding human genetics and reproduction are startling in their swiftness and impact on human health. In the last three decades, scientists in many nations have:

▷ discovered the biochemical basis of human genetic material
▷ introduced earlier and safer methods of prenatal diagnosis for inherited diseases
▷ found increasing evidence of strong genetic influence on some common diseases, e. g., cancer, heart disease, manic depression, Alzheimer's disease
▷ begun to map the contents of the human genome
▷ opened a window for research on the human embryo with *in vitro* fertilization
▷ advanced the understanding of the many causes of infertility

These exciting advances also raise complex ethical questions for every citizen, but especially for parents, health policy makers, geneticists and other scientists, e. g.,

▷ Can societies successfully guide the future of human genetics and reproduction in ethically desirable directions?
▷ How can individual freedom in reproductive choices be protected in a future where more genetic control will be possible?
▷ Should human embryos be fertilized solely for the purposes of research, e. g., to study diagnosis of disorders in the embryo and to understand infertility?
▷ Is universal pregnancy screening a socially desirable goal?
▷ Can genetic screening in populations remain truly voluntary?
▷ Who should have access to genetic information from screening? How can persons at higher risk be protected from genetic discrimination?
▷ Does the practice of prenatal diagnosis and abortion result in the loss of respect and compassion for the handicapped?

▷ How can society improve care of the genetically handicapped?
▷ Can public policies on these issues be formulated that preserve scientific freedom and allow co-existence of differing moral viewpoints about the application of genetic knowledge to human problems in different societies?

In many nations there is a great need for *independent* study of these questions, free
of excessive influence from government and special interest groups. Also, there is
a great need to promote *international* understanding of these issues, since they affect the well-being of all people, and since scientists are greatly influenced by the
collective wisdom of their international peers. No international organization exists
solely to advance study and shared understanding of these ethical questions. Also,
there is a need for an organization capable of funding sustained dialogue and research on these difficult questions. The dialogue needs to involve public and parent groups and ordinary citizens.

Therefore, we welcome ideas about an International Foundation for the Study
of Ethics in Human Genetics and Reproduction, as well as an impression of what
kind of support it would have in its mission.

The author gratefully acknowledges the help of William H. Boley with this
chapter as well as the constructive written comments of Mark J. Hansen and
Dorothy C. Wertz.

# References

Adler B, Kushnick T [1982] Genetic counseling in prenatally diagnosed trisomy 18 and 21: psy-
chological aspects. Pediat 69: 94–99
Aiken HD [1962] Reason and conduct. Knopf, New York
Anderson WF [1984] Prospects for human gene therapy. Science 226: 401–409
Anderson WF [1985] Human gene therapy: scientific and ethical considerations. J Med & Phil 10:
275–291
Andrews L [1987] Medical genetics. A legal frontier. American Bar Foundation, Chicago, p 138
Atkinson GM, Moraczewski AS [1980] Genetic counseling, the church, and the law. Pope John
XXIII Medical-Moral Research and Education Center. Franciscan Herald Press, Chicago
Beauchamp TL, Childress JF [1983] Principles of biomedical ethics, 2nd ed. Oxford University
Press, New York
Beecher HK [1966] Ethics and clinical research. N Engl J Med 274: 1354–1360
Berg K, Tranøy KE [1983] Research ethics. Alan R Liss, New York
Blumberg BD, Golbus MS, Hanson KH [1975] The psychological sequelae of abortion performed
for a genetic indication. Am J Obstet Gynecol 122: 799–808
Comings D [1980] Prenatal diagnosis and the "new genetics." Am J Hum Genet 32: 453
Donnai P, Charles N, Harris N [1981] Attitudes of patients after "genetic" termination of preg-
nancy. Br Med J 282: 621–622
Dove GA, Blow C [1979] Boy or girl parental choice? Br Med J 2: 1399
Dunstan GR [1984] The moral status of the human embryo. A tradition recalled. J Med Ethics 1:
38–44
Elias S, Annas GJ [1987] Reproductive genetics and the law. Yearbook Publishers, Chicago,
pp 48–49
Engelhardt HT [1986] The foundations of bioethics. Oxford University Press, New York
Etzioni A [1976] Issues of public policy in the USA raised by amniocentesis. J Med Ethics 2: 8–16
Fletcher JC [1978] Prenatal diagnosis. Ethical issues. In: Reich WT (ed) Encyclopedia of bio-
ethics. Free Press, New York, pp 1336–1346

Fletcher JC [1983] The evolution of the ethics of informed consent. In: Berg K, Tranøy KE (eds) Research ethics. Alan R Liss, New York, pp 187–228

Fletcher JC [1985] Ethical considerations in and beyond experimental prospective clinical trials of human gene therapy. J Med Phil 10: 293–309

Fletcher JC, Berg K, Tranøy KE [1985] Ethical aspects of medical genetics. Clin Genet 27: 199–205

Fletcher JC, Ryan KJ [1987] Federal regulations for fetal research: a case for reform. Law, Medicine & Health Care 15: 126–138

Fraser FC, Pressor C [1977] Attitudes of counselors in relation to prenatal sex determination for choice of sex. In: Lubs HA, DelaCruz F (eds) Genetic counseling. Raven, New York, pp 109–120

Gewirth A [1983] Ethics. In: Encyclopedia Britannica, 15th ed. University of Chicago Press, Chicago, p 977, vol 6

Gilligan C [1982] In a different voice. Psychological theory and women's development. Harvard University Press, Cambridge

Glover J [1984] What sort of people should there be? Penguin Books, New York

Gustafson JM [1984] Ethics from a theocentric perspective. University of Chicago Press, Chicago, pp 259–272, vol 2

Hamerton JL, Boue A, Cohen MM et al. [1980] Chromosome disease. In: Hamerton JL, Simpson NE (eds) Prenatal diagnosis: past, present, and future (Report of an international workshop) Prenat Diag (Special Issue), p 11

Hare RM [1981] Moral thinking. Clarendon Press, Oxford

Harris R [1988] Genetic counselling and the new genetics. Trends in Genet 4: 52–56

Harrison MR, Golbus MS, Filly RA (eds) Unborn patient, 2nd ed. Orlando, FL, Grune and Stratton (in press)

Hatch E [1983] Culture and morality. Columbia University Press, New York

Holtzman NA [1988] Recombinant DNA technology, genetic tests, and public policy. Am J Hum Genet 42: 624–632

Jones OW, Penn NE, Schucter S, et al [1984] Parental response to mid-trimester therapeutic abortion following amniocentesis. Prenat Diag 4: 249–256

Jonsen AR, Toulmin S [1988] The abuse of casuistry. University of California Press, Berkeley, pp 296–302

Kan YW, Dozy AM [1978] Antenatal diagnosis of sickle cell anemia by DNA analysis of amniotic-fluid cells. Lancet 2, 910

Kevles DJ [1985] In the name of eugenics. Knopf, New York.

Ladd J [1973] Ethical relativism. Wadsworth, Belmont CA

Ladd J [1978] Ethics. In: Reich WT (ed) Encyclopedia of Bioethics. Free Press, New York, p 402, vol 1

Ladd J [1982] The distinction between rights and responsibility: a defense. Linacre Quart 49: 121–142

Levine RJ [1985] Ethics and regulation of clinical research, 2nd ed. Urban and Schwarzenberg, Baltimore

Leschot NJ, Verjaal M, Treffers PE [1982]. Therapeutic abortion on genetic indications. A detailed followup study of 20 patients. In Verjaal M, Leschot JH (eds) On prenatal diagnosis. Rodopi, University of Amsterdam, p 85.

MacBeath A [1952] Experiments in living. MacMillan, London

McCormick RA [1981] How brave a new world? Georgetown University Press, Washington DC, p 200

McKusick VA [1986] Mendelian inheritance in man, 7th ed. Johns Hopkins University Press, Baltimore, p 1459

McLaren A [1985] Prenatal diagnosis before implantation: opportunities and problems. Prenat Diag 5: 85–95

Mareno J [1989] Ethics by committee: The moral authority of consensus. J Med & Phil (in press)

May WF [1983] The Physician's Covenant. Westminister Press, Philadelphia

Modell B et al [1985] WHO/Serono Meeting. Report: Perspectives in fetal diagnosis of congenital diseases. Serono Symposia

Murray T [1984] The social context of genetic screening. Hastings Center Rep 14: 21–23

National Commission for the Protection of Human Subjects of Biomedical and Behavioral Research [1979] The Belmont Report, Ethical principles for the protection of human subjects of research, GPO 887-809, US Government Printing Office, Washington DC

National Opinion Research Center (University of Chicago) [1987] General social surveys, 1972-1987: cumulative codebook. National Opinion Research Center, Chicago, July

Niebuhr HR [1963] The responsible self. Harper and Row, New York

Pappworth MH [1967] Human guinea pigs. Rutledge and Kegan Paul, London

Parsons T [1951] The social system. Free Press, New York, p 97

Powledge TM, Fletcher JC [1979] Guidelines for the ethical, social, and legal issues in prenatal diagnosis. N Engl J Med 300: 168-172

President's Commission for the Study of Ethical Problems in Medicine and Biomedical and Behavioral Research [1983] Screening and counseling for genetic conditions. US Government Printing Office, Washington, DC, p 58

Rawls J [1971] A theory of justice. Belknap Press, Cambridge, pp 107-108

Riskin T, Reilly P [1977] Remedies for improper disclosure of genetic data. Rutgers-Cambridge Law J 8: 480-483

Sladek JR, Shoulson I [1988] Neural transplantation: A call for patience rather than patients. Science 240: 1386-1388

Sorenson JR [1976] From social movement to clinical medicine: the role of law and the medical profession in regulating applied human genetics. In: Milunsky A, Annas GJ (eds) Genetics and the law. Plenum, New York, pp 467-485

Sorenson JR, Swazey JP, Scotch NA [1981] Reproductive pasts, reproductive futures: Genetic counselling and its effectiveness. Alan R Liss, New York

Toulmin S [1972] Human understanding. Princeton University Press, Princeton NJ

Toulmin S [1981] The tyranny of principles. Hastings Cent Rep 11 (Dec): 31-39

Tranøy KE [1983] Is there a universal research ethics? In: Berg K, Tranøy KE (eds) Research ethics. Alan R Liss, New York, pp 3-12

University of Colorado School of Nursing [1987] Genetics applications for health professionals (prepared by Forsman, I) Lerner Managed Designs, Lawrence KS

U.S. Congress, Office of Technology Assessment [1986] Technologies for detecting heritable mutations in human beings. US Government Printing Office, Washington DC, OTA-H-298, pp 6-19

US Congress, Office of Technology Assessment [1987] New developments in biotechnology. Background paper: Public perceptions of biotechnology. OTA-BP-BA-45 US Government Printing Office, Washington DC

US Government [1948] Trials of war criminals before the Nuremberg military tribunals. US Government Printing Office, Washington DC

Weatherall DJ [1985] The new genetics and clinical practice, 2nd ed, Oxford University Press, Oxford

West JD, Angell RR, Thatcher SS et al [1987] Sexing the human pre-embryo by DNA-DNA in-situ hybridization. Lancet ii: 1345-1347

White R, Caskey CT [1988] The human as an experimental system in molecular genetics. Science 240: 1483-1488

# 4  About the Authors

**Principal Authors** _____
DOROTHY C.WERTZ, Ph.D., is a medical sociologist with an interdisciplinary background in social ethics, social anthropology, and the study of religion and society. She received her Ph.D. degree from Harvard University in 1966. She is Research Professor in the Health Services Section at the Boston University School of Public Health, Boston, MA. Her publications include *Lying-In: A History of Childbirth in America* (Free Press, New York, 1977, enlarged ed., Yale University Press, New Haven, 1989); and articles on interpersonal communication and interpretation of risk in genetic counseling. She plans to continue the work begun in this volume by conducting an expanded survey in 30 nations that will also include patients.

JOHN C.FLETCHER, Ph.D., is Professor of Biomedical Ethics at University of Virginia School of Medicine and Professor of Religious Studies in the College of Arts and Sciences. An ordained Episcopal Minister and former Rector of the R.E. Lee Church in Lexington, Virginia, he founded Inter/Met, an interfaith seminary in Washington, DC, to offer theological education to students of Protestant, Catholic, and Jewish faiths. He subsequently became Chief of the Bioethics Program at the National Institutes of Health, Bethesda, MD, where he was responsible for research review and consultation on ethical problems in research and patient care. He is author of *Coping with Genetic Disorders* (Doubleday, Garden City, N.Y., 1982), a guide for clergy and parents, and of numerous publications on the ethics of fetal research, prenatal diagnosis and problems at the end of life. He is President of the Society for Bioethics Consultation, founded in 1986. He is currently developing a program in medical ethics at the University of Virginia.

**Australia** _____
JOHN G.ROGERS, M.B.B.S., D.C.H., F.R.A.C.P., is Acting Director, Department of Genetics, Royal Children's Hospital, Medical Geneticist, Monash Medical Centre, Melbourne, and Medical Geneticist to the Murdoch Institute for Research and Birth Defects. After 2 years of training in internal medicine he undertook training in paediatrics in Melbourne, Sheffield and London. After qualifying as a paediatrician he worked as a fellow in genetics with Victor McKusick at Johns Hopkins in Baltimore for 3 years. During this time he worked with S.H. Boyer IV on nerve growth factor and familial dysautonomia. On returning to Australia in 1976, he extended the existing genetic counselling services to cope with the increasing demand. He was Deputy Editor of the Australian Paediatric Journal 1979–1983 and Registrar of the Australian College of Paediatrics 1983–1986.

491

He is currently Secretary to the Human Genetics Society of Australia and the Board of Clinical Genetics. In addition he is a member of the Coordinating Committee for Genetic Services in Victoria and on the Commonwealth Department of Health Congenital Abnormalities Sub-Committee. His major clinical interests are in skeletal dysplasias, connective tissue disorders and mucopolysaccharidosis and approaches and techniques of counselling. He has developed particular interest in grief counselling in relationship to birth defects. His publications include:

*My Child is a Dwarf*, (JG Rogers and JO Weiss), published by the Little People of America Foundation, U.S.A., 1977, and articles on familial dysautonomia, fibrodysplasia, and genetic consequences of incest.

ANNA-MARIE TAYLOR, B. A. (HONS), M. A., Ph. D., is Consultant in Clinical Services, the Cairnmillar Institute, Melbourne, and Research Associate, Department of History & Philosophy of Science, University of Melbourne. She has taught Philosophy of Science at Melbourne, La Trobe, Monash, and Deakin Universities and was Community Liaison Officer for the Centre for Human Bioethics at Monash University. She has served as educator and facilitator/consultant to community and professional groups, including The Thalassaemia Society of Victoria; for the Department of Haematology and Oncology at the Royal Children's Hospital; the Victorian Council of Social Services; and the Spastic Society of Victoria. She has devised a model of moral problem-solving and conflict resolution to utilize in her work with health professionals. She is a member of the Clinical Board of the Australian Psychological Society and is currently working as a family psychotherapist. She has presented papers on ethical aspects of thalassaemia, employment for the disabled, adoption and A. I. D. Her Ph. D. thesis was entitled, "Facts and Values: Groundwork for a Theory of Moral Problem Solving" (University of Melbourne, 1984).

## Brazil _____

FRANCISCO M. SALZANO is Professor at the Departamento de Genética, Instituto de Biociências, Universidade Federal do Rio Grande do Sul, Porto Alegre, RS, Brazil. Born in 1928, he was educated at the University of Rio Grande do Sul (Sc. Lic., 1952) and Sao Paulo (Ph. D., 1955). He also has a Privat Docent degree obtained in Porto Alegre (1960). His graduate training was completed with one year of work at the University of Michigan, Ann Arbor, USA (1956-57) and one month at the MRC Population Genetics Research Unit, Oxford, England (1961). Past positions: Head of Department (1963-68; 1973-75) and Director, Institute of Natural Sciences (1968-71), Federal University of Rio Grande do Sul. He attended more than one hundred conferences both inside and outside Brazil, and organized two international symposia. A member of several Brazilian and international societies, he has been President, Brazilian Society of Genetics (1966-68), Secretary General, International Association of Human Biologists (1974-80) and Vice-President, International Union of Anthropological and Ethnological Sciences (1978-83; 1983-88). He was elected to the Brazilian Academy of Sciences in 1973, receiving in the same year the Medal of the Brazilian Society for the Advancement of Science for distinguished services to Brazilian science. His contributions to the scientific literature number more than 500 titles, including eight books, 20 chapters in books and 226 full scientific articles.

SERGIO D. J. PENA is Professor at the Departamento de Bioquimica e Imunologia, Instituto de Ciências Biologicas, Universidade Federal de Minas Gerais, and Head, Nucleo de Genetica Medica, Instituto Hilton Rocha, Belo Horizonte, MG, Brazil. Born in 1947, he was educated at the University of Minas Gerais (M. D., 1970) and Manitoba, Canada (Ph. D., 1977). His training also included internships and residencies in Pediatrics and Medical Genetics in Winston-Salem, USA and Winnipeg, Canada (1971–74). Past positions: Visiting Researcher, National Institute for Medical Research, Mill Hill, London, England (1977–78), Assistant Professor, McGill University, and Head of the Biochemical Genetics Laboratory, Montreal Neurological Institute, Montreal, Canada (1978–82). He attended several conferences inside and outside Brazil and received the Lafi Award in Medical Sciences [1984]. Dr. Pena has authored about 50 full scientific articles and five chapters of books, edited in the USA, England and Switzerland. In 1974 he and M. H. K. Shokeir described a syndrome that now bears their names.

## Canada

DR. DAVID J. ROY is founder and Director of the Center for Bioethics of the Clinical Research Institute of Montreal. In 1985 and again in 1986, he was one of Canada's three official representatives to the summit 'nations' international meetings on bioethics. He serves as consultant to doctors and health care professionals on ethical problems in medicine and clinical research, and devotes most of his time to research on ethical issues in clinical medicine and biomedical science. He is Editor-in-chief of the Canadian-based international *Journal of Palliative Care*.

JUDITH G. HALL is Professor of Medical Genetics at the University of British Columbia, and Director of the UBC Clinical Genetics Unit at Grace Hospital. She is an M. D., Fellow of the American Academy of Pediatrics, the American Board of Medical Genetics, the Royal College of Pediatrics (Canada), and the Canadian College of Medical Genetics. She has published widely in the area of clinical genetics with a special interest in congenital anomalies and the genetics of short stature. She has an ongoing interest in the natural history of genetic diseases and the provision of genetic services. She has worked extensively with patient advocacy and lay groups, serving as medical advisor to almost 20 such groups.

## Denmark

A. J. THERKELSEN, M. D., was born January 5, 1924. He has been Professor of Human Genetics at the University of Aarhus and Head of the Institute of Human Genetics since 1971. Member of the Danish Cancer Research Council for nine years and first President of the Danish Society of Medical Genetics. He has publications and research in radiation biology, cytogenetics, and clinical genetics.

493

LARS BOLUND, M.D., was born March 20, 1944. He is Professor of Clinical Genetics in the Institute of Human Genetics, University of Aarhus. He was a member of the Scientific Board of the Danish Medical Research Council from 1983 to 1987, and has been President of the Danish Society for Medical Genetics since 1986. He has publications and research in the fields of cell biology, developmental genetics, molecular genetics, and clinical genetics.

VIGGO MORTENSEN was born May 15, 1942. He is Lecturer and candidate in theology, Institute of Ethics and Philosophy of Religion, and former Dean of the Theological Faculty, University of Aarhus. He has publications in 19th and 20th century philosophy of religion, applied ethics and bioethics, including Viggo Mortensen and R.C. Sorensen (eds.): Free Will and Determinism (Aarhus University Press 1987). His work in progress on science and religion is entitled, Beyond Restriction and Expansion: On Naturalizing Epistemology, Anthropology, Ethics and Theology.

**Federal Republic of Germany** ⸺⸺⸺⸺

TRAUTE SCHROEDER-KURTH was born May 16, 1930, in Heidelberg, grew up in Northern Germany, studied Medicine at the University of Hamburg, and qualified in Human Genetics in 1971 at the University of Heidelberg. Since 1963, she has worked at the Institute of Human Genetics and Anthropology at the University of Heidelberg, specializing in genetic counseling and genetic diagnostics, predominantly prenatal and postnatal chromosome analyses. She is engaged in research on chromosome instability syndromes, mainly Fanconi anemia. Since 1979, she has been a member of the working group on "Ethics and Human Genetics" initiated by Prof. Huebner of the Protestant Institute for Interdisciplinary Research. She has written numerous papers concerning ethical problems of genetic counseling and prenatal diagnosis. She is consultant to numerous councils as an expert on genetic counseling and prenatal diagnosis.

JUERGEN HUEBNER, Professor, Dr. Theology, is senior research fellow at the Protestant Institute for Interdisciplinary Research (Forschungsstätte der Evangelischen Studiengemeinschaft, FEST) at Heidelberg, an institution supported by the Protestant Churches in the Federal Republic of Germany, and Professor at the Faculty of Theology at Heidelberg University. He has studied Biology and Theology. His doctoral dissertation was entitled "Theologie und biologische Entwicklungslehre" (Theology and the Biological Doctrine of Evolution), published 1966 in Munich. His main research interest is the dialogue between science and religion, its history, its philosophical foundations, and its ethical consequences. Further publications include: Biologie und christlicher Glaube (Biology and Christian Belief), Gütersloh 1973; Die Theologie Johannes Keplers zwischen Orthodoxie und Naturwissenschaft (The Theology of Johannes Kepler between Orthodox Confessional Theology and Science), Tübingen 1975; Der Dialog zwischen Theologie und Naturwissenschaft - ein bibliographischer Bericht (The Dialogue between Theology and Science - a bibliographical synopsis), München 1987; Die neue Verantwortung für das Leben - Ethik im Zeitalter von Gentechnologie und

Umweltkrise (The new responsibility for life: Ethics in the age of genetic engineering and environmental crisis), München 1986. His special interests are now medical ethics and bioethics. Works in progress are projects on the ethics of genetic counseling and the ethics of genetic engineering.

**France** ———————
JEAN-FRANÇOIS MATTEI, 44, M.D., Ph.D., is Professor of Pediatrics and Medical Genetics at the Medical University of Marseilles (France). Especially involved in genetic counseling, he is the Chief of the Department of Prenatal Diagnosis, which is the only one for a region of 4 million inhabitants. Head of a group for research in medical genetics (INSERM), he is especially involved in clinical cytogenetics (Trisomy 21 and origin of the nondisjunction, new syndromes, microcytogenetics, and mental retardation with fragile X site), gene mapping and DNA recombinant techniques applied in genetic diagnosis. President of a nonprofit association for both organization and research in prenatal diagnosis, he is an expert on medical genetics in the International Pediatrics Association.

MARC GAMERRE, 43, M.D., is Professor of Gynecology and Obstetrics at the Medical University of Marseilles (France). Interested in sterility (especially in surgical repair), in vitro fertilization and prenatal diagnosis, he is responsible for the unit of obstetrics in the Department of Prenatal Diagnosis in Marseilles. He is directly involved in the development of the new obstetrical techniques, such as chorionic villi and fetal blood sampling.

**German Democratic Republic** ———————
REGINE CH. WITKOWSKI, Dr. rer. nat. habil. (sc.), is professor of Medical Genetics and Director of the Institute of Medical Genetics, Medical School (Charité) of the Humboldt-University Berlin/GDR. She contributed to the establishment of Medical Genetics and genetic counseling services in the GDR. Since 1961, her special field of interest has been cytogenetics. She regards Dr. V. McKusick as one of her teachers, both through his publications and through direct contact at Johns Hopkins Medical School in Baltimore. The first edition of her most important publication appeared in 1974: Witkowski R, Prokop O, Genetik erblicher Syndrome und Missbildungen, Wörterbuch für die Familienberatung (Genetics of hereditary syndromes and malformations: a dictionary for genetic counseling), Akademie-Verlag, Berlin. The fourth edition of this three-volume work is in progress.

HANNELORE KÖRNER, Dr. sc. nat., is a biologist specializing in medical genetics. Dr. Körner's special positions of interest in research and practice are prenatal diagnosis, screening methods, extracorporeal fertilization and ethics. Dr. Körner is Head of the Department of Cytogenetics of the Institute of Medical Genetics at the Charité.

HERRMANN METZKE, Dr. sc. med., is a pediatrician, specializing in human genetics. He is the Head of the Department of Medical Genetics at the Medical

Academy in Erfurt/GDR and of the working group for genetic counseling of the Society of Human Genetics in the GDR. He has done much work in epidemiology, especially in hemophilia and Huntington disease, and in ethical problems of genetic counseling.

## Greece

LABRINI VELOGIANNIS-MOUTSOPOULOS received her law degree from the University of Athens, her M.A. in Philosophy and Bioethics from Georgetown University (U.S.A.), and her Ph.D. in History of Medicine and Social Medicine from the University of Ioannina, Greece. She practices law in Ioannina and teaches in the School of Medicine and School of Philosophy at the University of Ioannina. She has published articles on truth-telling to patients, the doctor-patient relationship, psychological approaches to seriously ill patients, and the rights of non-smokers. Her Ph.D. thesis [1984] was entitled "Ethics and public policy: ethical priorities for genetic services in Greece."

CHRISTOS S. BARTSOCAS received his M.D. (1960) and D.Med.Sc. (1963) from the University of Athens and his specialty training in Pediatrics at Yale University (1964–66) and Endocrinology-Genetics at Harvard University (1966–68). He is certified by the American Board of Pediatrics (1967) and the American Board of Medical Genetics (1982). His present position is Chair, Department of Pediatrics, "P. and A. Kyriakou" Children's Hospital and Associate Professor of Pediatrics, University of Athens. He is editor or co-editor of the following volumes: "The Management of Genetic Disorders", "Progress in Dermatoglyphic Research", "Skeletal Dysplasias" and "Endocrine Genetics and Genetics of Growth".

## Hungary

ANDREW (ENDRE) CZEIZEL, M.D., was born in Budapest in 1935. His Ph.D. thesis, entitled "Investigations on the pathogenesis of fetal anomalies," was written in 1965, while his academic M.D. thesis, entitled "Etiological studies of common isolated congenital abnormalities in Hungary," (1978) was published in 1982. In 1971, the Department of Human Genetics and Teratology was established at the National Institute of Hygiene and he was appointed head. Since 1986, this Department has been a W.H.O. Collaborating Centre for the Community Control of Hereditary Diseases. His main scientific interest is the epidemiological study of the etiology of congenital abnormalities. As head of a genetic counseling clinic, he is interested in its ethical problems.

GEORG ADAM has been writing on medical ethics and medical codes of law for 25 years. He received his doctorate of science in 1987. He is head of the Medical Ethics Group at Semmelweis Medical University, Budapest.

**India** _____

ISHWAR CHANDER VERMA is Professor in Pediatrics and Officer-in-Charge of the Genetics Unit at the All India Institute of Medical Sciences, New Delhi. Dr. Verma had residency training in pediatrics and internal medicine in Dar-es-Salaam, Tanzania and Liverpool, U. K. He received specialized training in genetics at the Divison of Medical Genetics, Kinderspital, University of Zurich, Switzerland and at the Genetics Unit, Massachusetts General Hospital, Boston, U.S.A. He is a fellow of the Royal College of Physicians, London; National Academy of Medical Sciences, India; International College of Pediatrics, and an honorary fellow of the American Academy of Pediatrics. He is past President of the Indian Society of Human Genetics.

He was the recipient of the Indian Council of Medical Research National Award for his investigations on "Genetic disorders in children" for 1987, and the Medical Council of India B.C. Roy National Award in 1985 for developing the specialty of genetics in India. He is Editor-in-Chief of the *Indian Journal of Pediatrics* and corresponding editor of the *American Journal of Medical Genetics* and *Neurofibromatosis.* He has written scores of scientific papers on pediatrics and medical genetics and is the author of three books on medical genetics in India. His current research interests include genetic disorders in pediatrics, medicogenetic problems of primitive tribal communities in the Andaman Islands, genetic causes of mental retardation, and prenatal diagnosis of genetic disorders. He has been a pioneer in the field of medical genetics in India and has represented India on the W.H.O. Advisory Committee on Hereditary Diseases and on the Permanent Committee of the International Congress of Human Genetics. He is a council member of the International Association for the Scientific Study of Mental Deficiency.

BALBIR SINGH obtained his M.A. degree from the University of Delhi in 1953, his Ph.D. from the Punjab University in 1962, and his D. Litt. degree from the University of Delhi in 1987. He taught Indian philosophy at Punjab University for five years, and has been teaching this subject for the last two decades at Hindu College, Delhi. He lectured extensively in four American universities and institutions in 1985 on various themes of Indian philosophy and religion. He has published over a dozen books and an equal number of research papers in various international journals.

**Israel** _____

JUAN CHEMKE was born in Germany in 1929. In 1939 he emigrated to Chile, where he obtained his M.D. in 1955. In 1957 he immigrated to Israel. He worked as a general practitioner during the first 4 years and later completed his internship and residency in Pediatrics at the Kaplan Hospital. In 1968-1969 he trained in Medical Genetics at the University of Colorado Medical Center, with Dr. Arthur Robinson. Since 1973 he has been Director of the Clinical Genetics Unit at Kaplan Hospital in Rehovot. Kaplan Hospital is affiliated with the Hebrew University and Hadassah School of Medicine. Dr. Chemke participates in teaching activities in the Medical School and in the Department of Genetics of the Faculty of Life

Sciences of the Hebrew University. His present academic position is Associate Professor at that University. Special studies have included research on very long-chain fatty acids at the Section of Biochemical Genetics at the National Institutes of Health, U.S.A. and the Laboratoire de Neurochemie at the Hôpital de la Salpetriere, Paris, France (INSERM). In 1985, he was a Visiting Professor in the Department of Medical Genetics at the Montreal Children's Hospital-McGill University. He was formerly involved in an epidemiological study of birth defects. His present research interests and publications are in clinical and biochemical genetics, and concern mainly ethical problems in Down syndrome, adrenoleukokystrophy, cystic fibrosis, prenatal diagnosis and ethical aspects of medical genetics.

AVRAHAM STEINBERG, M.D., is a graduate of the Hebrew University- Hadassah Medical School, Jerusalem, Israel, and the Rabbinical Academy, Mercaz Ha'Rav Kook in Jerusalem. His present positions are: (a) Attending Pediatric Neurologist, Division of Pediatric Neurology, Bikur Cholim Hospital, Jerusalem; (b) Attending Pediatric Neurologist, Department of Pediatrics, Shaare Zedek Medical Center, Jerusalem; (c) Head, Program of Medical Ethics, Hebrew University-Hadassah Medical School, Jerusalem; (d) Director, Center for Medical Ethics, Hebrew University, Hadassah Medical School, Jerusalem. His past positions include Director, the F. Schlesinger Institute for Medical-Halakhic Research, Shaare Zedek Medical Center, Jerusalem. His most important publications are Chapters in the Pathology in the Talmud, Jerusalem, 1975 (a book in Hebrew); Jewish Medical Law, Jerusalem, 1978 (a book in Hebrew and an English translation); and ASSIA, an Anthology on Jewish Medical Ethics, 4 Vols. His work in progress includes a book on the neurological manifestations of systemic diseases in childhood (which will be a volume of the International Review of Child Neurology series – an official publication of the International Child Neurology Association); Encyclopedia of Jewish Medical Ethics in 5 volumes; the attitude of Israeli physicians toward the defective newborn; and the attitude of Israeli cancer patients and Israeli physicians toward truth telling in malignant diseases. His major interests are in the comparative perspectives of secular and Jewish bioethics; education in bioethics; research on the attitude of Israeli care-providers toward issues in medical ethics.

## Italy ⸺

FAUSTINA LALATTA is a medical doctor. She is a Clinical Fellow in Genetics at the Department of Pediatrics, University of Milan. Her previous experience included a clinical fellowship in Medical Genetics, at the Department of Genetics, University of Milan (1981–83), a research fellowship in Medical Genetics at the Department of Pediatrics, University of Milan, and a research fellowship in Medical Genetics at the Department of Pediatrics, Mount Sinai School of Medicine, New York, N.Y. (1983–1984). She is a consultant for the Italian Association for the Study of Congenital Malformation, and a member of the European Association of Human Genetics, American Society of Human Genetics, and Italian Association of Medical Genetics.

498

GIANNI TOGNONI is a medical doctor, with previous degrees in philosophy and theology. He is head of the Laboratory of Clinical Pharmacology at the Mario Negri Institute of Pharmacological Research, Milan, where the main interests include large scale randomized clinical trials and epidemiological assessment of the benefit/risk profile of pharmacological and non-pharmacological interventions in various fields, including perinatal medicine and prenatal diagnosis.

## Japan

KOJI OHKURA, M.D., D.M.S., is Assistant Professor, Department of Human Genetics, Medical Research Institute, Tokyo Medical and Dental University. He is Executive Director of the Genetic Counseling Center, the Japan Family Planning Association, Inc., and President (1985-present) of the Japan Society of Medical Genetics. His publications include Ohkura K, Handa Y (eds.) Regional Genetic Counseling System: Its Views and Methods, (Genetic Counseling Center, Japan Family Planning Association, Inc., Tokyo, 1978), Ohkura K, Handa Y, and Matsuda T. Genetic Counseling: Present and Future, Medical Genetic Research (Rinsho iden kenkyu), 1981; Ohkura K, Handa Y, Principles of Genetic Counseling, 2nd. ed. (Nihon Ijishinposha, Tokyo, 1984), Ohkura K (ed.) Coping with Genetic Diseases (Kodansha, Tokyo, 1985), Ohkura K (ed.) Medical Genetics for Clinicians, (Nihon Ijishinposha, Tokyo, 1984), Ohkura K Introduction to Human Genetics, 3rd ed. (Igaku-shoin, Tokyo, 1987). Work in progress includes development of training programs for M.D. genetic counselors (1974-present) and public health nurses in medical genetics (1977-present) and organizing a regional and nation-wide genetic (counseling) service network system (1977-present). His research interests include 1) Genetic structures and relationships between East Asian populations; 2) Ethical and psychological attitudes of Japanese who face genetic problems; 3) Clinical classification of genetic diseases with heterogeneity.

RIHITO KIMURA, J.D., LL.M, is Professor of Bioethics and Law, Department of Health Sciences, School of Human Sciences, Waseda University, Tokorozawa, Japan. He is Director, International Bioethics Program, Joseph and Rose Kennedy Institute of Ethics, Georgetown University, Washington, D.C., U.S.A., and Adjunct Professor, Department of Family and Community Medicine, Georgetown University Medical School. His publications include "Rethinking Life-An Introduction to Bioethics" (Tokyo, 1987). He is a member of the Bioethics Panel, National Council of Churches of Christ, U.S.A. (1982–83), and Associate Director, Ecumenical Institute of Bossey, World Council of Churches, Geneva, Switzerland (1972–75). He is also a Steering Committee Member of the Council for International Organizations of Medical Sciences on Health Policy, Ethics and Human Values (1986-present).

## Norway

KÅRE BERG, M.D., Ph.D., is Professor of Medicine and Head of the Institute of Medical Genetics at the University of Oslo. He is Director of the Department of Medical Genetics, City of Oslo, and consultant in clinical genetics at University

Hospital, Oslo. He is editor of *Medical Genetics: Past, Present and Future* (Alan R. Liss, New York, 1985), *Human Gene Mapping 6* (Alan R. Liss, New York, 1982); *Genetic Damage in Man Caused by Environmental Agents* (Academic Press, New York, 1979); and of the journal *Clinical Genetics* (1970-present). He is associate editor of *Research Ethics* (Alan R. Liss, New York, 1983) and of the *Journal of Immunogenetics*. He is a member of the Permanent Committee for the International Congresses of Human Genetics and of the Steering Committee, European Advisory Committee on Health Research, W. H. O. He was appointed as a Fogarty Scholar at the National Institutes of Health, Bethesda, MD, U. S. A., in 1985.

KNUT ERIK TRANØY is Professor of Medical Ethics in the Medical Faculty of the University of Oslo. He was formerly Vice-President of the University of Oslo and Professor of Philosophy, and earlier was Professor of Philosophy at the University of Bergen. His interests include clarifying the relationship between the moral and the methodological foundations of science, especially in medical research as well as clinical practice. He is co-editor of *Research Ethics* (1983) with Kåre Berg. He has been a member of several important committees, most recently one that has proposed to the government guidelines for accepting priorities for medical care.

## Sweden _____

ERWIN BISCHOFBERGER, S. J., S. T. D. is a member of the National Medical Ethics Council in Sweden.

JAN LINDSTEN is Professor of Medical Genetics and Head of the Department of Clinical Genetics, and head physician at the Karolinska Hospital, Stockholm. He is a member of the Royal Swedish Academy of Sciences and secretary of the Nobel Assembly and Nobel Committee at the Karolinska Institute, Stockholm, Sweden.

DR. URBAN ROSENQVIST, M. D., Ph. D., is Associate Professor in the Department of Endocrinology, Karolinska Hospital, Stockholm, Sweden. He is a member of the Delegation for Medical Ethics of the Swedish Medical Society. Dr. Rosenqvists' interest in this field has focused on the ethical issues concerning the distribution of resources and patients' rights to information.

## Switzerland _____

ERIC ENGEL, Professor, is a Swiss national who earned his M. D. and Ph. D. degrees from the University of Geneva before spending some 20 years in the practice of medicine and medical genetics in the United States. He worked first for three years as research fellow and instructor in medicine at Massachusetts General Hospital and Harvard Medical School, then moved to Nashville, Tennessee, to become Director of the Genetics Division of Vanderbilt University, a unit which he built from a two-person laboratory to a full medical genetics center (offering laboratory, consultation and educational facilities). During these years, his group published numerous articles in the areas of dysmorphology, the syndromology of autosomal and gonosomal aneuploidies, and genetic counseling. In addition, he led a research team studying the genetics and cytogenetics of leukemias. In 1978, he returned to Switzerland to become Director of the Geneva University Institute of Medical Genetics, remaining active in all aspects of clinical genetics, particularly in the field of genetic counseling, and expanding prenatal diagnostic services as well as developing cytogenetic studies of leukemic processes. Professor Engel is an active or honorary member of such societies as the American Society of Human Genetics and the American Society for Clinical Investigation. He is the father of three and a recent grandfather as well.

C. DAWN DeLOZIER-BLANCHET, American-born and Swiss by marriage, holds a Ph. D. degree in medical genetics from Indiana University. For the past 10 years she has worked in the various clinical, teaching and research aspects of medical genetics with Professor Engel, first as clinical coordinator of the Genetics Division of Vanderbilt University (Nashville, Tennessee), and since 1979 as chief assistant at the University Institute of Medical Genetics in Geneva. Although the majority of her time and energy is spent in diagnostic, counseling and teaching activities in the medical genetics service, her research interests include cytogenetics of cancer (her Ph. D. thesis concerned testicular germ cell tumors), and various aspects of early human development and teratogenesis. She is active in various professional societies, including the European Societies of Human Genetics and of Human Reproduction and Embryology and the American Society of Human Genetics. She is the mother of a girl and twin boys.

## Turkey ————

IŞIK BÖKESOY, M. D., Ph. D., 42, is married and has two daughters. She graduated from the Medical Faculty of Ankara University in 1968, and worked in the Neurology Department for 2 years. In 1972 she joined the Genetics Department of Ankara University Medical Faculty. She received her Ph. D. in 1976 with a thesis entitled "Comparison of screening techniques for inborn errors of amino acid metabolism in the mentally retarded". She went to Denmark and worked with Dr. Mikkelsen and Professor Mohr with a scholarship from NATO in 1977. She received her Associate Professorship in 1981. She is now teaching at the Medical Faculty of Ankara University. She is interested in cytogenetics, mainly mutagenicity testing and syndromes. Her publications are in the areas of mosaicism, syndromes and reproductive failures.

FUAT AZIZ GÖKSEL, 60, M. D., is Professor of Psychiatry and Chair of the Department of Medical Ethics, Medical Faculty, University of Ankara. His interests include psychiatry, youth problems, and current psycho-social problems in Turkey. He is the author of Psychic Apparatus and Evaluation of Personality (Turkish), Ankara, 1970; and Medical Sociology (Turkish), Ankara, 1981.

## United Kingdom ————

RODNEY HARRIS qualified in medicine in Liverpool and trained originally as a general physician. He first became interested in genetics while doing an intercallated BSc, but it was in 1960 during a field trip to Nigeria that he became interested in human genetic resistance to disease. He became Head of the Department of Medical Genetics, St. Mary's Hospital, Manchester, in 1968. He is now Professor at the University of Manchester and has organised a multidisciplinary genetics service for a population of nearly four million.

**United States** ————

JOHN J. MULVIHILL, M. D., is Director of the National Institutes of Health Interinstitute Medical Genetics Program and Chief of the Clinical Genetics Section, Clinical Epidemiology Branch, National Cancer Institute, National Institutes of Health, Bethesda, Maryland. His research interests include the genetics of human cancer, epidemiology of childhood neoplasms and congenital defects, mutation epidemiology, and neurofibromatosis. His name appears on over 140 articles in scientific journals, and four books, including *Genetics of Human Cancer* (Raven Press, New York, 1977) and *Medical Genetics: 1987* (Foundation for Advanced Education in the Sciences, Bethesda, MD, 1987). He has participated in cooperative research programs on cancer and on environmental mutagenesis with Italy and Japan, and is the Secretary General of the Eighth International Congress of Human Genetics.

LEROY WALTERS, Ph. D. is Director of the Center for Bioethics at the Kennedy Institute of Ethics and Associate Professor of Philosophy at Georgetown University. He is co-editor of the annual *Bibliography of Bioethics* and of an anthology entitled *Contemporary Issues in Bioethics* (Belmont, CA, Wadsworth, 3rd edition, 1989). He currently serves as chairperson of the Human Gene Therapy Subcommittee of the Recombinant DNA Advisory Committee, National Institutes of Health.

# 5 Appendix: Survey Questionnaire

Card 1 I.D.
$\frac{}{1}$

$\overline{2}\ \overline{3}\ \overline{4}\ \overline{5}$

Country

$\overline{6}\ \overline{7}$

## International Survey of Medical Geneticists

We are conducting a cross-cultural survey of the approaches that medical geneticists take to some of the ethical problems that they and their clients face. Medical geneticists and ethicists in 19 countries are collaborating on this study, which will be published by Springer-Verlag in 1987 as a book, to be entitled *Ethics and Human Genetics: A Cross-Cultural Perspective*. Your responses to the following questionnaire will assist the representatives from your country to write their chapter describing the approaches of the medical geneticists in your country to current ethical problems. Answers will be reported only in statistically aggregate form.

Because this questionnaire requires careful thought, we are requesting you to complete it in two separate sessions. Please *stop* after question 8 on page 14. WAIT FOR AT LEAST ONE DAY, and then continue with question 9.

FIRST, WE WOULD LIKE SOME INFORMATION ON YOUR PROFESSIONAL ACTIVITIES AND PERSONAL BACKGROUND.

1. Which of the following degrees do you hold? (Check as many as apply)
   1. ( ) M. D. (specify):
   2. ( ) Pediatrician 3. ( ) Obstetrician-Gynecologist 4. ( ) Internist
   5. Other M. D. (specify) _____
   6. Ph. D. (specify field) _____
   7. M. S. (genetic associate) _____
   8. Other (specify field and degree) _____

$\overline{8}$

2. Do you have medical genetics certification, fellowship or licensure?
A. American Board of Medical Genetics
  1. No
  2. Yes
    If yes, which categories?
  3. clinical genetics
  4. genetic counselor

$\overline{9}\ \overline{10}$

503

5. cytogenetics
6. clinical biochemical genetics
7. other _____

B. Canadian College of Medical Geneticists
1. No
2. Yes                                             $\overline{\quad}$ 11

C. Other
1. No
2. Yes                                             $\overline{\quad}$ 12
    If yes, list _____

3. How long have you been working in medical genetics? _____     $\overline{\quad}$ $\overline{\quad}$
   year(s)                                                          13  14

4. Concerning medical genetics, approximately how many hours
   per week do you spend on the following?
   a. Seeing patients                    _____ hours/week
   b. Clerical and administrative work   _____ hours/week        $\overline{15}$ $\overline{16}$
   c. Laboratory work                    _____ hours/week        $\overline{17}$ $\overline{18}$
   d. Reading professional journals      _____ hours/week        $\overline{19}$ $\overline{20}$
   e. Other (specify)                    _____ hours/week        $\overline{21}$ $\overline{22}$
   f. _____                           _____ TOTAL hours/week  $\overline{23}$ $\overline{24}$
                                                                   $\overline{25}$ $\overline{26}$

5. Approximately how many patients do you counsel per week? ___    $\overline{27}$ $\overline{28}$

6. Memberships in professional organizations (List).              $\overline{29}$ $\overline{30}$

7. Your age at last birthday _____ _____                           $\overline{31}$ $\overline{32}$

8. Sex
   1. M
   2. F                                                            $\overline{\quad}$ 33

9. Marital status                                                  $\overline{\quad}$ 34
   1. single (never married)
   2. married
   3. widowed/widower
   4. divorced or separated

10. Number of children _____ _____                                 $\overline{35}$ $\overline{36}$

11. Citizenship _____                                  $\overline{37}$ $\overline{38}$

12. Religious background
    1. Protestant    4. Buddhist    7. Other                       $\overline{39}$ $\overline{40}$
    2. Catholic      5. Hindu       8. None
    3. Jewish        6. Moslem

504

13. Approximate number of times you have attended or performed a personal religious observance within the past year

DO NOT WRITE IN THIS COLUMN

    1. 0
    2. 1
    3. 2–4
    4. 5–14
    5. 15–24
    6. 25–49
    7. 50 or more

$\overline{41}$

14. In most aspects of your *non-professional* life, do you consider yourself

$\overline{42}$

    1. more conservative than liberal
    2. equally conservative *and* liberal
    3. more liberal than conservative

15. Do you, or does your genetics unit, do chorionic villus biopsy?
    1. Yes
    2. No
    3. Plan to do so as soon as my lab has the resources
    4. Do not plan to do

$\overline{43}$

*WHY* or *WHY* not?

$\overline{44}$ $\overline{45}$
$\overline{46}$ $\overline{47}$

16. Do you, or does your genetics unit, do fetoscopy?
    1. Yes
    2. No
    3. Plan to do as soon as my lab has the resources
    4. Do not plan to do

$\overline{48}$

*WHY* or *WHY* not?

$\overline{49}$ $\overline{50}$
$\overline{51}$ $\overline{52}$

## Ethical Issues in Medical Genetics

The following questions describe situations that sometimes occur in the practice of medical genetics. Please answer all questions even if you are unlikely to encounter the particular situation in the course of your own professional duties. You should answer in terms of how *you* would respond to the situation *as a geneticist, not* in terms of official or organizational guidelines.

    Most questions will follow the format illustrated below. A case will be described briefly. First you will be asked to indicate WHAT you would do, from a list of possible alternatives. Then you will be asked to describe, in your own words, WHY you would do this.

505

## Sample Question

A child is diagnosed with cystic fibrosis. The parents do not want the diagnosis or relevant genetic information disclosed to their own siblings. In your professional capacity as a medical geneticist, what would you do?

1. respect the parents' desire for confidentiality
2. provide the information to the parents' siblings only after all reasonable efforts to persuade the client to consent to voluntary disclosure have failed.
3. provide the information to the parents' siblings, taking care to insure that only information *directly relevant* to their risks is provided, regardless of the parents' desire.

You should select the *one* answer that you find *most* appropriate *most* of the time, even though you might do otherwise under certain conditions. DO NOT CIRCLE MORE THAN ONE ANSWER.

REMEMBER, THERE ARE NO "RIGHT" OR "WRONG" ANSWERS TO ANY QUESTION.

The second part of each question asks you WHY you have selected "1", "2", or "3". In answering "WHY", please try to express the *ethical* reasoning behind your actions. For example, a geneticist might choose "1" for several different reasons, including
a. the patients' right to privacy
b. to avoid causing harm
c. confidentiality of the doctor-patient relationship.

A geneticist might choose "2" on the basis of
   a. the siblings' right to know
   b. preserving the family unit
   c. professional responsibility toward all members of the family
   d. protecting the health of unborn children
   e. protecting the health of future generations
   f. potential emotional burden of an affected child on the family
   g. potential economic burden of an affected child on society
   h. a combination of several or all these reasons.

A geneticist might choose "3" on the basis of
   a. refusal to lie
   b. obligation to make the truth known
   c. responsibility to society at large
   d. to avoid causing harm
   e. a combination of reasons

THESE LISTS ARE NOT EXHAUSTIVE. They are presented here simply to provide a few examples of the kinds of ethical reasoning that some geneticists may use.

In answering the "WHY" section of a question, please DO NOT elaborate on WHAT you would do. For example, the answer, "if I knew the parents' siblings as their physician or knew their physicians, then I would choose '3', if I had no relationships to the siblings I would persist in '1'," is *not* acceptable as a WHY answer because it merely elaborates the WHAT. In giving a WHY answer, this geneticist should instead have described the physician's responsibility toward patients.

Please do not use the WHY section to provide only technical justification for your decisions. For example, the answer "I selected '1' because there is no prenatal diagnosis now available," is incomplete because it does *not* give the *ethical* reasoning behind your decision. A more complete answer might be, "in the absence of prenatal diagnosis, I am not certain whether the siblings would use genetic information if I provided it. Therefore, in this situation, the parents' right to privacy outweighs any benefit to future generations that might result from my providing the information."

Other examples of answers that are incomplete because they do not provide *ethical* reasons "why" are "You need patients' cooperation to know how to contact relatives at risk," or "most patients will consent to disclosure after the initial shock of the diagnosis subsides."

In summary, a "WHY" answer should provide some *ethical* justification for your action, for example, "the parents have a right to privacy", "the siblings have a right to know", "I have an obligation to make the truth known", "it is my duty to provide health care for *all*, including the siblings," or "I may be doing *harm* by telling the siblings because I'll cause them needless anxiety," "potential parents of a child with cystic fibrosis should be informed, so that they can avoid the burden that the child would cause", "I treat others as I would choose to be treated myself."

*Some* of the keywords that *may* appear in ethical reasoning are

| | |
|---|---|
| rights | obligation |
| responsibility | duty |
| harm | benefit |
| burden | choices |
| should be | preserve |
| ought to be | protect |
| knowledge | confidentiality |
| autonomy | future |
| truth | dishonesty |
| decision | relationships |
| | allocation of limited resources |

Sometimes a geneticist works in a situation where there are organi- DO NOT
zational or legal constraints that prevent the geneticist from practis- WRITE IN
ing the choice he or she has indicated. *If* you believe that such con- COLUMN
straints apply to your situation, please feel free to include in the
"why" section your comments on the relationship between your own
beliefs about what is ethically correct and any constraints represented by your colleagues, chairpersons, hospital administrators, or
legal consequences.

PLEASE ANSWER ALL QUESTIONS IN ENGLISH

1. You identify a parent of a Down syndrome child as having a balanced translocation. What is your approach to disclosure of this information to the parents? Select the *one* that best describes your response.

I would choose to:
1. *Before* drawing samples of the parents' blood for karyotyping, tell
   them that tests may identify one of them as a carrier and ask them
   if they want to know who is the carrier. If both say they want to
   know, tell them. If both say they do not want to know, do not tell
   them.  53
2. Ask the parents whether they want to know *everything* about the
   source of the child's abnormality, including their own carrier status, and if they say yes, tell them which parent carries the extra
   chromosomal material. If they say "no", I would not tell them.
3. Wait for the parents to ask which of them is the carrier, and if they
   ask, tell them.
4. Provide full disclosure to the couple whether or not they ask for it
5. Provide full disclosure to the couple whether or not they ask for it,
   *and* also provide full disclosure to all of their relatives who are at
   risk for having a Down syndrome child.
6. Not disclose information about carrier status even if asked
7. Tell them they are *both* carriers
8. Tell them that *one* is a carrier, then give them the choice of whether or not they wish to be told which one.

*WHY* did you select this course of action?

54 55
56 57
58 59
60 61

508

2. A client recently diagnosed as having Huntington disease (HD) refuses to permit disclosure of the diagnosis and relevant genetic information to siblings who may be at risk for Huntington disease. In your professional capacity as a medical geneticist, what would you do?

DO NOT WRITE IN THIS COLUMN

1. respect the client's desire for confidentiality
2. provide the information to siblings, whether or not they ask for it, only after all reasonable efforts to persuade the client to consent to voluntary disclosure have failed.
3. provide the information to siblings *only* if they ask for it, and after all reasonable efforts to persuade the client to consent to voluntary disclosure have failed.
4. provide the information to siblings, taking care to insure that only information *directly relevant* to the relatives' risks is provided, regardless of client's desire.
5. send the information to the client's referring physician, and let that physician decide about disclosure.

62

*WHY* did you select this course of action?

63 64
65 66
67 68
69 70

3. A client with a child recently diagnosed as having hemophilia A refuses to permit disclosure of the diagnosis and relevant genetic information to her relatives who may be at risk for conceiving children with hemophilia A. The information could be useful to these relatives both because the female carrier can usually be detected and because hemophilia A is usually diagnosable prenatally. As a medical geneticist, what would you do about disclosure of this information?

71

1. respect the client's desire for confidentiality
2. provide the information to relatives whether or not they ask for it, only after all reasonable efforts to persuade the client to consent to voluntary disclosure have failed
3. provide the information to relatives, whether or not they ask for it, taking care to insure that only information directly relevant to the relatives' risks is provided, regardless of client's desire.
4. provide the information to relatives only if they ask for it and only after all reasonable efforts to persuade the client to consent to voluntary disclosure have failed.
5. send the information to the client's referring physician as part of the medical record and let that physician decide about disclosure.

*WHY* did you select this course of action?

72 73
74 75
76 77
78 79

509

4. Laboratory analysis of amniotic fluid cells suggests that the fetus may be a trisomy 13 mosaic. There is disagreement among the medical geneticists responsible for the analysis as to whether or not the laboratory results are artifacts of culture, in other words, false positives. Given the present state of knowledge, there is no way of resolving this disagreement scientifically within the legal time limit for termination of pregnancy, because the results of repeat tests will not be available until after 24 weeks gestational age. You were not responsible for the laboratory work in this case and have not taken one side or the other. You are, however, the medical geneticist responsible for dealing directly with the prospective mother. Do you

DO NOT WRITE IN THIS COLUMN

$\overline{2}$
$\overline{1}\ \overline{2}\ \overline{3}\ \overline{4}\ \overline{5}$

1. tell her that there is *no* abnormality
2. tell her that there *is* an abnormality
3. tell her that there *may be* an abnormality
4. tell her that your colleagues disagree about the test results, and that there *may be* an abnormality
5. avoid mentioning the results of this particular test at all

$\overline{6}$

*WHY* did you select this course of action?

$\overline{7}\ \overline{8}$
$\overline{9}\ \overline{10}$
$\overline{11}\ \overline{12}$
$\overline{13}\ \overline{14}$

5. You are evaluating a child with an autosomal recessive disorder for which carrier testing is possible and accurate. In the process of testing relatives for genetic counseling, you discover that the mother and half the siblings are carriers, whereas the husband is not. The husband believes that he is the child's biological father.

Would you

1. tell the couple what the laboratory tests reveal about the child's parentage
2. tell the couple that they are *both* genetically responsible
3. tell the couple that the origin of the child's disorder is not genetic
4. tell the couple that you have not been able to discover which of them is genetically responsible
5. tell the couple the facts about the child's parentage, and try to get the name of the child's biological father so he can be told that he is a carrier
6. tell the mother alone, without her husband being present

$\overline{15}$

*WHY* did you select this course of action?

$\overline{16}\ \overline{17}$
$\overline{18}\ \overline{19}$
$\overline{20}\ \overline{21}$
$\overline{22}\ \overline{23}$

6. Prenatal diagnosis has revealed an abnormal fetus. The prospective parents come to see you in genetics clinic. In this question you are asked how you would react to two different fetal conditions, Turner syndrome (XO) and XYY, in your *professional* capacity. PLEASE PUT ONLY *ONE* CHECK IN EACH COLUMN.

DO NOT WRITE IN THIS COLUMN

| If the disorder were XO   XYY | I would | |
| --- | --- | --- |
| | 1. advise them to carry the pregnancy to term | $\overline{24}$ $\overline{25}$ |
| | 2. advise them to have an abortion | |
| | 3. refuse to make any suggestions about what they should do | |
| | 4. provide complete information about the disorder, including prognosis, potential treatment and education, and possible problems the child may present for parents and society, taking care to present both sides of any topic that is controversial, and then let them make their own decision. | |
| | 5. give them the information described under "4" in an optimistic form so that they will favor carrying the pregnancy to term | |
| | 6. give them the information under "4" but stress costs and burdens so that they will favor abortion without your having suggested it directly | |
| | 7. give them the information under "4" but also describe the emotional difficulties associated with terminating the pregnancy, and then tell them to make their own decision | |

*Why* did you select this course of action?

$\overline{26}$ $\overline{27}$
$\overline{28}$ $\overline{29}$
$\overline{30}$ $\overline{31}$
$\overline{32}$ $\overline{33}$

511

7. Evaluation of a child produces findings consistent with a diagnosis of tuberous sclerosis. Upon examining the parents, you find evidence that the father is carrying the tuberous sclerosis gene, even though he is of normal intelligence. After a discussion of the risk of having another child with tuberous sclerosis who might be severely affected, the couple asks you whether recurrence of the disorder can be prevented. What course of action do you take with regard to telling the couple about EACH of the following options?

DO NOT WRITE IN THIS COLUMN

Please put *one* check in *each* column

| *Taking Their Chances* *A* | *Artificial Insemination Donor* *B* | *Vasectomy* *C* | *Adoption* *D* | *Contraception* *E* | *Course of Action* | |
|---|---|---|---|---|---|---|
| | | | | | 1. Advise them to do this | $\overline{34}\ \overline{35}$ $\overline{36}\ \overline{37}$ |
| | | | | | 2. Advise them *not* to do this | $\overline{38}$ |
| | | | | | 3. Explain that this is a possibility, without giving any advice | |
| | | | | | 4. Explain that this is a possibility, and describe the risks and potential problems involved | |
| | | | | | 5. Not discuss this | |
| | | | | | 6. Discuss this only if the clients ask you about it | |

*WHY* did you select this course of action?

$\overline{39}\ \overline{40}$
$\overline{41}\ \overline{42}$
$\overline{43}\ \overline{44}$
$\overline{45}\ \overline{46}$

512

8. Evaluation of a child produces findings consistent with a diagnosis of tuberous sclerosis. Upon examining the parents, you find evidence that the mother is carrying the tuberous sclerosis gene, even though she is of normal intelligence. After a discussion of the risk of having another child with tuberous sclerosis who might be severely affected, the couple asks you whether recurrence of the disorder can be prevented. What course of action do you take with regard to EACH of the following options?

Please put *one* check in *each* column

| Taking their Chances A | Contra- ception B | Tubal Ligation C | Surro- gate Mother- hood D | Adop- tion E | Donor egg and in- vitro fertil- ization F | Course of Action |
|---|---|---|---|---|---|---|
| | | | | | | 1. Advise them to do this |
| | | | | | | 2. Advise them *not* to do this |
| | | | | | | 3. Explain that this is a possibility, without giving any advice. |
| | | | | | | 4. Explain that this is a possibility, and describe the risks and potential problems involved. |
| | | | | | | 5. Not discuss this |
| | | | | | | 6. Discuss this only if the clients ask you about it. |

*WHY* did you select this course of action?

STOP HERE.

PUT THIS QUESTIONNAIRE
ASIDE FOR A DAY. THEN
CONTINUE WITH #9

9. A woman of 25 with no family history of genetic disorders and no personal history of exposure to toxic substances requests prenatal diagnosis. There are no genetic or medical indications for its use in this case. Nevertheless, she appears very anxious about the normalcy of the fetus, and persists in her demands for prenatal diagnosis even after being informed that in her case the potential medical risks for the fetus, in terms of miscarriage, may outweigh the likelihood of diagnosing an abnormality. Assume that your clinic has no regulations that would prevent your doing prenatal diagnosis for her. What would you do, as a professional?

DO NOT WRITE IN THIS COLUMN

1. perform prenatal diagnosis
2. refuse to perform prenatal diagnosis
3. try to dissuade her from having prenatal diagnosis, and if she still insists on it, refuse her request
4. refer her to another medical geneticist or genetics unit offering the service

$\overline{\phantom{00}}$
61

*WHY* did you select this course of action?

$\overline{62}$ $\overline{63}$
$\overline{64}$ $\overline{65}$
$\overline{66}$ $\overline{67}$
$\overline{68}$ $\overline{69}$

10. A woman undergoes diagnosis for infertility. Tests reveal that she is chromosomally male (XY). Would you

$\overline{\phantom{00}}$
70

1. tell her that the reason for her infertility is well understood, explain to her the biology of gender, and then explain that she is chromosomally male
2. give her reasons for her infertility without telling her that she is chromosomally male
3. tell her that you do not know the reason for her infertility.

*WHY* did you select this course of action?

$\overline{71}$ $\overline{72}$
$\overline{73}$ $\overline{74}$
$\overline{75}$ $\overline{76}$
$\overline{77}$ $\overline{78}$

11. A woman of 42 requests prenatal diagnosis for Down syndrome. She and her husband are already the parents of a Down syndrome child. She tells you that they are opposed to abortion and that she will carry the fetus to term even if it is diagnosed as having Down syndrome. They would like to have prenatal diagnosis, however, in order to give themselves additional time to prepare for the birth of another affected child. Would you

3
$\overline{1}$ $\overline{2}$ $\overline{3}$ $\overline{4}$ $\overline{5}$

1. grant their request for prenatal diagnosis
2. refuse their request for prenatal diagnosis

$\overline{\phantom{00}}$
6

514

DO NOT
WRITE IN
THIS
COLUMN

3. try to dissuade them from having prenatal diagnosis, and if they still insist on having it, refuse their request
4. refer them to another medical geneticist or genetics unit offering this service

*WHY* did you select this course of action?

$\overline{7}$ $\overline{8}$
$\overline{9}$ $\overline{10}$
$\overline{11}$ $\overline{12}$
$\overline{13}$ $\overline{14}$

12. A couple requests prenatal diagnosis for purposes of selecting the sex of the child. They already have four girls and are desperate for a boy. They say that if the fetus is a girl, they will abort it and will keep trying until they conceive a boy. They also tell you that if you refuse to do prenatal diagnosis for sex selection, they will abort the fetus rather than risk having another girl. The clinic for which you work has *no* regulations prohibiting use of prenatal diagnosis for sex selection. What would you do?

$\overline{15}$

1. grant their request for prenatal diagnosis
2. refuse their request for prenatal diagnosis
3. try to dissuade them from having prenatal diagnosis, and if they still insist on having it, refuse their request
4. refer them to another medical geneticist or genetics unit offering the service

*WHY* did you select this course of action?

$\overline{16}$ $\overline{17}$
$\overline{18}$ $\overline{19}$
$\overline{20}$ $\overline{21}$
$\overline{22}$ $\overline{23}$

13. Maternal serum alpha-fetoprotein has been elevated in your patient on two occasions, but level II ultrasound discloses no abnormality, despite careful examination of the fetal head, spine, abdomen, and kidneys. The fetal karyotype is normal. Amniotic alpha-fetoprotein is elevated and acetylcholinesterase is borderline. These results raise the possibility of a small neural tube defect. What do you tell the parents?

1. tell them that there *may* be a small neural tube defect, and advise abortion
2. tell them that there *may* be a small neural tube defect, and advise them to carry the pregnancy to term.
3. tell them that there *may* be a small neural tube defect, explain the imperfect state of our scientific knowledge and possible other explanations for the test results, but refuse to give any advice about what they should do

$\overline{24}$

515

4. *not* tell them that there may be a small neural tube defect
5. tell them that the tests have not revealed any major abnormality

DO NOT
WRITE IN
THIS
COLUMN

*WHY* did you select this course of action?

$\overline{25}\ \overline{26}$
$\overline{27}\ \overline{28}$
$\overline{29}\ \overline{30}$
$\overline{31}\ \overline{32}$

14. Repeated maternal serum alpha-fetoprotein tests reveal a value that is *below* the norm. Although some studies have found low maternal serum alpha-fetoprotein values to be associated with Down syndrome, geneticists are not in agreement about how a low value should be interpreted. What do you tell the family?

1. tell them that the tests indicate a possible Down syndrome fetus $\overline{33}$
   and urge them to have prenatal diagnosis
2. tell them that the maternal serum alpha-fetoprotein value is low, but that research on this topic is so new that we do not know how to interpret the test results
3. tell them that geneticists are not in agreement about the interpretation of test results, but that some geneticists think there may be a possibility of Down syndrome, explain the relative risks, and then let them decide whether or not to have prenatal diagnosis
4. not tell them about the test results

*WHY* did you select this course of action?

$\overline{34}\ \overline{35}$
$\overline{36}\ \overline{37}$
$\overline{38}\ \overline{39}$
$\overline{40}\ \overline{41}$

15. Now go back over the previous 14 cases and select the *one* where you experienced the greatest ethical conflict in choosing a course of action.

Case number _____

$\overline{42}\ \overline{43}$

*WHY* did this particular case present an ethical conflict?

$\overline{44}\ \overline{45}$
$\overline{46}\ \overline{47}$
$\overline{48}\ \overline{49}$
$\overline{50}\ \overline{51}$

16. Which of the 14 cases gave you the *least* ethical conflict in choosing a course of action?
Case number _____

$\overline{52}\ \overline{53}$

*WHY?*

$\overline{54}\ \overline{55}$
$\overline{56}\ \overline{57}$
$\overline{58}\ \overline{59}$

516

17. A large commercial laboratory plans to open soon in your area. This lab has announced that it will have associated board certified obstetricians on the premises and that it intends to perform prenatal diagnosis for anyone who desires it and who is willing to pay the fee. Should there be any regulations prohibiting this lab from performing prenatal diagnosis *routinely* for any of the following indications?

| Indication | Yes, regulations should prohibit 1 | No, no regulations 2 | |
|---|---|---|---|
| a. maternal anxiety, regardless of maternal age or history | | | 60 |
| b. sex preselection | | | 61 |
| c. parents who will not abort, but nevertheless want to know whether fetus has a defect | | | 62 |
| d. not associated with a medical genetics unit to interpret results | | | 63 |

WHY or WHY NOT?

64 65
66 67
68 69
70 71

18. Assume that an accurate, simple, and reliable mass screening test has been developed for alpha-1-antitrypsin deficiency. This raises the possibility that factory workers who will be exposed to dust and smoke could be screened. Assume that you are a member of an advisory group that will develop guidelines for mass screening of workers in your country. Do you believe that mass genetic screening of workers and prospective employees in potentially dangerous industries should be

1. mandatory for all who would be occupationally exposed
2. voluntary

72

*WHY* did you select this course of action?

73 74
75 76
77 78
79 80

517

19. Who should have access to the results of genetic screening for occupational susceptibility?

| | Yes | Yes, but only if worker approves | No | |
|---|---|---|---|---|
| | 1 | 2 | 3 | 4<br>1 2 3 4 5 |
| a. worker<br>Why?_____ | | | | 6<br><br>7 8 |
| b. employer<br>Why?_____ | | | | 9<br><br>10 11 |
| c. worker's physician<br>Why?_____ | | | | 12<br><br>13 14 |
| d. worker's insurer for life insurance<br>Why?_____ | | | | 15<br><br>16 17 |
| e. employer's insurer for workers' compensation Why?_____ | | | | 18<br><br>19 20 |
| f. government health department<br>Why?_____ | | | | 21<br><br>22 23 |

DO NOT
WRITE IN
THIS
COLUMN

g. worker's insurer for health insurance
   Why?_____

$\overline{24}$

$\overline{25}\ \overline{26}$

h. employer's insurer for health insurance
   Why?_____

$\overline{27}$

$\overline{28}\ \overline{29}$

20. Assume that a cheap and accurate test, reliable at all ages, has been developed for cystic fibrosis. It diagnoses both carriers and affected individuals, distinguishes between them, and also separates each of them from non-carriers. The test is now ready for application on a population-wide basis. Assume that a gradual introduction of screening has been proposed in your country. Also assume that accurate *prenatal diagnosis* has become available for cystic fibrosis. In addition to the relatives of patients with cystic fibrosis, to whom and at what age should the carrier test *first* be given?

1. to all newborns, required by law
2. available to all newborns, but only with parents' consent
3. available to newborns of Caucasian descent, with parents' consent
4. available to all children under 12, required by law
5. available to all children under 12, with parents' consent
6. available to children under 12 of Caucasian descent with parents' consent
7. available to all adolescents 13–17, required by law
8. available to all adolescents 13–17, with parents' consent
9. available to adolescents of Caucasian descent with parents' consent
10. should *only* be given to persons over 18 years, but should be required by law
11. should be available to all persons over 18 years
12. available to persons over 18 years of Caucasian descent who request it

$\overline{30}\ \overline{31}$

*WHY* did you select this answer?

$\overline{32}\ \overline{33}$
$\overline{34}\ \overline{35}$
$\overline{36}\ \overline{37}$
$\overline{38}\ \overline{39}$

21. When a 99 percent accurate pre-symptomatic test for Huntington disease is developed that applies to all families, who should have access to the results of the test?

DO NOT WRITE IN THIS COLUMN

| | access if requested 1 | should be informed 2 | access if patient approves 3 | no access 4 | |
|---|---|---|---|---|---|
| a. individual at risk only Why?_____ _____ | | | | | $\overline{40}$ $\overline{41}$ $\overline{42}$ |
| b. school Why?_____ _____ | | | | | $\overline{43}$ $\overline{44}$ $\overline{45}$ |
| c. medical insurance co. Why?_____ _____ | | | | | $\overline{46}$ $\overline{47}$ $\overline{48}$ |
| d. life insurance co. Why?_____ _____ | | | | | $\overline{49}$ $\overline{50}$ $\overline{51}$ |
| e. employer Why?_____ _____ | | | | | $\overline{52}$ $\overline{53}$ $\overline{54}$ |
| f. spouse Why?_____ _____ | | | | | $\overline{55}$ $\overline{56}$ $\overline{57}$ |

520

DO NOT
WRITE IN
THIS
COLUMN

g. relatives who may be at
risk for
   Huntington disease
   Why?_____
_____

$\overline{58}$

$\overline{59}\ \overline{60}$

22. Below are listed some future issues that medical geneticists may face. Please *rank in order* (starting with "1" as most important) which of these you think *SHOULD BE* of most concern to medical geneticists *IN YOUR COUNTRY* in the next 10 or 15 years.

$\overline{61}\ \overline{62}$

a. _____ genetic screening in the workplace$_1$
b. _____ screening for genetic susceptibility to cancer and heart disease$_2$
c. _____ sex preselection for sex desired by parents$_3$
d. _____ increased demand for genetic services$_4$
e. _____ research on the human embryo, zygote, and fetus$_5$
f. _____ long-range eugenic concerns$_6$
g. _____ development of new treatments for genetic disorders including treatment in utero, organ transplantation, and molecular genetic manipulation$_7$
h. _____ environmental damage to the unborn$_8$
i. _____ carrier screening for common genetic disorders$_9$
j. _____ allocation of limited resources$_{10}$

$\overline{63}\ \overline{64}$
$\overline{65}\ \overline{66}$
$\overline{67}\ \overline{68}$
$\overline{69}\ \overline{70}$
$\overline{71}\ \overline{72}$

$\overline{73}\ \overline{74}$
$\overline{75}\ \overline{76}$
$\overline{77}\ \overline{78}$
$\overline{79}\ \overline{80}$

23. Below are listed some future issues that medical geneticists may face. Please *rank in order* (starting with "1" as most important) which of these you think *should be* of most concern to medical geneticists *AROUND THE WORLD* in the next 10 or 15 years.

5
$\overline{1}\ \overline{2}\ \overline{3}\ \overline{4}\ \overline{5}$

a. _____ genetic screening in the workplace$_1$
b. _____ screening for genetic susceptibility to cancer and heart disease$_2$
c. _____ sex preselection for sex desired by parents$_3$
d. _____ increased demand for genetic services$_4$
e. _____ research on the human embryo, zygote, and fetus$_5$
f. _____ long-range eugenic concerns$_6$
g. _____ development of new treatments for genetic disorders, including treatment in utero, organ transplantation, and molecular genetic manipulation$_7$

$\overline{6}\ \overline{7}$

$\overline{8}\ \overline{9}$
$\overline{10}\ \overline{11}$
$\overline{12}\ \overline{13}$
$\overline{14}\ \overline{15}$
$\overline{16}\ \overline{17}$

$\overline{18}\ \overline{19}$

521

h. _____ environmental damage to the unborn[8]
i. _____ carrier screening for common genetic disorders[9]
j. _____ allocation of limited resources[10]

$\overline{20}$ $\overline{21}$
$\overline{22}$ $\overline{23}$
$\overline{24}$ $\overline{25}$

24. Professionals in genetic counseling may hold one or more goals for their counseling. In *your* opinion, how important is it that your counseling achieve each of the following: (Please check _____)

| | Absolutely Essential | Important But Not Essential | Somewhat Important | Of No Importance | |
|---|---|---|---|---|---|
| | 1 | 2 | 3 | 4 | |
| a. The prevention of disease or abnormality | | | | | $\overline{26}$ |
| b. The removal or lessening of patient guilt or anxiety | | | | | $\overline{27}$ |
| c. A reduction in the number of carriers of genetic disorders in the population | | | | | $\overline{28}$ |
| d. Improvement of the general health and vigor of the population | | | | | $\overline{29}$ |
| e. Helping individuals/ couples adjust to and cope with their genetic problems | | | | | $\overline{30}$ |
| f. Helping individuals/ couples achieve their parenting goals | | | | | $\overline{31}$ |

522

| | | | | DO NOT WRITE IN THIS COLUMN |
|---|---|---|---|---|
| g. Helping individuals/ couples understand their options and the present state of medical knowledge so they can make informed decisions | | | | 32 |

25. In *your* opinion, how appropriate do you think it is for you as a professional in counseling to do each of the following:

| | Almost Always Appropriate 1 | Sometimes Appropriate 2 | Rarely, If Ever Appropriate 3 | Never Appropriate 4 | |
|---|---|---|---|---|---|
| a. Tell patients that decisions, especially reproductive ones, are theirs alone and refuse to make any for them | | | | | 33 |
| b. Suggest that while you will not make decisions for patients you will support any they make | | | | | 34 |
| c. Inform patients what most other people in their situation have done | | | | | 35 |
| d. Inform patients what you would do if you were in their situation | | | | | 36 |
| e. Advise patients what they ought to do | | | | | 37 |

523

# Subject Index

## A

abnormalities, *see* birth defects

abortion  VIII, xxv, 170–72, 189–92, 196, 198–99, 218–19, 235, 256–57, 273–77, 289–90, 303–304, 324, 332, 343, 346, 350–51, 363–64, 399–400, 427, 430, 438–39, 446, 458, 484, 486, 487
- advice about  201, 204
- as birth control  209, 219, 256–57, 266
- and Catholics  93, 189–92, 289–91, 365, 424
- choices  458, 459, 463–65
- and cost-benefit analysis  136–37, 163, 238, 273–75, 323–24, 362, 397–99
- counseling after  219, 403
- for cystic fibrosis  275, 400
- decreased fertility after  198–99
- doctors' views of  183, 280, 291, 439
- after environmental exposure  289–90, 333
- and eugenics  137–39, 375
- for genetic reasons  VIII, 22, 87–88, 112–13, 123–24, 136, 146, 163–65, 183–85, 189–91, 196, 215, 219, 227, 239, 257–58, 266, 274–77, 289–91, 303, 305, 312, 323–24, 333, 343, 362–63, 375–77, 398–400, 411, 427
- and Greek Orthodox Church  219, 226
- grief after  93, 219, 402–403
- guilt after  403
- handicapped views of  445
- and Hinduism  266
- illegal  211, 219, 383
- and Judaism  278, 281–82
- laws  21–22, 94, 108–109, 115, 132–33, 148, 151–53, 163–65, 189–92, 196, 205–206, 209, 218–19, 227, 239, 256, 265–67, 275–76, 282, 289–91, 303,
- - laws, ambiguity  464
- - laws, restrictive  464 305, 312 324, 330–33, 338, 343, 346, 349, 363, 369, 372, 374–75, 383, 385, 399, 410–12, 446
- livebirth ratio  88, 123, 146, 153, 163–65, 184–85, 209, 218–19, 235, 256, 276–77, 285–86, 294, 303–304, 324, 343, 363, 383, 399–400
- for mental handicap  22, 363, 400, 411, 427
- and minorities  410
- and Moslems  93, 256, 266–67
- for mother's mental health  22, 87–88, 163–65, 266, 276, 291, 333, 375, 399, 410–11
- for neural tube defects  201, 275, 400
- for physical handicap  22, 27–28
- and Protestants  320, 346–47, 365
- psycho-social aspects  402–403, 413, 438
- and public opinion  446
- refusal of after prenatal diagnosis  215, 363, 365–66, 423, 426–27
- selective  463–65, 475
- - arguments against  464
- - arguments for  464
- - emotional trauma  465
- for sex chromosome abnormalities  27–31, 167, 180, 241, 275, 363, 376, 400, 427, 438
- for sex selection  22–24, 111–13, 128, 277–78, 439, 461, 484
- for social reasons  22, 163–65, 184–85, 239, 275–76, 282, 291, 303–305, 312, 324, 330, 333, 364, 375, 399, 411
- spontaneous  235, 361
- for Tay-Sachs  275
- for thalassemia  275
- *see also* anti-abortion movements, cost-benefit analysis, genetic counseling, prenatal diagnosis for parents who refuse abortion, sex selection

absolutism, *see* ethical absolutism

access to and adequacy of genetic services  458, 459, 462

access to health care, *see* equal access

access to test results, *see* disclosure

action research  xx, xxi–xxvi
- aim  xxi
- definition  xxi

adoption  15, 28–31, 46, 111–13, 151, 201, 204, 368–69, 383, 407, 437, 478, 486, 512–13

adult polycystic kidney disease  397, 406

advice, *see* genetic counseling, directiveness in

AFP, see alpha-fetoprotein

age
- of geneticists  10–11, 184, 439, 504
- of mothers, *see* maternal age
- *see also* paternal age

AID, *see* artificial insemination – donor

AIDS  IX, 110, 402, 436, 451

allocation of resources, *see* equality of access

alpha-fetoprotein  18–20, 123, 360–61
- *see also* maternal serum alpha-fetoprotein